AF183230

Technology Implementation and Teacher Education: Reflective Models

Junko Yamamoto
Slippery Rock University of Pennsylvania, USA

Joseph C. Kush
Duquesne University, USA

Ron Lombard
Chatham University, USA

C. Jay Hertzog
Slippery Rock University of Pennsylvania, USA

Information Science REFERENCE

INFORMATION SCIENCE REFERENCE

Hershey · New York

Director of Editorial Content:	Kristin Klinger
Director of Book Publications:	Julia Mosemann
Acquisitions Editor:	Lindsay Johnston
Development Editor:	Tyler Heath
Typesetter:	Gregory Snader
Production Editor:	Jamie Snavely
Cover Design:	Lisa Tosheff
Printed at:	Yurchak Printing Inc.

Published in the United States of America by
Information Science Reference (an imprint of IGI Global)
701 E. Chocolate Avenue
Hershey PA 17033
Tel: 717-533-8845
Fax: 717-533-8661
E-mail: cust@igi-global.com
Web site: http://www.igi-global.com/reference

Copyright © 2010 by IGI Global. All rights reserved. No part of this publication may be reproduced, stored or distributed in any form or by any means, electronic or mechanical, including photocopying, without written permission from the publisher.

Product or company names used in this set are for identification purposes only. Inclusion of the names of the products or companies does not indicate a claim of ownership by IGI Global of the trademark or registered trademark.

Library of Congress Cataloging-in-Publication Data

Technology implementation and teacher education : reflective models / Junko Yamamoto...[et al.].

p. cm.

Includes bibliographical references and index.

Summary: "This book present viewpoints of the international authors, who are teacher educators, highlighting their best practices in their own environments, and how it can relate and be applicable to the readers' environment"--Provided by publisher.

ISBN 978-1-61520-897-5 (hardcover) -- ISBN 978-1-61520-898-2 (ebook) 1. Educational technology. 2. Teachers--Training of. 3. Teachers--In-service training. I. Yamamoto, Junko, 1967-

LB1028.3T39692 2010

371.33--dc22

2009039669

British Cataloguing in Publication Data

A Cataloguing in Publication record for this book is available from the British Library.

All work contributed to this book is new, previously-unpublished material. The views expressed in this book are those of the authors, but not necessarily of the publisher.

List of Reviewers

Joellen Maples, *St. John Fisher College, USA*
Peter Albion, *University of Southern Queensland, Australia*
Mark Hawkes, *Dakota State University, USA*
Ellen Newcombe, *West Chester University of Pennsylvania, USA*
William J. Gibbs, *Duquesne University, USA*
Terry L. Herman, *Bowling Green State University, USA*
Jeremy Dickerson, *East Carolina University, USA*
Padma Anand, *Slippery Rock University of Pennsylvania, USA*
Timo Salminen, *University of Jyväskylä, Finland*
Catherine McLoughlin, *Australian Catholic University, Australia*
Lawrence Tomei, *Robert Morris University, USA*

Table of Contents

Section 5
Framework and Application: Learning Environment of Digital Age

Detailed Table of Contents

The School of Rock (SOR) expedition was a unique at-sea teacher education workshop that sought to introduce inservice teachers to scientific ocean drilling and collaborate in developing ways to extend this science content to K-12 classrooms. During the workshop teachers used an expedition website to communicate their learning and the "results" of the expedition to an onshore audience of students. While adventure learning/hybrid online education is common in K-12 classrooms, the SOR expedition was unique in that teachers were the explorers and the workshop sought to use technology to enhance both the learning of students onshore and the learning of the participants of the workshop (Niemitz et al., 2008). Here, we examine how the SOR expedition website enhanced the teacher education goals of the workshop and compare and contrast our reflections with the literature on integrating technology into teacher education programs. The SOR experience identifies two new elements to consider as teacher educators design ways to integrate technology into education programs: 1) situations where pre- or in-service teachers can use technology to communicate narratives of inquiry can lead to engaging and formative learning experiences for both teachers and students; and 2) using technology to communicate new content knowledge to students in real or near real-time can reinforce a mindset for applying this knowledge to student learning needs as the teacher learning is in progress. We identify two examples of how to scale this model for integrating technology into teacher education and provide recommendations on appropriate technologies for doing so.

Teacher educators preparing their students for 21st century schools are increasingly using online technologies in on-campus courses. While some teacher educators have used such activities for almost a decade and have migrated from learning management systems to wikis and blogs, others still struggle to structure and facilitate online activities effectively. Ten teacher educators' decisions to use online activities in 23 face-to-face courses based on several criteria (class size, instructional goals, course type, students' prior knowledge, and the content of classroom instruction) are described in this chapter. Faculty member's reflections on their decisions, practical examples from different courses that they taught, and strategies they refined over time illustrated their focus on pedagogy as they migrated to newer technologies. The structure, design, and implementation of online activities discussed in this chapter could be useful to beginning educators, teacher developers, and instructional designers engaged in the integration of new technologies in higher education.

Ten elementary education student teachers communicated with each other on an electronic discussion board for thirteen weeks. Despite being overwhelmed at times with the demands of student teaching, participants posted 283 messages offering each other ideas and support. Students were grouped into two different discussion boards based on the grade level they were assigned to student teach, resulting in very specific help and feedback from peers who were experiencing the same or similar teaching top-

A new teaching and learning experience is emerging thanks to the emanation of a new set of Web 2.0 tools. This experience is more inclusive where students are guided through a curriculum that better adapts to their individual learning styles, encourages collaborative teamwork, and facilitates critical thinking and problem solving through a variety of communication, visualization and simulation technologies. A discussion of providing a platform for reviewing and reflecting on shared learning experiences through the use of VoiceThread and digital video recording for all levels of learners is presented. The chapter highlights the power and barriers related to the application of educational technology for teacher candidates, teacher educators, teachers and students. The author proposed that teachers can become empowered, teacher educators and teacher candidates can reflect and connect curriculum with authentic activities through the application of VoiceThread, a Web 2.0 tool that will support learning and collaborating more effectively worldwide.

The success of any educational technology lies in how students interact with it in an educational setting. In the iLRN model (Lennex & Nettleton, 2009), the teacher provides instruction but through activity theory the students transform the learning to suit their own designs. The quality of teacher directions determines the extent to which students depend on the teacher for further feedback and technical assistance. If a teacher is perceived as not understanding even a small part of the technology, Lennex (2008) discovered that P-12 students are unlikely to ask for clarification of assignments or for any further assistance. Exploration and peer coaching replaced the teacher. Technologically literate teachers who interacted with their students and encouraged the scaffolding of knowledge discovered that final student projects demonstrated

This chapter focuses on the utilization of technology to enhance the learning outcomes of pre-service teachers in the context of post secondary four year teacher education program provided by higher education institutions. A brief description of technology in teacher education precedes the discussion on

This chapter describes one science teacher educator's attempts to integrate various educational technologies in an elementary science methods course, her students' responses to her attempts, and the tensions that emerged. The science teacher educator employed teacher action research as a means of systematic, reflective inquiry to examine critically how preservice elementary school science teachers think about, use, and reflect on educational technologies and how their developing professional identities intersect with adoption of these technologies. Tensions emerged from a dichotomy between what methods students perceived as "traditional" science teaching and science teaching using technology. Resulting problems of practice included: expertise in/with science and negotiating a new curriculum, control in the classroom, content coverage, and support and sense of community. We conclude our chapter with implications and recommendations for future research related to the significant role educational technology can play in science teacher education and science teacher identity development.

Pre-service elementary teachers are faced with numerous technology tools which can be incorporated into their mathematics lesson plans. However, these teachers may not be experienced in evaluating technology tools for mathematical learning prior to using them. This chapter presents a reflective model for mathematics teacher educators. In a three-part activity, pre-service elementary teachers identify their criteria for evaluating technology tools, evaluate several technology tools according to their own criteria, and make recommendations for or against those technology tools. As pre-service elementary teachers reflect upon the criteria they feel are essential for evaluating technology tools, they begin to identify the specific affordances and limitations of the technology tools. This chapter describes this three-part activity by placing it within the context of a model for mathematics teacher education.

Mathematics education is used as a context to demonstrate the types of learning experiences that can be provided to preservice secondary mathematics teachers as part of a teacher education program to encourage technology integration. Specifically, I reflect on the design, development, and implementation of a mathematics-specific technology course and consider the extent to which this course provides prospective teachers experiences to achieve the goals identified in the Mathematics TPACK (Technological Pedagogical Content Knowledge) Framework developed by the Association of Mathematics Teacher Educators. In its current form, the course addresses most of the identified guidelines; however, after reflecting on the extent to which this course might satisfy all of the indicators, I conclude that a single course on technology integration is not sufficient. Technology integration should be considered a programmatic teacher education goal across multiple courses, both content and pedagogy.

The Professional Handbook is a teacher education assignment that allows preservice teachers to use technology to connect theory and practice while also developing their reflective skills and professionalism. The assignment involves compiling information in an easy-to-use website that preservice teachers can access while engaged in their semester-long student teaching experience and once they are employed as inservice teachers. This chapter describes the Handbook's essential goals, discusses its use in an instructional methods course, and makes recommendations for modifying the Handbook's format for use in any teacher education course while preserving the framework provided by the assignment's essential goals. The chapter serves as a resource for teacher educators looking to use technology to enhance the quality of teacher preparation assignments

Children and young people today are introduced to the virtual world via video games, and the way that they interact with technology is changing ways of learning and the production of knowledge. The design of a learning environment based on the educational properties of games seems to be an ideal way of increasing learning. Digital games offer a very good example of the principles of successful learning environments; they are users-centered, and they promote challenge, co-operation, engagement and the development of problem-solving strategies. Games can help students learn to collaborate, solve problems, collect and analyse data, test hypotheses, and engage in debate. But there are differences between using digital games for play and using them in a formal context. For this reason, methodologies must be developed for their use in the classroom. In this chapter, we propose examples of methods that can be applied to the use of video games in formal education.

The success of any educational technology lies in how students interact with it in an educational setting. In the iLRN model (Lennex & Nettleton, 2009), the teacher provides instruction but through activity theory the students transform the learning to suit their own designs. The quality of teacher directions determines the extent to which students depend on the teacher for further feedback and technical assistance. If a teacher is perceived as not understanding even a small part of the technology, Lennex (2008) discovered that P-12 students are unlikely to ask for clarification of assignments or for any further assistance. Exploration and peer coaching replaced the teacher. Technologically literate teachers who interacted with their students and encouraged the scaffolding of knowledge discovered that final student projects demonstrated higher levels of critical thinking and creativity when compared to teacher-controlled projects.

Foreword

Today's youth cannot imagine a world without mobile computing, social networking sites, iPods, handheld games and camera phones. Multimedia surrounds them constantly and many of the technology innovations that amaze adults are as natural as air and water for these youngsters. Yet, the disconnect between the way today's youth use technology in their personal and academic lives continues to grow. In fact, many youth are unable and unprepared to use technology in ways that effectively support academic endeavors. While numerous factors contribute to this phenomenon, the need for teachers with the knowledge, skills and dispositions to facilitate 21st century teaching and learning is clear.

This book builds on the editor's international experiences in teacher education to share promising practices that will prepare teachers ready to address this challenge. Not surprisingly these promising practices are diverse in nature and view technology through different lenses. Two lenses became apparent to us as we read the chapters: technology as a conduit and technology as a tool. In addition, several chapters showcase research related to how technology can be used in teacher education.

When technology serves as a conduit for teaching and learning, it supports interactions between and among learners, instructors, and content. Examples within this book include online and blended learning opportunities for teachers and preservice teachers and address a variety of important topics in teacher education including multicultural education and bullying. Providing online and blended opportunities for teachers is essential given the prominence of virtual primary and secondary schools and extended learning time via blended experiences. For teachers to effectively facilitate and promote learning in these environments they must have rich, personal experiences within them. Likewise, these opportunities are essential for ongoing professional development. Given the rise in online professional development, teachers must be proficient learning in such environments to remain current on new pedagogies, practices and tools.

In some chapters, technology is used as a tool to promote student acquisition of content knowledge. Some tools highlighted within this book include science probes, graphing calculators, Web 2.0 and educational games. These technology tools enable students to use technology to communicate, create, collaborate, analyze, synthesize and evaluate; skills essential for success in the 21st century. The tools described in these chapters focus on different content areas thus highlighting the importance of using different tools for different learning purposes and of putting the curricular objectives at the forefront of technology integration.

Finally, this book also includes studies designed to determine the ways in which teachers design online and blended learning environments, chapters designed to provide frameworks or ideologies about how to conceptualize technology use by teacher educators and chapters examining specific aspects of technology use such as its impact of male and female students.

While incredibly diverse in nature, the chapters within this book contain many innovative ideas, highlight many important social and affective issues of technology use and provide a unique multi-national perspective on the ways in which technology may be used in teacher education. Teacher educators, professional development specialists and others with an interest in technology and teacher education will undoubtedly find gems of knowledge related to their educational context.

Kara Dawson
University of Florida, USA

Cathy Cavanaugh
University of Florida, USA

Kara Dawson *is an Associate Professor of Educational Technology in the School of Teaching and Learning at the University of Florida where she serves as Program Coordinator for traditional and online graduate programs. Her funded research includes studies of the impact of professional development, classroom technologies and K-12/university partnerships on teaching practices, student achievement and school culture. She has published over 40 refereed articles in journals such as the British Journal of Educational Technology and the Journal of Research on Technology in Education, over a dozen editor-reviewed articles in outlets such as the Chronicle of Higher Education and Educational Leadership, numerous book chapters and an edited book. In addition, she has secured over 1 million dollars in funding since 2002. She currently serves on editorial review boards of prominent journals including Educational Technology Research and Development and serves as a consultant for the Florida Department of Education and Florida school districts. Prior to working at the University of Florida, Dr. Dawson worked as a post-doctoral fellow at the Center for Technology and Teacher Education within the Curry School at the University of Virginia. She also taught elementary and middle school in Virginia Beach.*

Cathy Cavanaugh *is an Associate Professor of educational technology in the School of Teaching and Learning, where she teaches in the areas of instructional design and distance education. Her funded research includes studies of classroom technology and professional development in Florida schools, effective practices in virtual schools, and online course design. Her primary research interests are in indicators of quality in distance education. She has authored, co-authored or edited numerous books and chapters, in addition to articles and papers in educational technology. She serves as editorial board member or reviewer for several professional publications and leads research groups for online education organizations. Prior to her higher education appointments, Cathy worked in K-12 settings for 14 years, teaching grades 6-9 science and coordinating a school district professional development center for math, science and technology.*

Preface

HOW THIS BOOK CAME ABOUT

Technology Implementation and Teacher Education, along with Technology Leadership in Teacher Education, was born from professional dialogues among scholars around the world. I love going to international conferences and listening to ideas of experts from different areas. Ideas grow with interaction: sometimes I have coffee or lunch with scholars that I just met at a conference so I can learn more about their practices, teaching philosophies, and important issues in their environments. Such conversation causes me to ponder this question: how can I successfully apply practices in Austria, Netherlands, Japan, or Great Britain, to the context of the United States, the country in which I am teaching? This book aims to mimic the structure of such a process: international authors, who are teacher educators, present their best practices in their environments. They also imply how their cases can be generalized so that the audience can think about how to adapt and implement what worked in the authors' environments into those of the readers.

Technology changes rapidly. Since the time span from a book proposal to the publication is about two years, books that focus on pedagogical issues rather than technological how-to tend to attract teacher educators. Also, an editor of an instructional technology book needs to have a keen sense of current and emerging trends. To grasp the trends, I skimmed through over 500 journal articles and conference proceedings covering the most recent three years. I composed the draft for the book proposal after identifying critical issues and trends. Then a group of teacher educators exchanged ideas about the draft and finalized our book proposal. While doing so, we decided to publish books for two different strands. One was for leadership in teacher education and the other was for teacher educators as reflective practitioners.

During fall 2008, I sent out emails to scholars who already published in relevant topics. The response was very encouraging. I especially enjoyed the process of reading their ideas via email or listening to them over the telephone. Authors asking for my feedback often motivated me to look for recent publications on their topics. Hence, there was a constant active exchange between authors and myself. Furthermore, reviewers and authors had very productive interaction during the formative evaluation process: first during the chapter proposal stage, then during the chapter drafting stage. The process was double-blind reviewed, so I often acted as a mediator to pass on the comments and questions between the reviewers and the authors. Authors displayed a high degree of professionalism as they used formative feedback to make their chapters stronger. This is another example of professional dialogue refining ideas.

ORGANIZATION OF THIS BOOK

The first section of this book discusses online and blended learning. Charalambos Mouzakis and Constantinos Bourletidis show details and participants' perceptions about their blended learning course initiated by the Greek Ministry of Education. Matthew Niemitz, Scott Slough, Kristen St. John, R. Mark Leckie, Leslie Peart, and Ann Klaus present a case study about adventure learning, a type of hybrid inquiry-based learning. Swapna Kumar analyzes factors that influence teacher educators' choices of online activities. Karen J. Johnson reports how an electronic discussion board can support peer support among student teachers.

The second section of the book focuses on communication and collaboration. Hasan Tinmaz and İlker Yakin provide an application for a 3x3 two-dimensional matrix of technology perception framework in information and communication technologies (ICT). Phillip David Jones and Adrian Ting show how an ePortfolio can promote peer-supported reflection. Virginia McCormack argues that VoiceThread, a Web 2.0 tool, can support collaborative learning. Lesia Lennex and Kimberly Fletcher Nettleton share their findings about the implementation of hand held technologies.

The third section is structured around social and affective issues. Nor Aziah Alias and Nor Aiza Alias discuss how technology can support affective learning. Kati Vapalahti, Miika Marttunen , and Leena Laurinen showcase a blended role-play model that raises awareness about the use of intoxicants among youths. Judith Cramer and Margaret Crocco present gender issues in digital learning.

The fourth section goes into subject-specific teacher education. Irina Lyublinskaya and Nelly Tournaki share reflections of preservice elementary school teachers after they utilized probeware in an inquiry-based math and science methods course. Ronald MacDonald demonstrates effective use of a hand-held data logger in a science classroom. Brenda Capobianco and James Lehman investigate preservice science teachers' process of integrating educational technology into the science classrooms. Christopher J. Johnston describes how preservice elementary teachers evaluate technology tools for mathematics education. Gladis Kersaint narrates course development and changes for her mathematics-specific technology course. Manuel Santos-Trigo shows uses of graphic tools that promote a deep understanding of mathematics. Adam Friedman and Tina L. Heafner examine the impact of Web 2.0 tools including blogs, wikis, and podcasts on social studies education.

The fifth section addresses frameworks and applications for learning environments of the digital age. Chinwe Ikpeze shows elements for supporting reflection. Sara Winstead Fry demonstrates how a professional handbook can support the reflective process. Begoña Gros mentions general definitions for games as well as how games are used in schools. Chris Penny offers detailed accounts of implementing a podcasting project for teacher candidates. Kevin J. Reins shows a use of digital ink on tablet PCs for integrating notes and supporting interaction.

Acknowledgment

I would first like to thank my co-editors for their enthusiasm, professionalism, and support.

Technology Leadership in Teacher Education: Integrated Solutions and Experiences

Chris Penny, *West Chester University of Pennsylvania, USA*
Joanne Leight, *Slippery Rock University of Pennsylvania, USA*
Sally Winterton, *West Chester University of Pennsylvania, USA*

Technology Implementation and Teacher Education: Reflective Models

Ronald Lombard, *Chatham University, USA*
Joseph Kush, *Duquesne University, USA*
Jay Hertzog, *Slippery Rock University of Pennsylvania, USA (retired)*

They worked well as a team to co-develop the two books, and then to review and to fine-tune the respective books.

This book could not have been made possible without a group of dedicated reviewers. Their expertise and dedication ensured the quality and the integrity of the double-blind review process.

Joellen Maples, *St. John Fisher College, USA*
Peter Albion, *University of Southern Queensland, Australia*
Mark Hawkes, *Dakota State University, USA*
Ellen Newcombe, *West Chester University of Pennsylvania, USA*
William J. Gibbs, *Duquesne University, USA*
Terry L. Herman, *Bowling Green State University, USA*
Jeremy Dickerson, *East Carolina University, USA*
Padma Anand, *Slippery Rock University of Pennsylvania, USA*
Timo Salminen, *University of Jyväskylä, Finland*
Catherine McLoughlin, *Australian Catholic University, Australia*
Lawrence Tomei, *Robert Morris University, USA*

I would also like to thank Dr. Richard Altenbaugh of Slippery Rock University of Pennsylvania. This book and *Technology Leadership in Teacher Education: Integrated Solutions and Experiences* were the first books that I edited. I depended on his experience as a journal editor when I wrote rejection messages that encouraged authors to keep up with their scholarship even though their chapters did not appear in the books. Finally, I would like to thank Mr. Tyler Heath and Ms. Julia Mosemann of IGI Global for the tireless support they have provided.

Junko Yamamoto, Editor
August 2009, Slippery Rock University of Pennsylvania

Section 1
Online and Blended Learning

Chapter 1
A Blended Learning Course for Teachers' Ongoing Professional Development in Greece

Charalambos Mouzakis
National and Kapodistrian University of Athens, Greece

Constantinos Bourletidis
National and Kapodistrian University of Athens, Greece

ABSTRACT

The purpose of this chapter is to describe the design, implementation and evaluation of a professional development program for teachers initiated by the Greek Ministry of Education and Religious Affairs in cooperation with the National and Kapodistrian University of Athens. The course focused on multicultural education and bullying in schools as it was realized through blended learning whereas the methodology applied was a face-to-face meeting and 250-hour web-based learning. The evaluation process aimed to involved teachers' perceptions toward different aspects of the blended training process. The quantitative and qualitative results indicate that the teachers were satisfied both with the opportunity to learn at home at their own pace as with the opportunity to develop knowledge and skills in relation to their work. The results brought to light arguments, controversies, and problems related to the course. Finally, some recommendations that would improve the effectiveness of courses employing blended learning methodologies are given.

INTRODUCTION

Teachers' professional development is integrally related to the quality of education and is closely linked to improved learning outcomes and school environment (Meiers, 2004; Snoek, Uzerli, & Schratz, 2008). Recent studies offer compelling evidence that professional development offers skills and knowledge that enable teachers to improve their instructional and intervention practices and to deal effectively with local community needs (Darling-Hammond et al., 2005; OECD, 2005). Teachers' professional development encompasses different types of facilitated learning opportunities, ranging from a single workshop to a full-semester academic course, and varying widely in the content and the form of the learning experiences involved (Borko, 2004; National Professional Development Center

DOI: 10.4018/978-1-61520-897-5.ch001

Copyright © 2010, IGI Global. Copying or distributing in print or electronic forms without written permission of IGI Global is prohibited.

on Inclusion, 2008). The rapid development in Information and Communication Technology (ICT) has provided more flexible and effective ways for professional development for teachers, not possible in traditional in-class education (Dede, et al. 2006).

Recognizing the importance of ICT, the majority of the countries in the world have developed open and distance learning methods supported by (ICT) to facilitate teachers' networking and to provide online learning experiences (Jung, 2005). Academics, education researchers, political and policy driven motivators have also begun to support the development of online professional development not only in distance education settings, but also in courses, which combine features of online learning with traditional classroom-based learning (Owston, et. al., 2008; Simkins, et. al. 2009). These courses are often referred to as 'blended learning', combining various types of pedagogy with different tools for interaction and discussion (Lord & Lomicka, 2008). Research evidence suggests that blended learning courses reap the benefits of both face-to-face and online learning such as flexibility, convenience, scalability and adaptability, enabling teachers to become more directly involved in their own learning and their professional growth (Rovai & Jordan 2004).

Based on the assumption that professional development should be an integral part of daily practice for all teachers, the European Commission supports policies for improving teacher competences and qualifications under the 'Education and Training 2010' programme (European Commission, 2007; Zgaga, 2008). In this context, the Greek Ministry of Education and Religious Affairs with the support of the European Commission initiated a teachers' professional development course under the name "A Web-based teachers' training to enhance teaching and learning". The course was developed in cooperation with the National and Kapodistrian University of Athens and combined both a face-to-face meeting and web-based learning, supported by facilitators. A total of 187 teachers employed in state schools, primarily from the rural areas of northern Greece, participated in the course, which lasted from October to November 2008.

This chapter aims to describe the components of the teachers' professional development course and to investigate the teachers' personal experience of the blended learning process. The findings of this study offer further understanding of the specific contexts, conditions, and practices that contribute to the success of blended learning for teachers' professional development courses.

BACKGROUND

Current literature provides varying definitions of blended learning, reflecting the diversity of instructional practices, pedagogic approaches and technology modes (Stacey & Gerbic, 2009; Martyn, 2003). Although there are different points of view regarding the various components of blended learning, educational theorists and practitioners seem to agree that the essential nature of blended learning is the on-line delivery of instructional content with the on-site implementation of instructional strategies (Graham 2006; Osguthorpe & Graham 2003). In teachers' professional development setting blended learning is viewed generally as a combination of face-to-face and distance learning methods offered to develop teachers' knowledge and skills and provide them with additional qualifications (Hellmig, 2008). Research evidence suggests that the blended learning approaches increase teachers' access to training, improve teachers' flexibility and convenience, and facilitate effective pedagogical strategies to develop teachers' knowledge and skills (Fiege, Peacock & Geelan, 2004; Hojsholt-Poulsen, 2007; Samarawickrema, 2009).

To date, much of the research examining blended learning has been done with researchers who are involved in national projects designed to support teachers' on-going professional development (Makey, 2008; Polhemus & Jennings, 2005). Although several of these projects have commonalities regarding the instructional system design, the alternation and variation of delivery mechanisms, each project offers insight into course structuring and blended learning efficiency. In particular, Wideman, Owston, & Sinitskaya (2007) presented a comparative analysis of the evaluation findings from three major multi-jurisdictional teacher professional development projects that used a blended model for delivery incorporating both online and face-to-face components. Their findings revealed several factors which had an impact on the level of success of these blended initiatives including the substantial face-to-face contact, the reliability and the simplicity of the software tools employed in the project, the adequate support from the administrators, and the on-going mentoring provided by the facilitators.

Similarly, Sinclair & Owston (2006) described a two-year professional development course consisting of a day long face-to-face session, an eight-week online session, and a final face-to-face session at the end of the course. Their results concluded that the course affected teacher attitudes and knowledge positively and motivated them to transform their classroom practices. However, lack of cohesion in the online session and the failing rate of the participation suggest the need to rethink some aspects of the design of blended learning environments. Henderson (2007) on the other hand, explored the role of community of practice in sustaining teachers' participation in a blended learning professional development course which consisted of face-to-face and online learning components. He suggested that teachers' participation in the learning process can be sustained by supporting teachers to work in small groups.

Likewise, Berger, Eylon and Bagno (2008) outlined a blended professional development course designed for physics teachers. The course had nine face-to-face meetings as well as continuous online exchanges between facilitator and teachers through a Website. Results revealed that both, face-to-face meetings and the Web-based environment played different and complementary roles in the teachers' learning. Combining the findings of three teachers' professional development courses Owston, et al (2008) found that blended learning methodologies were effective in providing teachers with an opportunity for learning on the job and collaborating with other teachers. These findings revealed several of the factors which had an impact on the level of success of blended initiatives. Since evidence from professional development courses support the ongoing acquisition of knowledge, further research is needed to understand more specific factors affecting the teaching and learning effectiveness in courses employing blended learning models. As Stacey & Gerbic (2009) noted "the literature to date indicates that attention in the teaching and learning area of blended environments has focused on understanding the aspects of the virtual and physical environments which are valuable for learning and how to integrate them so that they work in complementary fashion" (p.10).

THE PROGRAM DESCRIPTION

Bullying is a significant pedagogic issue connected to education, psychological well being and the social behavior of the students as the negative consequences affecting the young victims of intimidation and bullying are multiple and long-lasting (Anderson, 2005). The role of the teacher is of utmost importance, on the one hand for the social development of the students and the conveyance of the principles and rules that permeate the acceptable social behavior and, on the other hand, for the management of the relationship among the students and the treatment of possible problems that might lead to a manifestation of derailing behavior (Houndoymani & Pateraki, 2001).

At the same time, the ever increasing attendance in Greek schools of foreign students creates new problems for the schools and renders certain requirements allowing equal opportunities to all students of all levels a necessity (Georgiadis, & Zisimos, 2005). Within this framework, the need to sensitize the educational society and train the teachers for the prevention and management of the problems to arise due to the co-existence of various cultural influences within the school environment is deemed necessary (Govaris et al, 2003; Demetriou, 2004). The access given to all teachers as regards the continuous improvement programs relevant to their qualifications and skills in a way that reflects their daily needs comprises the focal point for the scientific community and the bodies involved in the further education of the teachers.

Within the aforementioned framework, the adoption of methods for distance learning with the support of information technology and communication promises the creation of continuous education structures in an effective, flexible and reliable way irrespective of the teachers' residence and location of work. The training program which is presented in this study was a blended learning program targeting multicultural education and bullying in schools. The main objectives of the program were to: (a) Help teachers acquire knowledge, attitudes, and skills needed to interact, negotiate, and communicate with students from diverse groups;, and (b) Advise teachers on how to confront and prevent bullying in schools. A total of 187 teachers employed in state schools primarily from the rural areas of northern Greece participated in the course (see Figure 1).

The teachers' professional development program included four components: (a) the program's content, (b) the web-based environment, (c) the face-to-face meeting and (d) the online learning process. These components are described below.

The Programs' Content and the Material

In the preparatory phase of the program, the modification/formation of the analytic program's

Figure 1. Map showing the two regions northern of Greece engaged in the course: Iperous, East Macethonia-Thrace

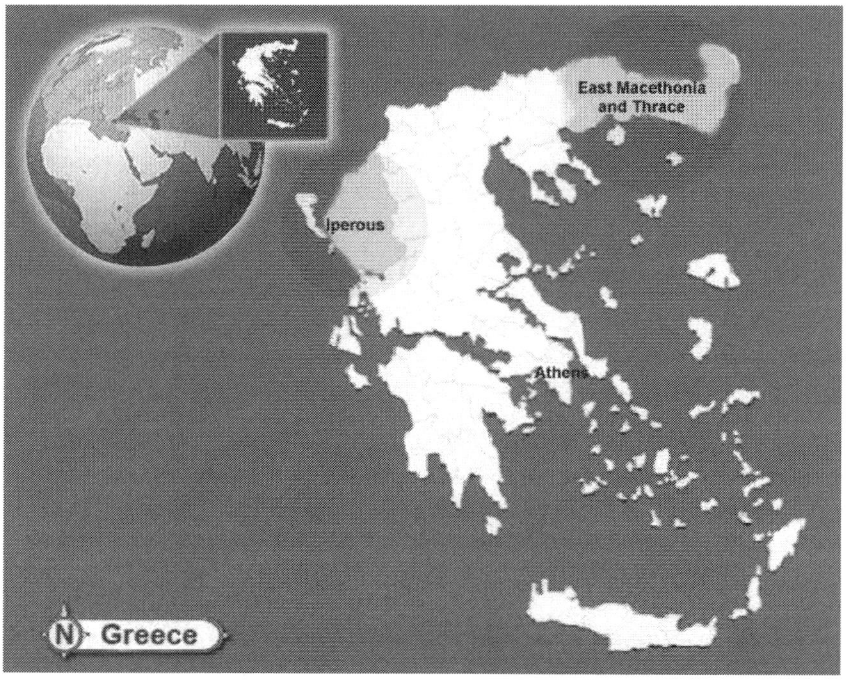

content was completed in addition to the writing of the material. The content of both the prevention of bullying and the management of multiculturalism in the school environment was divided into thirteen modules (Table 1).

The online learning material which was used to support the content was organized in lessons (5-7 lessons for each module). Each lesson included 10-15 pages of online text (Figure 2.)

The material was developed from the basic principles of open distance learning. In particular, the main features of the material were: (a) clearly stated objectives in each lesson, (b) examples and activities that illustrated functions and key issues of the subjects throughout every lesson, (c) self-assessment tests to help teachers check their own progress, (d) final tests and assignments to assess teachers' knowledge, and (e) resources including files in.pdf format and links to other resources. The material also included manuals and guides for the face-to-face meeting (see below). This material consisted of a study calendar, a prortfolio of programs' evidence and a web-based environment manual.

The Web-Based Environment

The second stage included the design of the web-based environment which was used to support the distance training process. The web-based environment was based on an open-code Learning Management System (www.istos.sch.gr) and the registered teachers had access to the lessons as well as a calendar (see Figure 3). The teachers

Table 1. The programs' subjects and modules

Subject	Modules
A. Prevention of bullying	1. Behavioral issues. 2. Bullying/ the bullying phenomenon. 3. Characteristics of children with behavioral issues. 4. Aggressive behavioral patterns at school. 5. Reasons and factors that enhance bullying. 6. Educational intervention for the prevention and management of bullying. 7. Intervention programs for the resolution of conflicts
B. Management of multiculturalism	8. Globalization and education. 9. Educational policy on multiculturalism. 10. Xenophobia, racism. 11. Analysis of experiences from countries with a history in the managements of relevant educational issues. 12. Principles of cross-cultural education. 13. Examples of educational application of the principles of cross-cultural education.

Figure 2. The structure of the online learning material

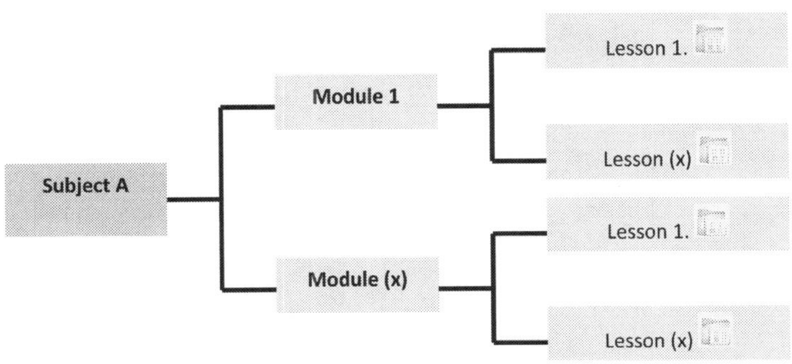

Figure 3. The user-interface of the web-based environment: (1) login account, (2) online users, (3) classes, (4) program's subjects, (5) material, (6) calendar

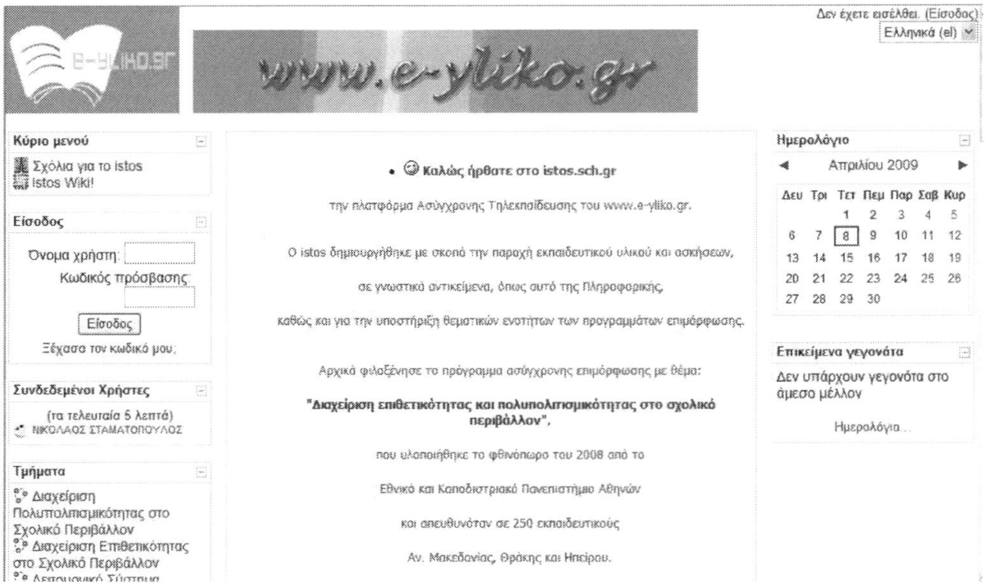

who participated in the program had their own personal account in the system and all program materials were available to them through login on the web site. All the interaction between the teachers and the facilitator took place through e-mails during the program.

Following this, the modification of the material according to the standard SCROM 1.2 was completed so as to be used in a web-based environment. The material modification in each of the program lessons was specifically structured and was divided in the following units/chapters: purpose, expected results, key concepts, introductory notes, contents of the lesson, summary, bibliography and tasks-activities (see figure 4.). In addition, the participants had the opportunity to download additional resources in.pdf files format.

Face-to-Face Meetings

The training process began with two six- hour face-to-face meetings held on the first two weeks of October, one for the teachers from the region of East Macethonia/Macedonia – Thrace held in Komotini and one for the teachers from the region of Ipirous held in Ioannina. During these face-to-face meetings the training process and the asynchronous distance learning platform were explained to the teachers as well as the purpose and the targets of the program. There followed a discussion where the teachers posed their questions concerning the administration of the educational process.

The Online Learning Process

The distance training process lasted for six weeks (October-November 2008). The trainees were grouped into 'classes' of between 16 and 25 teachers who each received support from their facilitators. Each teacher used his personal username and password to access the material and participate in the educational process. This process was based on the study of the contents by the teacher (self-directed learning). During the training process the teachers were engaged in online tests in order to confirm that the learning targets were met. In particular, these activities

Figure 4. The main features of the program's material in each lesson: (1) list of content, (2) title of subject, (3) title of module, (4) introductory notes, (5) examples and activities, (6) online text, and (7) recourses in.pdf format

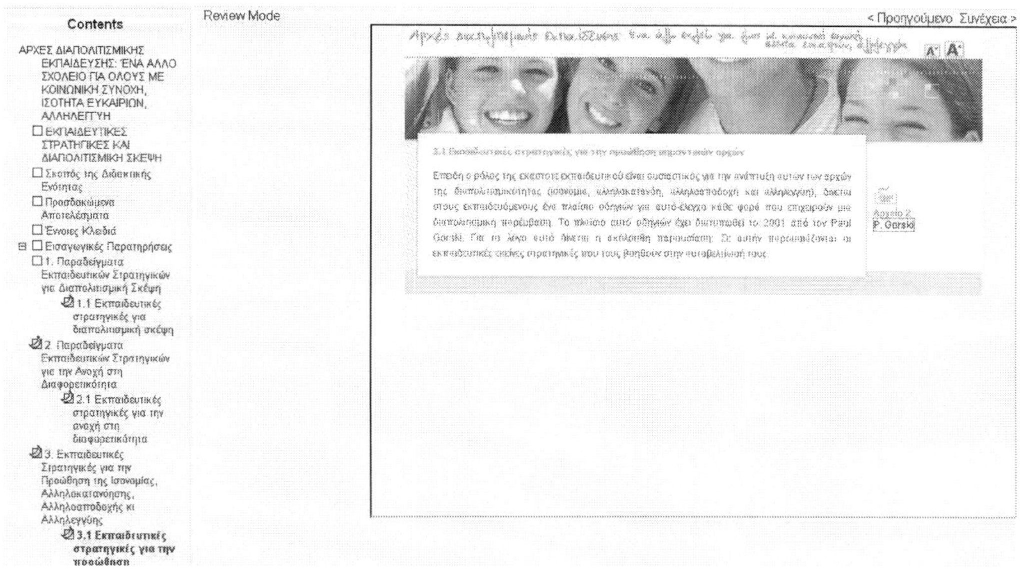

Table 2. The assignments

Prevention of bullying	Management of multiculturalism
Please describe a bullying case and suggest ways to manage the problem at a school level and through cooperation with the family and environment of the students.	Please describe an educational activity dealing with multicultural issues, defining the potential problems during the implementation phase and suggest ways for their resolution.

included:

- Self-evaluation tests which were given at the end of each lesson and a final test, where the teachers had to answer a group of questions that covered all the modules of the program. The tests included the following question and answer types (a) yes/no questions, (b) multiple choice questions, and (c) open-ended activities (submitted in.doc or.excel files format)
- A written assignment for each module of the training program (one for bullying in schools and one for multicultural education).

Throughout the educational process, a facilitator was responsible for monitoring and supporting each class of teachers while the teacher could address via electronic mail his facilitator for the resolution of questions as regards the lessons and the assessment exercises. In particular, the facilitator's responsibility concerned: (a) the informing of the teachers regarding the timetable of the educational activities, (b) the correction and assessment of the open-ended activities, (c) the support – elaboration of the assignments and their evaluation, (d) the communication with the teachers on a 24hour basis and the response to their messages providing instructions, advice and assistance, and (e) the reporting of the open-ended activities and assignments marks.

Figure 5. A multiple choice question in a self-assessment test

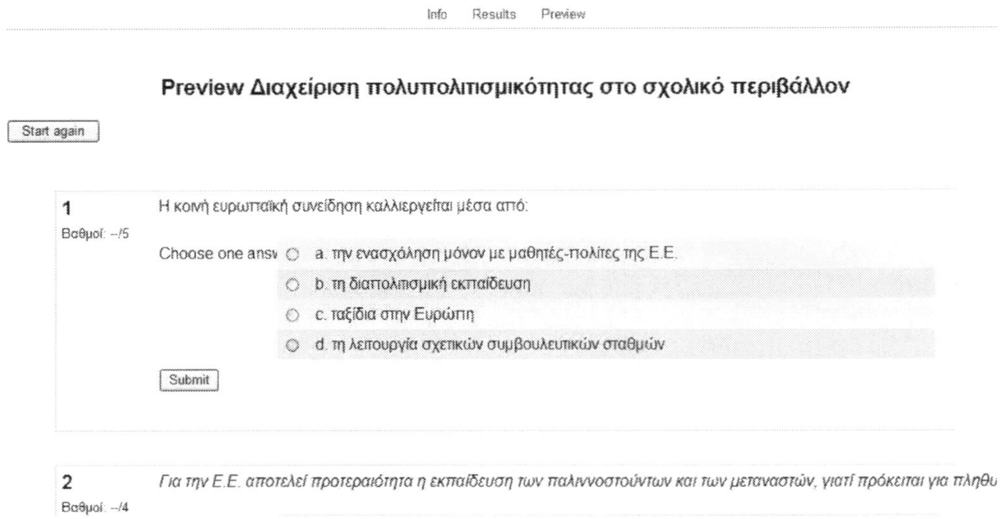

Figure 6. The pedagogy of the teachers' professional development program

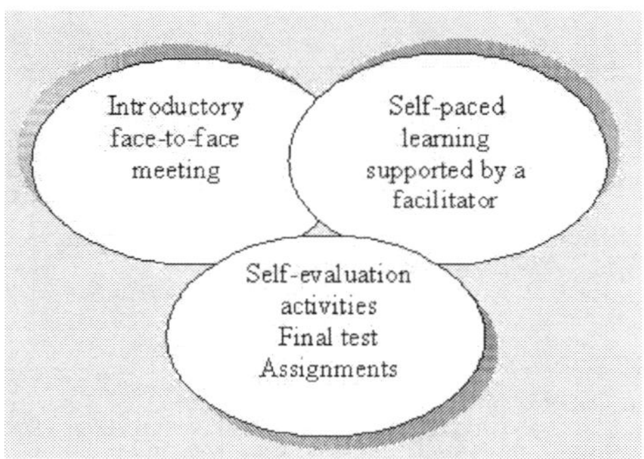

The Program's Evaluation

Sample

Of the 187 teachers initially enrolled in the training program, 132 participated in the evaluation process, resulting in a 70.6 percent participation rate. The gender and age profile of the sample is presented in Figure 7 and Figure 8 respectively. The majority of the teachers who participated in the evaluation process was secondary education teachers (64.4%, n=85) with primary education teachers comprising the remaining 35.6% (n=47). More than half of the respondents (n=76, 57.6%) reported that they already had more than 10 years of teaching experience, while 27.3% (N=36) reported that they had between 5-10 years, and 15.2% (N=20) reported that they had less than 5 years of teaching experience.

Instrumentation

A questionnaire was developed to investigate teachers' perceptions on the blended learning program. Apart from demographics and background information sections (i.e. gender, age, job status, and teaching experience in years) there were 7 scales, each containing from 3 to 7 items, in the questionnaire. All the scales and the items used to measure the participants' perceptions were adapted from prior studies with modification to fit the specific context of the teachers' professional development program. In particular, the scales of personal relevance, active learning, facilitator, and satisfaction were adapted from Walker's (2002) work on Distance Education Learning Environments Survey (DELLES) while the scales of the material was adapted from Clayton's (2007) work on online learning environment survey (OLLES) and the scale of web-based

Figure 7. Gender profile of the sample

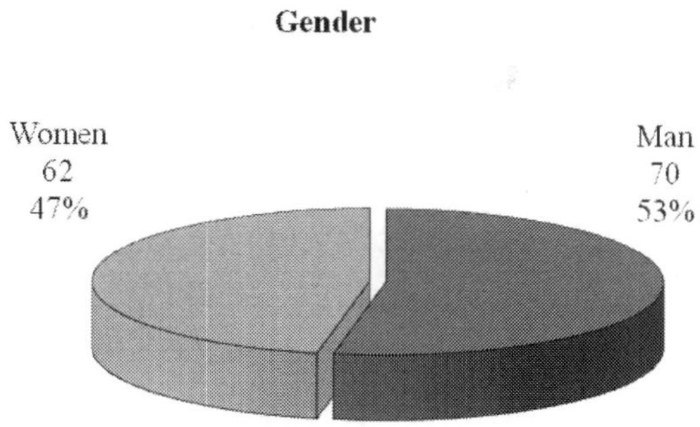

Figure 8. Age profile of the sample

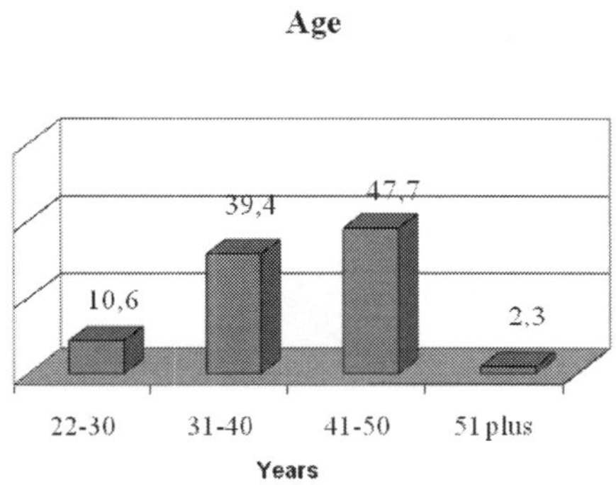

environment was adapted from Chang and Fisher's (2001) work on Web based Learning Environment Instrument (WEBLEI). In addition, three items were used to measure the teachers' perceptions toward the face-to-face meetings (Garrison & Vaughan, 2008). The description of the scales is presented in Table 3.

All items used a five-point Likert-type scale with anchors from 1 to 5 (1=strongly disagree, 2=disagree, 3=undecided, 4=agree, 5=strongly agree). Several of the items used negative undertones (i.e not) in order to detect acquiescent response sets that occur when the respondent supports items without regarding the actual content. Cronbach's coefficient test (*a*) was used to indicate if there was internal consistency of the questionnaire. The summary statistics of the item analysis for homogeneity and reliability indices reveal that the questionnaire reached a high alpha coefficient (*a*=.94) in all of the 34 intended items. The interval statistics concerning consistency reliability, ranged from.94 to.82 for the seven scales:.92 for personal development,.87 for active learning,.94 for the facilitator,.93 for the material,.91 for the web-based environment.82 for face-to-face meeting, and.88 for satisfaction. According to Kaplan & Sacuzzo (1993, 126) "it has been suggested that reliability estimates in the range of.70 to.80 are good enough for most purposes in basic research". Therefore, the alpha values will be considered acceptable for the objectives of this study.

Finally, the questionnaire included two open-ended questions to collect each teacher's perceptions about the blended learning program. These questions were:

Table 3. Description of the scales used to measure participants perceptions

Scale	Description	Number of Items	Example Item
Personal development	Extent to which teachers have opportunities for self-enhancement, development and knowledge achievement (Walker, 2002)	6	"I have the opportunity to work with authentic examples"
Active learning	Extent to which learners were engaged actively in the learning process (Walker, 2002).	4	"I am allowed to work during times I find convenient"
Facilitator support	The extent to which the facilitator guides teachers and provides comprehensive feedback and support (Clayton, 2007)	7	"The facilitator provides timely assessment on my assignment"
Material	Extent to which class materials are well structured and organised (Clayton, 2007)	5	"The content is well-organized and easy to follow"
Web-based environment	Extent to which the web-based environment is reliable and user friendly (Chang & Fisher, 2001)	4	"The web based learning environment held my interest throughout my course of study"
Face-to-face meeting	Extent to which face-to-face activities support students in their learning	3	"Face-face-meeting helps me to understand the concept and the goals of the course"
Satisfaction	Extent to which students enjoyed training and expressed positive attitudes toward the blended learning (Walker, 2002).	5	"I would better enjoy my professional development if more courses were offered through blended learning"

1. What did you like or dislike about the blended learning program?
2. Do you have any suggestions for improving the teachers' professional development program?

Data Collection and Data Analysis

The questionnaire was administered as an online form at the end of the training program. The teachers who agreed to participate in the evaluation survey completed the questionnaire anonymously. The researchers assumed that the participants in the evaluation study composed a representative sample of the program participants. It was further assumed that these participants provided truthful responses in the survey items. As far as the data analysis method is concerned, descriptive statistics methods were used for the quantitative data retrieved from the first and the second section of the questionnaire (frequency counts and percentages). In addition, content analysis method was used for the qualitative data retrieved from the open-ended questions of the questionnaire (teachers' comments analyzed and grouped according to similar responses).

ISSUES, CONTROVERSIES AND PROBLEMS

The results of the study highlight several issues affecting the teachers' perceptions regarding the main aspects of the blended training process. The results of the descriptive statistics regarding the items of personal development scale indicate that the majority of the teachers (75.8%) agree or strongly agree with the item that the program offered them the opportunity to work with cases drawn from their personal school experiences. A large percentage of the teachers also rated positively the items related to the opportunities they had to apply what they learned in their every day work (77.3%) as well as in their out-of-school life experience (75.5%). These findings are consistent with other studies demonstrating that teachers display readiness to learn when they have a perceived need, and they desire immediate application of new skills and knowledge (Nguyen and Katz, 2007). The results of this study also indicate that the teachers reported lower percentages of agreement in the items regarding the opportunities provided by the program's content to work with authentic examples and with realistic scenarios about practice of multicultural education and bullying prevention in schools (56.8% and 56.5% respectively). These findings reveal that further to the theoretical knowledge based on which the content was formed, the examples of school children behavioral problems and their treatment scenario at a school level did not fully cover the teacher's needs. As far as the organization of the training program are concerned, the results from the first open-ended question of the questionnaire indicate that the duration of the training process (the program lasted 6 weeks) was the most negative feature of the program. Many teachers responded that they did not have enough time to absorb the amount of information given (62 responses) and complete the online tests and assignments successfully (42 responses).

As far as the opportunities for active learning are concerned, the results indicate that the majority of the teachers appreciated the opportunity they had to explore their personal strategies for learning (79.5%). A majority of the teachers (77.7%) agree or strongly agree that the "anytime" and the "anywhere" features of the program provided them with the opportunity to plan their activities whenever and wherever it was most convenient for them. The results of this study also indicate that fewer teachers (60.6%) reported that during the program they felt confident of taking control of their learning as well as to incorporate their ideas into the learning process. A possible explanation for the relatively lower rate of teachers' confidence is that many of them did not have the appropriate required skills and attitudes to engage in self-directed learning. Previous research has shown that although online learning is a flexible and comfortable approach, many questions have been raised about the validity of self-directed learning for adults because many of them are not predisposed to take control of their learning and this is one important caveat regarding the distance learning process (Brookfield, 1995).

An examination of the first open-ended question demonstrates that some teachers (29 responses) claimed that although the program used some active learning approaches (open-ended activities, self-evaluation test and assessments), the nature of the program content, in general, demands teachers to take a more passive role in the acquisition of information on the web-based environment. As far as the teachers' perceptions of the material are concerned, the analysis of the quantitative data indicate that the majority of the teachers perceived that the assignments and the online tests were valuable for their learning (68.9% and 75.7% respectively). Many teachers also thought that the online texts were easy to read (61.4%) and the information was presented in a structured manner that was easy to follow (Figure 9).

In their comments on the first open-ended question, the teachers identified some negative features of the material regarding the self-evaluation tests. In particular, the teachers quite frequently commented that some questions in the self-evaluation tests presented errors or problems that affected the correct answers (29 responses). Some teachers also noted that the material would promote an active learning if the texts were designed carefully to integrate various media (textual and audiovisual) in an environment based on hypertext and hypermedia (27 responses).

As far as the role of the facilitator is concerned, although the 54.4% of the teachers appreciated the autonomy they had to ask the facilitator about issues they did not understand, the same percentage of teachers (55.6%) were neutral about or did not feel that the feedback they received from their facilitator was comprehensive. Similarly, 57.9% of

Figure 9. "The content information is well-organized and easy to follow"

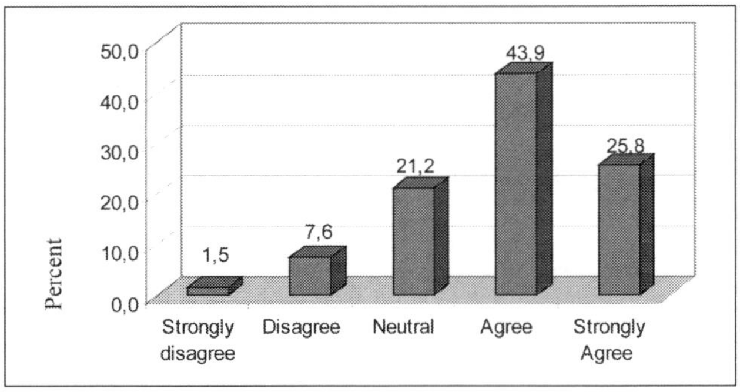

the teachers were either neutral or disagreed with the statement that the facilitator offered timely assessment on their assignments. About half of the teachers also strongly disagreed or disagreed with the item that the facilitator encouraged every teacher to participate by asking questions and exploring issues and ideas in depth (Figure 10). Relevant literature indicates the while participation is an obvious goal in face-to-face courses that include frequent discussions and small-group work, it is also important in a blended learning course (Garisson & Vaughen, 2008). In order to promote a learners' participation, the facilitator should encourage collaboration in small groups by utilising anywhere, anytime access to communication tools and facilitate the use of engaging assessment, utilising online web technologies for discussion, interaction, research, submission and/or reflection (Meyer, 2003; Webb et al., 2005).

In the open-ended questions of the questionnaire the teachers remarked frequently that their facilitator delayed evaluating their assignments and informing them about their scores (26 responses). Some teachers also expressed negative feelings about the absence of collaborative and cooperative learning during the learning process (21 responses). These findings confirm previous research on blended learning that emphasizes the ability of the facilitator to support learners through individual feedback in their written work (Wright et al., 2006). Equally important for the facilitator's role is to develop skills in facilitating online communities where peer-to-peer interactions provide a vital learning environment (Ziob and Mosher, 2006).

The results of this study reveal that the web-based environment held the teachers' interest throughout the program (71.2%) and enhanced their learning (69.7%). The results also indicate that a lower percentage of teachers claimed that they had no difficulty using the web-based environment (58.3%) and accessed the materials on their own (60.6%). The teachers commented on the first open-ended question of the questionnaire that many delays occurred in uploading the online texts (36 responses). Many teachers also complained that sometimes they were unable to open sources delivered through files in.pdf format (21 responses). Furthermore, the teachers also reported that the use of the web-based environment did not provide them with the necessary tools for real-time interaction and communication with their facilitator and other teachers (17 responses).

As far as the teachers' perceptions of the face-to-face meeting are concerned, the results of this study reveal that over half of the teachers reported that the meeting offered valuable information that helped them to understand the concept and the objectives of the program (Figure 11). A large percentage of teachers were neutral or disagreed with the idea that the introductory meeting did not provide them with the skills necessary to use the

Figure 10. "The facilitator encourages my participation"

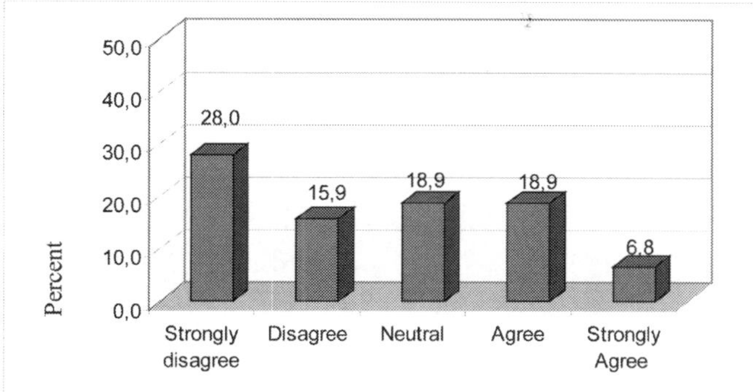

web-based platform effectively or that it did not provide them with specific directions on how to deal with the online test and complete the assessments (71.3% and 79.5% respectively).

In their comments on the first open-ended question the teachers suggested that during the face-to-face meeting a lot of time and effort was needed in order to get specific guidance on how to do their work in the web-based environment (27 responses). The findings of this study are consistent with results from other studies which indicate that blended learning must be supported by face-to-face interaction, especially at the early stages of the teachers' encounter with technology (Cashion and Palmieri, 2002). Evidence from these studies have shown that while the flexibility of the online environments allows learners to access the material most convenient to them, learners identify face-to-face interactions with their facilitators as the most desirable elements of blended learning courses (Kante, 2002).

Finally, the results of the descriptive statistics related to the scale of satisfaction indicate that the majority of the teachers expressed a strong interest in attending blended learning courses for their professional enhancement (91.7%). The vast majority of the teachers reported that they enjoyed their participation in the blended learning process (86.4%) and suggested that they would enjoy professional development better if additional courses were offered by blended learning methodologies (84%). The teachers also expressed a desire to participate in similar course in the future (78.0%) and expressed positive attitudes toward blended learning courses. The teachers' strong preference of the blended learning model is in agreement

Figure 11. "The face-to-face meeting helps me to understand the concept and the goals of the program"

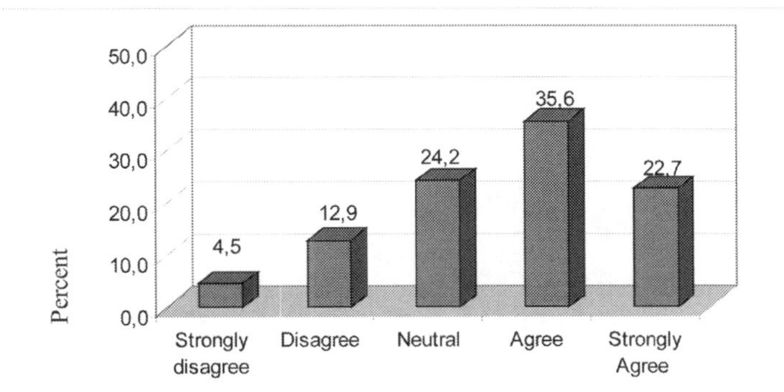

with reports from most current studies on online learning models (Bonk & Graham, 2006)

SOLUTIONS AND RECOMMENDATIONS

The goal of this section is to offer practical ideas and suggestions from the teachers' point of view on ways to improve the effectiveness of the particular professional development program. The teachers' comments on the second open-ended question of the questionnaire illustrate the need to adjust the content to the teachers' needs and their personal characteristics. Likewise, the timing and the duration of the training program should be reconsidered before deciding on the amount of information to be covered. The teachers very often noted that the present program could be restructured to last longer (10- to 15 months) in order to have enough time to study the material (45 responses) and to complete the tests and assignments effectively (32 responses). As regards the programs' structure, it should enable teachers to choose among different modules, those which meet their personal needs and interests (27 responses). Flexibility and choice in teachers' professional development courses are major issues for the majority of programs designers, namely to meet the diverse needs of trainee teachers and schools (Graham, Allen, & Ure, 2005).

Since the training program was offered mostly at distance, there were special challenges to meet in order to provide an effective pedagogical environment that motivate and support teachers to become self-directed learners (Merizow, 2004). According to the teachers' comments, the material should include additional scenario-based activities in relation to bullying in schools and multicultural education, which will lead to better learning results as well as effective professional development and reflection (25 responses). It is interesting to note that given the lack of many teachers' knowledge or experience in self-directed learning, an appropriate amount of face-to-face or online practice is needed before the main program begins. This practice will enhance all teachers' capability to understand the requirements of the program and thus sustain their interest, attitudes and efforts towards the program's objectives (17 responses). These findings corroborate the results of previous published research on what professional development course designers can do to promote the development of self-directed learning in distance learning environments (Garrison, 1997; Merriam, 2001;Song and Hill, 2007).

The received responses to the open-ended questions indicate that the material should include more activities catering for different learning styles, so that the teachers can select the appropriate activities based on their preferred style (29 responses). Teachers also commented that information should be presented in different formats such us textual, verbal and visual to improve their perception and attention for the learning process (21 responses). According to the teachers' views, the following modifications can improve the quality of the visual input:

- Important information and individual objects should become prominent by being placed in the centre of the screen and emphasizing different attributes of every visual object e.g. color, texture, or font (27 responses).
- Hypertext and hypermedia concepts should be used enabling teachers with diverse backgrounds and knowledge to establish their own path for learning (22 responses).
- Graphic design, tables and figures should be used to facilitate deep processing. In addition, the use of linear, hierarchical, or spider-shaped mind maps and concept maps would offer visual display of information and better understanding of relationships between objects (20 responses).
- The material should remain as reference material on the web helping other teachers

increase their knowledge in the fields of multicultural education and the prevention of bullying in schools (17 responses).

These findings of the current study are consistent with those of Ally (2004) who suggests that "information should be presented in different modes to accommodate individual differences in processing and to facilitate transfer to long-term memory. Where possible textual, verbal, and visual information should be presented to encourage encoding" (p.16).

One of the key issues which emerged from the teachers' comments on the second open-ended question pertains to the role of the facilitator and its possible suggestions for improvement. The teachers frequently noted that it would have been beneficial to them if they had more regular interaction with the facilitator (30 responses). Teachers also asked for improved timely interaction with their facilitator via the use of synchronous communication tools such as the Internet Relay Chat and the videoconference (25 responses). Interestingly, some teachers also reported needing telephone assistance available 24 hours a day (7 responses). Various improvements that were frequently noted by the teachers on the role of facilitators are the following:

- The facilitator should provide advice and guidance on tests and assignments regularly (22 responses).
- The facilitator should support collaborative and cooperative learning by giving teachers the opportunity to make use of the abilities of the other teachers (20 responses).
- The facilitator should provide prompt assistance and help the teachers spot the various online resources available (14 responses).
- The facilitator must be efficient to manage online activities effectively, support face-to-face and online contact and help teachers to complete tasks on time (13 responses).

These findings are consistent with other studies which suggest that effective facilitation skills include appropriate questioning and listening, engaging the learner in the learning process, providing direction and support to learners, and managing online discussion (Salmon, 2000). Thus, the facilitator must be knowledgeable in appropriate online support and have the ability to be innovative and experimental (Berge, 1995). The teachers' comments also demonstrate that the web-based environment should include synchronous communication tools such us chat, voice conferencing, and videoconferencing to improve timely interaction with the facilitator (31 responses). Relative research has shown that online learning activities are mediated by online learning tools (Lam, 2004). Thus, the development of interaction between the facilitator and the teachers is dependent on the facilitator's skills and features of the networked environment.

The results of this work also suggest that the web-based environment should include a forum for collaboration, conversation, discussion, exchange, and communication among the teachers (20 responses). This finding indicates the teachers' interest in collaborative learning components, such as discussion groups which is in agreement with other studies that explored the value of learners' engagement and interactivity in online groups and communities of practice (McConnel, 2006). As far as the web-based environment is concerned, the results of this work reveal that it should allow for uploading, downloading and printing of the materials without delays (29 responses). Relative literature confirms that for an web-based learning environment to be successful, learners must be able to easily focus on learning materials without having to make an effort to figure out how to access them (Chiu et al., 2005; Lohr, 2000).

Another area for improvement frequently asked for by the teachers is the need to increase face-to-face interaction with their facilitators and peers. The present findings reveal that the face-to-face meeting should increase the teachers' capability of using the web-based environment effectively so that teachers will achieve better results and improve their learning and reflection. Given the lack of experience in distance learning environments, teachers should be given an extra amount of time during the face-to-face meeting in order to become familiar with the web-based learning process. In consensus with prior literature, results of this work suggest that online learning needs to and must be supported by face-to-face interaction, especially at the early stages of teachers' encounter with technology (Kante, 2002). Furthermore, the results of this study indicate that the teachers recognized the need for some extra face-to-face meetings with their facilitator - apart from the introductory face-to-face meeting. These meetings would help the teachers identify barriers to their learning and provide them with effective solutions (24 responses).

In particular, the teachers would like to have two more meetings during the program of about three or four hours each in order to discuss with facilitators and peers, and create a feeling of togetherness (19 responses). According to the teachers, these meetings would be more effective if the facilitator creates small individualized or collaborative activities to fill the teachers' gaps and their personal interests (16 responses). This would reduce the teachers' personal anxieties about their ability to undertake the web-based activities (14 responses). Relative research has shown that face-to-face meetings in the blended learning process allow for social presence and collaboration to be established in blended learning courses (Wiesenberg & Stacey, 2009). As Stacey and Gerbic (2009) noted "the literature to date indicates that attention in the teaching and learning area of blended environments has focused on understanding the aspects of the virtual and physical environments which are valuable for learning and how to integrate them so that they work in a complementary fashion" (p.10).

FUTURE RESEARCH DIRECTIONS

This evaluation study provided information on teachers' perceptions about both pedagogical practices (online learning, face-to-face learning, material relevance, interactivity, etc.) and technical aspects of the web-based environment (reliability, user interface, access to the material, communication tools, etc.), enriched with teachers' satisfaction level of the blended learning program. In the future, further studies taking these findings into account will need to be undertaken in order to investigate how different approaches to the design and the implementation of blended learning models can affect teachers' satisfaction, engagement, and learning. Since many teachers would prefer the convenience offered by distance professional development program without sacrificing the social interaction and human touch evident in face-to-face environments, course designers face the challenge to achieve a right balance between flexible learning options available and high-touch interactive experience. From a pedagogical standpoint, there are various quality criteria that need to be considered to design effective professional development courses. Further research is needed to investigate on:

- The content or the interactions that are best delivered conveyed be online and face-to-face components of a blended learning course.
- The best combination of the pedagogical strategies and the media (synchronous and asynchronous) necessary to address the different needs of teachers.
- The conditions under which teachers are motivated to become actively involved in and take greater responsibility of their own learning in blended learning courses.
- The amount and the type of involvement on the part of the facilitator that can affect teachers' learning and participation in live and online options of a blended course.

> Since technology leads to a shift in the facilitators' role from one the sole source of knowledge to be a facilitator of self-paced teachers, many questions are raised on how the facilitator can enhance the quality of off-line and on-line learning and improve peer-to-peer interaction and collaboration.

In terms of the quality of course content and materials, more research is needed to investigate how the visual-textual layout, the navigation aids, and the interactive audio/visual components can be organised in a navigation hierarchy of hyperlinks (e.g., sequencing design, exploration design, indexed design, etc.) to take the advantage of the interactive properties of the Web. Although current learning management systems (LMS) provide us with a number of tools to develop learning environments based on principles of pedagogy, further research is needed to help us identify the strengths and weaknesses of the Web when used in such programs. In addition, blended learning provides us with the opportunity to reach large numbers of teachers from rural areas in a short period of time with consistent, semi personal content delivery, and thus it is essential to take into consideration all the costs associated with these approaches.

CONCLUSION

Blended learning approaches are increasingly transforming teachers' professional development worldwide. Owning to the newness of blended learning in teachers' professional development in Greece, this chapter aimed to identify some factors which may promote successful blended learning programs, drawing on both results of the current evaluation study and the literature on blended learning. The current study found the teachers' high satisfaction with the flexibility and convenience provided by the blended learning program. The training program provided them with the opportunities they needed to remain in their classrooms while using material and resources they might not have had access to in traditional face-to-face training modalities. Not surprisingly, the teachers expressed high levels of satisfaction with the training process and appeared to prefer blended learning modalities to fully face-to-face training programs.

From the pedagogical point of view, the results of this study indicate the program supported the development of the teachers' professional knowledge and skills in multicultural education and bullying in schools. The programs' content provided opportunities for teachers to apply theory and understand theory working with examples and problem-solving tasks. The content also provided opportunities for "hands-on" activities which are integrated into the daily life of the school. These results reinforce the widely-reported teachers' preference for content that meets their professional needs and makes their job more satisfying both professionally and personally (Kante, 2002).

The material of the blended learning program, it consisted of both texts which were related to the program's content and guides for the face-to-face meetings. As far as the material's quality is concerned, this study provides empirical confirmation of the literature regarding the features of materials for distance learning programs (Ally, 2004). The material should be developed according to the program's content and the specific needs of the teachers and also should be well-written and well-organized into the program's modules. Main principles of adult learning (work-related activities, activities that reflect teacher's interest etc.) and the learning theories (behaviorist, cognitive and constructivist strategies) should be taken into account to promote active learning and to foster higher-order thinking and meaningful knowledge (See Figure 12).

As far as the blended learning approach is concerned, the results of this study indicate that the mixture of online self-paced learning with a face-to-face meeting changed their traditional

Figure 12. Features of the material for blended learning

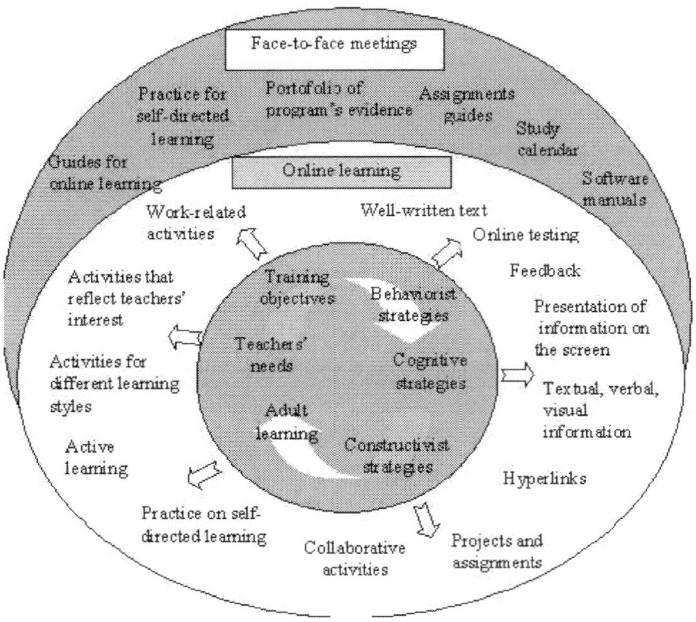

Figure 13. The model of blended training process

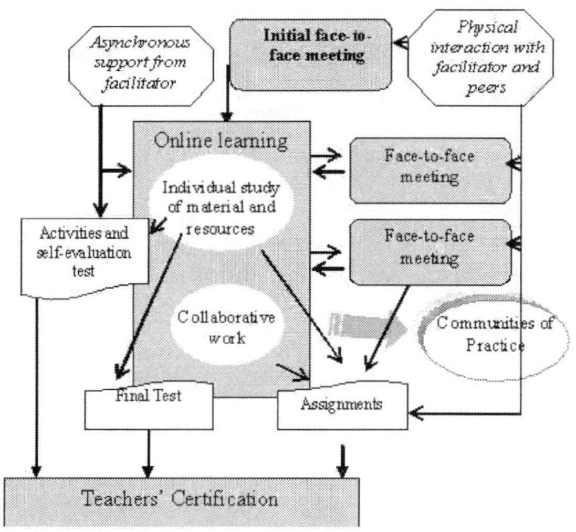

method of training and enhanced effective learning possibilities. The teachers who participated in the training program did not consider the face-to-face and the online components of the program separately, but as part of an integrated learning environment where the activity into the face-to-face setting have an influence on the online learning. Thus, the teachers emphasise the need for more regular face-to-face meetings which would help them to resolve issues that arise during the process.

Based on teachers' perspectives, this study provides a model of a blended learning to respond to local teachers' needs of their ongoing professional development. The model, which is presented in Figure 13, involves an introductory 6-hour face-to-face meeting followed by online learning with 2 intermediate face-to-face meetings. This model advice that the online learning should progress for a minimum of 4 months, integrating a combination of individual study of the material, active learning activities, self-evaluation tests, work-related assignments, assessment as well as cooperative learning and collaborative learning. Special emphasis is given in the interaction with facilitators during both face-to-face meetings (physical interaction) and online learning (asynchronous interaction). The importance of the establishment of communities of practices among teachers is also recognized (Garrison and Vaughan's, 2008).

Figure 14. Learning activities for the face-to-face learning environment and the online learning environment

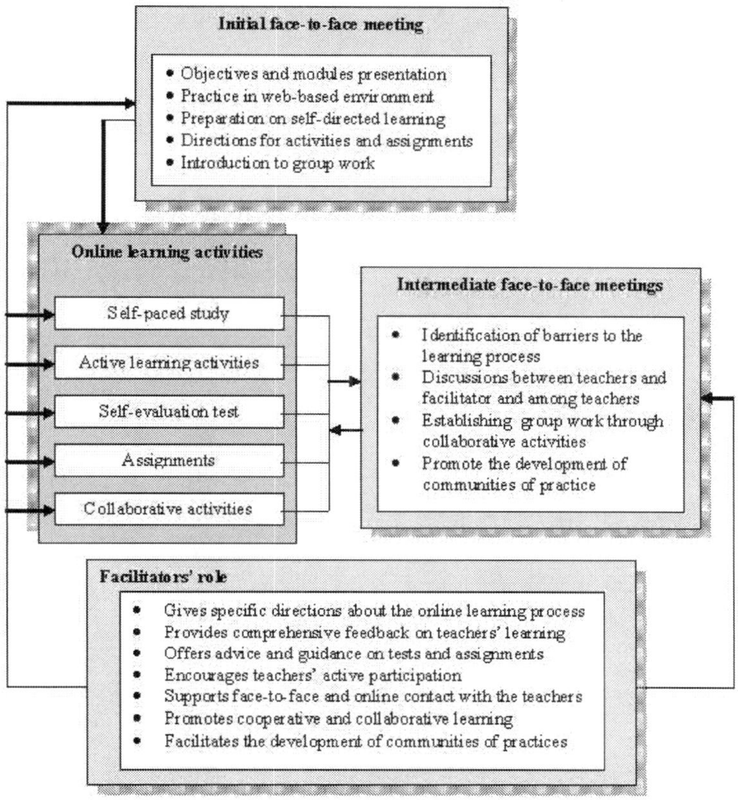

The results of this study provide also some recommendations for designing learning activities suitable for the face-to-face learning environment and the online learning environment. The activities presented in Figure 14, utilize the strength of each environment and add pedagogical value to the blended learning program. Special emphasis is given to facilitators' role. This study also indicate that the opportunity given to teachers to participate in an active and meaningful training process presupposes reliable network access, adequacy of links, pleasing and attractive layout, hyperlinks and hyper media options and synchronous and asynchronous communication tools that enhance various forms of interaction.

To conclude, this chapter explored the impact of blended learning on teachers' professional development through case study carried out by the Ministry of Education and Religious Affairs in cooperation with the National Kapodistrian University of Athens in Greece. As the need and demand for teacher professional development increase, future research is important to identify successful models of blended learning that can be adapted to create effective and flexible ongoing learning experiences in the field of ongoing teachers' professional development.

ACKNOWLEDGMENT

We would like to express our thanks to all the teachers who participated in the study. We would also like to thank Mr H. Maglogiannis, Assistant Professor, Dept. of Computer Science and Biomedical Informatics, University of Central Greece and Mr D. A. Bourletidis Assistant Researcher, National and Kapodistrian University of Athens for their valuable assistance in collecting the data for this study. Finally special thanks to Ms A. Zacharaki, teacher of English, for her editorial support and assistance in the study.

REFERENCES

Ally, M. (2004). Foundations of educational theory for online learning. In Anderson, T., & Elloumi, F. (Eds.), *Theory and practice of online learning* (pp. 3–31). Athabasca, Alberta, Canada: Athabasca University.

Anderson, J. (2005). *School bullying, a review of the research.* Crime prevention and criminal Justice policy, [CRIM 420], Amber MacDonald, Spring 2005

Berge, Z. L. (1995). The role of the online instructor/facilitator in facilitating computer conferencing: Recommendations from the field. *Educational Technology, 35*(1), 22–30.

Berger, H., Eylon, B., & Bagno, E. (2008). Professional Development of Physics Teachers in an Evidence-Based Blended Learning Program. *Journal of Science Education and Technology, 17*(4), 399–409. doi:10.1007/s10956-008-9109-3

Bleed, R. (2006, January). The IT leader as alchemist: Finding the true gold. *EDUCAUSE Review*, 33–42.

Bonk, C. J., & Graham, C. R. (Eds.). (2006). *Handbook of blended learning: Global perspectives, local designs.* San Francisco, CA: Pfeiffer Publishing.

Borko, H. (2004). Professional Development and Teacher Learning: Mapping the Terrain. *Educational Researcher, 33*(8), 3–15. doi:10.3102/0013189X033008003

Brookfield, S. (1995). Adult learning: An overview. In Tuinjman, A. (Ed.), *International Encyclopedia of Education* (pp. 265–269). Oxford, UK: Pergamon Press.

Cashion, J., & Palmieri, P. (2002). *The secret is the teacher. The learner's view of online learning. Australian National Training Authority.* Adelaide, South Australia: NCVER.

Chang, V., & Fisher, D. L. (2001). A new learning instrument to evaluate online learning in higher education. In Kulski, M., & Herrmann, A. (Eds.), *New horizons in university teaching and learning* (pp. 23–34). Perth, Western Australia.

Chiu, C.-M., Hsu, M.-H., Sun, S.-Y., Lin, T.-C., & Sun, P.-C. (2005). Usability, quality, value and e-learning continuance decisions. *Computers & Education, 45*(4), 399–416. doi:10.1016/j.compedu.2004.06.001

Clayton, J. (2007). *Development and validation of an instrument for assessing online learning environments in tertiary education: The Online Learning Environment Survey (OLLES).* PhD thesis, Curtin University of Technology.

Darling-Hammond, L., Holtzman, D. J., Gatlin, S. J., & Heilig, J. V. (2005). Does teacher preparation matter? Evidence about teacher certification, Teach for America, and teacher effectiveness. *Education Policy Analysis Archives, 13*(42), 1–48.

Dede, C., Ketelhut, D., Whitehouse, P., Breit, L., & McCloskey, E. (2006). *Research Agenda for Online Teacher Professional Development.* Cambridge, MA: Harvard Graduate School of Education.

Demetriou, O. (2004). Prioritizing ethnicities: the uncertainty of Pomak-ness in the urban Greek Rhodopi. *Ethnic and Racial Studies, 27*(1), 95–119. doi:10.1080/0141987032000147959

European Commission. (2007). *Improving the Quality of Teacher Education. Communication from the Commission to the Council and the European Parliament.* Brussels, Belgium: European Commission. Retrieved February 18, 2009, from http://ec.europa.eu/education/com392_en.pdf

Fiege, K., Peacock, K., & Geelan, D. (2004). Professional Development: A Rural School District's Experience with Videoconferencing. In C. Crawford et al. (Eds.), *Proceedings of Society for Information Technology and Teacher Education International Conference 2004* (pp. 2150-2157). Chesapeake, VA: AACE.

Garrison, D. R. (1997). Self-directed learning: Toward a comprehensive model. *Adult Education Quarterly*, *48*(1), 18–33. doi:10.1177/074171369704800103

Garrison, D. R., & Vaughan, N. D. (2008). *Blended learning in higher education - Framework, principles and guidelines*. CA: Jossey-Bass - A Wiley Imprint.

Garrison, R., & Kanuka, H. (2004). Blended Learning: Uncovering its transformative potential in higher education. *The Internet and Higher Education*, *7*(2), 95–105. doi:10.1016/j.iheduc.2004.02.001

Georgiadis, F., & Zisimos, A. (2005). Migrants', refugees' and minorities' children in European Education: the Greek experience. In *Proceedings from the Conference Diversity in Education in an International Context*, 20-23 April. (Verona, International Association of Intercultural Education (IAIE)).

Govaris, Ch., Kaplanoglou, M., Skourtou, E., & Vratsalis, K. (2003). The Construction of the Substantialist Obstacle in Education through promoting the 'Substance' of Culture. *International Journal of Learning*, *10*, 1219–1230.

Graham, C. R. (2006). Blended learning systems: definition, current trends, and future directions. In Bonk, C. J., & Graham, C. R. (Eds.), *Handbook of blended learning: Global perspectives, local designs* (pp. 3–21). San Francisco, CA: Pfeiffer Publishing.

Graham, C. R., Allen, S., & Ure, D. (2005). Benefits and challenges of blended learning environments. In Khosrow-Pour, M. (Ed.), *Encyclopedia of information science and technology* (pp. 253–259). Hershey, PA: Idea Group.

Hellmig, L. (2008). Blended Learning for Teachers' Professional Development. Paper presented in the conference E-Learning Baltics, Rostock, Germany.

Henderson, M. (2007). Sustaining online teacher professional development through community design. *Campus-Wide Information Systems*, *3*(24), 162–173. doi:10.1108/10650740710762202

Hojsholt-Poulsen, L. (2007). *Current Trends in Teachers' Professional Development - 21 Cst Teachers Need Digital Competences and Digital Learning Resources*. The Sixth Open Classroom Conference, Real Learning in Virtual Worlds, Stockholm, Sweden.

Holmes, A., Polhemus, L., & Jennings, S. (2005). CATIE: A blended approach to situated professional development. *Journal of Educational Computing Research*, *32*(4), 381–394. doi:10.2190/F97W-QUJ4-G7YG-FPXC

Houndoymani, A., & Pateraki, L. (2001). Bullying and Bullies in Greek Elementary schools: Pupils attitudes and teachers - parents' awareness. *Educational Review*, *53*(1), 19–26. doi:10.1080/00131910120033619

Huang, R., & Zhou, Y. (2006). Designing blended learning focused on knowledge category and learning activities. In Bonk, C. J., & Graham, C. R. (Eds.), *Handbook of blended learning: Global perspectives, local designs* (pp. 296–310). San Francisco, CA: Pfeiffer Publishing.

Jegede, O., Fraser, B. J., & Fisher, D. L. (1998). *The distance and open learning environment scale: Its development, validation and use.* Paper presented at the 69th Annual Meeting of the National Association for Research in Science Teaching, San Diego, USA.

Jung, I. (2005). ICT-Pedagogy Integration in Teacher Training: Application Cases Worldwide. *Educational Technology &Society*, *8*(2), 94–101.

Kante, C. (2002). E-training: The new frontier of the teacher professional development. *TechKnow-Logia*, *4*(4), 12–14.

Kaplan, R. M., & Sacusso, D. P. (1993). *Psychological testing: Principles, applications, and issues.* Belmont, CA: Wadsworth.

Lam, W. (2004). Encouraging on-line participation. *Journal of Information Systems Education*, *15*(4), 345–349.

Lohr, L. L. (2000). Designing the instructional interface. *Computers in Human Behavior*, *16*, 161–182. doi:10.1016/S0747-5632(99)00057-6

Lord, G., & Lomicka, L. (2008). Blended learning in teacher education: An investigation of classroom community across media. *Contemporary Issues in Technology & Teacher Education*, *8*(2), 158–174.

Mackey, J. (2008). *Blending real work experiences and virtual professional development.* Paper presented at ASCILITE 2008 conference, Institute of Teaching and Learning, Deakin University, Melbourne, Australia

Martyn, M. (2003). The hybrid online model: Good practice. *EDUCAUSE Quarterly*, *6*(1), 18–23.

McConnell, D. (2006). *E-learning groups and communities.* Berkshire, UK: Open University Press.

Meiers, M., & Ingvarson, L. (2004). *Investigating the links between teacher professional development and student learning outcomes. Australian Government Quality Teacher Programme over 2001–2003. Australia council of educational research.* Commonwealth of Australia.

Merriam, S. B. (2001). Andragogy and self-directed learning. *New Directions for Adult and Continuing Education*, *89*, 3–14. doi:10.1002/ace.3

Meyer, K. A. (2003). Face-to-face versus threaded discussions: the role of time and higher-order thinking. *JALN*, *3*(7), 55–65.

Mezirow, J. (2003). Transformative Learning as Discourse. *Journal of Transformative Education*, *1*(1), 58–63. doi:10.1177/1541344603252172

National Professional Development Center on Inclusion. (2008). *What do we mean by professional development in the early childhood field?* Chapel Hill, NC: The University of North Carolina, FPG Child Development Institute. Retrieved January 10, 2009, from http://community.fpg.unc.edu/resources/articles/NPDCI-ProfessionalDevelopment-03-04-08.pdf

Nguyen, T., & Katz, J. (2007). Learning Contract for Online Course Design. In C. Crawford et al. (Eds.), *Proceedings of Society for Information Technology and Teacher Education International Conference 2007* (pp. 2377-2380). Chesapeake, VA: AACE.

OECD. (2005). *Teachers matter: Attracting, Developing and Retaining Effective Teachers. Education and Training Policy.* Paris: OECD Publications.

Osguthorpe, R., & Graham, C. (2003). Blended learning systems: Definitions and directions. *Quarterly Review of Distance Education*, *4*(3), 227–234.

Osguthorpe, R. T., & Graham, C. R. (2003). Blended learning environments: Definitions and directions. *The Quarterly Review of Distance Education, 4*(3), 227–233.

Owston, R., Wideman, H., Murphy, J., & Lupshenyuk, D. (2008). Blended Teacher Professional Development: A Synthesis of Three Program Evaluations. *The Internet and Higher Education, 11*(3/4), 201–210. doi:10.1016/j.iheduc.2008.07.003

Ramsey, C. (2003). Using virtual learning environments to facilitate new learning relationships. *The International Journal of Management Education, 3*(2), 31–41. doi:10.3794/ijme.32.62

Rovai, A. P., & Jordan, H. M. (2004). Blended learning and sense of community: A comparative analysis with traditional and fully online graduate courses. *International Review of Research in Open and Distance Learning, 5*(2), 1–13.

Salmon, G. (2000). *E-moderating: The key to teaching and learning online*. London: Kogan Press.

Samarawickrema, G. (2009). Blended learning and the new pressures on the academy: Individual, political and policy driven motivators for adoption. In Stacey, E., & Gerbric, P. (Eds.), *Effective Blended Learning Practices: Evidence-Based Perspectives in ICT- Facilitated Education*. Hershey, PA: IGI Publishing.

Simkins, T., Coldwell, M., Close, P., & Morgan, A. (2009). Outcomes of In-School Leadership Development Work: A Study of Three NCSL Programmes. *Educational Management Administration & Leadership, 37*(1), 29–50. doi:10.1177/1741143208098163

Sinclair, M., & Owston, R. (2006). Teacher Professional Development in Mathematics and Science: A Blended Learning Approach. *Canadian Journal of University Continuing Education, 32*(2), 43–66.

Singh, H. (2003). Building effective blended learning programs. *Educational Technology, 43*(6), 51–54.

Snoek, M., Uzerli, U., & Schratz, M. (2008, February). *Developing teacher education policies through peer learning*. Paper presented at the TEPE conference, Ljubljana, Slovenia.

Song, L., & Hill, J. (2007). A conceptual model for understanding self-directed learning in online environments. *Journal of Interactive Online Learning, 6*(1), 27–42.

Stacey, E., & Gerbic, P. (2009). Introduction to Blended Learning Practices. In Stacey, E., & Gerbic, P. (Eds.), *Effective Blended Learning Practices: Evidence-Based Perspectives in ICT-Facilitated Education* (pp. 1–19). Hershey, PA: IGI Publishing.

Walker, S. L. (2002). *Development and Validation of an Instrument for Assessing Distance Education Learning Environments in Higher Education: The Distance Education Learning Environments Survey*. Unpublished doctoral dissertation, University of Curtin, Curtin.

Webb, E., Jones, A., Barker, P., & van Schaik, P. (2005). Perspectives of Faculty on the Use of e-Learning Dialogues. In P. Kommers & G. Richards (Eds.), *Proceedings of World Conference on Educational Multimedia, Hypermedia and Telecommunications 2005* (pp. 2354-2361). Chesapeake, VA: AACE

Wideman, H., Owston, R., & Sinitskaya, N. (2007). Transforming teacher practice through blended professional development: Lessons learned from three initiatives. In C. Crawford et al. (Eds.), *Proceedings of Society for Information Technology and Teacher Education International Conference 2007* (pp. 2148-2154). Chesapeake, VA: AACE.

Wiesenberg, F., & Stacey, E. (2009). Blended Learning and Teaching Philosophies. Implications for Practice. In Stacey, E., & Gerbic, P. (Eds.), *Effective Blended Learning Practices: Evidence-Based Perspectives in ICT-Facilitated Education* (pp. 204–221). Hershey, PA: IGI Publishing.

Wirght, N., Dewstow, R., Topping, M., & Tappenden, S. (2006). New Zealand examples of Blended Learning. In Bonk, C. J., & Graham, C. R. (Eds.), *The Handbook of Blended Learning: Global Perspectives, Local Designs* (pp. 169–181). San Francisco: Pfeiffer.

Zgaga, P. (2008). Mobility and the European Dimension in Teacher Education. In Hudson, B., & Zgaga, P. (Eds.), *Teacher Education Policy in Europe: a Voice of Higher Education Institutions*. Umeå, Sweden: University of Umeå, Faculty of Teacher Education.

Ziob, L., & Mosher, B. (2006). Putting customers first at Microsoft. In Bonk, C. J., & Graham, C. R. (Eds.), *The Handbook of Blended Learning: Global Perspectives, Local Designs* (pp. 92–104). San Francisco: Pfeiffer.

Chapter 2
Integrating K-12 Hybrid Online Learning Activities in Teacher Education Programs:
Reflections from the School of Rock Expedition

Matthew Niemitz
Adobe Systems Inc., USA

Scott Slough
Texas A&M University, USA

Kristen St. John
James Madison University, USA

R. Mark Leckie
University of Massachusetts - Amherst, USA

Leslie Peart
Consortium for Ocean Leadership, USA

Ann Klaus
Texas A&M University, USA

ABSTRACT

The School of Rock (SOR) expedition was a unique at-sea teacher education workshop that sought to introduce inservice teachers to scientific ocean drilling and collaborate in developing ways to extend this science content to K-12 classrooms. During the workshop teachers used an expedition website to communicate their learning and the "results" of the expedition to an onshore audience of students. While adventure learning/hybrid online learning is common in K-12 classrooms, the SOR expedition

DOI: 10.4018/978-1-61520-897-5.ch002

Copyright © 2010, IGI Global. Copying or distributing in print or electronic forms without written permission of IGI Global is prohibited.

was unique in that teachers were the explorers and the workshop sought to use technology to enhance both the learning of students onshore and the learning of the participants of the workshop (Niemitz et al., 2008). Here, the authors examine how the SOR expedition website enhanced the teacher education goals of the workshop and compare and contrast their reflections with the literature on integrating technology into teacher education programs. The SOR experience identifies two new elements to consider as teacher educators design ways to integrate technology into education programs: 1) situations where pre- or in-service teachers can use technology to communicate narratives of inquiry can lead to engaging and formative learning experiences for both teachers and students; and 2) using technology to communicate new content knowledge to students in real or near real-time can reinforce a mindset for applying this knowledge to student learning needs as the teacher learning is in progress. The authors identify two examples of how to scale this model for integrating technology into teacher education and provide recommendations on appropriate technologies for doing so.

In November of 2005, 13 educators, 6 staff members, and over 50 crew members embarked from Victoria, British Columbia aboard the scientific ocean drilling vessel *JOIDES Resolution* on the first School of Rock expedition (SOR). For 12 days at sea, the primary, secondary, and informal educators explored the world of scientific ocean drilling firsthand - conducting scientific experiments, interviewing members of the crew, participating in the life of the ship, and creating instructional resources that they could use in their own classrooms and museums. Meanwhile, thousands of miles away, in classrooms all across the United States, students logged onto an expedition website that connected them, in an authentic way, to the learning that these educators were experiencing. On its own, this unique professional development workshop held significant value in enhancing the content knowledge and teaching of the participants. But, coupled with an interactive virtual expedition, the learning was extended from a select few in the field to an unlimited number of learners at home in near real-time (Niemitz et al., 2008).

The concept of interactive virtual expeditions (part of a larger hybrid online learning model, adventure learning) is gaining traction in education for its exemplary approach to both experiential learning and inquiry-based learning (Doering, 2006; 2007). But, scholars have focused on the role this model has in enhancing student learning. Little consideration has been given to how this model can apply to pre-service and in-service teacher education. The SOR expedition affords a unique perspective on this question, as the educators were directly involved in the expedition, rather than guiding their students as they followed a third party online expedition. As the participants enthusiastically received instruction in the scientific topics they were deeply interested in (Leckie et al., 2006; St. John et al., in press), the interactive virtual expedition spurred them to immediately use the content they were learning to take action with their students' learning.

The goal of this chapter is to present the SOR expedition case study to help examine the use of distance communications technology in teacher education activities. How did the model of coupling teacher education with real-time teacher-to-student communication (usually separate activities) serve to influence both teacher education and student learning? What does this case study tell us about how this model could potentially be scaled to more widely available or more traditional pre- and in-service teacher education scenarios? This chapter will present a theoretical framework for adventure learning and technology integration into teacher education programs, describe and discuss the SOR expedition case study, and compare and contrast the theoretical framework with the case study to answer these questions. Our hope is that this case study and the ideas generated from it will encourage teacher educators to test these ideas and evaluate them in an empirical way.

THE THEORETICAL BASIS FOR INTEGRATING HYBRID ONLINE LEARNING ACTIVITIES INTO TEACHER EDUCATION PROGRAMS

The Adventure Learning Model

To consider the theoretical basis for coupling teacher education activities with real-time teacher-to-student communication, we must first examine the concept and qualify the effectiveness of hybrid online learning for student learning. We need not examine the entire landscape for online learning, other than to qualify hybrid online learning as that online learning which occurs in conjunction with face-to-face classroom instruction. This model may take many shapes, but differs from situations where online learning and face-to-face learning are separate pursuits (a model more common in higher education). In hybrid online learning, teachers assist, scaffold, and supplement student learning experiences that are delivered online.

One form of hybrid online learning is characterized by the term adventure learning. Doering (2006) defines adventure learning as "providing students with opportunities to explore real-world issues through authentic learning experiences within collaborative learning environments" (p. 198). The rationale for learning of this type is that it is experiential, inquiry based, authentic, and motivating (Doering, 2006, 2007; Niemitz et al., 2008). When students follow real-time exploration or adventure activities, they can create knowledge through a collaborative, constructivist, and transformative experience. Through transformative experiences, a student's conceptions of the world around them are synthesized and then transformed in relation to the new knowledge they are gaining (Mezirow, 1990, 1991; Palloff & Pratt, 1999).

Adventure learning also focuses on creating an inquiry-based learning environment. In science education in particular, creating situations for inquiry-based learning is critical (NRC, 1996; Duschl, Schweingruber, & Shouse, 2007). Adventure learning seeks to provide authentic, participatory environments for inquiry-based learning. Through their interaction and collaboration with explorers via the Internet and their participation in an expedition, students are able to learn in an authentic context. Participation opportunities allow learners to join the inquiry in a very real and timely way, by playing a role in an exploration community. While adventure learning does not afford learners a direct physical role in an exploration, it is designed to allow for academic and social participation. The learner's involvement – even at the rudimentary level of virtually asking a scientist a question – can be said to be part of the scientific inquiry experience (especially if the scientist has yet to or has only just discovered the answer to the question) (Niemitz et al., 2008).

Finally, the adventure learning model is highly motivating. By connecting students in classrooms with active scientists or explorers, students gain a picture of what it means to be a scientist or explorer and they form a mentorship connection (Niemitz et al., 2008). Both of these aspects of adventure learning have been shown to positively affect a learner's enthusiasm for learning science, satisfaction with the practice of science, attitudes about science as a career, and a more social (versus intellectual and academic) view of scientists (Abraham, 2002; Knox, Moynihan & Markowitz, 2003; Markowitz, 2004; Templin, Doran & Engemann, 1999).

With this theoretical background in mind, Doering (2006) has developed a framework for the design of adventure learning environments. This framework consists of seven, interdependent principles:

(a) a researched curriculum grounded in problem-solving, (b) collaboration and interaction opportunities between students, experts, peers, and content, (c) the utilization of the Internet for curriculum and learning environment delivery, (d) the enhancement of curriculum with media and text from the field in a timely manner, (e) synched learning opportunities with the adventure learning curriculum, (f) pedagogical guidelines of the curriculum and online learning environment, and (g) education that is adventure-based. (p. 200)

The extent to which the adventure learning model has impacted student learning has yet to be comprehensively quantified or qualified. However, early results indicate that adventure learning has a positive impact on students, across a number of metrics. Doering and Veletsianos (2008) have examined student responses to the way teachers integrated the GoNorth! adventure learning environment into their classrooms. Student reactions were generally positive – students were "excited, engaged, and motivated with the authentic and problem-based tasks employed within the adventure learning environment" (Miller, Veletsianos & Doering, 2008, p. 257). Additionally, the methods used to connect the students in the classroom to the explorers in the field were transformative in their ability to foster collaboration.

Bazler, Spokane, Ballard & Fugate (1993) conducted a small study of the student and teacher attitudes towards science after an early JASON project expedition, an early example of adventure learning. They concluded that participation in the JASON experience lead to positive emotional reactions towards science and intentional attitudes about science. A full scale evaluation of the JASON program revealed that students in classrooms participating in the JASON program achieved gains in scientific literacy – both in understanding key scientific concepts and in the process of scientific inquiry – that were not seen in classrooms where the JASON program was not used (Ba, Martin & Diaz, 2001; Ba, Admon & Anderson, 2002; Goldenberg, Ba, Heinze & Hess, 2003).

The previous work of the authors in the field of adventure learning has been largely reflective and theoretical. Niemitz et al. (2008) describe their SOR expedition as an interactive virtual expedition – a means of virtual communication that enables learners of all ages to experience and interact with the process of scientific exploration, in real or near real time and from a distance. Teacher-to-student interaction was made possible via a Q&A forum, teacher blogging, and interactive online activities all delivered using a simple website. The SOR expedition website was a unique example of an interactive virtual expedition, as it was coupled with a professional development workshop. The SOR expedition followed the adventure learning framework (Doering, 2006), but also differed from it in that the teachers were the explorers (along with active scientists) and were not in the classroom moderating the interaction between their students and distant third party explorers (this moderation was conducted by substitute or other teachers). Niemitz et al. (2008) argue that this model, while difficult to scale and implement, provides for a customized adventure learning experience that is most advantageous to the students of the participating educators. Who better to deliver adventure learning experiences from a distance than the teachers who spend nine months of the year in the classroom with their students?

Technology Integration in Teacher Education – Issues and Challenges

To more fully develop a theoretical basis for integrating hybrid online learning activities into teacher education programs, we must briefly examine the current landscape for technology integration in teacher education and preparation programs to determine where the adventure learning teacher education model may fit into the picture. A significant body of research has focused on the effect that integrating technology into teacher education programs has on the long-term integration of technology in classrooms. This research is informative for understanding how the SOR expedition technology integration model compares and contrasts with the overall field of study. With a comparative analysis, we can begin to use our experiences to form some ideas for technology use in teacher education programs.

Kay (2006) has completed an extensive review of the literature on strategies for incorporating technology into pre-service teacher education. She identifies ten strategies used by faculty to teach technology to pre-service teachers, and from this review of the literature, identifies a guiding model for designing an effective overall strategy for technology integration into pre-service teacher education. Access to software, hardware, and support at the university and in the field of placement must preclude the use of any other strategies. Instructors must "model and construct authentic teaching activities," (Kay, 2006, p. 394) regardless of which of the ten identified strategies are used. And finally, pre-service and in-service teachers, faculty, and mentor teachers must collaborate in order to ensure that the teacher candidates will be able to translate their technology use in the pre-service environment to the in-service environment (Fulton et al., 2003; Kay, 2006). Otherwise, teachers will not continue to gain the skills they need and will become frustrated.

In the in-service teacher education environment, scholars have qualified parallel pathways of technology use fostering a constructivist approach over time and teacher comfort levels with technology increasing over time (Matzen & Edmunds, 2007; Sandholz et al., 1997; Valdez et al., 1999). Teachers may at first be uncomfortable with technology and, lacking the skills and confidence to use it effectively, they integrate it into a traditional teacher-centered, transmission approach to teaching. This approach has limited effect and does not take advantage of the technology. Over time, as comfort increases, they use technology in ways that emphasize a learner-centered and constructivist approach. In one study, Matzen and Edmunds (2007) found that teachers tend to use technology in line with the their instructional beliefs (corroborating evidence from Dexter, Anderson, & Becker, 1999; and Ertmer, Addison, Lane, Ross, & Woods, 1999). Further, they found that teachers "tend to implement [technology] in the ways in which they have been shown" (p. 427). They conclude that rather than teaching technology skills, teacher education programs would be more successful if they model instruction by showing technology in the context of instructional practice, notably that of a learner-centered constructivist approach.

In another study, Brinkerhoff (2006) found that a long-duration professional development academy could be instrumental in overcoming the barriers to technology integration in the classroom. The study informed the design of technology integration in professional development programs, notably, that curricular materials need to be provided for post-program, in classroom use; instruction should be centered on participant's interests; participants should work individually, in pairs, and in groups during the program; participants should be held accountable for creating curricular materials that integrate technology; participants should be held accountable for following through with technology integration; and the goal of the technology professional development should be clearly defined and evaluated based on that goal.

In a study that did not deal directly with technology integration in teacher education programs but has important implications for our purposes here, Johnson and Golombek (2002) investigated teachers' narrative inquiry as a form of professional development. In the process of inquiry related to professional development activities, teachers frame their experiences through the connections they make between them and through their social and relational surroundings. They use narrative as a way to link their experiences to each other and provide the context for the experiences. As Johnson and Golombek (2002) state: "teachers' stories of inquiry are not only *about* professional development; they *are* professional development. Narrative inquiry becomes a means through which teachers actualize their ways of knowing and growing that nourish and sustain their professional development throughout their careers" (p. 6). During professional development programs, teachers who engage in narrative inquiry are better able to communicate what they know and their beliefs about teaching and being a teacher, and this affects change in the way they teach. It follows that activities that encourage narrative inquiry alongside communication of newfound knowledge and abilities would be advantageous in a professional development setting. It is our belief that technology can play an important role in the communication of these narratives and deliver powerful learning experiences to students in real or near real-time.

The literature on adventure learning substantiates the use of real-time teacher-to-student distance communications as an effective learning mechanism for students. In addition, the literature on technology integration in teacher education programs provides some recommendations of best practices in this field. Theoretically, we can draw connections between the body of literature and a case study of technology integration into a teacher education program that utilized real-time teacher-to-student distance communications. This exercise will then allow us to establish some recommendations for such integration and apply those recommendations to other teacher education settings. But, we must first take an in depth look at the SOR expedition case study and consider how this unique adventure learning experience enhanced the professional development of the participants.

THE SCHOOL OF ROCK EXPEDITION CASE STUDY

The Consortium for Ocean Leadership (formerly Joint Oceanographic Institutions) and the Integrated Ocean Drilling Program (IODP) – United States Implementing Organization sponsored the School of Rock expedition, a seagoing pilot teacher professional development workshop on board the scientific drilling vessel *JOIDES Resolution* during a transit from Victoria, B.C., Canada, to Acapulco, Mexico in the Fall of 2005. The Integrated Ocean Drilling Program (IODP) is an international marine research program that explores Earth's history and structure recorded in seafloor sediments and rocks and monitors subseafloor environments. IODP builds upon the earlier successes of the Deep Sea Drilling Project (DSDP) and Ocean Drilling Program (ODP), which revolutionized our view of Earth history and global processes through ocean basin exploration.

During this workshop, active IODP scientists, the Consortium for Ocean Leadership education staff and shipboard technical staff mentored and instructed thirteen educators. The instructional process modeled and supported open inquiry exercises based on authentic shipboard activities with the dual emphases in a community of learners of handling/processing authentic ocean core samples in the same labs as the scientists and of accessing archival data from the entire breadth of the scientific ocean drilling programs. Participants were also exposed to the legacy of scientific ocean drilling through shore-to-ship lectures and the IODP scientific plan. Ship-to-shore communications and on-shore interactive learning via an interactive virtual expedition was one of the key deliverables for the program.

Professional Development Aspects of the School of Rock Expedition

As a teacher research field experience blended with an inquiry-based in-service professional development workshop, the SOR expedition was a unique opportunity for a select group of educators. Ten grades 5-12 teachers with progressive, inquiry-focused philosophies and demonstrated track records of curriculum development and/or peer teaching were selected from an applicant pool of more than 60. Educator familiarity and comfort with the use of technology was also considered, but was not one of the primary qualifying factors. Three additional spots on the expedition were assigned to informal education partners from the Smithsonian's National Museum of Natural History and the Science Museum of Minnesota, and a K-12 textbook publishing representative.

While the SOR experience was one that sought to meet the content learning desires of in-service science teachers in a very novel learning environment, the overall goal of the expedition was to extend the scientific knowledge gained through the ODP and IODP programs to a wide audience of teachers and students. (For more details on the science content and instructional models of the SOR expedition, see Leckie et al., 2006 and St. John et al., in press.) So, integrated within the content instruction of the expedition were strategically designed tenants that sought to influence the teaching of the expedition participants, as well as that of non-participating educators:

- The SOR curriculum should be data-rich, integrating authentic ocean drilling practices that are fundamental to all IODP science....
- The teachers need access to curriculum that is based on actual scientific data and discoveries for use in their classrooms.... The participating educators themselves would be responsible for adapting and developing SOR curriculum for their classrooms during and after the SOR expedition.
- The educators need time in the field to communicate with their schools, students, and museum audiences.... We recognize that during professional development programs educators are constantly thinking "how can I use this in my own teaching?"
- The educators need time to make connections between and among the new things they are learning and experiencing in the field and their classrooms and museums, as well as their prior experiences and knowledge.... (St. John et al., in press)

Given this program design, the opportunities for traditional professional development (i.e. content learning with future face-to-face classroom teaching applications) were vast. The evaluation of the SOR expedition confirms that the workshop was incredibly valuable for the expedition participants (St. John et al., in press). The workshop was evaluated during the expedition and short-term and long-term outcomes were measured post-expedition. During the expedition, we used a design-based research approach that relied on participant's daily Connections journals. By collecting feedback from the participants during the expedition, we were able to adjust the workshop as needed to more adequately meet the needs of the participants. A summative evaluation included post-expedition interviews and questionnaires focused on determining the value of the workshop activities and the use of the developed curriculum in participant classrooms. Participant feedback during the expedition indicated "overwhelming enthusiasm and productivity...in spite of 12-14 hour workdays plus "homework" for eleven straight days in a shipboard environment" (St. John et al., in press). In their evaluation of the professional development aspects of the expedition, participants were very positive. One representative reflection sums up the experience for the participants:

My previous experience with professional development was about 90% useless and 10% valuable. Most professional development for teachers (at least in my experience) is designed and conducted by people who maybe don't quite understand teaching or students. As a result, it is often irrelevant to what actually goes on in the classroom... The School of Rock was clearly designed around a need... The key to the success of the School of Rock is that it was a responsive program – instead of creating something in a void, and then cramming it down our throats, the organizers sought to respond to an existing need; and during the program, they listened to our feedback and made adjustments as necessary. (St. John et al., in press)

In the long-term evaluation, three themes emerged. First, the participants, staff members, and crew have continued to engage with one another and remain a community of professionals who are regularly in communication with each other, sharing knowledge and experiences, and working collaboratively. Second, the SOR experience has lead several expedition participants to pursue new career opportunities that are more directly related to the activities they participated in during the expedition. Finally, the participants and staff have continued to use and develop curricular materials focused on the workshop content. These resources have taken many shapes and forms and have been implemented in K-12, university, and informal education settings all over the world.

Technology Aspects of the School of Rock Expedition

While we initially recognized that real-time or near real-time communication between the expedition participants and their students (and other teachers and students) onshore would be important, the means by which we sought to meet that need were limited in this pilot program. The SOR expedition website (http://www.oceanleadership.org/schoolofrock2005/default.html) was the expedition communication portal to the onshore audience thousands of miles away. Because the SOR expedition took place during the school year, it presented a unique opportunity to engage the students of the expedition participants in near real-time. Through ship-to-shore communication, facilitated by the expedition website, teacher-to-student and student-to-teacher communication pathways could be formative activities for both parties.

The website sought to influence the learning of the different constituents and was crucial to the success of the expedition in three key ways (Niemitz et al., 2008). The ship-to-shore communications via the website were designed to engage the students of the participants as well as other students in classrooms across the world. We hoped that the expedition would engage students "with the simple question of 'what is my teacher doing today?' In this way, students could be just as interested in what the teachers were learning about and participating in as the teachers themselves" (Niemitz et al., 2008, p. 568). Second, the website sought to engage non-participating teachers onshore. Since we were limited in the number of participants we could bring on the expedition, we sought to provide a way for the experiences of the participants to be shared with those unable to sail.

Finally, and most important for our purposes here, the website sought to benefit the participants of the expedition. In line with the design tenants of the expedition (St. John et al., in press), the daily ship-to-shore communication activities were part of the Communication, Curriculum, and Connections (C^3) time.

"The daily communication time was intended to slightly push participants away from their personal learning and bring them back into the realm of the average student. It was hoped that this would help the participants be in the right "frame of mind" for applying the new concepts that they were learning to their own individual classrooms" (Niemitz et al., 2008, p. 568).

Coupled with the connections and curriculum time, these periods of the expedition were collectively geared toward the educators immediately applying what they were learning to make connections to their classrooms back on shore, directly communicate with their classrooms, and/or create curricular materials that they could use in their classrooms. The intense schedule, complex science, ambitious learning agenda, and stimulating environment provided the unique opportunity to give the participants time to think of their students potential learning in the same enthusiastic and excited manner in which they were thinking about their own learning.

Despite the significant goals of the ship-to-shore communication aspect of the expedition, the expedition website was decidedly low-tech. The challenges of updating a website from a ship in the middle of the ocean were many and given the pilot nature of this expedition, much of what we sought to build and update during the expedition was experimental. The website was divided into six major sections, which we will describe only briefly here. (For more extensive details on the structure and motivation of the expedition website, see Niemitz et al., 2008.)

1. *The Classroom* – a listing of the daily schedule of the expedition complete with pictures of daily activities to showcase the *JOIDES Resolution* as a unique "classroom" for learning.
2. *Expedition Blog* – a daily chronicle of the activities, events, highlights, connections, and anything else the expedition participants were thinking and doing. The blog was written by a different participant each day, providing website viewers with thirteen different perspectives on the expedition.
3. *Where in the World?* – an inquiry-based, online activity to plot the daily location of the *JOIDES Resolution* on our journey southward toward Acapulco. Website viewers were given a map and daily longitude and latitude coordinates and encouraged to plot the movement of the ship.
4. *Video Q&A* – a near real-time online forum for asking question and reading answers. Participants answered the questions that came in from their students and each day one question was selected to be answered in video form, resulting in a number of videos that enabled students to see what the participants were learning.
5. *Participant/Staff Bios* – short biographical sketches of each participant and staff member designed to provide information about the diverse and talented community of learners involved in the expedition.
6. *The Library* – a catalog of all the activities, curriculum materials, background reading, and other resources used or developed on the expedition.

Using the same evaluation methods as described above, we determined that the expedition website was a valuable and critical part of the professional development workshop. The participants considered the ability to communicate back to their classrooms through the website as invaluable and essential to their participation in the workshop. In hindsight, many participants said they needed more C^3 time.

The engagement of the onshore audience was clear. Many students submitted questions through the *Video Q&A* section of the website that were in direct response to blog postings, pictures, weather data, or other information that informed the students of what their teachers were doing. The expedition participants were excited to be able to answer their student's questions about their experience while thousands of miles away. A few sample questions and teacher responses reveal that the students were interested in various aspects of the expedition and the participants took the opportunity to capitalize on teachable moments:

Question: *I understand that you are viewing some fossils, but what base rock material are you finding these in?*

Answer: *Hi Shelby, The fossils are in sediment samples called cores, not in rocks. The ship takes both sediment and rock cores, we just happen to be studying sediment at this time. A hollow pipe is pushed into the sea floor sediments then brought* *back to the surface. Later in the trip we will look at hard rock cores.*

Question: *How many people are there on the ship and where are they from?*

Answer: *Hi Jeremy, Just as the JOIDES Resolution sails all over the world, there are people on it that are from all over the world. Right now there are 99 people on board, which is about 11 less than the number that they usually have on board during scientific expeditions. Today, we had a BBQ outside for lunch and the crew hung up flags from all the nations that were represented on board. There were flags from South Africa, the United States, Taiwan, Australia, the Philippines, the United Kingdom, Canada, and Portugal. There are also people from the Netherlands, Japan, and Mexico.*

Given our modest goals for the expedition website, we considered this experimental pilot of ship-to-shore communication to be a success (Niemitz et al., 2008). Nearly 300 questions were submitted to the *Video Q&A* section of the website, from eleven different states and two countries other than the United States. The expedition participants recounted their students use of the website as a significant learning activity while they were at sea – some through the question and answer process and others through the *Where in the World?* activity. Some participants had set up learning activities that were based on the content on the website, so while students may not have been asking questions, they were consuming the content on a regular and intentional basis. Though we do not have page view data for during the expedition, views of the website were steady long after the expedition ended. The participants and non-participants have returned to the website for lesson plans and access to data and background resources.

Perhaps the most significant outcome of the ship-to-shore communication was the enthusiasm with which the teachers viewed the means of ship-to-shore communication and the desire to extend those means beyond what we had planned for. Despite very long days (10-12 hours of instruction plus "homework") the participants went above and beyond to communicate with their classrooms. Three participants filmed and edited instructional videos and interviews of crew members to send back to classrooms and be played on school websites or on the morning video announcements. While one participant had planned on sending videos ahead of time, the other two participants saw what the one was doing, recognized the value of using this type of communications technology, and asked us to help them do the same. Several of the participants maintained their own blogs and communicated with students outside of the means that we had set up through the website.

The ship-to-shore communication experience of one participant is especially informative for our purposes here. His experience illustrates the power that communication technologies can have in enhancing professional development opportunities like the SOR expedition. The participant has been (and continues to be) a high school science teacher at a very large school in Texas for over 30 years. During his long and successful tenure, he had made little to no use of technology in his classroom – *"prior to the trip my technology expertise consisted mostly of management, administrative, mundane tasks and procedures."* But, when accepted for the expedition, he immediately recognized that:

Sharing the personal enthusiasm for an experience like this is like describing a travel location. Unless they have been there, much is lost in the translation. Involving people somehow, someway during the trip was a high priority… My personal twist was to use technology as the key to bringing the experience home.

He approached the information technology department in his district and worked with them to design and set up a website on his school's server where he could post daily videos of his experience. His videos were also to be broadcast over his school's video announcement system every morning. In addition, his students were frequent contributors to the SOR expedition website by asking questions. Despite having never been trained in video production, he spent numerous hours on the expedition, (regularly the last one to go to bed and the first one up in the morning) outside of the instructional activities, to plan, film, and edit 15 videos. We were able to work through significant technical and bandwidth limitations to send his videos back to shore where the IT personnel in his district posted and distributed the videos to his website. Through these videos, the participant reached over 3200 students a day in his own school and many more in other schools in his district. The response from both students and district staff has been universally positive.

Since the SOR expedition, his use of technology has only increased.

The trip experience was the catalyst which redirected my focus for integrating technology into my Science classroom. Learning to share the use of the technology with my peers, and using the appropriate technology for the level of instruction was the real challenge. As a result of my experience I have increased my technology focus not just in the classroom but school wide with state mandated tests. I am always looking for a way to use the available technology in the 'regular labs.'

It is remarkable to see how communicating to students through such novel means from the middle of the ocean, thousands of miles away, could turn a technology adverse teacher into an innovator in the use of technology in his school. This experience underscores the value of our expedition for the participants. Without the valuable content being taught, the teachers would have had little to communicate to their students. And without the means with which to communicate ship-to-shore, the transmission of the wealth of new knowledge would have been delayed for weeks. The students would have missed the unique experience of learning *with* their teachers, as opposed to *from* their teachers. If nothing else, it is apparent from our experience that the practice of communicating and teaching about content concurrently with learning that content is a powerful model to consider using in other teacher education situations.

SCALING THE ADVENTURE LEARNING MODEL TO VARIED TEACHER EDUCATION SETTINGS

We have repeatedly stressed that the SOR expedition model is rare and difficult to implement and scale. Few in-service teachers have the ability or can get the approval to take a two-week mid-year hiatus from their classrooms for professional development purposes. (It is a testament to the quality and value of the SOR program that ten administrators were willing to allow their teachers to participate in the program.) Even without this challenge, the opportunities to experience adventures or explorations of this kind are also rare. But, from the SOR expedition case study we have also seen the value in these activities. This begs the question – how can we apply the lessons learned from the SOR expedition case study to more traditional teacher education programs, both in- and pre-service?

A Framework for Technology Integration into Teacher Education Programs – Applying Reflections from the School of Rock Expedition

Several themes emerge when we draw parallels between our reflections and case study of the SOR expedition and the review of the literature on the integration of technology in pre- and in-service teacher education. Given our in-service teacher education focus, it is somewhat difficult to compare and contrast the SOR expedition and the literature on technology integration in teacher education in pre-service settings. We believe that many of the same principles apply to in-service teacher education and putting the SOR expedition side by side with this literature is fair, but should be approached with caution.

Kay (2006) calls for modeling authentic learning activities through technology use. The SOR expedition website effectively modeled a constructivist approach to learning. Students were able to scan the website for information, ask questions based on their response to the information they collected, and receive answers. In the process, the students governed their own learning (with support and scaffolding from teachers in the classroom). The participants of the expedition played an important role in this process as they answered their student's questions and saw how students can be engaged in their learning through the ship-to-shore communications technology.

Kay (2006) and Fulton (2003) suggest that partnerships between teachers, faculty, and mentors are crucial to ensure pre-service teachers follow through with integrating technology once they enter the in-service classroom environment. The Consortium for Ocean Leadership has continued to work with and support the SOR expedition participants since the expedition. They have provided curricular materials that showcase ways to integrate technology, access to IODP science data and *JOIDES Resolution* personnel, and the means for participants to share their post-expedition experiences and successes. Not only has the success of the SOR expedition lived on through these partnerships, but the participants have also been able to continue their personal learning process and how to apply the science and technology aspects of the at-sea workshop in their classrooms.

Our reflections from the SOR expedition cannot speak to the issue of technology support and access to technology resources (hardware and software), as it was not within our purview to provide solutions to those potential problems. We recognize that this is a major issue for teachers and one that often precludes use of technology in the classroom. We also cannot corroborate the need for mentorship and partnership during the transition from pre-service to in-service settings, as the participants were exclusively in-service teachers.

The comparisons between the SOR expedition and the literature on technology professional development are more apt, as in-service teachers were the exclusive focus of the workshop. Matzen and Edmunds (2007) call for modeling a learner-centered, constructivist approach to teaching using technology in the classroom. As discussed above, the SOR expedition successfully modeled this approach. Brinkerhoff's (2006) findings would suggest that the SOR expedition was too short to effectively transform teacher use in technology in the classroom. Our reflections agree and disagree with this recommendation. Some of our participants were very enthusiastic about using technology on the expedition, but it is not apparent that their teaching practices and beliefs regarding technology were fundamentally altered due to the expedition. So, perhaps a longer program would have done more to encourage long-term changes in technology use in the classroom. However, we did have a significant case where the use of technology on the expedition has permanently changed a participants teaching practices, despite the short nature of the professional development workshop.

Brinkerhoff (2006) also recommends centering technology professional development on teachers' interests. It is our belief that the workshop science content and unique setting of the SOR expedition were primary reasons for the use of ship-to-shore communication technologies during the expedition. The simple fact is that the teachers were eager to share their experiences and communicate about the amazing things they were learning and seeing to their students back onshore. The quality of the learning experience and the immediate applicability to the participants' classroom almost demanded that they share the experience immediately.

An interesting parallel between the existing research on teacher education and the SOR expedition is the process of narrative inquiry as defined by Johnson and Golombek (2002). The SOR expedition provided a unique and formative setting for learning and in order for the participants to frame their experiences, they needed to reflect on the narratives of their inquiry. We provided time for them to accomplish this through the C^3 component of the program. This narrative of learning was so rich and engaging and it was clear that the stories would be ones that many others would respond to. The reflections of the participants affirm the fact that the C^3 time was essential to the overall value of the expedition. During this time, the teachers were able to frame their experiences, connect them with their prior learning and teaching, and transfer them to curricular materials that would take advantage of the inquiry. In addition, by enabling the participants to communicate their stories through a blog and by answering their student's questions on the website, the narratives could have the same formative effect on the students as they did on the participants. We believe this aspect is a key takeaway from our experience integrating technology into a teacher education workshop. We do not believe that the technology aspects of the expedition would have been nearly as successful without the unique setting and thoughtful format for the professional development. And we believe that the value for students was enhanced by the fact that teachers were immediately able to tell their stories using the technology.

One final aspect of the SOR expedition sets it apart from the existing literature. The real-time communication back to classrooms was unique in that it bridges the gap between teacher education and classroom instruction. Rather than having a teacher education program that focused on learning how to integrate technology in the classroom or modeling technology integration, the SOR expedition sought to seamlessly integrate technology into the program as a means to an end that did not necessarily focus on future technology integration in the classroom. The participants saw the power of the technology not because it was novel or unique, because it was integrated with curriculum, or because they felt they could use it in their classrooms in the future. They valued it because it enabled them to communicate with their students about their learning. We have already discussed the importance with which they viewed this activity during the expedition and we also conclude that it was this near real-time communication that most directly influenced the observed participant enthusiasm with using the technology. So, the question we need to answer is how much value does using communication technologies add to the development of teachers who are able to connect what they are learning in all types of situations back to their classrooms. In this way, a technology-based teacher education experience could become the basis for a mindset and belief about teaching rather than a new strategy. While we value the contributions of the literature on this topic (as discussed), we see this final point as another key to the success of the technology portion of the SOR expedition and the contribution the expedition can make to the overall field of technology integration in teacher education. We propose that by combining these two key takeaways of the SOR expedition with the recommendations of the literature, a technology-based teacher education program might accomplish much more.

Applications to Specific Teacher Education Settings

Based on our reflections on the SOR expedition case study and the parallels we have drawn between them and the literature, we can suggest settings and situations where communications technologies may be a value added proposition for teacher education programs. As previously stated, these recommendations are purely theoretical and empirical research and evaluation of them is necessary to establish the efficacy of implementing them on a non-experimental basis. Our hope is that this study will encourage teacher educators to experiment with these recommendations and evaluate them.

Our framework for identifying these settings and situations is as follows: 1) they should model authentic, constructivist teaching situations that use technology; 2) they should provide long term support in the form of mentorships, curricular materials, and/or partnerships; 3) they should be centered around the teaching and content interests of participants; 4) they should be situations where participants form a narrative inquiry that can also be engaging to students; and 5) they should help teachers connect with their classrooms in real or near real-time and, moving forward, push teachers towards making considering student connections a mindset. Using this framework, the research and reflections tell us that it is more likely that teacher attitudes and practices about technology integration in the classroom will change and a mindset about technology as a connection tool to students will be born. We identify only the most applicable settings for pre-service and in-service teacher education environments here, but we believe that, with some creativity, the solutions identified could scale to a number of other settings.

The adventure learning model could be more conveniently scaled to the pre-service environment, as pre-service teachers are completing teacher education programs at the same time as students are learning in K-12 classrooms. Possibly the most appropriate setting to integrate this kind of technology use is through an interdisciplinary combination of education/teaching courses and second major, minor, or elective courses. Many undergraduate education majors are double majoring or taking a minor in a second subject, which often corresponds to the subject they plan to eventually teach. We believe this is particularly applicable for physical and biological science courses, and to a lesser degree history, anthropology, art, music, sociology, and modern language courses. Schools of education could set up partnerships with local or distant classrooms and, using appropriate technology tools, pre-service teachers could communicate with their partner classroom as they learned new content. For example, a pre-service teacher enrolled in an environmental science course on sustainable water use might learn about the water usage in their town, region, or state through a field trip to a reservoir, dam, or water treatment facility. In addition to fulfilling the requirements for the environmental science course, the pre-service teacher might also receive education course credit for taking pictures, notes, and/or interviewing water treatment facility personnel, creating curricular materials around this topic, and communicating, through online or virtual means, what they saw and learned to an environmental science class at a local or distant high school. The class would in turn complete learning activities using the materials and new knowledge provided from the pre-service teacher. A second example might be a pre-service teacher enrolled in a biological anthropology course that is studying ancient hominid origins and has access to view and study the remains of ancient hominid species. Through the use of technology, the pre-service teacher could virtually take middle school students into the laboratory with them and let them see the skeletal remains. With proper curricular materials and learning support from the pre-service teacher, the students could learn alongside the pre-service teacher through a dialogue made possible by communications technologies. Teachers can describe their narrative inquiry through the use of communications technologies and have the opportunity to teach about subjects that interest them, all while learning how to reach students in classrooms and getting education credit for their coursework. Both these examples model a constructivist teaching environment, can be supported by mentorships, partnerships, and peers, is centered on teacher interests, allows for stories of inquiry to be told, and provide opportunities for connecting to classrooms in real-time.

These example settings take advantage of the extensive resources of colleges and universities to give K-12 students in classrooms access to learning opportunities they could never have where they are. It also overcomes the extreme difficulty teachers have in taking students on field trips that are often more hassle than they are worth. There are many other examples of this kind too numerous to go into detail here, though the popular study abroad experience would be another setting of this kind that would be particularly applicable. This solution would require proper vetting of non-education courses, setting up the infrastructure for technology use, and determining or creating the right education courses with which to integrate activities of this kind. But, this could be a relatively simple and quick way of using our framework for integrating formative and unique technology use into pre-service teacher education.

In the in-service teacher education environment, the challenges for integrating the adventure learning model of technology use are more difficult. The primary challenge is that most significant content-focused professional development programs take place during the summer months when students are not in the classroom. However, there are still opportunities for in-service teachers to attend professional development workshops or programs during the school year. For example, many teachers attend subject-matter conferences that focus on teaching methods, practices, new content, and resources for different subjects. These events can be opportunities for in-service teachers to integrate communications technology into the experience and communicate with their classrooms from a distance. To be sure, some conferences and events may be better suited for this kind of communications technology integration. One exemplary example is the National Association of Geoscience Teachers (of which several of the authors are members), which regularly holds regional two to three day conferences that include field trips to view and discuss the geology of the area where the conference is held. These events are relatively easy for teachers to attend and could provide valuable opportunities to extend the learning of the teachers directly and immediately into their classrooms. Prior to the conference, teachers could set up their desired means of communication back to their classrooms, along with assignments, homework, and learning activities that supplement the virtual experience for the students. During the professional development workshop, students could follow from the classroom and their homes and complete the assigned course work in the process. Schools and districts could set up partnerships with conference or event sponsoring organizations that could provide support for implementing communications technologies of this kind. And schools could link in multiple teachers and classrooms to leverage the attendance of one individual at an event. Multiple teachers could work together to create appropriate curricular materials for their classrooms and one or two teachers attending the event could deliver the distance communication element of the experience back to multiple classrooms in their school.

As with the pre-service application, this example also follows the framework we have identified as potentially advantageous for technology integration in teacher education programs. This example models authentic, learner-centered instruction that uses technology as teachers are reflecting on what they are learning at a conference or event and making inferences that lead to a more complete understanding of a subject matter. As mentioned above, partnerships between schools, event sponsoring organizations, and other teachers or mentors could be set up to ensure the maximum output of such an experience and that teachers would be more likely to integrate technology into their classroom in the future. Conference events and workshops are always linked to teacher interest, so as the in-service teachers learn content they are enthusiastic about, the students could learn alongside them. These unique experiences provide an ideal platform for telling stories about inquiry and framing the experiences in a way that is engaging for students. And finally, this is all done in real or near real-time, ensuring the teacher immediately puts what they are learning into practice and reinforces the mindset that all teacher learning can translate to student learning.

We recognize that attendance at these conferences is often at the discretion of administrators and the opportunities to attend are not always amply provided. However, with the added value that integrating communications technologies into participation in these events can provide for students in the classroom, perhaps this bolsters the rationale for increased participation in professional development conferences.

An Overview of the Technology Solutions and Challenges

Thus far we have not addressed the specifics of what we term communication technologies. We believe that this term can encompass many different technological solutions that would meet the needs for the adventure learning hybrid online model, but in the interest of providing some guidance and suggestions, we outline several possible options here.

Real-time interaction and communication is ideal, as there is evidence that this provides a more engaging and meaningful learning experience for students than near real-time communication (Goldenberg et al., 2003; Niemitz et al., 2008). Standard video conferencing equipment would be difficult to support in field based situations and we assume that most schools are not equipped to handle videoconferences. However, web conferencing can fulfill many of the same needs, including video and audio (VoIP) feeds, screen and document sharing, and collaboration tools. Web conferencing tools can be used to conduct virtual classes, lessons, and/or simply chat and interact with students. The most common web conferencing tools in education include Adobe Acrobat Connect Pro, Elluminate *Live!*, Wimba Classroom, Webex, GoToMeeting by Citrix, and Dimdim. Some of these solutions have versions that are free (Adobe ConnectNow or Dimdim Free) but have limits on the number of participants. Some are hosted solutions, others onsite, and some offer either hosted or onsite solutions. Costs are often calculated on a per-month or per-user basis and can vary depending on the maximum number of participants expected in virtual meetings.

In addition, teachers can use their computer's built-in tools like Apple iChat or Windows Live Messenger, or free downloadable applications like Skype to communicate virtually. These solutions offer video and audio communication capabilities, but lack the document, screen-sharing, and collaboration tools that web conferencing applications all contain.

While not real-time, online social networking tools offer free or low-cost ways to communicate virtually and quickly. Teachers can set up Facebook, MySpace, or Bebo accounts and share pictures, videos, news, events, quick status updates, and notes with students. Students (or "friends") can post questions and get responses and comment on pictures, events, and/or status updates. The viral nature of these tools also ensures that word can spread quickly and users outside the original target audience may also benefit from the virtual communication (or privacy can be maintained by restricting usage to predefined users). Additionally, Twitter provides an opportunity to share short 140 character or less updates on what a teacher may be learning during a teacher education program. All of these social networking applications can be updated using smart phones, such as the Apple iPhone, Palm Treo, Research in Motion Blackberry, Nokia E71, or the T-Mobile G1, making for a truly mobile and flexible communication solution.

Teachers can use blogs to communicate more detailed stories of their learning and provide large images, videos, documents, and links to their readers. Students can comment on blog posts with questions and teachers can subsequently respond in later blog posts. Blogging tools abound on the Internet and almost all are free. Blogger, WordPress, Moveable Type, LiveJournal, and TypePad all offer simple, easy-to-use features and setup. All these blogging tools can be completely private and restrict access to certain individuals. Depending on the blog hosting service, blogs can usually be updated via a smart phone like those listed above. Advanced users can set up their own blogs with a hosting server (for a minimal cost) to create a more custom experience.

Finally, a basic website (much like the SOR expedition used) can be a relatively easy and low-cost way of communicating virtually. Websites can be custom designed and developed to create the features and structure most desired. A custom website allows for the most flexibility in posting documents and creating custom learning activities and collaboration mechanisms. This solution also allows for integration with a school or district website and teachers can also utilize existing web based course management systems that may already be in use.

It is our belief that a combination of many of these tools would be most ideal, provided any solution follows the adventure learning design framework outlined by Doering (2006). The real-time nature of web and video conferencing and collaboration adds a novel experience for both teachers and students. Social networks are already heavily used by students (and some teachers), and meeting students where they already are has value. Students are familiar and comfortable with all these tools and in the end, the choice of which tools to use depends on the specific goals of the communication experience.

FUTURE RESEARCH NEEDS AND DIRECTIONS

While the reflections recounted from the case study and the recommendations posited here are theoretically sound, additional research is needed to test and affirm these positions. As stated, no empirical studies have been completed on whether activities like those described here successful transform teacher attitudes and beliefs about using technology in the classroom over the long term or create the mindset that teacher education can always be connected to student learning. Testing the two examples outlined here and qualifying the teacher experience with using technology in the short and long term would provide information on unforeseen challenges and results, help refine the framework for implementing communication technologies into teacher education programs, and possibly help identify additional settings where this kind of technology use may be most advantageous and formative.

SUMMARY

We have described the SOR expedition as a unique case study for the integration of technology in a teacher education program. This example is unique in that it did not focus on increasing teacher comfort with technology or ensuring that teachers used technology in their classrooms in the long term. Rather, we sought to provide a means for teachers to tell their stories of inquiry as they learned and connect those experiences back to their classrooms in near real-time.

These experiences add new ideas to the school of thought on technology integration into teacher education programs. First, teacher education experiences that provide opportunities for teachers to form an engaging narrative of their inquiry are powerful platforms for using technology to tell those stories to students and other readers from a distance. Second, by using technology as a tool for immediately communicating what teachers are learning back to their classrooms, a technology-based teacher education experience can become the basis for a mindset and belief about teaching with technology rather than merely a new strategy of teaching.

While this model is difficult to implement in teacher education settings, we see two possible ways it can contribute to pre- and in-service teacher education programs. Pre-service teachers can use communications technologies to link their content courses in fields other than education with partner classrooms in local or distant communities. In-service teachers can use opportunities for attending subject-matter conferences or field-based workshops to connect new knowledge acquisition back to classrooms in their school or district. Both of these examples focusing on pushing learning content to students immediately and helping teachers learn how to communicate new content to their students in an engaging way.

REFERENCES

Abraham, L. M. (2002). What do high school science students gain from field-based research apprenticeship programs? *Clearing House (Menasha, Wis.)*, *75*(5), 229–232. doi:10.1080/00098650209603945

Ba, H., Admon, N., & Anderson, L. (2002). *A quantitative investigation of teachers and the JASON Multimedia Science Curriculum: Reported use and impact: Year Two Evaluation Report.* New York: Center of Children and Technology, Education Development Center.

Ba, H., Martin, W., & Diaz, O. (2001). *The JASON Project's Multimedia Science Curriculum Impact on Student Learning: Final Evaluation Report Year One.* New York: Center of Children and Technology, Education Development Center.

Bazler, J. A., Spokane, A. R., Ballard, R., & Fugate, M. S. (1993). The Jason Project Experience and Attitudes Toward Science as an Enterprise and Career. *Journal of Career Development*, *20*(2), 101–112.

Brinkerhoff, J. (2006). Effects of a long-duration, professional development academy on technology skills, computer self-efficacy, and technology integration beliefs and practices. *Journal of Research on Technology in Education*, *39*(1), 22–43.

Dexter, S. L., Anderson, R. E., & Becker, H. J. (1999). Teachers' views of computers as catalysts for changes in their teaching practice. *Journal of Research on Computing in Education*, *31*(3), 221–239.

Doering, A. (2006). Adventure learning: Transformative hybrid online education. *Distance Education*, *27*(2), 197–215. doi:10.1080/01587910600789571

Doering, A. (2007). Adventure learning: Situated learning in an authentic context. *Innovate* *3*(6).

Doering, A., & Veletsianos, G. (2008). Hybrid online education in the K-12 classroom: Identifying integration models using adventure learning. *Journal of Research on Technology in Education*, *41*(1), 101–119.

Duschl, R. A., Schweingruber, H. A., & Shouse, A. W. (Eds.). (2007). *Taking Science to School: Learning and Teaching Science in Grades K-8.* Washington, DC: The National Academies Press.

Ertmer, P. A., Addison, P., Lane, M., Ross, E., & Woods, D. (1999). Examining teacher's beliefs about the role of technology in the elementary classroom. *Journal of Research on Computing in Education*, *32*(1), 54–72.

Fulton, K., Glenn, A. D., & Valdez, G. (2003). *Three preservice programs preparing tomorrow's teachers to use technology: a study in partnerships.* Retrieved April 2, 2009, from http://www.learningpt.org/pdfs/tech/preservice.pdf

Goldenberg, L., Ba, H., Heinze, J., & Hess, A. (2003). *JASON Multimedia Science Curriculum Impact on student learning: Final Evaluation Report.* New York: Center of Children and Technology, Education Development Center.

Johnson, K. E., & Golombek, P. R. (2002). Inquiry into experience: Teachers' personal and professional growth. In Johnson, K. E., & Golombek, P. R. (Eds.), *Teachers' Narrative Inquiry as Professional Development* (pp. 1–14). Cambridge, UK: Cambridge University Press.

Kay, R. H. (2006). Evaluating strategies used to incorporate technology into preservice education: a review of the literature. *Journal of Research on Technology in Education, 38*(4), 383–408.

Knox, K. L., Moynihan, J. A., & Markowitz, D. G. (2003). Evaluation of short-term impact of a high school summer science program on students' perceived knowledge and skills. *Journal of Science Education and Technology, 12*(4), 471–478. doi:10.1023/B:JOST.0000006306.97336.c5

Leckie, M., St. John, K., Peart, L., Klaus, A., Slough, S., & Niemitz, M. (2006). The School of Rock Expedition: Education and Science Connect at Sea Aboard the U.S. Scientific Drilling Vessel: A model for integrating cutting-edge ocean-going science with educational initiatives. *EOS, 87*(24), 240–241.

Markowitz, D. G. (2004). Evaluation of the long-term impact of a university high school summer science program on students' interest and perceived abilities in science. *Journal of Science Education and Technology, 13*(3), 395–407. doi:10.1023/B:JOST.0000045467.67907.7b

Matzen, N. J., & Edmunds, J. A. (2007). Technology as a catalyst for change: the role of professional development. *Journal of Research on Technology in Education, 39*(4), 417–430.

Mezirow, J. (1990). *Fostering critical reflection in adulthood: A guide to transformative and emancipatory learning*. San Francisco: Jossey-Bass.

Mezirow, J. (1991). *Transformative dimension of adult learning*. San Francisco: Jossey-Bass.

Miller, C. V., & Doering, A. (2008). Curriculum at forty below: a phenomenological inquiry of an educator/explorer's experience with adventure learning in the Arctic. *Distance Education, 29*(3), 253–267. doi:10.1080/01587910802395789

National Research Council [NRC]. (1996). *National science education standards.* Retrieved January 10, 2006, from http://www.nap.edu/readingroom/books/nses/

Niemitz, M., Slough, S., Peart, L., Klaus, A., Leckie, M., & St. John, K. (2008). Interactive Virtual Expeditions as a Learning Tool: The School of Rock Expedition. *Journal of Educational Multimedia and Hypermedia, 17*(4), 561–580.

Palloff, R., & Pratt, K. (1999). *Building learning communities in cyberspace*. San Francisco: Jossey-Bass.

Sandholz, J., Ringstaff, C., & Dwyer, D. (1997). *Teaching with technology: Creating student-centered classrooms*. New York: Teachers College Press.

St. John, K., Leckie, M., Slough, S., Peart, L., Niemitz, M., & Klaus, A. (in press). *Field Geoscience Education – The Pilot School or Rock Program at Sea for Teachers.* Geological Society of America Special Paper.

Templin, M. A., Doran, R. L., & Engemann, J. F. (1999). A locally based science mentorship program for high achieving students: Unearthing issues that influence affective outcomes. *School Science and Mathematics, 99*(4), 205–211. doi:10.1111/j.1949-8594.1999.tb17475.x

Valdez, G., McNabb, M., Foertsch, M., Anderson, M., Hawkes, M., & Raack, L. (1999). *Computer-based technology and learning: Evolving uses and expectations*. Oak Brook, IL: North Central Regional Educational Laboratory.

Chapter 3
Faculty Reflections on Decision-Making and Pedagogical Use of Online Activities in Teacher Education

Swapna Kumar
University of Florida, USA

ABSTRACT

Teacher educators preparing their students for 21st century schools are increasingly using online technologies in on-campus courses. While some teacher educators have used such activities for almost a decade and have migrated from learning management systems to wikis and blogs, others still struggle to structure and facilitate online activities effectively. Ten teacher educators' decisions to use online activities in 23 face-to-face courses based on several criteria (class size, instructional goals, course type, students' prior knowledge, and the content of classroom instruction) are described in this chapter. Faculty members' reflections on their decisions, practical examples from different courses that they taught, and strategies they refined over time illustrated their focus on pedagogy as they migrated to newer technologies. The structure, design, and implementation of online activities discussed in this chapter could be useful to beginning educators, teacher developers, and instructional designers engaged in the integration of new technologies in higher education.

Teacher educators preparing their students for the schools of tomorrow are constantly faced with the challenge of staying informed about new technologies. They not only experiment with new technologies in order to be able to find tools and strategies that fit their own teaching style and instructional goals, but also attempt to model thoughtful use of technology that will prepare their students to teach with the new technologies that are available in the schools. Notwithstanding time constraints and the rapid changes in technology, teacher educators would like to communicate proven pedagogical strategies to their students, while immersing them in the technology of the time. Text-based online communication is currently used widely by faculty in courses in higher education (e.g. in learning management systems, blogs, wikis, and more recently social networking sites), but many faculty still

DOI: 10.4018/978-1-61520-897-5.ch003

Copyright © 2010, IGI Global. Copying or distributing in print or electronic forms without written permission of IGI Global is prohibited.

struggle with how to put online communication to best use for student learning. Even as they integrate online activities into their on-campus courses, they constantly experiment in order to make informed decisions about best practice.

The focus of this chapter is on faculty planning, guidance, and facilitation using online communication tools for student learning and student interaction in face-to-face courses, which can be transferred to other online technologies that are being introduced in teacher education courses. Online bulletin boards, discussion boards or forums have been used for over a decade to facilitate student interaction in higher education. An increasing number of teacher education faculty routinely use such tools in on-campus courses, and are now attempting to design similar activities with newer technologies like blogs, wikis, and social networking tools. Although most research studies explore the use of new technologies in education before those technologies become part of the mainstream, the purpose of this study is to focus on best practice by studying faculty members who have used both old and new online technologies in multiple courses over a period of time. On the one hand, their reflections on their practice and the changes in their teaching can inform other educators who are not as experienced in using these technologies. On the other hand, best practice from the use of online discussion boards and online collaborative activities can be adapted and transferred to newer technologies.

The chapter presents the experiences of ten teacher education faculty members who experimented with online student activities in different ways to model technology use as well as achieve their instructional goals in 23 courses. It provides practical examples of online activities by teacher educators, but also empirical data in the form of faculty reflections on their use of those technologies and how they made changes in consequent iterations of a course based on experience. A description of faculty use of online activities as well as the identification of the factors that play a role in their decisions to modify or change these activities in each course will benefit practitioners and teacher educators who would like to apply new technologies. Researchers seeking to understand why and how faculty members use online technologies for instruction might also find the results informative. The chapter begins with an overview of the research on teaching with online communication tools and a description of the research methodology, followed by a description of the ways in which faculty used online communication tools for pre-class, post-class, and supplemental instruction. A discussion of faculty considerations when implementing and adapting online activities in each course that they taught, and guidelines for practitioners seeking to integrate online activities are provided at the end of the chapter. The term 'online interactions' in this study refers to asynchronous online interactions between students and the professor or among students while using a discussion board within a learning management system, a wiki, or a blog to supplement classroom instruction.

RESEARCH ON ASYNCHRONOUS ONLINE COMMUNICATION IN HIGHER EDUCATION

Garrison, Anderson and Archer (2000) posited that communities of inquiry, both face-to-face and online, consist of three elements: cognitive presence, social presence, and teaching presence, all three of which, they argue, are "crucial prerequisites for a successful higher education experience" (p. 87). In studying the effective use of online interactions for student learning, they also asserted that a participant's cognitive presence is the most important factor that influences his/her learning. They defined cognitive presence as "… the extent to which the participants in any particular configuration of a community of inquiry are able to construct meaning through sustained communication" (p. 89) and stated that learners construct experiences and knowledge by analyzing the subject matter, raising questions, challenging assumptions, and integrating diverse ideas. In a later article, Garrison and Kanuka (2004) claimed that just as oral critical discourse can facilitate critical thinking, the reflective and explicit nature of online text-based communication is extremely conducive to higher-order cognitive learning. The process of writing helps to facilitate reflective thinking about problems, to formulate and clarify ideas, to organize thoughts, and to develop critical thinking, which is fundamental to communities of inquiry (MacArthur, 2006).

Benefits of Asynchronous Online Communication in Higher Education

The use of asynchronous online discussions or computer-mediated communication (CMC) in on-campus courses has been reported to increase student participation and interaction, to provide increased opportunities for engaging with course content, expose students to multiple perspectives, contribute to a better understanding of course concepts, and facilitate the application of new and existing knowledge (Angeli, Bonk, & Valanides, 2003; Biesenbach-Lucas, 2003; Dietz-Uhler & Bishop-Clark, 2002; Fauske & Wade, 2003; Gorski, Heidlebach, Howe, Jackson, & Tell, 2000; Hara, Bonk & Angeli, 2000; Kumar, 2007; Meyer, 2002; Schaff, 2003; Slavit, 2002; Vaughan & Garrison, 2005; Young, 2002). Teacher education researchers have concluded that asynchronous online communication fosters reflection on teaching and learning, student engagement with course concepts, and increased student communication (Barnett, 2006; Ferdig & Roehler, 2004; Kian-Sam & Lee, 2008; Hough, Smithey & Evertson, 2004; Jenning, 2005; Jetton, 2004; Lee-Baldwin, 2005; Lord & Lomicka, 2007; Maher & Jacob, 2006). In addition to enabling students to reflect on their teaching beliefs and teaching styles, and exposing them to multiple perspectives, integrating asynchronous online discussions in teacher preparation provides pre-service teachers with technology skills that can be useful to them later in their teaching practice (Jetton, 2004; Lord & Lomicka, 2007). Further, Ferdig and Roehler (2004) stated that, "students who used discussion forums... were more likely to achieve understandings of teaching and learning that went beyond just a surface level" (p. 131).

The research reviewed also indicated that interactions in the classroom can be positively influenced by online interactions (Vess, 2005). While Dietz-Uhler and Bishop-Clark (2001) concluded that online discussions can be beneficial to "subsequent face-to-face discussions with the same people, assuming that the two discussions are temporally close" (p. 271-272), Kumar (2007) reported on a professor's creation of a synergy between online and classroom discussions leading to enhanced student understanding of course topics in an undergraduate course. Garrison and Anderson (2003) argued for a blended learning environment that has a creative and well-designed discussion board. They claimed that instructors can best achieve higher-order learning by combining the energy and social interaction in a classroom with the increased response time and the resultant reflective dialog of an online discussion environment.

Factors Influencing Outcomes of Online Activities in On-Campus Courses

As with any use of technology in teaching practice, reflection or increased student engagement are not innate in the technology that is used but come about due to the strategies that faculty employ when using the technology. The question is how asynchronous online activities can be planned or structured by faculty to achieve the benefits described by the researchers cited above. Ferdig and Roehler (2004) suggest that the success of an online asynchronous discussion is influenced by multiple factors, including the relationship of discussion content to the course goals, and the modeling of discussion by the instructor. According to other researchers, the frequency and quality of student participation in online activities as well as the resulting knowledge construction are influenced by:

a. Instructor prompts or the nature of instructor questions
b. The subject-matter of the course or online activities
c. Instructor participation and guidance in online activities
d. Provision of structure and guidelines
e. The mandatory or optional nature of online activities
f. The task-related and non-task-related nature of online activities

(Angeli, Valanides, & Bonk, 2003; Christopher, Thomas, & Talent-Runnels, 2004; Fauske & Wade, 2003; Gilbert & Dabbagh, 2005; Kumar, 2007; Oliver & Trigwell, 2005; Schellens & Valcke, 2006; Overbaugh, 2002; Wu & Hiltz, 2004).

Similar factors have been found to influence student participation and learning when faculty use freely available blog and wiki software instead of the discussion board feature in learning management systems in higher education. Phillipson and Hamilton (2004) highlighted the importance of well-defined parameters to the success of a wiki that they designed, in which college students responded to annotations from poems using images, links, and author information. On experimenting with two different wikis that had different learning designs, tasks, and projects, Bower, Woo, Roberts and Watters (2006) concluded that task authenticity influences student contributions to wiki activities in a course. The content-centeredness and structure of a wiki as well as planning by the instructor have been reported to contribute to the success of a wiki in graduate education (Engstrom & Jewett, 2005; Raman, Ryan & Olfman, 2005).

Discussion of Research on Online Interactions in Higher Education

It follows that the ways in which an instructor structures, guides and participates in online activities contributes significantly to the success of such activities for student engagement and student learning. Course goals as well as the choices that instructors make when designing and participating in online activities could also be important. How do faculty members decide or plan their use of such online activities in teacher education courses? Do they use online activities in one particular way because it works for them, or do they adapt their activities according to the technology of the time and according to their prior experiences? Although the benefits and outcomes of computer-mediated communication or online interactions have been studied in the past, as have faculty perceptions and attitudes toward such technologies for instruction, the criteria that instructors consider when making choices and decisions to use online activities or use them in a certain way were not identified. Understanding how teacher education faculty currently use online technologies, the ways in which they have modified or adapted their use of the technology or their curriculum along the way and their perceptions of the resulting benefits to students can provide valuable insight for other educators who are also experimenting with asynchronous communication tools or online activities. This research was conducted to answer the following question:

What factors influence teacher educators' decisions to structure and facilitate online student activities (e.g. collaborative online assignments, online discussions) in their on-campus courses?

Faculty who use discussion boards, wikis, or blogs in more than one course are faced with decisions to structure and implement those technologies according to their course goals in each course. Teacher educators who use online discussions or online group activities in multiple courses that they teach were identified as an ideal sample to study this question, because it would be important to determine if they use online discussions or assignments in the same way or different ways in their teacher education courses.

METHODOLOGY AND DATA COLLECTION

Thirty-four teacher education faculty members in a large private university who had more than one course website listed each semester were contacted by email and provided with a description of the study. In order to exclude courses that used a learning management system, wiki, or a blog solely for presenting information and course materials to the students, faculty members were asked whether they included online discussions or activities by their students in their courses, whether they had done so for at least two years and in more than one course, and whether they used such activities in different ways. Fourteen faculty members who replied in the affirmative were contacted for semi-structured interviews. Ten faculty members who have their students interact in online discussion forums, blogs, and wikis finally participated in this research.

The ten faculty members had between four and twenty-six years of teaching experience and had been using online activities for two to four years in their undergraduate and graduate teacher education courses. They teach courses in foundations of education, educational policy, educational reform, physical education, history education, reading and writing education, special education, deaf studies, and instructional technology. At least one 60-minute semi-structured interview was conducted with each professor guided by the following topics:

- Faculty goals in integrating online activities into their on-campus courses
- The ways in which faculty have used/are using online activities in their on-campus courses
- Faculty reflections on the factors that influenced that use or on the ways in which they changed their use of online activities based on each experience.

The interview data were transcribed and managed using qualitative research software. Two interviews coded by two doctoral students in addition to the researcher were compared for inter-rater reliability. Cohen's kappa was between 0.6 and 0.8 before discussion, indicating a reasonably high agreement.

FACULTY USE OF ONLINE ACTIVITIES IN TEACHER EDUCATION COURSES

The teacher education faculty interviewed in this study cited several reasons for their initial use of online discussions in their courses: ensuring that students completed the readings (n=8); wanting students to think about and be "engaged with course topics" when not in the classroom (n=8); ensuring that all students participate and that "nobody hides" (n=5); gauging student understanding of course material (n=6); getting students to talk to one another instead of just to the professor (n=5) and keeping students "connected" and "less isolated" during student-teaching (n=4).

The faculty interviewed in this study used online discussion or online group activities in a learning management system, wiki, or blog in three ways: Pre-class (activities completed by students online before they met face-to-face weekly), Post-class (activities completed by students after they met face-to-face weekly), or as a supplement to classroom instruction (e.g. Online journals, online communications during student-teaching).

Pre-Class Online Activities

Nine of ten faculty members interviewed in this study had used online activities (group tasks or online discussions) prior to weekly class meetings in undergraduate or graduate courses. In some cases, these activities were initiated by the instructor – professors provided a prompt, a question about readings, or a resource (online video/ online link) to which students reacted. In other cases, students were required to post a prompt or lead the discussion for that week. For group activities, professors often provided clear instructions to students about what they should prepare in the group and present to the rest of the class in the online space. Four professors had students participate in online group activities related to the readings. For example, each group found an online video related to a topic from the readings, and posted it in the online discussion area along with a short summary of its relevance to the course. The group then prepared to answer questions from the instructor or peers in the classroom. In another instance, each group was asked to find an online research report with data pertaining to the weekly topic and post it along with a comment on its relevance.

The professors interviewed reflected that online discussion or group activities before a classroom session were extremely beneficial to them and to the students in several ways. Eight of them found that it helped both them and their students to prepare for classroom activities. One professor found it a good way to "break the ice" during the weeks when the course dealt with sensitive topics that students "got fired up about." He especially referred to one student who was very confrontational and whose participation in online discussions before a class had been helpful in preventing potential confrontations that could have taken up valuable class time. Another professor teaching a universal design course was able to provide students with easy contexts for problem-solving online and then raise the difficulty level of the problem in the class. Professors reflected that discussions could be taken to another level and that course topics were "initiated" online and "cemented" in the classroom.

Six professors reported being able to plan their classes better because the online activities exposed them to gaps in student knowledge. One professor said,

I tweak my lecture according to their comments, questions and concerns so that I am not second-guessing but really lining myself up with where they are at in their reading. It also gives me some sense of where we need more attention and more

Figure 1. Pre-class online activities

Students	Students	Professor	In the Classroom
- Complete readings - View online resources	- Discuss readings online - Post a resource along with a summary individually or in groups - Complete an online problem or case study in a group	- Prepares for class sessions based on student contributions - Clarifies problematic terms or topics - Steers "off-course" discussions - Gauges student understanding of course topics - Identifies and helps individual students with problems	- Solve tougher case studies/ problems - Results in deeper discussion

time and where they seem to be doing just fine. I pull out ideas that I want to encourage or discourage and I try to use them in the class.

Other professors similarly steered "off-course" discussions online, prepared comments or a summary of students' online discussions, and clarified problematic terms or topics that had arisen online, in the classroom. Three professors mentioned that they were able to identify and help students who had individual problems but who did not express themselves in the classroom.

Post-Class Online Activities

Three of the ten faculty interviewed reported using online activities to engage students after a classroom session. One professor provided additional resources or summarized classroom discussion, "If we've spent a week talking about how students learn new vocabulary, that you know, we've spent the class session talking about that. Then I give them an article to extend their understanding of the topic, to further their thinking about other aspects of it." Another professor used questions and prompts to encourage students to "contextualize" and "apply" material that had been discussed in the classroom, sometimes getting students to work in groups on specific cases where different meanings could be attributed to the same word.

One of the benefits of post-class online discussions, according to one professor was that "Often times when it worked well, students were really able to make connections between the weeks. They began to see all the different topics in the context of educational policy, with basic elements that recurred." She used post-class activities to connect with students and synthesize topics in a class where a large number of lectures by guest speakers prevented student discussion of course topics. All three professors observed that some students who did not speak much in class took the opportunity to "make themselves heard" by taking notes in class and either posing questions or commenting online.

Supplementing Classroom Instruction with Online Activities

Four of the professors interviewed used a blog, a wiki, or an online discussion board for students to share and report on their field experiences or student teaching. These were courses that did not meet every week in the semester or where professors did not feel that the class meetings addressed students' individual challenges or concerns, so they used online space in the following ways:

- The professor created a password-protected wiki where each student had his/her own

Figure 2. Post-class online activities

Students	In the Classroom	Professor	Students
- Complete readings - View online resources	- Initial discussion on topics - Professor /Guest speaker presentations - Students watch video /analyze cases or analyze classroom situations / solve cases in groups	- Provides additional resources - Reflects and comments on classroom content and interactions - Provides prompt for application/ synthesis of weekly topic	- Discuss additional resources in the context of classroom work and readings - Make connections between several course topics - Synthesize/ summarize

page to document and share his/her experiences teaching with technology. Students could comment and provide advice to each other.

- The professor created a password-protected blog where students posted weekly about their student-teaching experiences.
- Students posted their weekly comments in an online discussion forum on: a) how their field experiences corresponded to course topics, b) how they observed application of concepts in the school classroom they were visiting, c) how teacher leaders they observed demonstrated certain behaviors or not.
- Students kept an online journal about their pre-practicum experiences that was password-protected to only the professor and that student.

The professors reflected that these activities were more challenging to implement as student-student interactions because students were looking to the professor or teaching assistant to provide guidance and support. Nevertheless, they found these online activities extremely valuable because they could help, guide, and support individual students through their field experiences, and also received feedback that students felt less isolated as a result.

FACULTY DECISIONS WHEN USING ONLINE ACTIVITIES IN TEACHER EDUCATION COURSES

Whether the online activities were pre-class, post-class, or supplemental to class instruction, all ten faculty members interviewed in this study reflected that they had to take the following decisions when a) first using online activities in a course, b) adapting online activities for a different online tool (e.g. moving from an online discussion board to a blog) or c) adapting online activities for a different course that they taught.

How Should Online Activities Be Structured?

All the professors interviewed considered it important to structure the online communication space and provided substantial structure for online activities. Six of the ten faculty interviewed always provided a discussion prompt or a question when using online discussions in their courses. They posed a question that they found crucial to student understanding of the course topics and provided a resource e.g. an online video or podcast that they asked students to discuss. Two faculty members experimented with letting students post discussion questions for the week and act as discussion leaders. While one professor found that very satisfying, the other professor decided against it in future offerings of the course, because she thought that students should discuss topics that she considered important in the course.

The remaining four faculty members interviewed preferred to allow students to either post reactions to readings or find resources to post on the blog, and allowed pairs of students to lead the discussion or summarize the discussion. One professor provided a format to students – they had to name the reading, formulate a question, and summarize their reasons for asking the question. Professors who required groups to find and present resources online also provided a clear format for the group, sometimes providing an example as a model. One professor who used a blog to have students share their project ideas and comment on each others' projects, created specific areas on the blog and provided a template-like structure where students could do so.

In moving from online discussion boards within a learning management system to a wiki and to a blog, two professors initially tried to replicate what they had done before. While the professor who used the wiki moved to a less-structured and more student-driven format in subsequent offerings of the course, the professor who used a blog found the sequential nature of the blog irritating and difficult to structure. She reverted back to using an online discussion board in her courses because she could structure activities for each week in advance.

How Should Online Groups be Formed?

The decision to form groups or have students contribute individually was another dilemma faced by the professors, because they could not initially conceive of all the students interacting with one another online. Four professors preferred to use online groups because students would then interact closely with each other - "they might get to know people they wouldn't normally know that are outside of their program and who in class, they might not normally sit with or talk to." To this end, two professors assigned the groups very "deliberately" but differently. While one chose students from different programs or who were preparing to teach different grades for each group, the other professor grouped together students with similar interests and backgrounds. The first professor reasoned that students would have exposure to other subject-matter and grades:

I assign students to a group... it's very intentional. There are students from different programs – from the special education program, from early childhood, from elementary education, some who are interested in the primary grades, some who are interested in the intermediate grades. I set them up very deliberately with one from each of the specializations to the extent possible so that the groups are meant to be diverse in terms of their teaching interests, their disciplines of study, etc.

Two professors who initially asked graduate students to form their own groups in the first course where they included group activities decided against it in later courses. They found that not only was it time-consuming when students formed the groups, but that some students were left out, or were dissatisfied with the groups, which affected student participation.

Should Online Activities be Mandatory and Graded?

Eight of the ten professors interviewed in the study required online activities as part of the course assessment and allotted between 10% and 40% of the course grade to online activities. Students sometimes had the option of participating in online discussions for a certain number of weeks or could choose their "best six weeks out of ten" to be graded. Students in groups were always given the same grade, except for those taught by one professor, who required peer evaluation as part of the grade to determine participation and contribution by students in a group. Although the mandatory nature of online activities "raised the level of discussion," professors found it more time-consuming to grade these activities than to read them.

What Guidelines Would Help Students Succeed Online?

All the faculty members who were interviewed asserted that very clear instructions on the syllabus, on the course website, wiki, or blog, as well as explanations in class were very important to students' completing online activities properly individually or in groups. All the professors provided instructions about acceptable use of language and many of them set expectations by providing a model posting, a grading rubric, and examples of unacceptable contributions. Eight out of ten professors set a deadline for postings, including a day of the week and the time. One professor stated,

You're going to have to make students extremely accountable every week, and you're going to have to find some way to hold them accountable. So what I did was I set a deadline. And the reason I did that was that everyone in class knew that after that time, they could go to that thread and see everybody's response that was going to be there, if they were going to respond or...Having that knowledge ahead of time gave the course a nice structure.

Deadlines ensured that professors had time to read student contributions, that other students could comment on peer contributions, and that a student or group could summarize the contributions for the face-to-face class.

How Often Should the Professor Participate Online?

Four of the ten faculty members interviewed never participated in the online activities although they answered student questions that were addressed to them in the online discussion board, wiki, or blog. They reasoned that it was a space for students to interact with each other and not with them – "I didn't want to interpose myself between the students. I wanted it to be their own thing." Two professors reflected that they found it difficult at first, but they learned over time to let the students talk to each other or explain concepts to each other online. They found this satisfying because in the classroom, students always addressed their comments to the professor, and the professor found it difficult not to "sway the discussion the way I want it to go." Nevertheless, they made it very apparent to the students that they were reading or "watching" their online interactions, and often referred to the online activities in class. All the other professors "jumped in" to clarify terms and concepts that students did not understand or had misinterpreted. One professor described it as,

I could really hone in on what they were getting right and what they were getting wrong and say, let's pick up on this point. Now I'd really like you to think about how x, y, and z relates to Professor A's presentation on this and the classroom in the video we watched two weeks ago, and what does this all mean?

FACTORS INFLUENCING FACULTY DECISIONS WHEN USING ONLINE ACTIVITIES

Faculty members in this study reported changes in their instruction as they gained experience using online activities and as they migrated to new technologies. While they continued to provide structure and guidelines to students, they found that as they continued to use online discussions, wikis, or blogs for student interaction, they "controlled" the interactions or "intervened" less and less, allowing students to "take it and run with it." They solicited student feedback and were gratified that students perceived the same benefits of online activities to classroom instruction that they did. In addition to their own experiences using these technologies, the factors that formed the basis of the professors' decisions to use online activities in different ways were ***class size***, the ***course level*** (undergraduate or graduate), and the ***content and format of classroom sessions*** in a course.

Class Size

The number of students in a class was a decisive factor in the professors' decisions about whether students would do individual or group work, whether students would be required to comment on each others' work, and whether the professor participated online. One professor participated often in a small class with 20 students, where students posted individually and were required to post comments or resources weekly, but decided to only read students' contributions in a large class of 80+ students where she required students to post only seven out of 14 weeks in the semester. Describing the responses in the larger course as "overwhelming", in a subsequent offering of the course the professor designed group activities that required students to solve only four problems in groups during the semester instead of responding to readings individually. Another professor divided up the discussion groups according to the Teaching Assistants' sections in a class of over 100 students, where the Teaching Assistants interacted intensively with the individuals in the group and the professor commented once a week on each group's work online.

Course Goals and Course Level

One professor described the difference between his undergraduate and graduate courses as the students' prior knowledge of a subject and "the life experience" they brought to course activities. He is comfortable discussing the format of his online activities with students in a doctoral seminar, and designing collaborative writing activities online that "the students drive." However, in his Master's level courses he provides clear structure and deadlines for activities that are very focused on weekly course content. Another professor stated that she participated more and was "looking for higher-level thinking" in online activities in her graduate courses whereas she wanted students to apply course content and "situate readings in a broader context" in her undergraduate courses. Professors thus designed online activities differently and set different expectations depending on the course level, course goals and course content.

Content and Format of Classroom Instruction

The amount of time that was needed and available for professor-student interaction or student-student interaction influenced many professors' decisions to use online activities or virtual space for interaction. In lecture-based classes, or classes with guest speaker presentations, professors required students to post their reflections or responses online in order to "know that they are thinking." One professor stated that it bothered him that he "delivered" content in the classroom so he exploited the online discussion board to allow students to talk, ask questions, and relate the content to a bigger context. In contrast, two professors reflected that in discussion-based seminars where students interacted a lot in the classroom, they were challenged to come up with online collaborative projects that were worthwhile for students to complete and that deepened or broadened students' understanding. They wanted to integrate online activities because they considered online collaboration and group work to be valuable to students in real life, where students were increasingly required to work individually and as members of a team in a virtual environment. They also wanted their students to be exposed to online activities that could be used in their future classrooms.

Four professors struggled with deciding which parts of the curriculum students should engage with online and which topics should be reserved for the classroom. One professor pointed out that when she first used online discussions, students were discussing the same topics online and in class, which was not very useful. In the last couple of years she has consciously worked towards choosing topics for online activities or problem-solving, and topics that she feels require classroom time. Another professor experimented with asking students to complete a group task online as well as in the classroom during different weeks in the semester and asked for student feedback on the usefulness of each medium. Three professors reported changes in their classroom instruction as a result of the online activities. They began asking students to complete some of the activities they had been doing in the class online, thus freeing up time for new activities in the classroom.

DISCUSSION AND IMPLICATIONS FOR EDUCATORS

Out of the 23 courses included in this research, 16 used online discussion boards or group discussion areas in learning management systems, four used blogs, and three used wikis. Faculty commented on several benefits of online activities that were discussed in previous research – increased participation by all students, exposure to different aspects of course content, continuation of course topics and conversations outside the classroom, and reflection (Angeli, Bonk, & Valanides, 2003; Barnett, 2006; Ferdig & Roehler, 2004; Kian-Sam & Lee, 2008; Hough, Smithey & Evertson, 2004; Jenning, 2005; Jetton, 2004; Lee-Baldwin, 2005; Lord & Lomicka, 2007; Maher & Jacob, 2006). In addition, they reported increased familiarity with students' understanding of course content and individual problems. The professors in this study especially found online group activities useful to make it possible for students to "think with each other" and to take the attention away from the professor – "it's not about me anymore, it's about them and the readings." Furthermore, they consider it extremely important for their students to participate and succeed at such activities in order to better prepare them for the real world where virtual collaboration and communication are now ubiquitous. Due to these perceived benefits, faculty continue to find ways to use online discussions and online group work as means to engage students, migrating to new technologies but retaining the structure and goals of their online assignments.

All ten professors in this study began using online activities within the learning management system provided to them at their university. Four of those professors later tried to apply the same strategies that they had used in an online discussion board or in online group spaces to wikis or blogs. Although the attributes of the technology (e.g. the wiki) caused the professors to adapt their strategies and instructions to students, the types of online activities they used and the scaffolding that they provided to students did not change. It follows that the different examples provided in this chapter can largely be adapted to newer technologies in courses with similar instructional goals or content. In experimenting with online activities, the faculty members moved from a professor-controlled environment to a more student-controlled environment, and became more comfortable allowing the students to lead the discussion or restructure the virtual space. Provision of structure and guidelines, as well as professor monitoring of online activities, however, remained very important regardless of the student-centered nature of online activities.

Professors in this study leveraged their pedagogical knowledge and skills as well as their prior experiences with technology to structure online activities to supplement their on-campus courses. They took several decisions when combining online components and classroom instruction. The analysis of the qualitative data highlighted the importance of four main factors for decisions made by faculty members in the different courses they taught – the number of students, the type of course (e.g. course level, content, and goals), students' prior knowledge of course content, and classroom activities. The time taken to read, provide feedback, and integrate students' online work into classroom instruction can be a challenge for professors in courses with a large number of students. Online group work, lesser number of activities or giving students the option of completing activities only for a certain number of weeks during the semester could be considered by educators teaching large courses. Appointing discussion leaders or discussion groups who are responsible for different topics can also be an effective way of engaging large numbers of students. Discussion leaders or discussion groups can be asked to summarize and synthesize resources or discussion content either online or in the classroom. Students in smaller courses can take on specific roles in online activities, can carry out peer evaluations and provide feedback to one another, and can also contribute new resources about course topics.

The goals, the subject matter, and the level of courses (basic or advanced; undergraduate, graduate, or doctoral) influence the ways in which faculty structure and participate in online activities. If professors want students to engage with certain concepts e.g. universal design, at a beginner's level, they can provide easier scenarios that students can analyze and solve in groups online whereas in a doctoral seminar, students can be expected to introduce a scenario for their peers to analyze and discuss. While students are completing a practicum, online journals, blogs, or activities based on field experiences can be far more helpful than online discussion threads, especially if students are not comfortable sharing their experiences with all their peers. Topics that require students to identify types of instruction or skills can benefit from activities where students analyze and discuss online videos or podcasts. When students have prior knowledge of topics or have already worked in schools e.g. as in-service teachers or administrators, it is easier for professors to implement online activities that involve application of course content to real-world environments. Online activities that involve student contribution of resources like videos or podcasts work especially well for courses where the professor expects students to tie the instruction to a larger context, or relate it to trends, standards, or policies.

When deciding to use online student interactions in face-to-face courses, educators should review their plans for classroom instruction, thus deciding whether students would learn best by completing the activities before or after each classroom session. The format can be varied depending on the format for a class session. For example, during a week when there is a guest speaker, the professor can decide to have a post-class online activity. If the professor uses class time to lecture, he/she can decide if students should discuss readings online before the class, thus allowing her/him to prepare and adapt his/her lecture. The professor may also decide that after a lecture, the students should comment on the lecture and describe how the content connects to course topics. Dividing up course topics for discussion and interaction online and in the classroom can be an effective use of both online and classroom time, because students can easily become bored or weary of repetitive topics online and in the classroom.

DIRECTIONS FOR FUTURE RESEARCH

This research highlights ways in which a small group of teacher educators use current technologies as integral to the pedagogy of a course and course activities, thus modelling certain strategies and decisions that are not dependent on the technology used for online activities but on the outcomes that they hope to achieve. Teacher educators' use of online activities or online discussions in their courses acquaints students with the use of online tools for teaching and exposes them to the experience of working online individually or in a group before they design and use online activities in their classrooms. Pre-service or in-service teachers are thus better prepared to use similar tools in their teaching, and become more sensitive to students' participation or problems as a result of their participation in online activities. The combination of online and classroom activities in higher education can yield substantial benefits to students and their learning.

As the Web-based component of on-campus courses in higher education increases, the choices that instructors make when using online activities in their courses become more important, as do the strategies that they employ when using online technologies. Teacher educators are experts at pedagogy so future research should focus on identifying: (a.) the ways in which they use online technologies, (b.) the activities they design for students to interact online, (c.) the types of guidelines and structure that they provide when teaching with online technologies and the outcomes thereof, and (d.) how they evaluate student participation in those online activities. The ways in which online activities are used by faculty when teaching online courses could also inform educators seeking to integrate such activities into face-to-face instruction. Notwithstanding the value of individual case studies, studying the evolution and refinement of online activities by faculty members in multiple courses, when they use different technologies for online activities, and use these over a period of time could also be beneficial for beginning educators.

Each professor in this study reflected on lessons learned from his/her experiences, for example, with using online discussions or structuring online groups in a certain way, providing examples from different courses. The professors stressed the importance of pedagogical strategies that could leverage the capabilities of new technologies and yet be applied when using multiple technologies. The identification of such activities and strategies that can be adapted and applied when using newer technologies could inform other faculty and teachers wishing to use new technologies in teaching other disciplines. As online technologies become more sophisticated, educators will continue to adapt and apply these strategies to podcasting, audio or video communication tools, and virtual environments. Studying how much they learn from past experiments with online technologies, and what factors influence their decisions to use certain technologies over others would be useful to teacher developers and instructional designers engaged in the integration of new technologies in higher education.

REFERENCES

Angeli, C., Valanides, N., & Bonk, C. J. (2003). Communication in a web-based conferencing system: The quality of computer-mediated interactions. *British Journal of Educational Technology*, *34*(1), 31–43. doi:10.1111/1467-8535.00302

Barnett, M. (2006). Using a web-based professional development system to support preservice teachers in Examining Authentic Classroom Practice. *Journal of Technology and Teacher Education*, *14*(4), 701–729.

Biesenbach-Lucas, S. (2003). Asynchronous discussion groups in teacher training classes: Perceptions of native and non-native students. *Journal of Asynchronous Learning Networks*, *7*(3), 24–33.

Bower, M., Woo, K., Roberts, M., & Watters, P. (2006). *Wiki Pedagogy – A Tale of Two Wikis*. Paper presented at the 7th conference on Information Technology based Higher Education and Training, Sydney, Australia.

Christopher, M. M., Thomas, J. A., & Talent-Runnels, M. K. (2004). Raising the bar: Encouraging high level thinking in online discussion forums. *Roeper Review*, *26*(3), 166–171. doi:10.1080/02783190409554262

Dietz-Uhler, B., & Bishop-Clark, C. (2002). The psychology of computer-mediated communication: Four classroom activities. *Psychology Learning & Teaching*, *2*(1), 25–31.

Engstrom, M. E., & Jewett, D. (2005). Collaborative learning the wiki way. *TechTrends*, *49*(6), 12–15. doi:10.1007/BF02763725

Fauske, J., & Wade, S. E. (2003). Research to practice online: Conditions that foster democracy, community, and critical thinking in computer-mediated discussions. *Journal of Research on Technology in Education*, *36*(2), 137–154.

Ferdig, R. E., & Roehler, L. R. (2003). Student uptake in electronic discussions: Examining online discourse in literacy preservice classrooms. *Journal of Research on Technology in Education*, *36*(2), 119–136.

Garrison, D., Anderson, T., & Archer, W. (2000). Critical inquiry in a text-based environment: Computer conferencing in higher education. *The Internet and Higher Education*, *2*(2-3), 87–105. doi:10.1016/S1096-7516(00)00016-6

Garrison, R., & Kanuka, H. (2004). Blended learning: Uncovering its transformative potential in higher education. *The Internet and Higher Education*, *7*(2), 95–105. doi:10.1016/j.iheduc.2004.02.001

Gilbert, P. K., & Dabbagh, N. (2005). How to structure online discussions for meaningful discourse: a case study. *British Journal of Educational Technology*, *36*(1), 5–18. doi:10.1111/j.1467-8535.2005.00434.x

Gorski, P., Heidlebach, R., Howe, B., Jackson, M., & Tell, S. (2000). Forging communities for educational change with e-mail discussion groups. *Multicultural Perspectives*, *2*(4), 37–42. doi:10.1207/S15327892MCP0204_8

Hara, N., Bonk, C. J., & Angeli, C. (2000). Content analysis of online discussion in an applied educational psychology course. *Instructional Science*, *28*(2), 115–152. doi:10.1023/A:1003764722829

Hough, B. W., Smithey, M. W., & Evertson, C. M. (2004). Using computer-mediated communication to create virtual communities of practice for intern Teachers. *Journal of Technology and Teacher Education*, *12*(3), 361–386.

Jenning, H. (2005). Increasing value without increasing effort? The use of WebCT in accompanying face-to-face lectures under the constraint of low budget. *Journal of Distance Education*, *20*(2), 78–84.

Jetton, T. L. (2004). Using computer-mediated discussion to facilitate preservice teachers' understanding of literacy assessment and instruction. *Journal of Research on Technology in Education*, *36*(2), 171–191.

Kian-Sam, H., & Lee, J. C. (2008). Postgraduate students' knowledge construction during asynchronous computer conferences in a blended learning environment: A Malaysian experience. *Australasian Journal of Educational Technology*, *24*(1), 91–107.

Kumar, S. (2007). Professor Use, Facilitation, and Evaluation of Asynchronous Online Discussions in On-campus Courses. In C. Montgomerie & J. Seale (Eds.), *Proceedings of World Conference on Educational Multimedia, Hypermedia and Telecommunications 2007* (pp. 2855-2863). Chesapeake, VA: AACE.

Lee-Baldwin, J. (2005). Asynchronous discussion forums: A closer look at the structure, focus and group dynamics that facilitate reflective thinking. *Contemporary Issues in Technology & Teacher Education*, *5*(1), 93–115.

Lord, G., & Lomicka, L. (2007). Foreign language teacher preparation and asynchronous CMC: Promoting reflective teaching. *Journal of Technology and Teacher Education*, *15*(4), 513–532.

MacArthur, C. A. (2006). The effects of new technologies on writing and writing processes. In MacArthur, C. A., Graham, S., & Fitzgerald, J. (Eds.), *Handbook of writing research* (pp. 248–262). New York: Guilford.

Maher, M., & Jacob, E. (2006). Peer computer conferencing to support teachers' reflection during action research. *Journal of Technology and Teacher Education*, *14*(1), 127–150.

Meyer, K. A. (2002). *Quality in distance education: Focus on on-line learning*. Hoboken, NJ: Jossey-Bass.

Oliver, M., & Trigwell, K. (2005). Can 'Blended Learning' be redeemed? *E-learning*, *2*(1), 17–26.

Overbaugh, R. C. (2002). Undergraduate education majors' discourse on an electronic mailing list. *Journal of Research on Technology in Education, 35*(1), 117–139.

Phillipson, M., & Hamilton, D. (2004). *The romantic audience project: A wiki experiment.* Retrieved November 22, 2007, from http://www.rc.umd.edu/pedagogies/commons/innovations/rap/toc.htm

Raman, M., Ryan, T., & Olfman, L. (2005). Designing knowledge management systems for teaching and learning with wild technology. *Journal of Information Systems Education, 16*(3), 311–320.

Schaff, M. (2003). Student perceptions of technology and how it impacts their learning: A technology integration experience. In *Proceedings of World Conference on Educational Multimedia, Hypermedia and Telecommunications* (pp. 1764-1768). Chesapeake, VA: AACE.

Schellens, T., & Valcke, M. (2006). Fostering knowledge construction in university students through asynchronous discussion groups. *Computers & Education, 46*(4), 349–370. doi:10.1016/j.compedu.2004.07.010

Slavit, D. (2002). Expanding classroom discussion with an online medium. *Journal of Technology and Teacher Education, 10*(3), 407–423.

Vaughan, N., & Garrison, D. R. (2005). Creating cognitive presence in a blended faculty development community. *The Internet and Higher Education, 8*(1), 1–12. doi:10.1016/j.iheduc.2004.11.001

Vess, D. L. (2005). Asynchronous discussion and communication patterns in online and hybrid history courses. *Communication Education, 54*(4), 355–364. doi:10.1080/03634520500442210

Wu, D., & Hiltz, S. R. (2004). Predicting learning from asynchronous online discussions. *Journal of Asynchronous Learning Networks, 8*(2), 139–152.

Young, J. R. (2002). Hybrid teaching seeks to end the divide between traditional and online instruction. *The Chronicle of Higher Education, 48*(28), A33.

Chapter 4
Peer to Peer:
Using the Electronic Discussion Board During Student Teaching

Karen J. Johnson
West Chester University, USA

ABSTRACT

Ten elementary education student teachers communicated with each other on an electronic discussion board for thirteen weeks. Despite being overwhelmed at times with the demands of student teaching, participants posted 283 messages offering each other ideas and support. Students were grouped into two different discussion boards based on the grade level they were assigned to student teach, resulting in very specific help and feedback from peers who were experiencing the same or similar teaching topics or situations. Results indicate that 70% of the participants used an idea that had been posted on the discussion board by a peer and 100% of the participants stated that the discussion board was a means of support during student teaching. Although an electronic discussion board is not a new technology, it is underutilized, especially as a means to connect geographically distant student teachers so they can offer each other support and ideas for teaching.

INTRODUCTION

Student teaching is the culminating activity in teacher education preparation programs (Anderson, 2007; Spooner, Flowers, Lambert, & Algozzine, 2008). Student teachers are used to spending many semesters taking courses together, often collaborating with peers on many group projects and assignments. Then, during student teaching, a student teacher may find himself or herself as the sole college student in an elementary school building. In order to stay connected daily to peers, especially those student teaching at the same time and at the same grade level, student teachers can use an electronic discussion board (EDB). This kind of technology can be a valuable tool for students to take advantage of as they work through the many issues and emotions that accompany student teaching. Peers who are set-up on the same discussion board and who are student teaching in the same

DOI: 10.4018/978-1-61520-897-5.ch004

Copyright © 2010, IGI Global. Copying or distributing in print or electronic forms without written permission of IGI Global is prohibited.

grade level can provide a constant connection for each other that can be a means of support that often cannot be found in the student-supervisor or student-cooperating teacher relationship. This chapter will focus on why student teaching supervisors should provide this electronic tool to their student teachers, how this author has already utilized it with two different groups of students teachers, and issues for supervisors to consider when setting up an electronic discussion board for their student teachers. This chapter can also be applicable to the coordinator of field experiences since the coordinator may choose to set up multiple discussion boards for all of the different grade level or subject placements within his/her department or college of education.

BACKGROUND

Hey everyone, I was just wondering... Is anyone else incapable of relaxing and thinking about other things (other than school)? Lately I cannot think about anything but what lessons I have to make, how I can reach my students better, how I can incorporate different ideas and methods into lessons, etc! My social life has officially flown out the window, as a result. I feel constantly stressed about students and the amount of work I have. Is anyone else in the same boat?? I guess I just want to know I'm not alone...! Best of luck! (Posted on 10/26/08)

The above quotation from a student teacher in the middle of her elementary education student teaching placement is a reminder that students often feel isolated from their peers and without a social or emotional group to connect with during this very stressful time in their lives. After studying and preparing for many semesters, teacher education majors who are now student teaching are asked to take everything that they learned and apply it to an actual classroom. Thankfully they are not alone. They are placed in a classroom with an experienced teacher who will hopefully model good teaching practices and provide advice, ideas, and helpful feedback. In addition, student teachers often have a university supervisor observing several lessons each semester, and are available for questions and support. Having the support and advice of peers, however, can be a much-needed and often lacking part of the student teaching equation (Assaf, 2005; Nicholson & Bond, 2003). Although many universities do require their student teachers to attend a seminar on-campus during student teaching, there are often too many things for the group to discuss and individual questions and advice between peers may not fit the time frame. Student teaching supervisors at several colleges of education (Assaf, 2005; Pena & Almaguer, 2007) are beginning to use computer-mediated communication to overcome this obstacle and keep students connected to each other.

Definition of Terms

Computer-mediated communication is a term that refers to the communication that is transmitted via the computer such as email, list serves, and electronic discussion boards. The terms, web-based discussion board, asynchronous discussion board, electronic discussion board, and online discussion board are used interchangeably in this chapter. They are referring to a website that will give students access to a place where they can read, post, and respond to messages exchanged among student teaching peers. The discussion board is threaded which means different topics will be separated from each other, rather than one long discussion that lasts for the duration of the semester. Threaded discussions also allow preservice teachers to read and respond to specific posts. The asynchronous nature of the electronic discussion board means that students do not have to be online at the same time to read messages, post messages or reply to messages.

Student Teaching and Computer Mediated Communication

Student teachers are often placed in field settings that are quite far apart from their preservice teacher colleagues. If a preservice teacher is the only student teacher in the building, feelings of isolation from the university community can follow (Schlagal, Trathen, & Blanton, 1996; Smeaton & Waters, 2000). In fact, the two major problems that universities often experience with their preservice teachers who are completing their student teaching semester are: not feeling they are a part of the university community and not being able to get support from peers and professors during student teaching (Smeaton and Waters, 2000).

Computer technology, specifically computer-mediated communication (CMC) has been the tool chosen by many colleges to attempt to overcome those problems. A number of universities have set up email groups, listservs, and discussion groups for their student teachers to stay connected to their cooperating teacher (Stegman, 2007) or the university faculty and peers (Devlin-Scherer & Daly, 2001; Edens & Gallini, 2000; Ferdig & Roehler, 2004; Mayer, 2002; Paulus & Scherff, 2008; Smeaton and Waters, 2000). In addition, some colleges provide laptops to ensure that student teachers have access to technology so that they can stay connected to their university supervisor as well as to make sure that they can have a working computer to use for lesson planning and other curricular tasks (MacKinnon, Aylward, & Bellafontaine, 2006; Thomas, Larson, Clift, & Levin, 1996). All of these examples demonstrate ways that keep student teachers in touch with those who can offer support.

Internationally, electronic discussion boards are being utilized by teacher education programs for various purposes including helping to form teacher identities in Italy (Grion & Varisco, 2007), building in ways for more substantive discussions online for teacher educators who also meet face-to-face in Canada (MacKinnon, Aylward, & Bellafontaine, 2006), gaining a virtual connection to peers and supervisors in Australia (Mayer, 2002), and setting up a shared display system for teacher education majors in Norway (Morken, Divitini, & Haugalokkent, 2007).

Teacher candidates who have been involved in asynchronous, web-based discussions have spoken of the importance of having both opportunity and place where they can access ideas and share their reflections and reactions to what they are seeing or doing in their field placements (Biesenbach, 2004) while sharing ideas and offering support to one another (Wilkerson, 2003). The use of electronic communication helped to facilitate belonging to a group (Singer & Zeni, 2004) and to reduce the isolation felt by many student teachers.

More recently, Assaf (2005) examined how student teachers in a reading specialist program used an electronic discussion board. The four participants communicated with each other during their student teaching semester and were then interviewed about it the following year, well after they had completed their semester and had moved on to their first year of teaching. Assaf (2005) found that three of her four participants felt the support of their peers through the use of the EDB. The three main themes found in these results were support, relationships, and learning from each other (Assaf, 2005). Similarly, Paulus & Scherff (2008) evaluated fifteen secondary education English majors participating in EDB during their internship experience. These researchers found that student interns talked about six major topics during the fifteen week semester: student issues, university concerns, curriculum, relationships with others, organization/time management, and classroom ownership (Paulus & Scherff, 2008). More and more universities are implementing some type of computer-mediated communication for the benefit of the students (Bulger, 2006; MacKinnon, Aylward, & Bellafontaine, 2006) and student teachers are reporting that this tool helps them to feel an important connection to their peers (Assaf, 2005; Mayer, 2002; Poole, 2000). In fact, in one study in the United Kingdom where tutors informally set up peer support groups for student teachers, at the end of the semester, seventy percent of the participants indicated that there should be a more formal system in place for peer support (McCarthy & Youens, 2005). The author of this chapter has set-up a more formal system of peer support during student teaching which will be described in the next section.

USING THE ELECTRONIC DISCUSSION BOARD

Issues, Controversies, Problems

In this section, information about two studies involving an electronic discussion board for two different groups of student teachers will be reviewed. This author has previously conducted research in this area and has made adjustments to the requirements of using a discussion board during student teaching to better meet the needs of the student teachers. In order to make sense of the results, some details of the first study need to be shared. In the initial version of the research I conducted with elementary education student teachers at a small college in the Northeast United States, I organized an asynchronous discussion board for a group of twenty-six student teachers using WebCT, which was provided by the university. The participants in this group were required to post one message each week and to reply to three peers each week. They were told that the only topic for discussion was computer use during student teaching since the first version of the study sought to determine in what ways student teachers can support each other's efforts at including computers in their teaching through the use of the electronic discussion board. For their one posting each week, the student teachers could either describe how they had used computers in a lesson or ask a question to their group of peers about computer use in an upcoming lesson. Despite those specific guidelines, it was obvious as the semester was progressing as well as at the end of the semester when the data was analyzed fully, that student teachers wanted to use the electronic discussion board not only as a place to share computer use ideas but also to vent, share stories, offer support and encouragement. Seventy percent of the messages involved computers while the other thirty percent were non-computer use messages. In other words, they were using the electronic discussion board for more than just the required topic discussion of computer use.

When the analysis was completed it was apparent that student teachers had a need for connecting with their peers on many areas of student teaching, not only how to include computers in their teaching. Specifically, the other areas that were frequently discussed topics were offering emotional/social support, sharing a teaching idea, and requesting help that did not involve computer use. Since almost one-third of the messages that pertained to student teaching were not specifically about using computers in teaching, it seemed that student teachers should be encouraged to use an electronic discussion board in the future to discuss any and all student teaching topics of their choice.

Unlike many of the other studies in this area, there were no postings or replies by the instructor that had to be specifically responded to by the student teachers. In fact, there were no postings of any kind by the instructor during the semester. The student teachers knew that the author would be eventually reading and analyzing their posts for a research project, but they also knew that when a peer posted a request for help, it would not be answered by an instructor or supervisor. All postings and replies to postings were done only by the student teachers.

In order to better address the needs of student teachers, I modified the study and conducted a second version at a larger university in a different state. The second version of the study again involved elementary education student teachers, however, there were some specifically targeted changes were incorporated. In this revision, ten student teachers, who were all part of the same on-campus student teaching seminar group, were asked to communicate on the electronic discussion board weekly. The requirement was for each of them to post one message a week and reply to two messages each week. This represents one of the lessons learned from the first study. The student teachers were too busy to be required to post and reply frequently each week, so the requirement was cut down slightly. A second change was to group the participants into two separate discussion boards-one for those student teaching in grades one and two and the other for those student teaching in grades four and five. All students had access to post, read and reply in either discussion board but separating the groups by grade level was intended to allow for peers to give each other more specific help and feedback during student teaching. A third change was to allow student teachers to discuss any relevant topic, not just computer use.

In order to demonstrate the benefits of using this discussion board with your student teachers, the author will describe the second study in more detail. Implementing this kind of discussion board is very easy to do and with the details following, a similar design can be replicated or revised and used with the group of student teachers you may be supervising.

Methodology

The ten elementary education student teachers from a mid-size Mid-Atlantic university in the United States communicated with each other for thirteen weeks of a fall semester. They were using Blackboard as the host for the electronic discussion board, which was housed on the university server, and used in many courses to post documents for students. These ten student teachers were all in the same seminar group that met once a week on campus for two hours. At the conclusion of the semester they were asked to complete an eleven question survey (see Appendix A). Their thirteen weeks of messages were then analyzed as was their day and time usage and number of times accessing the discussion board (whether just reading or reading and posting). Mixed methodology was utilized in the analysis of the surveys, the posts, and the day/time usage. The posts were read, reread, and categorized using the constant comparative method (Lincoln & Guba, 1985). The survey results were quantitatively analyzed where appropriate and open-ended questions were coded and classified into categories. The background information retrieved from Blackboard about the frequency of hits on the discussion board, the day and time use, were all analyzed quantitatively.

Results

The results of this second version of the study overwhelmingly support the use of an electronic discussion board for student teachers. All ten participants (100%) reported that the electronic discussion board was a means of support during student teaching. One survey comment from a participant went as follows, "It was great networking with the other student teachers. It also provided a sense of comfort knowing there are others going through the 'same' exact thing. Giving pointers and heads-up with material".

Over the course of thirteen weeks, these ten elementary education student teachers posted 283 messages. More importantly, they had 2,612 hits on the discussion board during those same thirteen weeks. Although they did not post the required number of posts and replies, they did utilize the discussion board often, reading posts more than purely posting. The nature of the elementary student teaching semester is extremely busy and stressful so the researcher chose not to send frequent emails reminding participants to post. They received two reminder emails spread throughout the thirteen weeks. After categorizing and analyzing the postings, it was apparent that the student teachers posted messages in four main categories: classroom teaching ideas (46%), emotional/social support postings (26%), issues with their students (15%), and informational posts (13%). Each of these categories will be subsequently described in detail and examples of actual posts for each category will also be shared so that they reader can get a flavor for the type of messages that the student teachers were posting.

The most common topic for a new thread on the discussion board was classroom teaching ideas (46%). The student teaching survey responses corroborate with their actual usage. Grouping the students into two different groups based on their grade level was of some benefit since the sharing of teaching/lesson ideas and suggestions was the most commonly discussed topic. An example of a post from this category is as follows, "My coop had shown me a few math books that are great. They are fun to do with the kids during core extension or fun Friday. They are by Greg Tang. The one book I was looking through is called The Grapes of Math. They are great for the younger students and allow for something a little different rather than the instructor book. Just a thought for everyone."(Posted on 11/16/08). This is one of many examples where students shared ideas with each other. In that case, the student teacher was sharing a teaching idea that she has not used but had learned of it from her cooperating teacher. The next example is representative of the many times when a student teacher described a lesson she had taught with enough depth that someone else could replicate it.

In science, we have been learning about parts of trees and the functions of each part. I came up with a lesson last week that the kids really enjoyed and thought I would share it with all of you. After they came back in from lunch, I had a video projected onto the screen and it was of tree sounds. The volume was turned up and I had the kids come in and get settled so they could hear the video. I told them to get into the mindset of a tree...think about any thoughts, feelings or actions you would have on a daily basis. I let them sit there for a minute or two with their eyes closed and listen to the video. I then passed out a graphic organizer I made in the shape of a tree with bubbles at the top as branches. The children were encouraged to brainstorm and write down any ideas they might have. We shared with the class after allowing them some time to brainstorm and I was really surprised at some of the great ideas they came up with! We began the actual writing piece this past Thursday, so I am very anxious to see what the kids come up with...they seem to be really enjoying it:) (posted on 10/4/08)

A third example in the category of teaching/lesson ideas demonstrates that student teachers were not only sharing lesson ideas but asking for suggestions for lesson ideas from their peers who were teaching in the same grade level. This post, from the primary grade discussion board focuses on seeking help for social studies. "We haven't done much social studies so far. I was curious to see what you have been doing in your classroom? We are trying to do immigration but it's hard without text books. Would love to have a little insight on what's been going on with you girls. Thanks!" (Posted on 10/8/08) There were three replies to this post offering ideas. This category of posts was clearly the most common in this study. Having the electronic discussion board allowed this group of student teachers the opportunity to share ideas and ask for teaching ideas from peers who were teaching the same grade level.

Emotional/social support postings (26%) were the second most common grouping of posts. A fourth of all topics posted were about issues, situations, feelings, and emotions where student teachers were able to share those comments and respond to each other about those delicate issues. A common discussion in that area was the overwhelming nature of student teaching and asking if others were just as overwhelmed. Other posts in this category were describing a situation and asking if others feel the same way. In other words, looking for confirmation that the student teacher is not the only one who feels this way or is not the only one experiencing something. One posting reads as follows,

I noticed I have a sort of "stagefright" when there are adult teachers watching me. Whether I am being observed or I just have my co-op in the room. The other day we had a substitute in the room who graduated a year ago and I taught the whole time, she just assisted. All of a sudden my fears were gone and I had the whole morning running smoothly. Does anyone else feel a little intimidated or nervous in front of adult teachers, yet when there is someone else your age around, you actually teach better? (Posted on 9/25/08)

Since one-fourth of all posts were in this category, it lends support to the idea that student teachers need a place to vent and to compare how they are feeling with others who are going through similar experiences.

The third most common type of posting were made by the student teachers about the elementary students they were working with (15%). These were typically postings about an individual elementary student in the class where they were student teaching. No names of students or cooperating teachers were ever used by the student teachers. Many times, the person who started the thread was describing something unusual that a student was doing and then asked for suggestions from peers about what she could do about this situation with this student. Many of those pertained to behaviors of a student but occasionally it pertained to something other than a student's behavior. An example of such a post follows.

Even though this is our last week I wasn't sure what I was going to write. Then I had a student that has been somewhat...annoying. haha. He was the student I picked for my journals because he is extremely smart and will be getting tested again for gifted. However, the last couple of days he has just been out of control. He won't stop talking, he is making noises and always fooling around. We keep giving him warnings and actually taking some recess time away but that doesn't seem to help. I thought that it was just because it was Friday last week but today he has already lost some recess and it wasn't even ten o'clock and he was gone for gym for forty minutes. I am wondering if he is goofing off because he knows he is getting tested again for gifted and doesn't need to do work or he is just trying to be the class clown. Any suggestions? (Posted 12/8/08)

These kinds of posts received several responses since most students were able to relate to the student being described and share what they were already doing with students who were difficult to handle.

Informational posts (13%) were the fourth most common kind of post made by these student teachers. In these posts student teachers were sharing information or asking for information about things that were not lesson/teaching ideas or student issues. Some of the topics posted were about technology workshops at the university, the teacher discount weekend at a local bookstore, cap and gown and graduation rehearsal, and interviewing/job search. All ten of these student teachers were graduating at the conclusion of student teaching so finding a job was very much on their minds as they were in their last few weeks of student teaching. An example of one of the informational posts follows.

I just got this today from the librarian at my school. I thought some of you would be interested...

I don't know if anyone is interested in this as it is a bit of a drive, but this is a special event that I am going to attend and I wanted everyone else to be aware of just in case. {Name of bookstore} hosts an author/illustrator night every year and the lineup is rather impressive this year. It's this Friday (short notice, I know) and this store is not a huge place, but WOW! What a lineup! I've attached the lineup and directions if you are interested. (Posted on 11/6/08)

Table 1.

Day of the Week	Percent of Hits
Sunday	17.63%
Monday	12.86%
Tuesday	19.26%
Wednesday	14.59%
Thursday	14.59%
Friday	11.07%
Saturday	10.00%

Certainly these student teachers could have emailed their group of ten when they had an informational item to share or to ask a question about but whether or not they would take the time to do so is what makes the discussion board the easiest method to share informational items.

The data from the electronic discussion board corroborate what the students reported in their surveys. One hundred percent of the participants reported that the electronic discussion board was helpful to them and examining the days and times that they used the tool would confirm that they certainly did spend a great deal of time reading and/or posting. The study lasted for thirteen weeks (91 days). During that time, there were only six days when none of the ten participants were on the electronic discussion board. There were several weekends when there was a great deal of participation, especially the weekends prior to their "full-time" weeks of teaching. There were even 24 hits on Thanksgiving Day from three participants! The breakdown by day of week was as follows:

Tuesday received the most hits throughout the semester with Sunday seeing the second highest number of hits. Friday and Saturday had the fewest hits, as is not a surprise. In thinking about the set-up of the week, students were meeting with me and each other on-campus in a seminar on Thursday afternoons. As students were preparing lessons plans and coming across issues earlier in the week, they were perhaps relying on the discussion board to connect with each other. Late in the week they met face-to-face on-campus and could ask more questions and share stories in person during seminar.

As an asynchronous tool, the participants had access to the electronic discussion board 24 hours a day. Unlike videoconferencing or live chats, these students could take advantage of posting or reading posts when it was most convenient for them. Upon examination of the usage each day, there were only two one-hour time-slots in the day when the electronic discussion board was never used: 12-1am and 2-3am. As the table below indicates, the student teachers utilized the discussion board throughout the entire day and night, something that cannot be done with live chatting or live video conferencing.

It would seem from that data that students took advantage of the asynchronous nature of the electronic discussion board. If this were only seen as a requirement for student teaching/seminar, one would not expect to find the electronic discussion board being used over such a wide range of days and times throughout the semester. This is one of the most important results for supervisors to consider. If students felt as if this was just another requirement that had to get done, one would have expected many days when there was no activity, or many weeks when each student logged on only once during the week to make the required one post and two replies. However, data analysis reveals that these participants were using the discussion board frequently throughout the semester, not always posting but often reading posts. In all thirteen weeks, more than one person logged in to the discussion board on more than one day in a week. Specifically, there were two weeks of the thirteen weeks of the study when two participants logged in more than one day during the week. The other eleven weeks saw at least three participants logging on at least two different days of the week and six of those thirteen weeks saw at least half (five) of the participants logging on for at least

Table 2.

Time of day	Percent of hits
Midnight-12:59am	0.00%
1:00-1:59am	0.39%
2:00-2:59am	0.00%
3:00-3:59am	0.39%
4:00-4:59am	0.55%
5:00-5:59am	0.61%
6:00-6:59am	0.29%
7:00-7:59am	1.61%
8:00-8:59am	3.00%
9:00-9:59am	1.97%
10:00-10:59am	2.94%
11:00-11:59am	6.03%
12:00-12:59pm	7.03%
1:00-1:59pm	2.45%
2:00-2:59pm	4.94%
3:00-3:59pm	10.97%
4:00-4:59pm	6.49%
5:00-5:59pm	3.39%
6:00-6:59pm	8.13%
7:00-7:59pm	10.07%
8:00-8:59pm	9.33%
9:00-9:59pm	8.81%
10:00-10:59pm	6.81%
11:00-11:59pm	3.81%

two different days in a week. These results are encouraging and lend support to the survey results that this electronic tool was very beneficial to student teachers. Some utilized it much more than others. For example, one participant logged in three or more days of a week for twelve of the thirteen weeks in the study, including five or more days in a given week for seven of those thirteen weeks. Clearly this was more than was merely "required". It is not known the exact purpose of all of those logins. Perhaps some of those were to re-read someone's supportive post to her from a previous day after having had another difficult day. Perhaps it was checking to see if a peer had replied to a post she had made previously. Others did not utilize the discussion board nearly as much with one student ignoring it for the entire month of November.

Solutions and Recommendations

Being part of the electronic discussion board community provided participants with a strong feeling of support and connection during student teaching as has been found by others (Assaf, 2005; Paulus & Scherff, 2008). One of the benefits of creating an electronic community through a discussion board for student teachers is that they can feel more connected with their peers who are student teaching at the same time. In this second study I conducted, Lydia (a pseudonym) noted, "It {the EDB} allowed me to communicate with other student teachers who were experiencing the same issues and could perhaps give me feedback since they are in the classroom as well". The asynchronous nature of the electronic discussion board allowed for students to post and read replies from peers when it was convenient to them. Following is a quotation from the discussion board at the end of the semester.

Hey Ladies, Just wanted to write one last post about my student teaching experience and how much it's meant to me. I am in the post-bacc program, so I have been in the "real world" for about 2 or 3 years and have had all sorts of jobs. After completing student teaching, I finally realized my purpose in life. I am here to teach. There is nothing else in the world that I can imagine doing. It's like a light went off inside of my head and I have finally found my spot in this world. I have been searching for so long for that intrinsic motivation and sense of purpose and I have finally found it....it's an incredible feeling. I am just so happy and can't wait to begin my career in education. Does anyone feel the same way I do? (Posting on 12/13/08)

Issues to Consider for Implementation

There are three main areas that student teaching supervisors should consider when implementing an electronic discussion board with their group of student teachers: Purpose, Participants, and Posts. All three areas are important for supervisors to reflect on before implementing this type of tool with student teachers.

Purpose

If a supervisor wants to implement an electronic discussion board for his/her student teachers, the purpose needs to be clear to the student teachers. The students should be informed of the purpose at the start of the semester. For this author's first study, the entire purpose was to use the electronic discussion board as a place to share ideas and get help specifically focused on using computers in teaching elementary students. The second version of the study had a broader focus: Using the electronic discussion board to discuss issues of interest and/or concern during student teaching. I recommend that the student teachers be allowed to discuss any topics relevant to student teaching, rather than restricting their topic discussions.

Participants

The second recommendation is to consider the participants. Some supervisors develop their discussion board with the plan of being an active participant themselves along with their student teachers. Others, like this author, chose to allow the student teachers to be the only participants on the discussion board. My recommendation is to allow the students to use the electronic discussion board without comments from their supervisor so that they can feel free to be more honest and open in their responses. More importantly, when the students know that there is no teacher or supervisor responding, they will be more likely to respond to each other when someone needs advice. When students have areas of concern that need a supervisor's advice, they will most likely initiate an email or phone call with their supervisor. In addition, another issue to consider regarding participants is which grade levels the students will be student teaching in when setting up the discussion board(s). The first study that this author conducted did not consider this factor. The results from the surveys as well as the interviews were that the help that a student teacher received from a peer (in the form of a reply to a post on the EDB) was not specific enough to be useful. Those student teachers were teaching in grades 1 through 5. Although there were topics that could transcend all grade levels, participants noted that most times when help was sought, there were not specific suggestions offered that could be useful at their particular grade level. This second version of the study corrected that problem by setting up two separate forums (one for grades one and two and the other for grades three and four) within the discussion board. Not one of the participants in this version of the study had an issue with not receiving detailed help or advice in their peers' posts.

Setting up these forums within Blackboard's discussion board is relatively easy. Supervisors need to make sure that each separate forum is labeled with the appropriate grouping so that student teachers know which one to enter. For example, if a supervisor chooses to set up a discussion board by grade level of the student teaching placements, there may be one labeled "Grade Two Student Teachers". When the student teachers enter the discussion board they will see the different listings and can choose the one that fits their placement. Supervisors can also inform student teachers that they can read posts in other grade level forums as well. Sometimes there are general topics discussed that everyone may want to read. Additionally, if there are many students in your group and many different grade level forums, student teachers may request to have an additional forum set up by the supervisor for general posts.

Posts

The third recommendation is to decide up front if the supervisor will require a minimum number of posts and replies each week or month, or if using the electronic discussion board will be optional. Both versions of this author's study were performed using required postings; however no student actually posted the full required number of times. One possible solution is to require using the electronic discussion board during the first half of student teaching and then make it optional during the second half of student teaching. Another possibility is to require just one post and one reply each week. Those who are interested will likely reply more often but are not obligated to do so.

Other Issues

There are several other issues that were not experienced in either university by this researcher but could be issues at other institutions and are worth mentioning. When you set up an electronic discussion board for your student teachers, you would want to make sure that the courseware program that you are using is familiar to the student teachers. If it is not, you would want to offer a brief training session for them. Student teaching is a busy semester as it is and to ask students, especially if you have any digital immigrants (Prensky, 2001), to navigate through something they have never used before, would be detrimental to them. At both universities I used something that was already used by students in their previous education courses so they were familiar with it. However, your students may need to participate in a brief training session with you just before the semester begins. A second issue to consider is whether or not the discussion board postings are backed-up by the university's IT department or if you will need to save them some other way. In this study, the university's IT department conducted a back-up every 24 hours. Those are two main technological issues to consider in addition to the other issues described above.

FUTURE RESEARCH DIRECTIONS

Unlike five or ten years ago, the student teachers who will be in our programs in the next few years have grown up with computers, the web, and email. These digital natives (Prensky, 2001) are accustomed to checking several email accounts as well as other websites on a daily basis, making the use of the electronic discussion board potentially more familiar and part of their routine. Future research in this area could include offering the electronic discussion board to student teachers as an optional activity during student teaching, rather than a stated requirement. Within this optional model, student teachers could still be placed into groups based on the grade level they are assigned to teach. Another area that this research topic could extend to would be connecting our graduates when they are surviving their first year of teaching with their peers who are also first-year teachers. Many school districts have mentoring programs for first-year teachers, but the electronic discussion board could link first-year teachers with each other, many of whom would already know each other from their education classes and seminars during student teaching.

The potential for a learning community to be formed during student teaching and then continued into the first year of teaching with the same group of participants would also be an interesting area of research to pursue. Many strong peer relationships are built during student teaching that could be continued as the graduates conduct their job search, interviews, and then begin their teaching careers.

Examining the ways in which student teachers at other levels or situations utilize the electronic discussion board during student teaching would also be interesting. How do early childhood or secondary education student teachers use the discussion board and is that different from how elementary education majors use it? How do physical education or music education student teachers use the electronic discussion board that might be the same or different? Perhaps there are certain areas or majors that would utilize the discussion board in very different yet still meaningful ways due to their content areas or grade levels. All of these are areas that need to be examined in detail.

CONCLUSION

The job of the student teaching supervisor is complex and important. Providing support to the student teacher throughout the semester is certainly one of the many requirements of a university student teaching supervisor. However, it is also important for students to have access to their peers who are also student teaching at the same time and preferably in the same or similar grade levels or situations. These peers can provide each other with advice, support, and suggestions during the stressful semester of student teaching. Providing an asynchronous discussion board for students who are student teaching at the same grade level would be a worthwhile task for university supervisors to consider for the benefit of their student teachers. The small amount of time involved in setting it up is well worth it for the benefits that the student teachers will get when they participate in discussions with their peers.

REFERENCES

Anderson, D. (2007). The role of cooperating teachers' power in student teaching. *Education*, *128*(2), 307–323.

Assaf, L. (2005). Staying connected: Student teachers' perceptions of computer-mediated discussions. *Teacher Educator*, *40*(4), 221–237. doi:10.1080/08878730509555363

Biesenbach-Lucas, S. (2004). Asynchronous web discussions in teacher training courses: Promoting collaborative learning - or not? *AACE Journal*, *12*(2), 155–170.

Bulger, S. (2006). A web-enhanced approach to undergraduate internship supervision. *Physical Educator*, *63*(3), 114–125.

Devlin-Scherer, R., & Daly, J. (2001). Living in the present tense: Student teaching telecommunications connect theory and practice. *Journal of Technology and Teacher Education*, *9*(4), 617–634.

Edens, K. M., & Gallini, J. K. (2000). Developing a discourse community of preservice teachers in a technology-mediated context. *Teacher Educator*, *34*(4), 64–82. doi:10.1080/08878730009555238

Ferdig, R. E., & Roehler, L. (2004). Student uptake in electronic discussions: Examining online discourse in literacy preservice classrooms. *Journal of Research on Technology in Education*, *36*(2), 119–136.

Grion, V., & Varisco, B. (2007). On line collaboration for building a teacher professional identity. *PsychNology*, *5*(3), 271–284.

Lincoln, Y. S., & Guba, E. G. (1985). *Naturalistic Inquiry*. Beverly Hills, CA: Sage Publications.

MacKinnon, G. R., Aylward, M. L., & Bellafontaine, J. (2006). Electronic discussion: A case study of the range of applications in a laptop university. *Computers in the Schools*, *23*(1/2), 59–71. doi:10.1300/J025v23n01_06

Mayer, D. (2002). An electronic lifeline: Information and communication technologies in a teacher education internship. *Asia-Pacific Journal of Teacher Education*, *30*(2), 181–195. doi:10.1080/13598660220135685

McCarthy, S., & Youens, B. (2005). Strategies used by science student teachers for subject knowledge development: A focus on peer support. *Research in Science & Technological Education*, *23*(2), 149–162. doi:10.1080/02635140500266377

Morken, E. M., Divitini, M., & Haugalokkent, O. K. (2007). Enriching spaces in practice-based education to support collaboration while mobile: The case of teacher education. *Journal of Computer Assisted Learning*, *23*(4), 300–311. doi:10.1111/j.1365-2729.2007.00235.x

Nicholson, S. A., & Bond, N. (2003). Collaborative reflection and community building: An analysis of preservice teachers' use of an electronic discussion board. *Journal of Technology and Teacher Education*, *11*(2), 259–279.

Paulus, T., & Scherff, L. (2008). Can anyone offer any words of encouragement? Online dialogue as a support mechanism for preservice teachers. *Journal of Technology and Teacher Education*, *16*(1), 113–136.

Pena, C. M., & Almaguer, I. (2007). Asking the right questions: Online mentoring of student teachers. *International Journal of Instructional Media*, *34*(1), 105–113.

Poole, D. M. (2000). Student participation in a discussion-oriented online course: A case study. *Journal of Research on Computing in Education*, *33*(2), 112–130.

Prensky, M. (2001). Digital natives, digital immigrants. *Horizon*, *9*(5), 1–2. doi:10.1108/10748120110424816

Schlagal, B., Trathen, W., & Blanton, W. (1996). Structuring telecommunication to create instructional conversations about student teaching. *Journal of Teacher Education*, *47*(3), 175–183. doi:10.1177/0022487196047003003

Singer, N. R., & Zeni, J. (2004). Building bridges: Creating an online conversation community for preservice teachers. *English Education*, *37*(1), 30–49.

Smeaton, P. S., & Waters, F. H. (2000). Keeping connected: An asynchronous communication system to support student teachers. *T.H.E. Journal*, *28*(2), 106–115.

Spooner, M., Flowers, C., Lambert, R., & Algozzine, R. (2008). Is more really better? Examining perceived benefits of an extended student teaching experience. *Clearing House (Menasha, Wis.)*, *81*(6), 263–270. doi:10.3200/TCHS.81.6.263-270

Stegman, S. (2007). An exploration of reflective dialogue between student teachers in music and their cooperating teachers. *Journal of Research in Music Education*, *55*(1), 65–82. doi:10.1177/002242940705500106

Thomas, L., Larson, A., Clift, R., & Levin, J. (1996). Integrating technology in teacher education programs: Lessons from the teaching teleapprenticeship project. *Action in Teacher Education*, *17*, 1–8.

Wilkerson, T. L. (2003). A triad model for preparing preservice teachers for the integration of technology in teaching and learning. *Action in Teacher Education*, *24*(4), 27–32.

ADDITIONAL READING

Anderson, D. (2007). The role of cooperating teachers' power in student teaching. *Education*, *128*(2), 307–323.

Assaf, L. (2005). Staying connected: Student teachers' perceptions of computer-mediated discussions. *Teacher Educator*, *40*(4), 221–237. doi:10.1080/08878730509555363

Bulger, S. (2006). A web-enhanced approach to undergraduate internship supervision. *Physical Educator*, *63*(3), 114–125.

Cook-Sather, A. (2007). Direct links: Using email to connect preservice teachers, experienced teachers, and high school students within an undergraduate teacher preparation program. *Journal of Technology and Teacher Education*, *15*(1), 11–37.

Doering, A., Johnson, M., & Dexter, S. (2003). Using asynchronous discussion to support preservice teachers' practicum experiences. *TechTrends*, *47*(1), 53–55. doi:10.1007/BF02763337

Duffy, T. M., & Jonassen, D. H. (1992). *Constructivism and the technology of instruction*. New Jersey: Lawrence Erlbaum Associates.

Edens, K. M., & Gallini, J. K. (2000). Developing a discourse community of preservice teachers in a technology-mediated context. *Teacher Educator*, *34*(4), 64–82. doi:10.1080/08878730009555238

Ferdig, R. E., & Roehler, L. (2004). Student uptake in electronic discussions: Examining online discourse in literacy preservice classrooms. *Journal of Research on Technology in Education*, *36*(2), 119–136.

Jonassen, D. H., Peck, K. L., & Wilson, B. G. (1999). *Learning with technology: A constructivist perspective*. Upper Saddle River, NJ: Prentice Hall.

Kamens, M. W. (2004). Student teacher support: Collaborative experiences in a technology training partnership. *Action in Teacher Education*, *22*(2A), 39–44.

McCarthy, S., & Youens, B. (2005). Strategies used by science student teachers for subject knowledge development: A focus on peer support. *Research in Science & Technological Education*, *23*(2), 149–162. doi:10.1080/02635140500266377

Nicholson, S. A., & Bond, N. (2003). Collaborative reflection and community building: An analysis of preservice teachers' use of an electronic discussion board. *Journal of Technology and Teacher Education*, *11*(2), 259–279.

Paulus, T., & Scherff, L. (2008). Can anyone offer any words of encouragement? Online dialogue as a support mechanism for preservice teachers. *Journal of Technology and Teacher Education*, *16*(1), 113–136.

Pena, C. M., & Almaguer, I. (2007). Asking the right questions: Online mentoring of student teachers. *International Journal of Instructional Media*, *34*(1), 105–113.

Poole, D. M. (2000). Student participation in a discussion-oriented online course: A case study. *Journal of Research on Computing in Education*, *33*(2), 112–130.

Singer, N. R., & Zeni, J. (2004). Building bridges: Creating an online conversation community for preservice teachers. *English Education*, *37*(1), 30–49.

Smeaton, P. S., & Waters, F. H. (2000). Keeping connected: An asynchronous communication system to support student teachers. *T.H.E. Journal*, *28*(2), 106–115.

Stegman, S. (2007). An exploration of reflective dialogue between student teachers in music and their cooperating teachers. *Journal of Research in Music Education*, *55*(1), 65–82. doi:10.1177/002242940705500106

Weisner, J., & Salkeld, E. (2004). Taking technology into schools: A dialogue between a preservice teacher and university supervisor. *TechTrends*, *48*(3), 12–16. doi:10.1007/BF02763350

KEY TERMS AND DEFINITIONS

Asynchronous Discussion Board: A discussion board that allows participants to access the messages from other participants at any time, regardless of whether any other participants are online at the same time or not.

Cooperating Teacher: A classroom teacher (K-12) who hosts a student teacher

Electronic Discussion Board: A web-based tool where individuals can post, read, and reply to messages to each other at anytime.

Student Teaching: Culminating semester of supervised teaching at the end of the preservice teacher's university teacher training.

University Supervisor: A University faculty member (full-time or adjunct) who is assigned to supervise a preservice teacher during his/her student teaching semester. This supervision includes observing lessons, offering advice and support, and evaluating the preservice teacher.

APPENDIX A

Survey for Student Teachers

1. On a scale of 1 to 5, how useful was the Electronic Discussion Board during your student teaching semester?
2. What specifically was useful for you? Please provide details. If it was not useful for you, why not?
3. Which topics were the most important for you to discuss on the discussion board with your peers (if any)?
4. If you had the choice to student teach with or without the addition of the discussion board, which would you prefer?
5. Did you ever use an idea or suggestion that a peer posted? If yes, how often did you use an idea from a peer?
6. The Electronic Discussion Board was a means of support for me during student teaching.
   Agree Disagree
7. The Electronic Discussion Board was a valuable place for me to obtain helpful ideas for teaching.
   Agree Disagree
8. The Electronic Discussion Board could be eliminated from student teaching.
   Agree Disagree
9. Did you ever post or reply to a peer with ideas for using computers in your teaching? If yes, how often?
10. Circle the answer for the next question. Who provided you with the most support for including computers in your teaching? Peers on the discussion board; computer teacher; peers in class; co-operating teacher; other (please list)
11. Do you have any suggestions for including the discussion board with future student teachers?

Section 2
Communication and Collaboration

Chapter 5
Technology Perception Framework for Education Faculties

Hasan Tinmaz
Educational Technologist, Turkey

Ilker Yakin
Middle East Technical University, Turkey

ABSTRACT

Technological innovations have strongly influenced our routines. Instructional activities have been also reshaped in parallel to the latest developments in Information and Communication Technologies (ICTs). For the adaptation to those indispensable changes, Faculty of Education in Higher Education Institutions must be reformed fundamentally. What is essential and initial for Education Faculties is to comprehend the technological perception of stakeholders within their organizations. These stakeholders are managers, teacher educators and preservice teachers who require certain knowledge, skills and abilities (KSAs) in relation to educational sciences and ICTs. This chapter offers "3 X 3 two-dimensional matrix" framework for Faculties of Education concerning the technology perception of the stakeholders. In the first dimension the authors reveal the KSAs as software, hardware and peopleware, in the second dimension stakeholder groups are listed. In each intersection of the dimensions, the authors provide adaptable hints and factors to increase the possibility of favorable technology perception in Faculties of Education.

INTRODUCTION

In every second, humanity is faced with innovations. Every day we wake up to a different world. When we go for shopping, we realize new companies and their new products. Every night, the anchormen of different television channels inform us about new developments in health sciences, security products, computer tools and so forth. On the other hand, we feel that the pace of the technology overcomes the pace of humanity. In other words, we suffer from adapting these innovative efforts in our daily lives which have been altered from inner dynamics. For instance, if you need money from your account, you should know how to deal with ATMs, or if you change your mobile phone with an extremely-

DOI: 10.4018/978-1-61520-897-5.ch005

Copyright © 2010, IGI Global. Copying or distributing in print or electronic forms without written permission of IGI Global is prohibited.

functionalized one, you ought to sit down and look at the mobile phone for hours. We have been experiencing a reality that integration of innovations into our daily routines demands as equivalent efforts as the development of those innovations.

Innovation is anything which represents newness in the minds of the users (Rogers, 1995). Yet, when we speak the word "innovations", the majority of the community assumes that they are about developments in "Information and Communication Technologies (ICTs)". In the last decade, we have realized the different reflections of ICTs in our lives. We started to use satellite or cable systems for TV, mobile phones for communication, Magnetic Resonance Imaging (MRI) systems for diagnosis of sickness, eye-sensitive security systems for entrance permission, etc... Vrasidas and Glass (2007) reflect on the advantages of ICTs on offering new opportunities for personal and professional developments in addition to enabling access to the knowledge we demand. All these different ICTs and their integration shows us that inevitably, we cannot run away from their effects on different aspects of human lives where education is one of them. Jimoyiannis and Komis (2007) refer to that integration by commenting that ICTs have emerged to alter the innate structure of instructional activities. On the other hand, as Roger (1995) noted those innovations require extensive time to be adapted within the society.

Starting from the late thirties, different scholars from a variety of disciplines have intended to functionalize different technologies for learning and/or teaching activities. Instructional Films and Radios, Teaching Machines, Personalized Learning Systems, and Computer Aided Instruction (CAI) are the examples of these technology infusions into education (Reiser, 2007). In parallel with those theoretical and practical attempts with technology and education, scholars have also discussed about the future of teachers regarding educational policies, practical decisions and implementations, and the philosophical aspect of the profession. Some scholars agreed with each other about the idea that these innovations would replace teachers and we would not need the teachers anymore. This argument suggested that we should focus more on technologies than teachers. Fortunately, both scientific studies and scholars are convinced that teachers are major actors of our educational systems where they can still take advantage of ICTs for instruction. To this end, different actors of educational systems have commenced to identify the ways of ICTs integration into teaching and learning activities. This multi-faceted revolution has affected educational sciences and ICTs. New philosophical reconstructions have appeared in the educational sciences (such as constructivism) in competition to user-friendly and learner adaptable ICT tools. Historically, Reiser (2007) points out that instructional tool development and instructional design activities have occurred in parallel.

Although the scholars of educational sciences and ICTs spend their effort and time on their disciplines separately, they have recognized the importance of collaboration between their fields of studies. This realization of cooperation leads the scholars to create new and multi-discipliner studies. This newly occurring and rising discipline has been called Instructional (or Educational) Technology which concentrates specifically on effective infusion (macro level) and integration (micro level) of different ICTs into different learning and teaching activities. Well-known scientists of the Instructional Technology field, Seels and Richey (1994), delineate Instructional Technology "… as theory and application of design, development, utilization, management and evaluation of processes and resources for learning and teaching" (p.1). When this definition is scrutinized, we realize that different levels of education have been introduced with a variety of resources both theoretically and practically. This essential evolution of educational activities has placed a lot of work and pressure on the shoulders of teacher training institutions. These faculties of education not only focus on scientific research about the ICTs in education but also train the academicians, managers or preservice teachers about how to implement instructional technology processes.

Educational faculties possess innate responsibilities in relation to the entire education system of a country. There emerges a long list of duties for educational faculties, for example, (a) conducting scientific research on the effects of different technologies on different levels of schooling, (b) designing and developing new technology supported learning environments, (c) following the innovations in different countries and their adaptation to their own country, (d) training of both preservice and inservice teachers in the national system, (e) supporting continuous professional development of the teacher trainers, and etc… For all these different missions, educational faculties benefit from different ICT tools. In order to initialize the realization of ICTs in the educational faculties, the stakeholders of faculty must perceive the ICTs as beneficial and effective for themselves. Therefore, the perception of stakeholders is highly crucial and indispensable for scholars. For that reason, this chapter offers a framework about the realization of the fundamental factors affecting the perception within a faculty of education.

Briefly, the framework includes a 3 x 3 two-dimensional matrix for explaining the certain elements about technology perception. The first dimension occupies the stakeholders referring to the group of people who can possibly be affected by the actions within the organization. We have clustered the stakeholders under three groups; preservice teachers, teacher educators and managers. In the second dimension, we concentrate on three deep-seated features; software, hardware and peopleware. Peopleware is related to the personal and professional characteristics of stakeholders about the utilization of software and hardware and their integration into instruction. Therefore, this chapter aims to inform the readers about important dimensions of an educational faculty in relation to the utilization of ICTs in the instructional activities.

BACKGROUND

As frequently reported, our world has been reshaped by the impact of the latest improvements in ICTs (Angeli & Valanides, 2009). This exponential growth has projected itself on the field of education as well (Mouzakis, 2008). For example, computers have been situated in the teaching-learning activities for more than three decades (Baron & Bruillard, 2007). Moreover, the world has started to anticipate a reformation of education with the utilization of ICTs which enhanced their roles much further than the concept of learning materials (Wong & Li, 2008).

In parallel with the advancements in ICTs, the center of attention in relation to ICTs in education has also altered (Baron & Bruillard, 2007). While ICT was considered as a tool for teachers and an alternative form of education, the notion and practical implementation of the ICT in instructional settings, and also philosophical approaches to ICT have been changed with the development and dissemination of constructivist philosophies. Therefore, ICTs in education have been used, implemented and approached more than as tools or as alternative models of education. Hence, a long research history on the effects of ICTs in education has already been available. As Wong and Li (2008) argued it is obvious that students have been influenced by ICTs and their roles in education. This influence has lead scholars to invest the role of ICTs in different instructional contexts. Angeli and Valanides (2009) emphasize that proper utilization of different technologies possesses immense power for altering instructional context. For instance, Vrasidas and Glass (2007) listed some factors affecting the integration of ICTs into education such as "…the availability of the necessary technology infrastructure, support for teachers, accessible change models, teachers' practices, curriculum constraints, assessment practices, education policies, and professional development" (p. 87). Furthermore, some scholars, as in the paper of Phelps and Graham (2008), note that ICTs offer advantages to the teachers for their activities.

In different research studies, scholars have identified a range of variables in relation to the "ICTs in education" phenomenon. As Wong and Li (2008) argued that these different variables which have been obtained from different schools demonstrate that "ICTs in education" is a multi-level concept to be taken into consideration. In one dimension, the ICT covers both software (as the all programs), hardware (as the all tangible elements), and people (as the all entities using the software and hardware). In the other dimension, framework considers the major groups (students, their instructors and the mangers) in a faculty environment. On the other hand, this multi-level structure must be assessed with a holistic and flexible approach to comprehend the entire framework (Phelps & Graham, 2008). Therefore, this chapter proposes a dynamic and multi-level framework for understanding the technology perception in the faculties of education which aims to prepare teachers for the entire national educational system for a country.

Increasing the qualifications of inservice teachers is one of major priorities for any country. Especially their adaptation to highly developing ICT systems is a pressing objective. Moreover, in the last decades, the use of different ICT tools in the practical contexts has transformed the innate structure of the teacher training systems (Bigum & Rowan, 2008). For instance, there are a lot of attempts to offer teacher training with blended learning - online and in-class education together (Mouzakis, 2008). Additionally, the affective standpoints of both inservice and preservice teachers toward organizations (schools or higher education faculties) and ICTs are highly fundamental for their professional developments (Phelps & Graham, 2008). Wong and Li (2008) recommended that perceived impact of ICTs on instructional context is an important topic for research studies.

In Figure 1, this chapter delineated a framework under the roof of the faculty of education. Within the multi level structure, we have concentrated on preservice teachers, teacher educators and managers. It is a fact that all these members of the faculty represent different subject matter areas. Therefore, their needs and demands about ICTs deviate from each other. The framework values that differentiation and provides an adaptable structure. Moreover, the framework notifies that ICTs have three overlapped stages; software as the programs, hardware as the tangible parts and peopleware as the end-users of software and hardware. The framework lists certain knowledge, skills and abilities for a better perception toward technologies.

THE PROPOSED FRAMEWORK FOR POSITIVE TECHNOLOGY PERCEPTION

In the previous section, we gave a general picture of our 3 X 3 two-dimensional framework. In the first dimension, we cluster the stakeholders of an education faculty under three broad groups; preservice teachers, teacher educators and managers. As a second dimension, we create three

Figure 1. The general structure of 3 x 3 two-dimensional matrix of technology perception framework

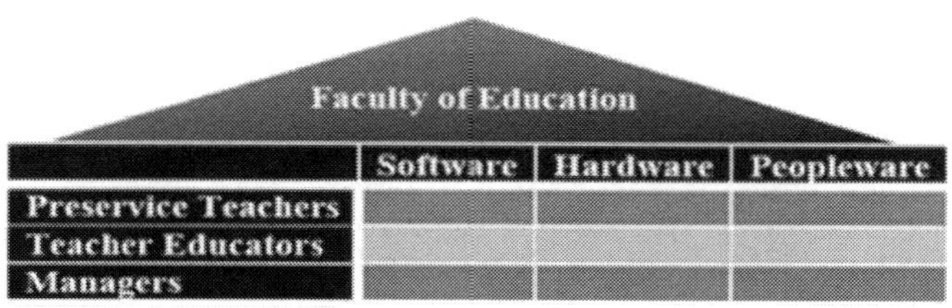

groupings of important knowledge, skills or abilities (KSAs) for the stakeholders in the faculty of education; software, hardware and peopleware. In that section, we will explain each intersection of our two-dimensional framework. It is essential to comprehend each intersection holistically so that we reveal every factor affecting the technology perception.

Stakeholders vs. Software

The initial group of stakeholders should be preservice teachers in the sense that they will create the future of new generations. Today's preservice teachers will be the teachers of tomorrow. We need to furnish our preservice teachers with the KSAs of today and tomorrow. To this end, preservice teachers must possess the fundamentals of each and every KSA in the dimension including software, hardware and peopleware because new technologies lead us to use, implement and think new teacher roles, pedagogies, and new approaches to teacher training (United Nations Educational, Scientific and Cultural Organization [UNESCO], 2008a). Afterwards, stakeholders must be life-long learners so that they adapt themselves within that dimension. Flexibility, adaptability and being open to all innovations are the essential characteristics a preservice teacher has to possess to fulfill the needs of tomorrows.

Today, most of the preservice teachers cross the threshold of the university entrances with certain KSAs in relation to computer, especially on software. That's why it is significant to delineate their entry KSAs before they assign to certain ICT oriented courses. On the other hand, to what extent or to what last point, preservice teachers move from their entry KSAs is challenging. If we make a basic search on the Internet about software, we can identify an enormous number of different software from different companies serving for different purposes. To simplify the situation, we offer to move from general toward specific software KSAs for preservice teachers whereas there is no predefined list. What is general or what is specific is up to the characteristic of both country-wise and globalized requirements. The general or the specific types of software must be revealed by each faculty in accordance with scrutinizing the needs of current era, current curriculum, current level of KSAs and etc...

When we read the certain literature on general software KSAs for preservice teachers, we can identify a long range of different KSAs in relation to different software. Here we make a generalization for the general KSAs under the following points;

- Language of software KSA,
- Operational software KSAs,
- Utility software KSAs,
- Internet oriented software KSAs,
- Life reflected software KSAs.

As an initial point, preservice teachers must understand the language of ICTs to a certain extent. Most of the times, "free-from-jargon" concept is emphasized in literature; yet, we express the importance of understanding ICT jargon for preservice teachers. To become a life-long learner, to understand what is written in an installation guide, to solve the ICT related problems as defined in the booklets, or to adapt themselves to innovations, preservice teachers should speak the ICT language. In addition to learning the foreign language of ICT, preservice teachers must know how to initialize a computer in order to make it ready for use. In other words, the KSAs on operating systems are important. Here, we must point out a general mistake that our preservice teachers must know all possible alternatives regarding operating systems including their advantages or disadvantages, their problem-solving alternatives and their load on the current computer infrastructure. Otherwise, our preservice teachers will become the sympathizer of an operating system and will be addicted to using it for years and every situation.

In addition to the operational initialization of our computers, preservice teachers must be capable of using certain general programs called as utility software. The utility software consists of word-processors, spreadsheets, presentation programs, pdf readers and zipping programs. Different companies offer different names for those programs; yet, the logic for their work is nearly the same. At least, preservice teachers are expected to use basic and advanced functions of utility software and transfer data between applicable programs. For more communication oriented purposes, it is vital for our preservice teachers to realize the power of the Internet. They should have the ability to evaluate the quality, credibility and adaptability of Internet resources quickly and efficiently. To serve that purpose, our preservice teachers must know the alternatives within Internet browsers, Internet service providers, search engines, email and chatting providers and Internet related utility programs; flash players. After all these wide-range alternatives on general software, preservice teachers must recognize the reflection of this software on the real life. This unfolds ethical, legal, and privacy concerns of ICTs. Copyright laws and fundamental principles in the access and use of information from different technologies and resources comprise these concerns about knowledge and understanding of the legal and ethical issues (Murphie & Potts, 2003). Unfortunately, the last item on our list is the mostly neglected standpoint on technology literacy.

As notified earlier, preservice teachers must indispensably direct themselves to the discipline-oriented software. It is a reality that teachers demand different tools with respect to their subject matter area. For instance, a geography teacher needs different maps whereas a music teacher needs a musical instrument like a flute. This is also true for the software KSAs. For instance, a literature teacher might learn more about word-processors and a mathematics teacher might know how to use graphing calculators while an economy teacher might learn more about spreadsheets. In short, specific KSAs stem from the innate structure of the discipline, which preservice teachers attend to. The important aspect of the process is to recognize software applications which are related and appropriate to a specific discipline. Here, we suggest to all preservice teachers be on familiar terms with some audio-visual programs as the specific software (picture or music editing, visualization tools and etc…). In fact, they should be familiar with the developing instructional activities and design models such as simple hypermedia and multimedia products which are based on basic instructional design principles. In the multimedia dominant era, it is inescapable to manage certain basic operation within those audio-visual programs (Mayer, 2001).

The final point about preservice teachers and software connection is the level of KSAs. Here the question of "how much a preservice teacher must know about software" will be answered by some levels of KSAs, known as taxonomy. When we look for technology taxonomies on the Internet, we could find a variety of different levels about ICT KSAs. Some scholars divide them into four stages starting from beginner users to advanced users. In each level, they define certain characteristics of a preservice teacher in that level. It is not easy to download these levels and utilize them in our cases. What an appreciable endeavor is to create our ICT taxonomies within our organizational structure and to reveal the number of preservice teachers stand in what levels. This taxonomy compartments will assist us to see the big picture about our preservice teachers and to realize the possible requirements to take them one level upper than their current levels.

To guide our preservice teachers, the roles of teacher educators are highly crucial. It is essential to remember the proverb saying that "what creates the difference in the classroom is not what we say, but what we do". Therefore, teacher educators should help students to acquire ICT skills within the context of their courses and instructional activities. That's why what our teacher educators do in and out of the classrooms will profoundly affect how much time our preservice teachers will deal with software. As Löfström and Nevgi (2008) stated that teacher educators should know how to use ICT in teaching in addition to using that knowledge in their own classroom activities. The same structure for preservice teachers is also valid for our teacher educators. Teacher educators must also know all the general issues about software. Nonetheless, the items under the general software KSAs might not be enough for teacher educators. Here we will make some editions to the list above;

- Distance education software KSAs,
- Management systems software KSAs,
- Computer aided instruction software KSAs,
- Web 2.0 software KSAs.

The teacher educators are always the models for the utilization of different ICTs for the preservice teachers. Therefore, teacher educators must follow the innovation regarding both ICT and educational sciences. Distance education is one of those innovations which has affected teaching-learning processes. Under this general "distance education" term, there are some important concepts related to education; e-learning, online learning, virtual learning communities, m-learning, e-portfolio and so on. As Löfström and Nevgi (2008) noted teacher educators face demanding challenges when they try to take teaching online. In that sense, teacher educators must know at least the basic usage of the software related to distance education tools and modes. Matching teacher educators' specific curriculum needs with particular software packages and applications should support the innovations of the distance education concepts (UNESCO, 2008b). The delivery of lecture notes, online syllabus or online assessment tools, e-mail and web browser applications for communications and for research to support instruction is some examples of KSAs under this item.

In parallel with distance education software, the KSAs on the tools of different management systems are very important for teacher educators. Learning management, course management, content management, or web based assessment are some exemplars of management systems. They offer advantages to teachers for completing their tasks during the learning-teaching process effectively. Moreover, these systems could offer alternative methods of designing, constructing, and supporting communities of teachers to give an opportunity for their professional developments (Vrasidas & Glass, 2007). The teachers who avoid using those management systems will be at disadvantage. Especially, KSAs' about information collection, analysis and management in instructional settings are the important features of these systems. Using common communication and collaboration technologies in social environments to support increased knowledge and understanding of their subject matter can be seen as an activity in management systems. Therefore, teacher educators must know posses the KSAs of using them then utilize them for their instruction and foster them so that their preservice teachers can learn and use them for their prospective classrooms.

The teacher educators must be knowledgeable about Computer Aided Instruction (CAI) and its tools; tutorials, drill-and-practice, education games and so forth… The software KSAs on how to install these tools, how to solve problems, how to use them effectively and how to integrate them into educational activities to support preservice teachers' acquisition of knowledge of different subjects are important for education faculties. The integration of ICT into curriculum and teaching activities has been promoted in recent years (Lin, 2008). Since the teacher educators are the models for preservice teachers, their uses will inevitably facilitate preservice teachers. CAI tools are somewhat the eldest modes of computer in education phenomenon whereas the Web 2.0 technologies are the newest modes. Web 2.0 technologies (even they are called as Web 3.0) include social networking, blogging, wikis, social bookmarking (Velden, 2008), which mainly concentrates on the social/human aspect of web technologies. In order to adapt themselves to innovations in the

Internet technologies, teacher educators must be acquainted with those Web 2.0 technologies. Web 2.0 tools have potentials for teachers creating collaborative learning environments and learning communities (Teaching and Learning Research Programme, 2008).

The teacher educators are the mediator force between preservice teachers and managers. They are the models for preservice teachers and workers (or colleagues) for faculty managers. Teacher educators realize all the missions with the support of faculty managers; dean, vice-deans, and head of departments. This support could be tangible or intangible because administrative support for ICT has been considered as one of the major components of teacher education (Clausen, 2007). Managers could support the teacher educators with necessary software or could encourage them to use the computer programs. To serve these purposes, teacher educators have the chance to experiment with new and different software products which to be used in instruction to meet their individual needs about specific curriculum needs. Therefore, the managers should possess all the KSAs which have been described before. At least, managers must be knowledgeable about the software jargon of ICT and ICT in education. Otherwise, some communication problems could occur among the stakeholders in the faculty.

The managers are the key people in the adaptation of new technologies. In that manner, they must follow the innovations in ICT field. Whenever there appears a need of learning new software, managers should know what to do. If necessary, they should organize trainings for either preservice teachers or teacher educators. The managers should know how to assess the effects of using different software in their faculties. To achieve this task, they must know how to use statistical programs or some qualitative transcribers or data analyzers.

As a last recommendation, we think that the managers must take advantage of databases for their work routines or executive activities. Databases are situated in most of the office software packages; on the other hand, they are not well-known or utilized as much as other software. The managers can learn the basic concepts and use of this database software for their personal and professional efficiency.

Stakeholders vs. Hardware

Software works effectively and appropriately if and only if it is installed on the required hardware. Hardware is the tangible part of ICTs where all stakeholders touch daily. Hardware is somewhat the nightmare of most people. Yet, people are afraid of the things that they do not know. Therefore, the extension of hardware KSAs depends on the perception or attitudes of faculty stakeholders toward ICTs.

The preservice teachers face with hardware in different contexts; in classrooms, in faculty and in real life where the KSAs must fold them. To address the general hardware KSAs requirements, we propose the following list;

- The language of hardware,
- The basic parts of computer case,
- The peripherals (screen, keyboard, printer…),
- The basic elements of computer network,
- The basic solutions of hardware problems.

The language of the hardware is indispensably fundamental for the rest of the list. Moreover, it is helpful for preservice teachers when they want to buy a personal computer. If they realize that they understand what the computer seller offers, they will be more satisfied and will develop more favorable attitude toward the computer technologies. In addition to the jargon, preservice teachers must know what a computer case is and what parts it includes. Here, we do not imply that preservice teachers should be knowledgeable about how each part of the case works. Preservice teachers must be aware of what is going on in the computer case.

Afterwards, preservice teachers must learn about the fundamental KSAs about how to functionalize peripherals such as printers, scanners, keyboards and etc... At least, they should recognize basic system components and connections for peripherals. On the last step, preservice teachers should learn the fundamental KSAs on networking concept. Especially, how to develop a wired or wireless network, and shared printers could be beneficial for them in their lives. For more permanent KSAs, we propose preservice teachers to learn hardware under problem oriented situations. Contrary to software KSAs, hardware KSAs do not come to the surface too often. We utilize our hardware KSAs mostly when need them, in other words, when we face with a computer problem. Therefore, we believe that hardware KSAs should be situated on a problem-solving context.

Similar to software, the preservice teachers might need specific hardware KSAs in accordance with their subject matter expertise. For instance, a preservice teacher might need to learn how to connect a projector to a laptop, or to a television, or to a special technological tool, such as an epidiascope, might be installed for a presentation. Therefore, it is significant to delineate specific hardware KSAs and embed them into courses of technology literacy. Most of the times, preservice teachers underestimate the hardware KSAs in a way. Therefore, most of them could be grouped under the name of "novice" in the hardware KSAs taxonomy. The mission of teacher educators is to assist them move forward in the steps of the taxonomy.

The teacher educators must be educated about general or specific KSAs so that they can help, foster or motivate their preservice teachers utilize different hardware for their prospective classrooms. The teacher educators are the role models for their students. Hence, their way of overcoming hardware related problems will definitely affect the cognitive and affective standpoints of the preservice teachers. With this role, teacher educators should also furnish with the similar hardware KSAs of hardware. They should have an experience to describe and demonstrate the use of common hardware technologies. Additionally, they must utilize their KSAs in front of their students so that they reshape the students' perception, attitude and KSAs. Moreover, teacher educators must be acquainted with the domain-specific hardware and their usage and also should show a capacity to learn new features of hardware systems independently.

For fulfilling the necessities of their job, teacher educators must be supported by their managers, deans or head of departments. From our perspective, the managers' hardware KSAs are highly important in a way that they lead the acceptance of the ICTs within their faculty. First of all, when the rest of the faculty stakeholders (preservice teachers, teacher educators or clerks) wants to talk about a hardware issue (either a problem or a need), the manager should understand their language. In other words, what they refer to is to create the same sense in managers' minds, too. For that purpose, managers must know the basic list we provided above. Moreover, managers are the ICT providers of the faculty. Therefore, they should place, organize and integrate computers and other digital resources to be used by teacher educators and preservice teachers in learning activities. In that role, they must have an inventory of ICT infrastructure because one of the main challenges of ICT education is the availability of the ICT infrastructure (Altun, 2007). Moreover, managers' role within the whole networking is also important for the faculty. Wherever needed, the managers must create wireless Internet access points for ICT revolution in their faculties. What they offer for the instructors and students will lead to a more accepted, favorably perceived and utilized ICT in the faculty.

Stakeholders vs. Peopleware

Up to that point, we have framed the important factors about software and hardware and their importance on affecting the perception of stakeholders (preservice teachers, teacher educators and managers) toward ICT. We always take into consideration that any ICT tool is useless without a person who functionalizes that tool. The uncontrollable development in ICTs over last decades has influenced the teaching profession. So, it is expected that professional organizations, academicians, and community policy makers have recognized the imperative and pressing need to integrate technology in all levels of educational efforts. While the efforts on effective use of ICTs in instruction increase, educators are dealing more with offering adequate preservice teacher education to prepare new teachers to adapt into the modern era.

Without hesitation, today's contemporary teachers are expected to be competent users of technology and be the experts of technology integration. As being a necessity, teachers must primarily master ICTs in order to be able to integrate them into their teaching. As Lockyer and Patterson (2007) noted technology use in teacher education programs should be well-planned and integrated so as to create positive impact on the technology practices. Through the trainings, managers will support the teacher educators with infrastructure and motivation so that teacher educators will be the role model for their preservice teacher. Therefore, actual usage of the ICT in teaching is strictly related with the mastery of the teacher educators' ICT competences (Valcke, Rots, Verbeke & Braak, 2007). This makes the teacher training programs as being a matter of concern and interest internationally as well as in development policy. The high expectations and demands associated with education, at all levels, in the context of ICTs must be handled with adequate efforts in the development of teachers' competence and perception. The need to train preservice teachers about technology is a long-term issue.

Professional development of teachers is a dynamic framework and it will only be updated in accordance with new research, educational theories, and responses from preservice and inservice teachers and teacher educators. Accepting our preservice teachers as our prospective teachers, their ideas will make a great contribution to understand the current teacher training programs and more generally our current educational system. Therefore, both general cognitive and technical capabilities for ICT literacy should be taken into consideration (Markauskaite, 2007).

Technology training and integration in preservice teacher education is a current research concern. It is believed that by exploring the perceptions of preservice teachers regarding technology integration experiences toward their professional development can provide essential and fundamental knowledge for preservice teacher education programs. Considering the increase in the number of research concerning technology (or in) education, the pace of innovative diffusion into teacher training has increased. As further researches will be conducted in the area of teacher training and technology, better utilization and investment could be planned which will lead to increased teacher computer competencies and favorable teacher perception towards computer and related technologies.

Teachers with favorable technology perception believe that ICTs make their teaching more pleasant and interesting for both the teacher and their students. They will be more willing to overcome the barriers relating to deficiencies of resources, technical problems and a lack of technical support. They will be eager to spend their personal time on developing their competencies and their integration into classrooms. Moreover, they will be interested in helping their colleagues to develop their competencies as well.

For the development of positive ICT perception for preservice teachers, two aspects of teacher training program should be emphasized; ICT literacy and its implementation into teaching-learning processes. To possess positive perception, initially preservice teachers must have the KSAs described earlier and also understand the meanings of terms and terminology associated with ICT. Afterwards, preservice teachers should realize how ICT is utilized in education. They must experience that ICT offers opportunities for instruction, in addition to learning how ICT could be integrated into instruction. In those efforts, they should have a chance to experience with ICTs via accessing and sharing resources to support and use their instructional activities and their own professional development. These two overlapped learning processes will finally yield a positive perception for our prospective teachers at the end of their teacher training program. Through different courses, the preservice teachers will develop several psychological constructs which will affect their perception of ICT in education. For instance, as they learn how to manage ICT in their teaching activities, they will be more motivated, satisfied, self-esteemed, and excited about them. We should always remember that affective changes are not as quick as cognitive learning. That's why all these psychological changes will take time to shape the positive perception. In short, the preservice teachers will learn about ICT and ICT in education, and then they will believe that ICT could be utilized in education effectively. In addition to positive belief, preservice teachers will begin to value the ICT in education. At the last stage, preservice teachers will have positive perception toward ICT in education.

The major actor for yielding positive perception is the teacher educators. They are the role models for their students with their knowledge and practice. The teacher educators are teaching ICT, ICT in education, or other courses. Their instructional strategies have a major impact on the effective usage of ICT (Cox & Marshall, 2007). It will be useless if the teacher educators talk about them in their courses but do not apply them in the classroom. The creation of multimedia presentations in planning, designing and implementation of instruction process and using non-computer technologies to support instruction might be examples that sustain role models for preservice teachers. Teacher educators should use ICT as a model expert in their teaching activities and their courses (Vrasidas & Glass, 2007). Hence we repeat the phrase "what the teacher does will create a difference in students' minds rather than what they say". The repertoire of teaching activities supported by different ICTs will initialize new learning opportunities and facilitation for preservice teachers to acquire the skills of reasoning, planning, designing, reflective learning, knowledge building, and communication (Gagné, Wager, Golas, and Keller, 2005).

The willingness of the teacher trainers about innovations in ICT and education is indispensably significant for better quality in the entire education system of a country. For instance, through Web 2.0 technologies, teacher trainers can create a learning community in their faculty where all stakeholders can learn from each other. As other example, teacher educators can create a content-management system where they can share reusable learning objects which can easily be adapted to different courses or sessions. The third example is a central web-based assessment tool which can make the assessment activities easier for teacher educators.

Flexibility and adaptability are also vital for teacher educators. Flexibility is about how much a teacher educator can change his/her teaching activity in accordance with students' needs or behaviors. Adaptability is to what extent a teacher educator can settle a learning activity to the other one with the assistance of a technological tool. Both flexibility and adaptability can be maintained by different ICT tools.

When the teacher educators and preservice teachers feel the support and motivation of the faculty managers, they will be more eager toward using ICT both personally and professionally. Within the boundary of fiscal budget, managers suppose to provide all opportunities for keeping ICT up-to-date. Management of the supplemental ICT resources for this purpose is also important both for teacher educators and preservice teachers for instructional purposes. Moreover, managers are also responsible for updating the current KSAs of teacher educators and preservice teachers. To this end, new trainings or seminars could be designed for the faculty. Managers should be the early adapters of innovations for the all stakeholders.

Managers should establish an ICT facilitated learning assistance center where both teacher trainers and preservice teachers will be supported for their instructional activities. Whenever they need a help for overcoming a problem in relation to ICT, this center could assist them. When they overcome the barriers, all stakeholders will have a tendency toward more ICT in education which finally turns out to be a positive perception in their minds.

FUTURE RESEARCH DIRECTIONS

This chapter has attempted to provide a descriptive framework concerning technology perception for education faculties. This framework has been designed by considering the effective usage of ICTs for stakeholders so that its implementation can be generalized to the other faculties of higher education. It is essential that this framework does not offer a list of predefined KSAs to guarantee its flexibility. By design of the framework, we have avoided attempting to generate predefined lists for each KSA in factors. Our framework 3 X 3 two-dimensional matrix attempts to overlay a framework on technology perception research to better understand and investigate ICT in education. As we offer, the dimensions dealing with integration, design, implementation and innovation of ICT could be investigated holistically. In further studies, researchers might conduct specific nature of technology perception studies with whole important factors rather than investigate single section of perception process.

As new technologies have emerged, new pedagogy, instructional strategies, knowledge construction and representation have gained importance in ICT researches. Therefore, various approaches about teaching process should be more concentrated by researchers. As Angeli and Valanides (2009) noted that the effectiveness of different approaches to ICT training has not been conducted rarely because contexts of research situation and process vary. Beside experimental researches, qualitative and mixed research methodologies might be effective to point out these different contexts. Especially, grounded theory, action researches, and case studies can be used to explore new relationships, models and frameworks of ICT in education in further studies. Naturalistic research methodologies enable researchers to grasp meanings and understandings people make on the studied phenomena (Denzin & Lincoln, 2000). To with this advantage, in-depth examination of KSAs in software, hardware and peopleware for stakeholders of education faculty can be conducted in further researches. Triangulation and embedded research designs, as the types of mixed methodologies, can be used for conducting prospective research. The researches that include the topic of technology access, developmental and instructional support, innovations of both in ICT and educational sciences for managers are some examples of further research directions with new perspective.

As for teacher educators, KSAs about integrating, designing and implementation of ICT tools in teaching activities, developing socially active classrooms, designing collaborative learning and cooperative interactions via the newest modes of computer technologies, and distance education concepts are the other research orientations considered under this approach. As a future direction, dynamic ICT standards reflecting adaptable and broad usage for new technologies may be investigated with both dimensions for preservice teachers. The effectiveness of social networks, cooperation tools, management systems in preservice teachers' education and their KSAs for ICT tools are still major topics that require to be investigated for ICT research.

Table 1. 3 X 3 two-dimensional matrix of technology perception framework for stakeholders

	Software	Hardware	Peopleware
Preservice Teachers	• Language of Software o ICT Language o ICT Jargon • Operational Software • Utility Software o Basic and Advanced functions o Data transfer • Internet Oriented Software o Power of Internet o Copyright laws o Ethical, legal, and privacy concerns • Life Reflected Software o Discipline-oriented software o Hypermedia and Multimedia products	• Language of Hardware • Basic Parts of Computer Case • The Peripherals o System Components o Connections • Computer Network o wired or wireless network o Shared printers • Solutions of Hardware Problems	• ICT Competencies • ICT Literacy • Professional Development • Diffusion of Innovation • Barriers • Experiences • Curriculum • Psychological Constructs • Valuing the ICT
Teacher Educators	• Distance Education Software o ICT Language o ICT Jargon o e-learning, online learning, virtual learning communities, m-learning, e-portfolio o online syllabus, online assessment tools, e-mail, web browser applications • Management Systems Software o Social environments o LMS, CMS • Computer Aided Instruction Software o Tutorials, drill and practice, education games • Web 2.0 Software o Social networking, blogging, wikis, social bookmarking o Learning communities	• Language of Hardware • Common Hardware Technologies • Basic Parts of Computer Case • The Peripherals o System Components o Connections • Domain-Specific Hardware • Computer Network o wired or wireless network o Shared printers • Solutions of Hardware Problems	• Integration o Instruction • ICT Competencies • Perception • System • ICT Literacy • Professional Development • Diffusion of Innovation • Barriers • Curriculum • Experience • Valuing the ICT • Role Models • Flexibility and Adaptability • Trainings • Life-long learners
Managers	• Software Jargon • Administrative support • Databases, statistical programs	• Language of Hardware • Common Hardware Technologies • Basic Parts of Computer Case • The Peripherals o System Components o Connections • Resources • Inventory of ICT Infrastructure • Networking	• Support • Policies • System • Diffusion of Innovation • Valuing the ICT • Management • Trainings • Life-long learners

Lastly, it is possible to conclude that ICT training in education faculties should be considered as continuous process. The role of stakeholders in faculties shapes not only ICT training strategies but also technology management issues. Therefore, understanding of organization culture and change management processes should be concentrated on the researches. In order to successful and effective usage of ICT in teaching activities for faculties, instructional technology plans should be generated with all stakeholders' contributions, and also this strategic planning should be followed step by step.

CONCLUSION

Teacher educators, preservice teachers and managers, as stakeholders, are essential agents for the process of utilization of ICTs in instructional activities. Therefore, software, hardware and peopleware KSAs for them are the other essential perspectives that should be taken into consideration not only for academic studies but also for practical implementations of ICT in education faculties. The intent of this chapter is to share an adaptable and flexible framework to be utilized in instructional settings for the professionals in education faculties. Table 1 summarizes the major points about this two dimensional framework. While ICT language, ICT jargon and specific software related with educational and instructional purposes emerge as common required KSAs for software perception, language of hardware, common hardware technologies and solutions of hardware problems appear as mutual hardware perceptions for whole stakeholders. ICT competency and literacy, diffusion of innovation, and valuing the ICT can be summarized as for common perceptions among stakeholders about peopleware, ICT, KSAs for ICT, ICT literacy, ICT competencies, technology perception, ICT integration, and innovation are the words that compel professionals and researchers in teacher education. Successful use of the framework and offered strategies in this chapter depends upon a careful planning and implementation policies that stakeholders involve in and also this process could be thought as an on-going project.

ACKNOWLEDGMENT

When we start to write this chapter, Mr. Yakin welcomed his son, Deniz, who became the internal motivation source during the writing process with all his smiles, cries and beauty. Hence, we dedicate this chapter to Deniz, who is the hope for a better future.

REFERENCES

Altun, T. (2007). Information and communications technology (ICT) in initial teacher education: What can Turkey learn from range of international perspectives? *Journal of Turkish Science Education, 4*(2), 45–60.

Angeli, C., & Valanides, N. (2009). Epistemological and methodological issues for the conceptualization, development, and assessment of ICT–TPCK: Advances in technological pedagogical content knowledge (TPCK). *Computers & Education, 52*, 154–168. doi:10.1016/j.compedu.2008.07.006

Baron, G. L., & Bruillard, E. (2007). ICT, educational technology and educational instruments. Will what has worked work again elsewhere in the future? *Education and Information Technologies, 12*, 71–81. doi:10.1007/s10639-007-9033-9

Bigum, C., & Rowan, L. (2008). Landscaping on shifting ground: Teacher education in a digitally transforming world. *Asia-Pacific Journal of Teacher Education, 36*(3), 245–255. doi:10.1080/13598660802232787

Clausen, J. M. (2007). Beginning teachers' technology use: First-year teacher development and the institutional context's affect on new teachers' instructional technology use with students. *Journal of Research on Technology in Education, 39*(3), 245–261.

Cox, M. J., & Marshall, G. (2007). Effects of ICT: Do we know what we should know? *Education and Information Technologies, 12*, 59–70. doi:10.1007/s10639-007-9032-x

Denzin, N. K., & Lincoln, Y. S. (2000). Introduction: The discipline and practice of qualitative research. In Denzin, N. K., & Lincoln, Y. S. (Eds.), *Handbook of qualitative research* (2nd ed.). Thousand Oaks, CA: Sage Publications.

Gagné, R. M., Wager, W. W., Golas, K. C., & Keller, J. M. (2005). *Principles of instructional design.* Belmont, CA: Wadsworth/ Thomson Learning.

Jimoyiannis, A., & Komis, V. (2007). Examining teachers' beliefs about ICT in education: Implications of a teacher preparation programme. *Teacher Development, 11*(2), 149–173. doi:10.1080/13664530701414779

Lin, J. M. (2008). ICT education: To integrate or not to integrate? *British Journal of Educational Technology, 39*(6), 1121–1123. doi:10.1111/j.1467-8535.2008.00825.x

Lockyer, L., & Patterson, J. (2007). Technology use, technology views: Anticipating ICT use for beginning physical and health education teachers. *Issues in Informing Science and Information Technology, 4*, 261–267.

Löfström, E., & Nevgi, A. (2008). University teaching staffs' pedagogical awareness displayed in ICT-facilitated teaching. *Interactive Learning Environments, 16*(2), 101–116. doi:10.1080/10494820701282447

Markauskaite, L. (2007). Exploring the structure of trainee teachers' ICT literacy: The main components of, and relationships between, general cognitive and technical capabilities. *Educational Technology Research and Development, 55*, 547–572. doi:10.1007/s11423-007-9043-8

Mayer, R. E. (2001). *Multimedia learning.* New York: Cambridge University Press.

Mouzakis, C. (2008). Teachers' perceptions of the effectiveness of a blended learning approach for ICT teacher training. *Journal of Technology and Teacher Education, 16*(4), 459–481.

Murphie, A., & Potts, J. (2003). *Culture & Technology.* New York: Palgrave Macmillan.

Phelps, R., & Graham, A. (2008). Developing technology together, together: A whole-school metacognitive approach to ICT teacher professional development. *Journal of Computing in Teacher Education, 24*(4), 125–134.

Reiser, R. A. (2007). Trends and issues in instructional design. In R. A. Reiser, & J. V. Dempsey, A history of instructional design and technology (2nd ed., pp. 27-45). Upper Saddle River, NJ: Pearson.

Rogers, E. V. (1995). *Diffusion of innovation* (4th ed.). New York: The Free Press.

Seels, B. B., & Richey, R. C. (1994). *Instructional technology: The definition and domains of the field.* Bloomington, IN: Association for Educational Communications and Technology.

Teaching and Learning Research Programme – TLRP. (2008). *Education 2.0? Designing the web for teaching and learning.* Retrieved March 20, 2009, from http://www.tlrp.org/tel/files/2008/11/tel_comm_final.pdf

United Nations Educational, Scientific and Cultural Organization. (2008a). *ICT competency standards for teachers, policy framework.* London: UNESCO.

United Nations Educational, Scientific and Cultural Organization. (2008b). *ICT competency standards for teachers implementation guidelines.* London: UNESCO.

Valcke, M., Rots, I., Verbeke, M., & van Braak, J. (2007). ICT teacher training: Evaluation of the curriculum and training approach in Flanders. *Teaching and Teacher Education, 23*, 795–808. doi:10.1016/j.tate.2007.02.004

Velden, M. (2008). *Usability of web 2.0 functionalities for information dissemination organizations.* Unpublished Master Thesis. Erasmus University Rotterdam.

Vrasidas, C., & Glass, G. (2007). Teacher professional development and ICT: Strategies and models. *Yearbook of the National Society for the Study of Education*, *106*(2), 87–102.

Wong, E. M. L., & Li, S. C. (2008). Framing ICT implementation in a context of educational change: a multilevel analysis. *School Effectiveness and School Improvement*, *19*(1), 99–120. doi:10.1080/09243450801896809

KEY TERMS AND DEFINITIONS

Faculty of Education: The faculty of a higher education institution which is mainly responsible for the training of teachers and offering master and PhD degrees in graduate level.

Hardware: The common name for the physical parts of Information and Communication Technologies.

Information and Communication Technologies (ICTs): The technologies for creating, processing and transmitting of information, such as satellites, laptops, wireless networks and so forth…

Innovation: The general expression for any modernized or new technology.

Management Systems: The computer programs for managing different instructional activities for teaching-learning activities, such as learning management system (LMS) or content management system (CMS).

Managers: The personnel from the faculty of education who are generally responsible for administrative issues in the organization, such as deans or head or department.

Peopleware: The broad term for the user characteristics of Information and Communication Technologies.

Preservice Teachers: The students of a faculty of education who are prospective teachers for the education system of a country.

Software: The general name of the programs for utilization of Information and Communication Technologies.

Teacher Educators: Or teacher trainers are the academic personnel within a faculty of education who are responsible for furnishing the preservice teacher with the necessary knowledge, skills and abilities in relation to teaching profession.

Technology Perception: The affective perspective of a person in perceiving different technologies.

Chapter 6
Using Free Source ePortfolios to Empower ESL Teachers in Collaborative Peer Reflection

Adrian Ting
Hong Kong Institute of Education, Hong Kong

Phillip David Jones
Hong Kong Institute of Education, Hong Kong

ABSTRACT

This chapter reviews literature in the domain of collaborative peer reflection and the concept of voice for English teachers and puts forward three stages that need to be followed when selecting a suitable free source technology to create ePortfolio networks that are sensitive to the local environment. This is achieved by comparing twelve free source technologies against ten separate criteria to aid the reader in selecting a free source technology for ePortfolio use. The chapter then goes on to put forward five stages for facilitating collaborative peer reflection and the dissemination of ePortfolio use. This is presented together with sound advice that is applicable worldwide to ensure that success at each stage is achieved. The authors also draw attention to the future direction of research in this field.

OVERVIEW

With the realization of the importance that ePortfolios play in the development of professionals clashing with the current global financial crisis, a need has arisen for systems that are readily available and affordable that can meet this new demand.

Globally, with many educational systems being government maintained, they are historically slow to react to changes and new needs as they arrive. This chapter accepts the challenge in the conclusion of Jones (2008) that for language teacher development, a school or government responsibility need be no greater than *"providing teachers with a webfolio and that this responsibility will soon be usurped by free source technologies such as MSN, MySpace, Facebook and Xanga"* (p. 58). Therefore, this chapter is founded on the premise that the use of free source technologies is the solution to the problem of inadequate infrastructure within educational settings and can provide solutions that promote collaborative reflection that are generalizable for teacher educators across the world.

DOI: 10.4018/978-1-61520-897-5.ch006

Copyright © 2010, IGI Global. Copying or distributing in print or electronic forms without written permission of IGI Global is prohibited.

In this chapter, we define free source technologies as all technologies that are available to the user free of charge. Examples would include the majority of networking sites such as Facebook and MySpace but would also include software and programs that are available as free downloads. Further, we define readily available technologies are technologies that are expected to be readily available to most users but which at some point in the products history will have had some financial compensation attached. A good example of this would be Microsoft word. Almost all users will already have access to this software but at some point it will probably have been purchased even if it was purchased as part of a package when the hardware was initially bought.

As free source technologies are seen as providing an internationally generalized solution, it raises the question of which free source technologies educators should select, at either the organizational, national or international level. To address this issue, the first part of this chapter reviews collaboration in the process of reflection and reports upon an analysis of readily available and free source technologies that have the potential to create ePortfolios that can be used as learning tools to promote collaborative reflection. For this analysis, a total of 12 free source technologies were subjected to comparative analysis against 10 criteria that are essential for the facilitation of collaborative reflection.

The second part of this chapter then reports upon a case study that details the use of a free source technology to create ePortfolios with English language teachers in Hong Kong. The case study considers the concept of a community of teachers all supporting one another on the world wide web by using free source technologies. More specifically the case study examines the issue of voice - gaining the floor, speaking acceptably and being heard by others (Bailey, 1996) in collaborative reflection which can often be a debilitating factor for non native speakers of English when engaging in collaborative reflection in English.

Finally, this chapter provides recommendations for those who wish to exploit free source technologies for the creation of collaborative ePortfolios and assists readers in selecting a free source technology which is most suited for their context. This allows the reader to overcome educational bureaucracies that, although well intentioned, are not always able to provide adequate technological solutions. In turn, this enables the reader to join a global community of reflective practitioners.

Collaborative Reflection for ESL Teacher Development

Teachers have always been encouraged to be reflective in their practice, and therefore the use of portfolios for reflection is of high importance (Lyons, 1998). Biggs (2003) emphasizes the importance of reflective practice. He believes that being reflective is a learning cycle for teachers who should always strive to update and improve their current teaching practice. In regards to collaborative reflection, Vygotsky (1978) takes us further with his belief that all human learning takes place through interacting with other people. His Zone of Proximal Development (ZPD) theory advocates that social interaction is most beneficial to learners as it allows peer learning between people with lower and higher ability to take place. These theories provide a peer learning cum collaborative framework for our studies. There is further support for this from Bailey (1996). However, Bailey adds to this within an ESL context, as English language teachers that are non-native speakers of English can find it difficult to fulfill his three criteria for voice, that being gaining the floor, speaking acceptably and being heard by others. ePortfolios allow ESL teachers to fulfill these three criteria for the purposes of collaborative peer reflection through the medium of asynchronous communication.

Social Networking Sites for Professional Development

According to Boyd and Ellison (2007), social network sites are "*web-based services that allow individuals to (i) construct a public or semi-public profile within a bounded system, (ii) articulate a list of other users with whom they share a connection, and (iii) view and traverse their list of connections and those made by others within the system.*" The authors further commented on the benefits of social networking sites:

What makes social network sites unique is not that they allow individuals to meet strangers, but rather that they enable users to articulate and make visible their social networks. This can result in connections between individuals that would not otherwise be made... (p.211)

Scholars in the field of education constantly advocate and emphasize the importance of social networking websites in relation to teaching and learning. Due to all the potential benefits of social networking websites, studies were carried out on how they could be used in teaching and learning. Griffith and Liyanage (2008) conclude in their paper that because of the popularity of social networking sites, schools and universities are finding that social networking sites are now used to help group and team based work with the social structure of the social networking site aiding additional interaction. Dudeney and Hockly (2007) provide insights into how social networking sites can be used for continuous professional development such as "*involv[ing] a collection of people, all working towards shared goals*" (p.152).

Choosing a Free Source Technology

There are many criteria one can choose to form the basis of a comparison depending on the purposes these free source technologies are to be used for. For exploiting it as a tool for professional development such as an ePortfolio, it is necessary to consider the functionality that users would wish the system to possess. In general, users would probably want to create a profile, upload videos and photos, keep a blog and comment on other users' blogs and participate in group discussions.

Ten criteria were selected on the basis that they catered to the needs of ePortfolio creators. Hence, we focused primarily on functionality. The criteria included: video clips, photos, Word files, chat rooms, instant messaging, discussion forums, blogs, groups, personal profiles and the ability to post comments.

There is little doubt about the benefits Computer Mediated Communication (CMC) tools such as blogging, discussion groups and instant messenger (IM) bring to learning. Therefore it was important to consider its role in ePortfolio use. According to Lavooy and Newlin (2007), CMC can be broadly categorized into two categories for web based teaching and learning. They are synchronous and asynchronous CMC. Asynchronous CMC transcends the traditional barriers such as time zones and geographical location. This includes email, bulletin boards and discussion forums. Users can send or post messages and communicate with other people from anywhere in the world. Because of their asynchronous nature, they offer little interaction between users, and the sender has no control on when the recipient will read the message or when the message will be responded to. Synchronous CMC offers similar services to users but different in a sense that communication is in real time and spontaneous. Users engaging in this kind of communication are expected to give instant responses and there is often little time to think, as opposed to composing an email, where there is less time pressure and allows for reflection and proofreading before a message is sent. Examples of such CMC include chat rooms and instant messenger. It is therefore not beyond the realm of possibility that these functions would promote collaborative peer reflection during the ePortfolio review process. It was believed that, because most of the ePortfolio creation process was to be completed in the participants' own time, and they may be using technologies like video cameras and files in digital formats for the first time, they may have questions. Having a discussion forum or a group serves as a social support network. If participants have questions that need to be answered urgently, they can make use of the IM tool, to see whether anyone online would be able to offer assistance instantaneously.

Other essential criteria for the selection of free source technologies for ePortfolio use were the ability to upload video clips, photos and Word documents. The reason for this is that they are beneficial in creating artifacts to be archived and displayed in the ePortfolio. Of course, the use of video playback in teacher education has been in practice for well over 30 years, as can be evidenced by the work of Fuller and Manning (1973). What is new is the ability to provide feedback online at anytime and from anywhere in the world. Photos that could be included by teachers may be examples of student work such as drawings or sculptures. Additionally, the physical environment may be photographed to facilitate a discussion on classroom layout or to capture board work. Documents may be included as jpegs, such as certificates, observation reports or teaching materials.

Selection Process for Free Source Technologies

The comparison table in Social Networking Websites Review provided a good starting point for our quest for a suitable free source technology (http://social-networking-websites-review.toptenreviews.com). As there are hundreds of social networking sites, it would be impossible to evaluate all of them. Although in principle they are very similar in terms of features, they are oriented towards different domains, such as music videos or businesses. In the end, the twelve most widely used sites were short listed and researched from the user's point of view. The results are as follows:

Affordances and Constraints of Free Source Technologies

When searching for a suitable free source technology for ePortfolio use, each free source technology was compared against the 10 criteria that were considered necessary for the creation of ePortfolios. There was no particular order in which these technologies were looked at. Of course, these 10 criteria should by no means be considered as exclusive, but they are rather the minimum features that an ePortfolio creator may require.

Friendster, Xanga and, to a certain extent, Facebook, are probably the three most well known free source technologies in the Asia Pacific region. Friendster in particular has many Asian members. According to Lipsman (2007), visitation of Friendster by users aged 15 or above from the Asia Pacific to selected social networking sites in June 2007 reached 88.7%. Further, these three technologies allow users to choose a Chinese language interface. However, although they are useful, they are perhaps more oriented towards making acquaintances with people. The lack of an instant messaging function was also problematic. If a participant encountered a problem, they would not be able to solve the problem instantly by asking other participants on IM but would need to resort to asynchronous CMC like email or forums. Since users are often on IM, they will be able to answer any queries or offer assistance to participants online.

Other technologies like Bebo, Zorpia, Hi5, Orkut and Windows Live are considered easy to use and are likely to be the least problematic for beginners. However, they all lack one or more essential requirements for ePortfolio creation, such as video and discussion forums. It is interesting to see that none of the twelve free source technologies allow users to upload Word or PDF files. However, one solution is to scan a hard copy of a Word or PDF document and save it as a jpeg file so it can be uploaded as a photo.

From Table 1, it is clear that MySpace, MyYahoo and AOL appear to suit ePortfolio creation best. They all meet 9 out of 10 criteria needed. Based on the above discussion, the three technologies were then further trialed to investigate the user's experience and impression of each of these three free source technologies. The general impression from this investigation was that MySpace had a better layout, resulted in less spam and was generally far more user-friendly than the other two.

CASE STUDY

Rationale and Objectives for Using Free Source Technologies

One barrier of using technology in education often cited by teachers is the lack of infrastructure and support. This is particularly true of developing countries and with the current economic environment, it is perceived to be likely to be a significant problem in developed countries for the next decade. The use of free source technologies provides a solution to this problem and empowers teachers and teacher educators to integrate technology into teaching and professional development without recourse to centralized funding.

This project is at the forefront of ePortfolio use as it provides a collaborative ePortfolio network that is readily available to all teachers that have a computer with internet access. More importantly this network is available at no cost to the individual, their school or their government and works as an excellent example of the benefits that free source technologies can bring to the world of ePortfolios.

Another reason for using free source technologies for this project is that currently there is no ePortfolio system at the Hong Kong Institute of Education. Although some participants have their own ePortfolio system at their school, they are not open or freely available to external parties. This means a teacher from school A might have an ePortfolio, but they cannot interact with a teacher from school B as the systems are not compatible and cannot be accessed by anyone who is not a member of that school.

Table 1. Free source technology selection criteria

	MySpace	Bebo	Hi5	Facebook	Friendster	Xanga	Zorpia.com	LinkedIn	My Yahoo	AOL	Orkut	Windows Live
Types of files user are allowed to post												
Video	✓	✓		✓	✓	✓			✓	✓	✓	✓
Word files												
Photos	✓	✓	✓	✓	✓	✓	✓	✓	✓	✓	✓	✓
Personal profile	✓	✓	✓	✓	✓	✓	✓	✓	✓	✓	✓	✓
Availability of CMC Tools												
Chat room	✓		✓						✓	✓		
IM	✓								✓	✓	✓	✓
Discussion forum	✓			✓	✓		✓		✓	✓		
Groups	✓	✓		✓	✓	✓	✓	✓	✓	✓	✓	
Blog	✓		✓		✓	✓	✓		✓	✓	✓	✓
Post comments	✓	✓	✓	✓	✓	✓	✓		✓	✓	✓	✓

The lack of communication between teachers and students from different schools around Hong Kong due to individualized ePortfolio solutions or the lack of any system at all is a barrier in creating collaborative professional networks. This minimizes collaborative reflection and the sharing of new ideas, which in turn inhibits teachers from becoming better teachers through portfolio learning.

In Hong Kong, the high school curriculum is going through major changes. One of these changes is that from 2009, all high school students will be required to keep an ePortfolio. It will be used not only to store personal information but also their assignments, which count toward their school leaver exams (Education and Manpower Bureau, 2004). However, there is a panic among school teachers that not enough training is provided and they are not comfortable to grade students based on their professional judgment in a high stake public exam for the first time in history.

A keystone of this project was that not only would the participants develop professionally as English language teachers but the course would also help prepare teachers to better meet student expectations when ePortfolios are introduced into the secondary school system from 2009 onwards. This project was predicated on the basis that in order to successfully teach with technology, teachers must first know about its affordances and constraints by becoming a user themselves and experience the challenges and frustrations so that they will be better able to empathize with their students. (Kolaitis et al, 2006)

Therefore, the objectives of the project were as follows:

- To enable secondary school English language teachers to create and manage ePortfolios using free source and readily available technologies.
- To create an online professional network of collaboration and support.
- To enable participants to become better language teachers.
- To provide participants with an understanding of the theoretical educational rationales of ePortfolio use for teaching, learning, assessment and professional development.
- To allow participants to gain practical first-hand experience of the benefits and frustrations of creating and maintaining an ePortfolio to help inform the introduction of ePortfolios into Hong Kong secondary schools

OVERVIEW

This project was funded by the Sir Robert Black trust fund in Hong Kong and involved 50 in-service secondary school English language teachers from 50 different government maintained schools in Hong Kong. Their level of IT competency varied. While all participants reached 'basic' level of IT competency in the education bureau's framework on IT proficiency for teachers, five reached 'intermediate' level and two reached 'upper intermediate' – the highest level on the scale.

To broadly describe the profiles of the participants in Mark Prensky's term (2001), it was assumed that most teachers in the group would be digital immigrants (people who did not grow up using technologies and who only adopted the use of technologies later in life) as opposed to tech savvy digital natives (people who grow up using computers or digital technologies like MP3 players and mobile phones). Although in reality there is often no clear cut distinction between the two terms, a large proportion of teachers have, according to Prensky, displayed traces of "accents". Prensky provides some examples of a digital immigrant accent. One example is that that when a digital immigrant edits a Word document, he will need to first print it out and do the editing physically rather than having it done directly on screen; another example is if he comes across an interesting website, he will share this with people by inviting them to go to his office and view it on his computer screen while a digital native will just send people the URL of that website. From our observation of the participants over the duration of the project, they could indeed be described as digital immigrants as we had hypothesized. However, the group did contain perhaps one or two digital natives.

Course Structure

The project ran for 9 months and included 3 workshops. The first workshop was merely an introduction to ePortfolios but importantly also provided instruction in the use of the free source and readily available technologies that were to be used during the project.

The second workshop was performed after the first 3 months of the course had been completed and provided an opportunity for reflection. During the second workshop the participants were encouraged to compare their experiences of creating and maintaining an ePortfolio with the educational theory of ePortfolio use.

The third workshop towards the end of the course encouraged participants to reflect upon their experiences of ePortfolio use and required participants to formulate a plan of how they could implement ePortfolio use within the secondary school where they work. This was to encourage ePortfolio use within the Hong Kong secondary school system as a key professional development tool.

In between workshops, participants were asked to complete a number of tasks designed to: build their ePortfolio, share their good teaching practice, view and comment upon other people's work, reflect upon their own practice, share their experiences of using ePortfolio and build a professional network. (See Table 2)

Analysis of Achievement against the Objectives

The first objective was to enable secondary school English language teachers to create and manage ePortfolios using free source and readily available technologies. The advantage in asking participants to use free source technologies for the creation of e-Portfolios was that it provided participants an opportunity to use technology, which is similar to Fuchs' project (2005) which aims to provide future language teachers the opportunity to experience CMC-based learning. This experience in turn is potentially useful for teaching in the future, as participants will have to teach their students how to use this kind of technology. Here is an example of a comment received from a participant regarding their ability to use, create and manage an ePortfolio using free source technologies:

After the course, I feel more confident to use free source technology, like MySpace, Xanga or Facebook, in my classes... We teachers can "exploit" these platforms for developing ePortfolio.

The second objective was to create an online professional network of collaboration and support. It was felt that online environments would be particularly helpful in allowing participants to fulfill Bailey's (1996) three criteria for voice. Take blogging as an example, CMC related studies (Warschauer, 2004; Warschauer and Meskill, 2000; Campbell, 2004; Ellison and Wu, 2008) show the effectiveness of using blogs for learning. The asynchronous nature of the blogging environment provides participants a more level playing field, which is important in Hong Kong and China, where collectivism is often an issue. Individuals are often shy or even reluctant to contribute to discussions because of factors like the fear of making mistakes and thus losing face in front of an audience. However, they are often less inhibited when working in groups because individual mistakes do not stand out and affect

Table 2. Tasks for the project

Task	Description of task
1	Attend workshop one
2	Post one photo of a lesson you have taught along with a short description of the lesson and an explanation of why this lesson was so successful. If you have problems visit the help area on the Group page and post a message for help. One of the other participants or facilitators will be able to help you. Alternatively, use MySpace's IM function as covered in the workshop.
3	Review the postings for task 2 from *two* of the other participants on the ePortfolio program, make one comment, and ask one question about their lesson.
4	Respond to the questions you have been asked (if any) for task 3 by posting a response in your ePortfolio under the question asked.
5	Post one video clip of a school activity you have facilitated or a video clip of part of a lesson you have taught. Also, post a short description of the activity or lesson and an explanation of your feelings regarding the activity or lesson.
6	Review the postings for task 5 from *two* of the other participants on the ePortfolio program, make one comment, and ask one question about their lesson. The comment and question should be posted to their ePortfolio not yours, and should be posted under the description and explanation they have provided.
7	Respond to the question you have been asked (if any) for task 6 by posting a response in your ePortfolio under the question asked.
8	In your ePortfolio post a reflection of a lesson that you have taught recently that didn't go as well as you had hoped. In your post write at least 2 questions that will stimulate the other participants to provide suggestions that may help you.
9	Review the postings for task 8 from *two* of the other participants on the ePortfolio program, and provide suggestions
10	Attend workshop two
11	• Choose *one* other social networking site from the list posted inside the group function on MySpace. • Sign up as a user and explore its features. • Think about how this compares with MySpace. Which would be better for your students to use? Post comments in the appropriate forum under the groups function.
12	Read the paper concerning teacher's pedagogical beliefs in regards to technology integration that has been emailed to you. Answer the discussion questions in the appropriate forum under the groups function.
13	• Reflect on your experience as an ePortfolio user. How would you promote this as a professional development tool at your school? • As an ePortfolio user, how can you help your students to use ePortfolios as an effective learning tool? Be prepared to share your views with your group mates
14	Attend workshop three

their personal image (Salili, 2001). Therefore, as Jones (2008) states in reference to Bailey's three criteria for voice in asynchronous discussions in ePortfolio are thought to be able to "*ease the problematic and complicated nature of gaining the floor, speaking acceptably and being heard by others for non-native speakers of English*" (p.57).

It was predicted that by reading each other's postings on blogs and discussion boards, it would enhance participants' understanding of the subject matter or issues being discussed. Further, if constructive feedback is given, it would also enhance their analytical as well as critical thinking skills (Ellison and Wu, 2008).

Participants on the course specifically made reference to how this collaborative network is successful:

It is good for nurturing a sharing culture and developing professionally.

Provides an opportunity for interaction among teachers.

I now understand the importance of peer support and participation.

I feel I have the support from other people.

Teachers compose their lesson plans on the topics they are familiar with and post them on the forum for other teachers to use in their lesson. After reading the lesson plans, other teachers can add/modify the plan and post in on the forum for revising before using it in class.

Collaboration among the department of English, project learning team and Humanities (implementation plan).

The third objective was to enable participants to become better language teachers. This objective was included as we did not want participants to lose sight of the main impetus behind the project, which was to ultimately make the participants better language teachers by engaging in the processes facilitated by the course activities. However, we did not necessarily intend to provide evidence of their development at the outset of this project but rather wanted to show evidence of the participants engaging in the processes that bring about teacher development, such as sharing and learning new ideas and reflecting. There was indeed evidence of this found within the comments given by participants.

I have... new teaching techniques which worked in my class.

The tasks made me more reflective about my teaching. I rarely plan my lesson in so much detail (not since my teacher training days!)

Keeping an ePortfolio can help a teacher to be more reflective. It is also a good way to organize the teaching materials, plans and successful experience. It helps the teacher to grow professionally and may further improve teaching.

I enjoyed the reflection part and reading about other people's lessons and their comments on my lessons

The fourth objective was to provide participants with an understanding of the theoretical educational rationales of ePortfolio use for teaching, learning, assessment and professional development. To facilitate this process, the participants were provided background reading with a series of questions which were discussed online in groups. It was felt that after this process, the participants had a much better idea of what an ePortfolio is and the theory behind how the system can be constructed for learner growth and the value of eportfolios as professional development tools.

I liked this project as it gave me an insight of what ePortfolio is.

A matrix-based system offers another edge in which learners assume more responsibilities of their learning. There could be a constant flow of reflections and ideas for growth

E-portfolios is definitely a means of improving learning and assessment in teacher education... E-portfolios can enhance professional growth of teachers because the lesson samples and various artifacts such as video, audio, text etc. indicate a pre-service teacher's learning progress in a continuous manner. All these help the teacher to reflect on each piece of work, focus on strengths, weaknesses and changes made in teaching, which can be used for self-evaulation or external review. It is something we cannot avoid, but to do what is best for professional as well as school improvement.

The fifth objective was to allow participants to gain practical first-hand experience of the benefits and frustrations of creating and maintaining an ePortfolio to help inform the introduction of ePortfolios into Hong Kong secondary schools.

In terms of frustration, the participants expressed:

It is very time consuming to use.

I received some spam.

My IT skills aren't good.

Once you have added someone as a friend, it's difficult to keep your profile private.

However on the whole, the participants seemed to be supportive of using free source ePortfolios to introduce a collaborative learning process and even reflected upon how current practices may be enhanced by the use of ePortfolios created by free source technologies.

Both students and teachers can learn collaboratively through sharing resources and regular feedback.

To prepare students for the new senior secondary curriculum, our school has started a Life Building Scheme in S1 & S2 (Grades 7 & 8) Students have to keep a record of their Other Learning Experiences (OLE) and reflect on them. However, the students are not doing their work very systematically. To make the scheme more comprehensive, I propose changing it into an ePortfolio system for every student... maybe they can always use the MySpace.com website which is readily available.

Other Observations

In general, we believe that most participants regarded their experience of using and keeping an ePortfolio as a positive one. For many, this was the first time they collaborated with their counterparts from other schools on professional development, let alone in an online environment. Three of the fifty participants had serious concerns over safety issues such as being contacted by strangers and receiving spam. Internet privacy was another concern. Their concerns are legitimate given the bad reputation of MySpace in the media. Butterfield (2005) highlights the danger to teenagers' safety posed by sexual predators in chat environments, both synchronous and asynchronous, as well as publishing information about themselves on the internet such as their contact information. In a study Dwyer et al (2007) show that users of Facebook and MySpace expressed worries over internet privacy. There have also been numerous reports of sexual offences carried out by online predators exploiting MySpace to prey on their victims (Williams, 2006; Chiaramonte and Martinez 2006, Schrobsdorff, 2006, Haas 2006, Mintz, 2005, Read 2006, cited in Dwyer et al, 2007). To protect social networking site users, legislators in the state of New York are working with social networking websites to expose the online aliases and email addresses of sexual offenders in hope to combat this problem. (Bauman, 2008). However, legislation in other parts of the world might not offer the same protection to users.

As for formulating an action plan for their schools, approximately 80% of the participants expressed that they would ask their colleagues to do the same tasks as they were asked to complete. They thought the best way to promote the use of technology in the classroom is to get teachers to use the technology themselves based on the learning by doing principle, assign manageable tasks each time and make sure they have enough technical support when needed. Having experienced using something new in isolation, all participants recognized the importance of support. They also appreciated the importance of creating a culture of using technology in order to make it work – it is necessary to get all teachers involved, otherwise it will not make any significant impact.

As to what they can do to help students use ePortfolios as learning tools, because this was a homogenous group of English teachers, the focus of their discussion was mainly around the use of ePortfolio in helping students improve English. Teachers thought students could engage in projects making use of video clips and photos, e.g.

give them a topic to research and investigate in, interview people, conduct surveys and present findings in English. Their peers can then view and comment on their project and think about what they can learn from their classmates. Regarding motivation, as mentioned in Jonassen (1996), teachers thought students would try their best in producing these artifacts, since they know other people will view and critique their work. This will be a major change in the teaching and learning paradigm as students have always wanted to remain competitive and are not willing to help each other, which is understandable when one's future is shaped upon the results of one major public exam in the current system. This competitive culture is predicted to disappear when students are required to work together once the school reform is implemented.

RECOMMENDATIONS

How to Select a Free Source Technology for ePortfolio Use

When selecting a free source technology to replicate this study within different environments or contexts, we believe that there are three key considerations. Firstly, the technical resources available need to be evaluated, as this places the biggest constraint on the functions that will be available to be exploited. Second, once you know which functions technologically speaking are available for use, it is necessary to consider which functions are desirable for your ePortfolio network and to compare this functionality with the free source technologies available. A good starting point may be to refer to Table 1 of this chapter. Once you know which free source technologies could be used, it is necessary to consider affective factors which may lead you to select one free source technology over another. Table 3 summarizes some examples that may need to be deliberated upon for each of the three stages. Figure 1 is a pictorial representation of the stages.

How to Facilitate Collaborative Peer Reflection and the Dissemination of ePortfolio Use

We surmised from evaluation of and reflection upon the project that in this case study, the process from initial meeting to the dissemination of ePortfolio use within a secondary context consisted of five stages as shown in the flow diagram below (Figure 2). The first stage was training which involved setting up a user account and generally becoming familiar with the technology that would be used. Step by step demonstrations were provided. The second stage provided online activities designed to facilitate an exploration of the systems functions and collaborative peer reflection. The third stage was conducted as a workshop where participants shared their experiences so far and helped offer solutions to one another with the problems they had. The fourth stage was really teacher education with materials on the subject being provided together with questions for online discussion. The fifth stage was conducted as a workshop where participants created an implementation plan to disseminate ePortfolio use in their school. This is represented graphically in Figure 2.

Advice for the Five Stages

Before the commencement of stage one, it is probably useful to know as much as possible about the participants, especially their IT competency. It is suggested before the first workshop, that the participants complete a self evaluation form. It is useful to know basic information such as their access to a computer and the internet, other hardware devices they may have such as digital cameras, video cameras and web cams. Additionally, some idea about which programs they have access to and their familiarity with us-

Table 3. Factors to consider when selecting a free source technology

Consideration	Examples
Technical resources	• Hardware (video camera, desktop, laptop, web cam, microphones) • Software (MS Word) • Internet connection (bandwidth, WiFi, reliability) • Computer access (home, work, internet cafe)
Functionality	• Area for reflection (blog, journal) • Artifacts (Photos, videos, word files etc.) • CMC tools (synchronous and asynchronous) • Language Interface
Affective factors	• IT competency • Local usage

Figure 1. Stages of consideration

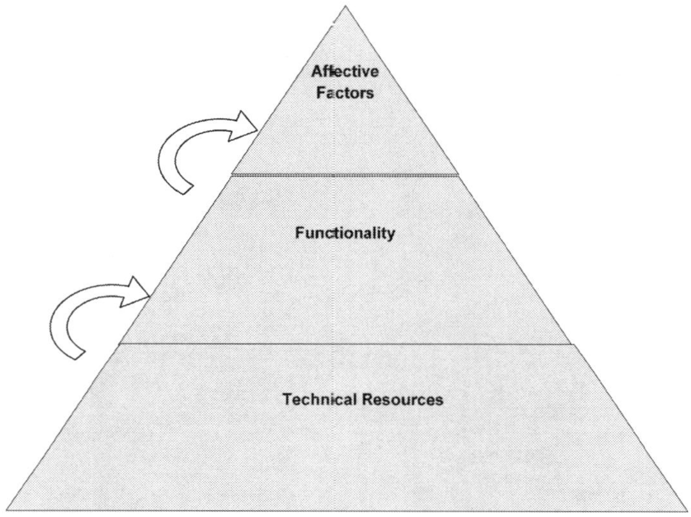

ing them will also be helpful. It is suggested that the questionnaire also include a section on free source technologies so you can have some idea of their previous experience of using the free source technology that you have selected, and also are aware of any other experience they may have. This preparation should help stage one be as painless and productive as possible and be an opportunity for participants to build confidence in using the ePortfolio network. During the workshop for the first stage, it is probably best to adopt a logical, coherent approach to instruction demonstrated via a projector with supporting instruction material so that the participants have a step-by-step manual to take away with them that will help them complete the activities for stage two.

Early on in stage two, to build confidence and relationships, set tasks that are easy to complete and that facilitate peer interaction. However, also ensure that during stage two, participants are introduced to the full range of functions that you will be using. This means a consideration of the complexity of each function should be undertaken so that not until the later stages are complicated functions attempted to be used. To ensure that workload is manageable, it is useful to issue

Figure 2. Steps of implementation

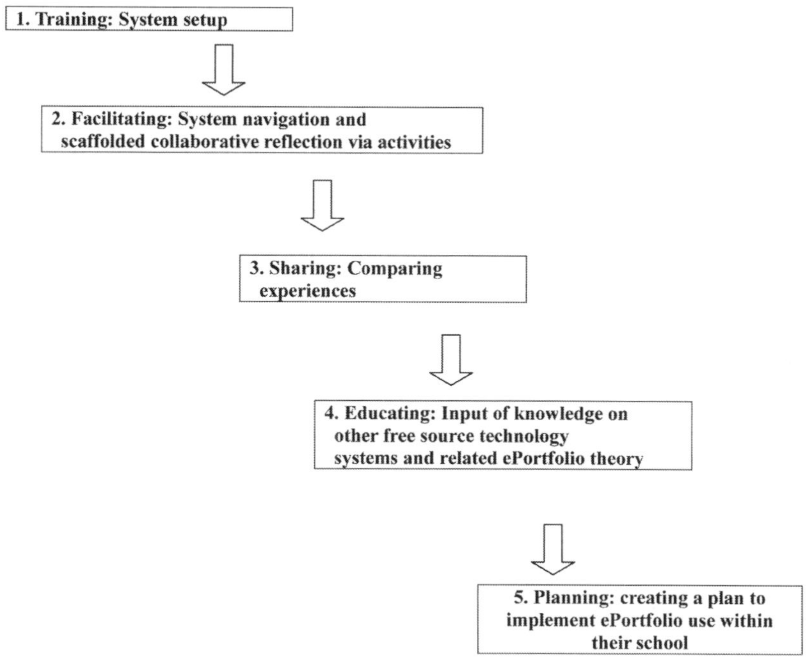

deadlines. Additionally, if you have a large number of participants, and they are required to comment on each other's contributions, it can be helpful to arrange students into groups during stage one.

When running the workshop for stage three, it is important to create an atmosphere that is conducive to allow negative comments to be shared and discussed. In stage four, it is essential to set questions for discussion to reinforce the literature input so that it helps participant conceptualize ePortfolio use within their context. Providing that stage four has been conducted adequately, stage five should be relatively straight forward, as stage five brings together their experiences from stages one, two and three and the content knowledge from stage four.

FUTURE RESEARCH DIRECTIONS

As this project in itself is really the first step in taking free source ePortfolio use in a new direction, replication of this study within varying contexts around the world and with teachers from different disciplines is required. It would be useful to know whether the five stages are sufficient in all contexts and how they can be improved. Additionally, a series of studies examining the proliferation of free source ePortfolio use generated by participants in secondary and tertiary contexts would be of interest.

CONCLUSION

This chapter has reviewed relevant literature in relation to collaborative peer reflection amongst ESL professionals with particular attention being given to the concept of obtaining voice by using ePortfolio in relation to Bailey's three criteria.

In total, this chapter compared twelve free source technologies against ten separate criteria.

The authors have also highlighted three distinct stages that need to be completed for the selection of a suitable free source technology to create ePortfolio networks that are sensitive to local constraints. Furthermore, it has put forward five stages for facilitating collaborative peer reflection and the dissemination of ePortfolio use, together with sound advice that is applicable in various contexts to ensure success at each stage.

REFERENCES

Bailey, F. (1996). The role of collaborative dialogue in teacher education. In D. Freeman & J.C. Richards (Eds.), *Teacher Learning in Language Teaching* (pp. 260-280). Cambridge: Cambridge University Press.

Bauman, V. (2008, January 29). N.Y. legislation targets Internet predators. *MSNBC.* Retrieved March 29, 2009, from http://www.msnbc.msn.com/id/22903731/

Biggs, J. (2003). *Teaching for quality learning at university – what the student does*. Buckingham, UK: The Society for Research into Higher Education and Open University Press.

Boyd, D. & Ellison, N. (2007). Social network sites: Definition, history, and scholarship. *Journal of Computer-Mediated Communication, 13*(1). Retrieved February 22, 2009 from http://jcmc.indiana.edu/vol13/issue1/boyd.ellison.html

Butterfield, L. (2005). Cybersafety: An intrinsic part of the online experience. In K.W. Lai (Ed.), *E-learning communities: Teaching and learning with the Web* (pp 179-197). Dunedin, New Zealand: University of Otago Press.

Campbell, A.P. (2004). Using LiveJournal for authentic communication in EFL classes. *The Internet TESL Journal, 10*(9). Retrieved February 22, 2009, from http://iteslj.org/Techniques/Campbell-LiveJournal/

Dudeney, G., & Hockly, N. (2007). *How to teach English with technology*. Harlow, UK: Pearson/Longman.

Dwyer, C., Hiltz, S. R., & Passerini, K. (2007). Trust and privacy concern within social networking sites: A comparison of Facebook and MySpace. In *Proceedings of the Thirteenth Americas Conference on Information Systems*, Keystone, Colorado. Retrieved on February 2, 2009, from http://csis.pace.edu/~dwyer/research/DwyerAMCIS2007.pdf

Education and Manpower Bureau. (2004). *Reforming the academic structure for secondary education and higher education- actions for investing in the future*. Retrieved March 5, 2009, from http://www.edb.gov.hk/FileManager/EN/content_4034/main.pdf

Ellison, N. & Wu, Y. (2008). Blogging in the classroom: A preliminary exploration of student attitude and impact on comprehension. *Journal of Educational Media and Hypermedia, 17*(1), 99-122.

Fuchs, C. (2005). CMC-based model learning in language teacher education: A German-American telecollaboration. In I. Thompson & D. Hiple (Eds.), *Selected papers from the 2004 NFLRC symposium: Distance Education, Distributed Learning and Language Instruction* (pp. 141-156). Honolulu. HI: University of Hawai'i, National Foreign Language Resource Center. Retrieved March 2, 2009, from http://nflrc.hawaii.edu/NetWorks/NW44

Fuller, F. F & Manning, B.A. (1973). Self-confrontation reviewed: A conceptualization for video playback in teacher education. *Review of Educational Research, 43*(4), 469-528.

Jonassen, D. (1996). *Computers in the classroom: Mindtools for critical thinking*. Engelwood Cliffs, NJ: Prentice-Hall Inc.

Jones, P. D. (2008). Using ePortfolios. *Modern English Teacher*, *17*(4), 53–59.

Kolaitis, M., Mahoney, M.A. & Pomann, H. (2006). Training ourselves to train our students for CALL. In P. Hubbard & M. Levy (Eds.), *Teacher Education in CALL* (pp 317-314). Philadelphia, PA: John Benjamins Publishing Company.

Lavooy M.J. and Newlin, M. H. (2003). Computer Mediated Communication: Online instruction and interactivity. *Journal of Interactive Learning Research, 14*(2), 157-165

Lipsman, A. (2007). *Social networking goes global*. Retrieved March 22, 2009, from http://www.comscore.com/press/release.asp?press=1555

Lyons, N. (1998). Reflection in teaching: Can it be developmental? A portfolio perspective. *Teacher Education Quarterly*, *25*(1), 115–127.

Prensky, M. (2001) Digital Natives, digital immigrants. *On the Horizon, 9*(5). Retrieved on July 13, 2006, from http://www.marcprensky.com/writing/Prensky%20-%20Digital%20Natives,%20Digital%20Immigrants%20-%20Part1.pdf

Salili, F. (2001). Teacher-Student interaction: Attributional implications and effectiveness of teachers' evaluative feedback. In D. Watkins & J. Biggs (Eds.), *Teaching the Chinese Learner: Psychological and Pedagogical Perspectives*. Comparative Education Research Centre, Hong Kong: The Chinese University of Hong Kong.

Vygotsky, L.S. (1978). *Mind in society*. Cambridge, MA: Harvard University Press.

Warschauer, M. (2004). Technology and writing. In C. Davison and J. Cummins (Eds.), *Handbook of English Language Teaching*. Dordrecht, Netherlands: Kluwer.

Warschauer, M. and Meskill, C. (2000). Technology and second language teaching and learning. In J. W. Rosenthal (Ed.), *Handbook of undergraduate second language education: English as a second language, bilingual, and foreign language instruction for a multilingual world* (pp. 303-318). Mahwah, NJ: Erlbaum

Williams, P. (2006). MySpace, Facebook attract online predators. *MSNBC*. Retrieved February 3, 2009 from http://msnbc.msn.com/id/11165576

Chapter 7
Utilizing VoiceThread to Increase Teacher Candidates' Reflection and Global Implications for Usage

Virginia McCormack
Ohio Dominican University, USA

ABSTRACT

A new teaching and learning experience is emerging thanks to the emanation of a new set of Web 2.0 tools. This experience is more inclusive where students are guided through a curriculum that better adapts to their individual learning styles, encourages collaborative teamwork, and facilitates critical thinking and problem solving through a variety of communication, visualization and simulation technologies. A discussion of providing a platform for reviewing and reflecting on shared learning experiences through the use of VoiceThread and digital video recording for all levels of learners is presented. The chapter highlights the power and barriers related to the application of educational technology for teacher candidates, teacher educators, teachers and students. The author proposes that teachers can become empowered, teacher educators and teacher candidates can reflect and connect curriculum with authentic activities through the application of VoiceThread, a Web 2.0 tool that will support learning and collaborating more effectively worldwide.

INTRODUCTION

The next level of learning and teaching has come about by the rapid progression and integration of technology in a time of growing global and cultural diversity affiliation. Curriculum development is being adapted to individual learning styles, encouraging collaborative teamwork, and facilitating critical thinking and problem solving through a variety of communication, visualization, and simulation technologies. Students, teacher candidates, and teacher educators should be familiar with and build competence around technological tools used in the classroom, online and in the world around them. The technology tools should support the increasing diversity in students' abilities, thoughts, perceptions, cultures and lived realities. By integrating technology-enhanced reflective practice into the

DOI: 10.4018/978-1-61520-897-5.ch007

Copyright © 2010, IGI Global. Copying or distributing in print or electronic forms without written permission of IGI Global is prohibited.

learning process contributes to students' continued growth.

The purpose of this chapter is to examine and discuss the reflective practice of teacher candidates and the implementation of VoiceThread, a Web 2.0 tool and the evolution of teaching and learning on teacher preparation. The key benefits of using VoiceThread in learning environments and educational content applications are explored to gain clarity. Furthermore, it identifies the global challenges, barriers, and limitations that inhibit the application of technology and describes how to address those barriers and limitations related to teacher preparation and professional development.

Although there are constraints related to technology use, VoiceThread and other Web 2.0 tool utilization can be essential for classroom teachers, teacher candidates, and students to encapsulate learning and evidence of understanding. These tools empower teachers, teacher candidates, and students by connecting curriculum with authentic activities. Samples of teaching and student work can be presented through the use of the digital modeling strategies, by capturing experiential learning for data collection and assessment, and providing a platform for reviewing and reflecting on shared learning experiences while exploring open problem solving solutions. VoiceThread was used as a potential stimulus to strengthening assignment responses comprehensively. After seeing how the teacher candidates responded to the VoiceThread-based assignments, the author suggests that much can be learned that will assist teachers in assimilating VoiceThread and other Web 2.0 tools into their learning environment.

Additionally, there are some obstacles related to access, fundamental beliefs, and cultural implications that may impede the integration of Web 2.0 tools. Teaching from a web-based learning tools perspective, suggests the necessity of examining the manner of how teachers instruct, how students learn and the cultural underpinnings. Traditional teaching focuses on increasing knowledge through the memorization of facts and the retention of this new knowledge. Some will argue that there is a disconnect between the way students live and the way they learn. In particular, educators are challenged with a new generation of students expecting a learning environment that accommodates their digital lifestyle that is global, multidisciplinary and reflective. The Partnership for 21st Century Skills, a leading advocacy organization focused on infusing 21st century skills into education endorsed helping students master core subjects and become skilled at communication, problem solving, critical thinking, global awareness, financial literacy and technology. Other constituents offered that mastering those skills means learning how to think critically and creatively, work collaboratively, use technology for research, and communicate clearly and effectively. For other educators, the integration of technology into teaching may seem complicated, particularly when current teaching or an educational policy may follow a more traditional curriculum. The use of digital technologies call forth a different manner of thinking that looks to future possibilities and a transformation that will complement teaching and provide a learning environment to access, teach, and support each student's learning needs and potential.

BACKGROUND

All countries have established institutions and processes dedicated to the education of teacher candidates and professional for teachers; however these institutions and processes differ in their composition, goals, and regulations all around the world. The trend is to refer to the preparation of teachers as professional development because it suggests a lifelong process of learning and development rather than teacher training. The transmission-oriented model of teacher education has been supplanted by a new paradigm of teacher education that is based on constructivism that considers professional development a collaborative process. With this movement toward teacher education and professional development, a teacher is deemed a reflective practitioner, who enters into the profession with an evident knowledge base and who builds additional knowledge and experiences grounded in that prior knowledge.

As beginning teachers experience and process new information during their initial acts of teaching, reflection is an inherent part of the process (Romano & Schwartz, 2005). Cornford (2002) argued that reflection requires prior thinking, reflection, and the ability to engage in critical thinking. That is, there must be content or coherent body of knowledge and logical processing skills. Technologies hold promise for eliciting and encouraging beginning teachers' reflective practice. The technology tools provided an avenue for reflection on teaching and a structure for thinking and talking about their work as teachers. Through these technology tools, beginning teachers can engage in reflection on their teaching practices and use these reflections to improve their teaching skills and knowledge (Hawkes & Rosmiszowski, 2001).

Educators must assess their needs, cultural beliefs and practices to decide which type of professional development may flourish in their unique context. Most nations recognize that initial teacher education is just the first phase in an extensive process of professional development. The emphasis on certain components of the curriculum, usually include courses and experiences that address content matter, foundations in education, child development, pedagogy and methods courses, and student teaching. In a number of developed and developing countries, the necessity for more teachers has been fertile ground for the creation of a number of alternatives that employ technology within the teacher education programs. Innovations in teacher education programs are deploying means to increase collaboration and student responsibility. With affordance ever in mind, free Web 2.0 tools are available to teachers, students and teacher candidates to create, share, and organize text and media, allowing individuals to reflect, collaborate and communicate in new ways with individual sustainable technologies.

Brent (2005) indicated that the world of learning technology today is radically different from that of just a decade ago. And a decade from now will be radically different from that of today. Learning technologies are in a state of "interpretive flexibility": the technology itself subject to change, as its application. However, learning technologies are affected not just by the possibilities of the technology but by our understanding of learning as well (Oblinger, 2005).

The New Media Consortium and the Educause Learning Initiative identify the trends for emerging technology in higher education in an annual Horizon Report (Serim & Schrock, 2007, 6-28). The predicted adoption timeframes includes:

1 year or less
- social computing
- social networking
- personal broadcasting
- user-created content-producers of information

2 or 3 years
- mlearning: mobile phones for usage, text, and visual communications, web resources and applications, any media
- virtual worlds-immersive environment, multi-user virtual environments (MUVE's)
- educational gaming

4-5 years
- augmented reality and enhanced visualization
- context-aware environments and devices
- The new scholarship and emerging forms of publication: digital and interactive blogs, wikis, videos, podcasts
- mass multiplayer educational gaming-increase oral and language skills

Information and communication technology is a part of our environment and growing rapidly. Some of the technologies mentioned by Serim and Schrock are already in active use, long before the projected timeframe in elementary schools, high schools and universities. Koehler & Mishra (2008) maintain that because of such interactivity, researchers increasingly view technology selection not as an inert decision, but as one where the intersections of technology, pedagogy, and content must be carefully considered. Freidhoff (2008) urged teacher educators to select technologies that best fit the learning task by identifying the learning task, evaluate the affordances and constraints and assess technology implementation according to the principles of practice. Using digital tools to create learning plans, manage educational content, providing a framework for reflection, and track student progress are ways in which technology can be applied to teaching and learning. New styles of teaching with technology include using more audio and video clips, data collection, MUVE with avatars, electronic excerpts from article and books, and podcasts..

VoiceThread offers a new venue for reflective discourse. Research by Hawkes & Rosmiszowski (2001) has shown that discourse through technology achieved a higher overall reflective level than do reflections generated by teachers in face-to-face interactions, therefore, recognizing the value of time independence for providing a greater chance to ask reflective questions. Reflection enables practitioners to analyze, discuss, evaluate and change their own practice, adopting an analytical approach toward their practice, and encourages them to appraise the moral and ethical issues implicit in classroom practices, including the critical examination of their own beliefs about effective teaching. In addition, it encourages them to take greater responsibility for their own professional growth and to seek ways of acquiring some degree of professional autonomy (Hussein, 2007).

Antstey and Bull (2006) contended that from reflections, teachers and students can deduce the knowledge, skills, and processes that are essential in order to function productively as citizens of the local and global community in the present-day and in the future. Students can participate in global events primarily or vicariously through the medium of technology. Various media platforms can be implemented such as Web 2.0 tools, phones with video and photograph capabilities, video cameras. Students and teachers can become cognizant of global events and more conscious of global trends. Communication and social skills will develop by interacting with different groups and cultures in a variety of settings from home to workplace. Reflection as an individualized practice mirrors preparation in teacher education programs that have traditionally focused on the development of knowledge, skills and dispositions of prospective teachers rather than on the socialization and establishment of communities for collaborative participation. With reflection as a social practice, emphasis is on interconnectedness with other teaching professionals as well as with peer involvement as a necessary component of reflection to push each individual's thinking beyond personal limitations according to Putnam & Botko (2000).

With the increase of technology integration such as VoiceThread into education settings, it is essential that teachers understand how to generate reflective learning opportunities using technologies to create optimal reflective learning environments. Oliver & Herrington (2001) suggested scaffolding as a means to assist student by modeling reflective behavior, identifying the processes used in reflective practice, providing feedback and promoting a supportive environment where students can identify areas of uncertainty and articulate their opinions to facilitate learning. Brigden (2004 communicated that through these reflective learning experiences, students can demonstrate that they are able to reconceptualize by synthesizing various quantities of information that they have received or obtained through resources to solve a problem.

Incorporating technology infused learning and teaching provides the context for global education across pedagogies, disciplines, and cultures that can stimulate rich contexts for critical reflection. Schools immersed in technology-based learning can increase the quality, relevance and amount of information that can be imparted and be more time-effective. Collaborating with all levels of classroom teachers and education programs that model technology can serve as authentic environments for teacher education and provide professional development for current teachers. User-friendly networking technologies have enabled students to collaborate in their own educational setting and connect with their peers around the world.

ISSUES, CONTROVERSIES, AND PROBLEMS

The Challenges, Barriers, Limitations and Rewards of Global Educational Technology Integration and Reflection

Educators endeavoring to integrate technology cope with an array of challenges. They must understand and view the broad context of technology, instruction, and curriculum. To comprehend the innovative possibilities, it is necessary to determine what possibilities subsist in the existing definitions of what constitutes teaching and curriculum (Cowan, 2008).

There are a number of impediments to the utilization of technology for educational and professional reflection. Institutional barriers are depicted as the lack of access to technology, inadequate technological support or deficient technology skills. In addition, using technology can be time-intensive for both the student and teacher. Another barrier may be related to intrinsic beliefs about teaching and learning in a global world.

Many challenges are faced by the African countries to transform the educational and social aspects of education and teacher preparation. The social, political and economic contexts have shaped the educational systems in Africa and many of these countries lack the resources to improve their educational systems and teacher education programs. Moja (2004) expressed that sub-Saharan African nation's grapple with low-quality education, limited technology access and inadequate funding.

The Wormnaes research study of Norwegian and Egyptian educator's interview data showed that an emphasis on reflection, exploration, and evaluation rather than on drills and repetition was both unexpected and unfamiliar to most Egyptian student teachers. Significant findings indicated that lecturers who wanted to pursue teaching methods that enhanced reflection needed to prioritize time for reflection even if the majority of the student-teachers asked for more information, more facts, and for more presentations of the "the right methods" for teaching learners with disabilities. Wormnaes (2008) urged that lecturers should be context sensitive, having an inquiring and accepting attitude, and experience challenges, encounters, and exposure in the project country over time rather than imposing their views and perspectives on teacher candidates.

Research findings indicated that teachers' beliefs may be an important element regarding the integration of technology. Studies have frequently stated that teachers teach the way that they have been taught. Other findings point toward exposure or improper usage that may deter the integration of technology. Chen (2008) disclosed that educational reform in Taiwan encouraged teachers to incorporate technology into instruction to engage students in activities of problem-solving and collaborative learning, but a culture emphasizing competition and a high-stakes assessment system can strongly discourage teachers from undertaking such innovative initiatives. Farrell, T. (2008) discovered the existence of a series that promotes reflections on practice in the Malaysian and other Asian contexts called the Sasbadi-MELTA ELT series. The English language teaching series addresses diverse practices, topics, qualitative tools, and features of English language teaching in Malaysia and worldwide.

The United Arab Emirates examined the development and implementation of a school based professional development program that aimed to encourage communities of practice (CoPs). Findings showed a disparity between the values of the school leaders and the aims of the project. Further research accentuated the lack of adequate scaffolding for technological and pedagogical supports to express represent and share practices or debate and reflect about the practices. The research also indicated limited opportunity to organize arguments and manage the reflection about the life of the community; develop, embody and attain knowledge bases; or facilitate engagement, participation and learning.

Instructional methods that are innovative and stimulating may also face resistance.

Disclosed by Rao (2008, 23-25), research in English foreign language teaching has revealed three problems:

1. Insensitivity to students' linguistic problems
   - Lack insight into typical problems Chinese students face learning English
   - Uneasy with hands-on approach or feeling pleasant and relaxed when involved in these communicative interactions, students feel teachers go to an extreme in organizing these teaching activities.
2. Mismatch between teaching and learning styles
   - Uncomfortable with global or top-down method of teaching English reading and listening.
   - They often ask students to use holistic strategies such as guessing or making inferences to search for a main idea, but seldom pay attention to the analysis of linguistic details.
   - It is impossible to infer meaning without possessing background knowledge of the topic.
   - Chinese students also identified the "open style" of learning as an incongruent instructional technique/ Chinese students are accustomed to receiving an accurate answer to each question, and when they receive multiple correct answers, which leaves them frustrated and unable to learn the concept. Creating an intuitive-random style of teaching that is friendly and relaxed atmosphere conflicts with their traditional way of learning.
3. Unfamiliarity with the local cultural and educational system
   - Unacceptable because of casual manner and failure to match their instruction to the school's expectations or the students needs.

Cultural patterns of behavior are fixed by mid-teens. Educators must be mindful of the types of methodology that have been most effective and to what students are accustomed and what constraints on the teacher's innovativeness might exist and what social, cultural, and academic adjustments the teacher candidates will have to fit into the existing setup (Rao, 2008). Before implementing new methodology, guided learning style-stretching will assist in encouraging a change in student behavior and acceptance. It is critical to respect the values as well as their cultures, educational systems, living conditions, and work ethics.

Global Educational Technology Applications and Traditional Instruction

Diverse educational points of view exist on the employment of technology in the classroom. Cross-cultural collaboration may have a unique potential to uncover the existence of a diversity of beliefs and perspectives, and to challenge both teacher educators' and student-teachers' understandings (Wormnaes, 2008). Exposure to cultural variation has been widely recognized as a learning opportunity for individuals and communities. For example, Rogoff (2003) has said that recognition of an array of approaches affords us with a chance to reflect on our own customary manner of thinking and accomplish things.

Teachers in Egypt were expected to give learners instructions rather than teach them to problem-solve, and that typical teaching method involved asking them to memorize, repeat and recall what the teacher said. Foreign lecturers put much effort into teaching them to ask questions, to reflect on their own situation, to inform when they did not understand and to request the student teachers to discuss matters. Some of the student-teachers graduates viewed having a foreign lecturer as a chance to share experiences, to learn from each other, to be confronted with opinions, to be shown new ways of facing particular problems and to learn about new teaching techniques. Self-reporting by the foreign lecturers questioned if the lecturers should have appreciated the student teachers' cultural background more and tried to take advantage of their strength in memorizing, instead of regarding this as an incorrect learning strategy (Wormnaes, 2008).

The research study went on to say that the lecturers and supervisors an awareness of their own frames of reference and how these were contextualized, in order to understand that they were not necessarily universal. In Egypt, to be self-sufficient is not necessarily highly valued as a goal of education. Lecturers who want to pursue teaching methods that enhance reflection must create an accepting atmosphere and dare to prioritize time for reflection and discussion, even if the majority of the students-teachers will ask for more information, more facts, and for presentations that described the correct methods for teaching learners (Wormnaes, 2008)

Developmentally Appropriate Educational Technology Applications through VoiceThread

The nature of teaching is changing because of the emerging technologies from Web 2.0. The Web 2.0 paradigm shift encourages communication and interaction through user-generated content. Borsheim, Merritt, and Reed (2008) posited that it increase recognition, sensibility and respect for differences of any kind; improves their skills and commitment to communication with others on a larger scale to share and exchange ideas, and builds knowledge collectively; and helps to gain deeper insight into and global understanding of learning. Educators, who implement these technologies in their educational setting, prepare their students with multiliteracies and for the actualities for the technological world. Developmentally appropriate educational technology applications should always be compatible with how students develop and learn as well as complement their specific stages of development. Instructionally sound, developmentally appropriate technology must be interactive, assist in meeting the prescribed courses of study and benefit student learning in ways that are essential to the curriculum.

There are hundreds of Web 2.0 tools that offer promising, free interactive tools with ways to interface through blogs, wikis, photographs, video sharing, bookmarking sites, and social networking. The growing collection of Web-based 2.0 tools focuses on practices such as sharing thoughts and information to increase the level of student engagement through self-publishing and harnessing the collective intelligence of all users to generate information and solve problems. These tools can be used to instruct students and support learning activities while enriching educational experiences.

I would like to highlight the use of VoiceThread; a Web 2.0 hosted service because it constitutes a free, simple tool that is suitable for any teacher or student to use. A VoiceThread is a collaborative, multimedia slide show that collects and retains images, documents, and videos. Individuals or groups can navigate the pages and comment through text, audio files, by voice using a microphone or a telephone, or using video by means of a web cam. There is no software to install and content can be shared worldwide. Identities can be created with the users name; users photograph or create a user avatar.

Security settings allow the creators or instructor to choose what tools the viewer's access. Users can select which comments are shared through comment moderation and can embed comments in other Web sites or export to MP3 players. The instructor may also choose to hide students' comments from one another. VoiceThread can be set up with restrictions that allow only your students to view the files. As the instructor, you have full moderation over your VoiceThread.

VoiceThread supports numerous standard file formats, along with PDF, Microsoft Word, Excel, and PowerPoint images, videos, and photos from Flickr, Facebook, or the web. A free VoiceThread account provides up to 75 MB of storage. VoiceThread technology provides an expanding knowledge of professional presence and engages the student, teacher or teacher candidate in the process of social and conceptual negotiation, conceptual and written revision, technological prowess, and professional communication (Borsheim et al., 2008).

How VoiceThread Can Be Put Into Practice

Uploading digital video into VoiceThread is a dynamic mode of communication in the context of new literacies and teacher education. My students considered VoiceThread uncomplicated to use and a fairly quick process. Handheld digital video recorders captured course lectures and lessons taught in the field that were uploaded to VoiceThread. The teacher candidate assessed their teaching and evidence of student learning through reflection and the instructor inserted comments in response to the teacher candidate reflection or as a means of beginning the dialogue of reflection. Successful and unsuccessful interactions were reviewed and explained to further digital communication assessment that presented evidence of learning over time. Video reflection is useful because it does not require an immediate response, affords the teachers the luxury of being able to engage in reflection on their teaching practice combined with the ability to see their teaching through the eyes of students in the classroom. It is essential to unpack teacher reflection through tools that complement and in some ways are derived from the teaching practice (Hawkes & Rosmiszowski, 2001). Beginning teachers appreciated the opportunity for instant reflection on their teaching practice combined with the ability to see their teaching reflection through tools that complement and in some ways are derived from the teaching practice (Romano & Schwartz, 2005).

Reading and studying a case study on VoiceThread furnished an opportunity for the teacher candidates to respond and complete sample assessments related to the case study. The teacher candidates viewed examples of a step-by-step procedure that they later implemented in a final case study project. The students commented that VoiceThread was thought provoking, challenged them to think outside of the box to respond to the case study questions and a great tool to gain extra practice formulating thorough responses. The majority of the teacher candidates indicated that completing the case study assignment increased their ability to reflect and to apply language related to the diagnosis, prescription and remediation rather than just reading about the processes.

VoiceThread was the platform used for diagnosing a child's reading through a miscue analysis.

The teacher candidates listened to an accompanying streaming audio file of a child orally reading a passage and recorded the miscues in VoiceThread that did not match the expected response. The miscues were analyzed and the teacher candidates were able to determine whether the

Figure 1. Case study. © 2007-09 VoiceThread. (used with permission)

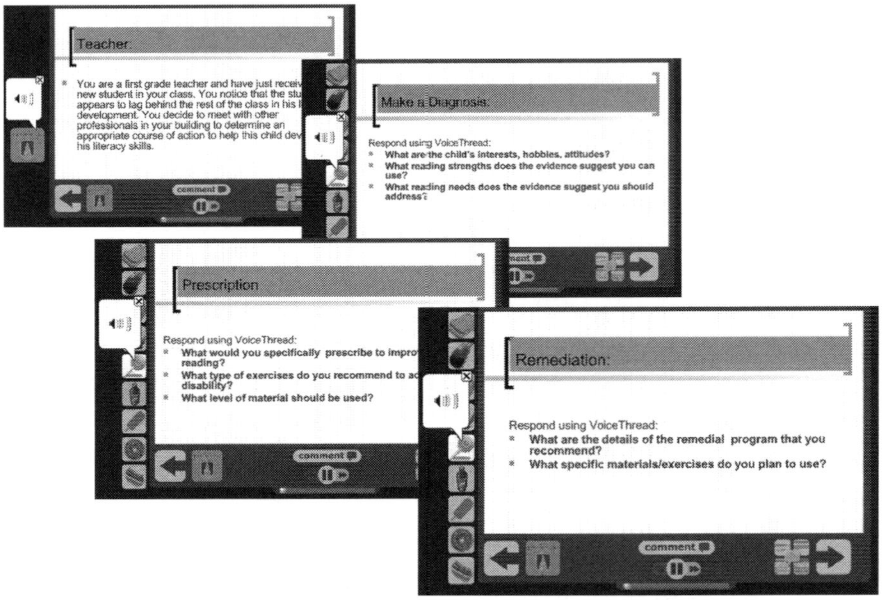

student understood the passage, had the ability to self-correct, or use strategies to aid comprehension. Many of the teacher candidates indicated that they listened to the oral reading passage several times to make sure that they identified all of the miscues and the responses of the teacher candidates was more extensive and some noted a greater confidence in their abilities to administer a miscue analysis. However, the pen feature is difficult to maneuver in a normal manner. When the assignment is reviewed legibility is a key concern and the time delay between documenting miscues that may occur if the miscues are not marked in a rapid mode. Once the pen feature is activated, the student must apply the pen to the screen otherwise there will be large gaps of time until the convention markings appear.

Authoring children's stories and content digital stories enabled teacher candidates to capitalize on increasing comprehension and also cast them as writer, publisher and producers by using computer-based tools to tell stories. The teacher candidates selected a particular topic and developed a high-interest, motivational children's story that contained a mixture of computer-based images, text, recorded audio narration, photographs, and some music. The length of the children's stories varied but typically lasted between two and a half minutes to three and a half minutes. The digital content stories emphasized the power of weaving digital images from digital libraries or YouTube, narrative, and voice related to a content area, concept, or historical event that were four to ten minutes in length. King (2007) asserted that the value and benefit of preparing teacher candidates with digital media skills empowered educators to use real life applications and invest in critical reflection to increase student learning.

VoiceThread can be used in all content areas. So, if you upload a PowerPoint, Word documents, Excel spreadsheets, video, photographs, or any file and ask you student's questions and have them respond by speaking, by typing, by webcam, by drawing on the slide, or by uploading an audio or music file. Students can also set up VoiceThread for content presentations and respond to other students asynchronously. There is also an extension of VoiceThread called

Figure 2. Miscue analysis. © 2007-09 VoiceThread. (used with permission)

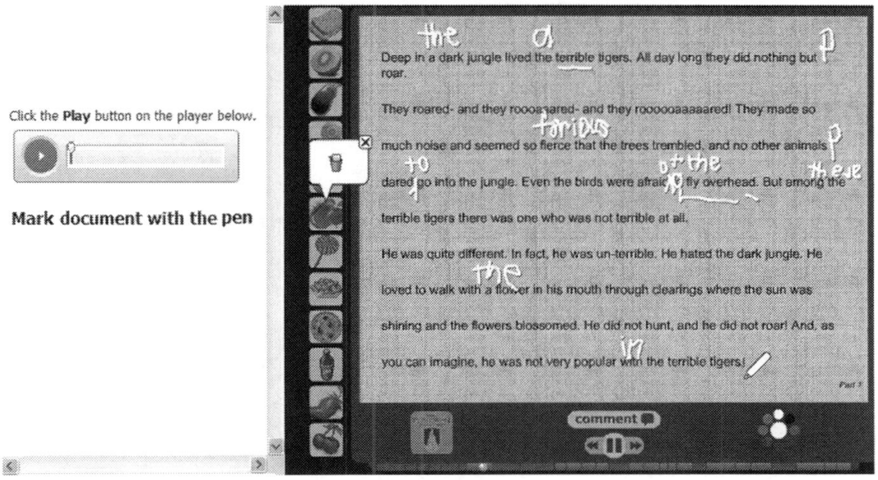

Ed.VoiceThread that is a free, transformative, digital tool for all teachers.

A myriad of content specific activities can be developed to give voice. In art, notable works of art can be displayed and discussed. Students can work with graphic design or animation to create projects. Learning standards can be applied and digital guides for museum visits can be created. Scrapbooking or photograph albums can be planned to illustrate watercolor techniques or a particular era of art design.

A language art curriculum can use VoiceThread to promote effective public speaking techniques or provide a vehicle for book talks. Simple games can be fashioned to match pictures to vocabulary words. VoiceThread can be used for creative writing to narrate stories or arrange collaborative writing assignments. Digital literature road trips can be devised to highlight supplementary information on historical and geographical orientations, biographical information, and cultural correlations related to the literature.

Students can attach personal meaning to mathematics by generating and solving problems by using digital tools rather than relying on recitation and memorization. Interactive mathematics concepts using the pen feature can be manipulated to record answers. Discussions of foods grown within a fifty-mile radius with digital images, and shared recipes related to the culture can be constructed through VoiceThread. Gesture counting may be recorded and uploaded to VoiceThread to provide a clear understanding. Mathematics concepts such as graphing and measures of central tendency can be taught through geocaching, a high-tech treasure-hunting game in which the participants equipped with a global positioning system receiver search for containers called geocaches and share their experiences online.

VoiceThread gives all music students the opportunity to express their creativity and to learn innovative skills by providing a venue for student compositions and digitized singing. Musical instrumentation can be uploaded to note the progression of skill and finesse. Multimedia portfolios that embed music and digital images show a correlation between music and core subject area standards.

Physical education content can be demonstrated by having the students create inexpensive strength training equipment and posting the project on VoiceThread. Teams of physical education students can assemble a first aid kit or sports medicine kit that can be assessed collaboratively for comprehensiveness and usefulness on VoiceThread. Teachers can upload and provide a simulation of disease with diagrams and digital images to enhance content materials. A survey of students about their nutritional habits can be given, data collected and the results analyzed.

Another example of integration would be the application of technology to science. The investigation of scientific methods and laboratory experiments can be clearly illustrated through VoiceThread where students apply the knowledge and skills to their learning to make natural connections. Digital notecards with facts about endangered animals, changes in properties in matter, or other concepts can be developed to provide a foundation to support theoretical referents. LEGO and robotics is a natural link for using a VoiceThread and acts as a catalyst for integrating content and curricula.

Second language teachers are using VoiceThread to assist their students to learn and practice speaking a second language. Oral reports or debates can be presented or cartoons can be captioned. The audio recording of book chapter or poetry can signal correct pronunciation and inflection while reading.

Map links with digital images or video of local landmarks around the world engage social studies students with VoiceThread applications. Student projects might include digital content area storytelling about the mysteries of history or global citizenship. Oral history projects can be uploaded and shared collaboratively.

Special education instruction can employ social stories with social cues and appropriate responses in VoiceThread. Students can view role-playing lessons for gestures, voice tone, proximity and emotions related to context. Developing conversion starters in VoiceThread allows the students to respond and adjust their responses, if necessary.

Infusing instructional technology requires teachers to be inventive, creative and committed to exploring new uses of technology for teaching and learning. Currently, there is a great demand for innovation in educational practice and global applications. A Web 2.0 tool such as VoiceThread can prove to be invaluable to teachers as they prepare their students for the future.

SOLUTIONS AND RECOMMENDATIONS

Bridging the Disparity

When you review educational technology use by regions, it is dominated by North Americans followed by Europe, the Middle East, Africa, and the Asia Pacific region with limited access in South America and Latin America. Efforts need to be made to advance capacities in countries at the individual, organizational, and societal levels by customizing educational experiences to specific national needs and priorities and by designing programs with long-term outcomes in mind. Further attention should be given to awareness and advocacy on the connectivity through the provision of hardware and software for building universal access.

The application of a digital tool such as VoiceThread can augment, extend and refine teacher reflection experience by facilitating and structuring the analysis process. Technology–enhanced educational innovations begin in the classroom but escalate into intercontinental contexts through repeated application. As enhanced instructional technology continues to develop and teachers continue to learn more about how to use it, students will gain the ability to identify and solve problems for which there is no routine solution. Teacher educators assist teacher candidates in cultivating more advanced mental models that correspond with problem-solving approaches by challenging students with ambiguity and contradictory perspectives. Teacher candidates need to have more opportunities for skill development and ability to infuse technology into course work, so faculty should meet and review course syllabi for technology integration.

Skill development requires repeated assessment of the skill, practicing and feedback. Formative and summative assessment is essential for the development of skills, because with these assessment methods, we can improve and support students' self-directed and shared learning. As teacher educators, we need to provide timely feedback, so that students' self-assessment will be fostered and students' learning will be supported during the whole process. Future practice ensuring technology-enhanced reflective learning activities consistently provide students with a reason and will to engage in and to support successful outcomes.

Teacher education programs can be instrumental in providing the opportunities to learn about technology and how to use it for educational purposes, so that disparities are overcome and teachers can collaborate within the culture of those who are creating the digital world of learning. Critical to this issue is bridging various problems that stem from access, partnerships funding and policy.

Improving Private and Public Sector Partnerships

Private and public sector partnerships are vital to bridging educational, economic and cultural barriers that are pervasive in the world. A number of partnership initiatives have been established such as the United States Higher Education Initiative Planning Grants, the Education Program of the World Bank Institute, the United States Agency for International Development (USAID), the Ed tech 20/20 Technology in Education Project, and U.S. Department of State's Middle East Partnership Initiative. Numerous foundations have made funding available such as the Sun Wah Education Foundation, the Gates Foundation, and the Longview Foundation. All of the partnerships and funding are intended to define needs, support planning and implementation, and the evaluation of education reforms while strengthening the capacity of education and teacher preparation.

Educational policy shapes the direction of education and teacher professional development. In Ireland, the Human Resources Operational Programme (HROP) of the European Union under the National Development Plan allocated over £35m for six years during 1994-1999 for collaborative research and professional activities for teacher education. This led to a consultative policy process in Irish education that re-appraised and analyzed policy formulation and legislation. Considerable advancement has been made in the assortment and value of continuing professional development activities available to teachers through these efforts.

The Australian Government has been focusing on improving the delivery of services, and building greater opportunities for education for indigenous families and individuals. This required the development of a range of different models for teacher education institutions and assessing mixed modes of delivery. Additional objectives included training sufficient numbers of teachers to be effective in Indigenous schools and using teaching methods that are known to be the most successful.

Traditional African teaching methods require memorization of the content provided and little or no time for inquiry. In southern African, a new transformative method called Critical Practitioner Inquiry (CPI) provided a framework to assist educators to look at matters holistically through action research and critical pedagogy. Critical Practitioner Inquiry (CPI) was introduced successfully in Ethiopia; however eliminating the traditional scheme of thinking and proceeding will take some time to transform educational policy, the educational systems, and teacher education programs.

Integrating VoiceThread and Other Web 2.0 Tools into the Curriculum

The strongest lesson learned from the sequence of studies discussed is the implications such research carries with multiple pathways into the application of technology. New technological tools can benefit the learning process but teachers must effectively contextualize the use of VoiceThread or other Web 2.0 tools by providing sustained practice. Clear and careful thought to creating the learning objectives for using the tools and the preferred learning outcomes must be evident to create a more meaningful learning experience for students.

After observing how the teacher candidates responded to the VoiceThread-based assignments, the author suggests that much can be learned that will assist teachers incorporate technology into their learning environment. The participants in this study have used VoiceThread before, so the technological aspects were familiar and they did not have problems undertaking these assignments. The author recommends that those inexperienced in using VoiceThread will require basic instruction and explicit guidelines before completing the assignments.

Cultural barriers may present a problem using online social networking tools and the community has an immense role in how organizations interact within themselves as well as with external associates. Developing a healthy community can initiate new education opportunities, improve collaborative relations, as well as, advance communications with the world. Some recommended steps to overcoming barriers are to empower educators through professional development, building relationships and cultural awareness, and modeling technology applications.

The adoption of a digital tool such as VoiceThread can augment, extend and refine teacher reflection experience by facilitating and structuring the analysis process. Educational technology can heighten our ability to access authentic teaching opportunities and provide a transition to daily classroom teaching by manipulating various forms of new media. There is the potential for broad application but the implementation will be determined by the curriculum and the needs of the educators.

Through careful investigation, the features of different applications of VoiceThread demonstrate the potential use to inform policy and practice. My recommendation is to be adventurous while cognizant of the cultural and accessibility aspects. Explore and sample VoiceThread and the other Web 2.0 tools that are available and you may be surprised at the response and endorsement of the students and teachers.

Implications for Teacher Preparation and Professional Development

There are many pedagogical advantages such as motivating students, supporting higher-thinking and extending scope, and facilitating learning in areas of speaking, listening and reflecting. The current Voice Thread application and collection of data incorporated video from a handheld digital video recorder that recorded teaching, teaching reflections and evidence of student learning. The teacher candidate assessed their teaching and evidence of student learning through reflection and the instructor inserted comments in response to the teacher candidate reflection or as a means of beginning the dialogue of reflection. King (2007) asserted that the value and benefit of preparing teacher candidates with digital media skills empowered educators to use real life applications and invest in critical reflection to increase student learning.

The application of educational technology has increased in intensity and complexity and requires teacher candidates to acquire a wide range of abilities and competencies. New contexts need to be investigated, so that teacher candidates and teacher educators develop proficiency with the tools of technology. Our world is becoming more global and we are becoming inextricably linked in building relationships to design and share information in global communities. Teacher candidates will need to have learning experiences that promote reflective practice and work collaboratively in virtual environments that immerse them in solving problems collaboratively and cross-culturally. Tillma, H. (2000) stressed that reflection is interactive and that reflection and experiences lead to a greater openness of beliefs. In doing so, teacher candidates are encouraged to question and view the realities in which schools and classrooms are situated and the impacts of diverse personal and collegial perspectives on educational issues. Reflective collaboration then, becomes a social process that elaborates and connects the implicit knowledge. Flores-Marti, I. (2008) suggested that teacher candidates ought to understand the purpose of reflection and be guided through the reflective experience in order to know how to shift their reflective focus as their experience progresses.

Technology–enhanced educational innovations begin in the classroom but escalate into intercontinental contexts through repeated application. As enhanced instructional technology continues to develop and teachers continue to learn more about how to use it, students will gain the ability to identify and solve problems for which there is no routine solution. So by challenging students with ambiguity and contradictory perspectives, teacher educators assist teacher candidates in cultivating more advanced mental models that correspond with problem-solving approaches.

FUTURE RESEARCH DIRECTIONS

Future research directions advocate for approaches that build on the synergy of technological concepts and well-established pedagogical principles. VoiceThread and the wide variety of Web 2.0 tools provide a service and give us a new worldview through a range of free, participatory, shared and disseminated resources that educators can use in their classroom or online. Current research trends in technology-enhanced learning aim at addressing the multiplicity and complexity of the needs of students, teacher candidates and teachers. Some research has suggested that a platform for modeling educational technology integration would be the methods course in teacher education. I envision the advantages of infusing Web 2.0 tools in all courses where student can utilize video, web-cam, image, and voice technologies for communicating, reflecting, and collaborating in electronic constructivist learning settings. However, educators should select technology that best fits the learning task and complements the culture, should evaluate the affordance and constraints of implementation, and the impact on pedagogical goals.

Educators perceive reflective tasks as significant, based on the results of earlier studies that indicated reflection improved student achievement and involvement. A multiliterate teacher understands the many ways that technology interacts and intertwines with reflection, and actively ascertains how to manage those aspects impacting teaching and professional development. Russell, McPherson, and Martin (2001) expressed that innovative teacher programs include some commonalities such as establishing dialogue so that student teachers' experiences and issues tie in theory to reflective practice; collaborative environments with student cohorts, with schools boards and university, within university departments, between teachers, mentors, and student teachers with inquiry practice; and explicit explanations of teachers' actions, thinking while planning, implementing and evaluating.

Mc Gee and Diaz (2007) stressed that this multifaceted approach involves determining needs and wants and preferences, capturing current practices, and matching the pedagogical value of the tools as it relates to teaching and learning behaviors.

- Do emerging and innovative technologies actually result in an improved educational model?

- How are these technologies implemented and sustained?
- How do these technologies map instructional problems?
- Which technologies actually improve learning?
- Assist learners to become active engaged learners and information evaluators.
- Do not create media that plays for so long that students would not finish a module.
- Prescribed timeline.

Teacher candidates and teachers expand their knowledge base through professional development, reflection, and application of VoiceThread and other Web 2.0. tools. Instructionally sound, developmentally appropriate technology must be collaborative, assist in meeting the prescribed courses of study and benefit student learning in ways that are essential to the curriculum. So, educators must assess their needs, cultural beliefs and practices to decide which type of professional development may flourish in their unique context.

CONCLUSION

Changes in the contour of teacher preparation and professional development through the use of VoiceThread, a Web 2.0 tool will not be easy. Teacher educators have been proposing reflective journals as instruments of sharing experiences and thinking, now have the electronic means to do so. Most teacher candidates' are adept at utilizing technology and seem to prefer assignments that are concentrated on their needed skills preferably that they can self-select. They are comfortable with collaborating and can create projects and presentations that can be posted in course management systems and on Web pages. Educators now and in the years ahead, will need to understand and have access to digital tools, greater amounts of information, and multiple data streams to create learning plans, manage educational content, and track student progress.

The nature of teaching is being transformed because of emerging technologies and educators impassioned to integrate technology, must manage an assortment of challenges. Educators must understand and view the broad context of technology, instruction, and curriculum. The application of a digital tool such as VoiceThread can augment, extend and refine teacher reflection experience by facilitating and structuring the analysis process.

REFERENCES

Antstey, M., & Bull, G. (2006). *Teaching and learning multiliteracies: Changing times, changing literacies*. Kensington Gardens, Australia: International Reading Association and Australian Literacy Educator's Association.

Borsheim, C., Merritt, K., & Reed, D. (2008). Beyond technology for technology's sake: advancing multiliteracies in the twenty-first century. *Clearing House (Menasha, Wis.)*, *82*(2), 55–59. doi:10.3200/TCHS.82.2.87-90

Brent, D. (2005). Teaching performance in the electronic classroom. *First Monday*, *10*(4).

Brigden, D. (2004). Becoming a reflective practitioner. *The Newsletter of Itsn-0*. Retrieved March 29, 2009, from http://www.medev.ac.uk/newsletter/01.6.html

Chen, C. (2008). Why do teachers not practice what they believe regarding technology integration? *The Journal of Educational Research*, *102*(1), 65–75. doi:10.3200/JOER.102.1.65-75

Cornford, I. R. (2002). Reflective teaching: Empirical research findings and some implications for teacher education. *Journal of Vocational Education and Training*, *54*, 219–235. doi:10.1080/13636820200200196

Cowan, J. (2008). The Strategies for planning technology–enhanced learning experiences. *Clearing House (Menasha, Wis.)*, *82*(2), 55–59. doi:10.3200/TCHS.82.2.55-59

Farrell, T. (2008). *Reflective practice in the professional development of teachers of adult English language learners*. Washington, DC: Center for Applied Linguistics. Retrieved February 3, 2009, from http://www.cal.org/caelanetwrok/pd_resources/reflectivepractice.html

Flores-Marti, I. (2008). Reflection as a critical component in the preparation of teacher candidates. *Strategies*, *21*(6), 15–18.

Freidhoff, J. (2008). Reflecting on the affordance and constraints of technologies and their impact on pedagogical goals. *Journal of Computing in Teacher Education*, *24*(4), 117–122.

Hawkes, M., & Rosmiszowski, A. (2001). Examining the reflective outcomes of asynchronous computer-mediated communication on inservice teacher development. *Journal of Technology and Teacher Education*, *9*(2), 285–308.

Hussein, J. (2007). Experience gained through engaging student teachers in a developmental reflective process. *Teacher Development*, *11*(2), 189–201. doi:10.1080/13664530701414852

King, K. (2007). *New technology to revolutionize teaching and learning*. Charlotte, NC: Information Age Publishing.

Koehler, M. J., & Mishra, P. (2008). Introducing TPCK. In AACTE Committee on Innovation and Technology (Ed.), Handbook of technological pedagogical content knowledge (TPCK) for educators (pp. 3-29). New York: Routledge.

Mc Gee, P., & Diaz, V. (2007). Wikis, and podcasts and blogs! Oh, my! What is a faculty member supposed to do? *Educause*, *42*(5), 28–41.

Moja, T. (2004). Policy responses to global transformation by African higher education systems. In Zeleza, P. T., & Olukoshi, A. (Eds.), *African universities in the twenty-first century* (*Vol. 1*, pp. 21–41). Dakar, Senegal: CODESRIA.

Oblinger, D. (2005). Learners, learning and technology. *EDUCAUSE*, *40*(5), 66–75.

Oliver, R., & Herrington, J. (2001). *Teaching and learning online. Mt. Lawley*. Perth, Australia: Centre for Research in Information Technology and Communication, Edith Cowan University.

Putnam, R. T., & Botko, H. (2000). What do new views of knowledge and thinking have to say about research on teacher learning? *Educational Researcher*, *29*(1), 4–15.

Rao, Z. (2008). Reflecting on Native-English-speaking teachers in China. *Essential Teacher*, *5*(1), 23–25.

Rogoff, B. (2003). *The cultural nature of human development*. Oxford, UK: Oxford University.

Romano, M., & Schwartz, J. (2005). Exploring technology a s a tool for eliciting and encouraging beginning teacher reflection. *Contemporary Issues in Technology and Teacher*, *5*(2), 149–168.

Russell, T., McPherson, S., & Martin, A. K. (2001). Coherence and collaboration in teacher education reform. *Canadian Journal of Education*, *26*(3), 14.

Serim, F., & Schrock, K. (2007). *The Horizon Report*. Stanford, CA: The New Media Consortium.

Tillma, H. (2000). Belief change towards self-directed learning in student teachers: Immersion in practice or reflection on action. *Teaching and Teacher Education*, *16*, 575–591. doi:10.1016/S0742-051X(00)00016-0

Wormnaes, S. (2008). Cross-cultural collaboration in Special Education: An arena for facilitating reflection? *International Journal of Disability Development and Education*, *55*(3), 205–225. doi:10.1080/10349120802268305

Chapter 8
The Golden Apple:
A Quest toward Achievement

Lesia Lennex
Morehead State University, USA

Kimberely Fletcher Nettleton
Morehead State University, USA

ABSTRACT

The success of any educational technology lies in how students interact with it in an educational setting. In the iLRN model (Lennex & Nettleton, 2009), the teacher provides instruction but through activity theory the students transform the learning to suit their own designs. The quality of teacher directions determines the extent to which students depend on the teacher for further feedback and technical assistance. If a teacher is perceived as not understanding even a small part of the technology, Lennex (2008) discovered that P-12 students are unlikely to ask for clarification of assignments or for any further assistance. Exploration and peer coaching replaced the teacher. Technologically literate teachers who interacted with their students and encouraged the scaffolding of knowledge discovered that final student projects demonstrated higher levels of critical thinking and creativity when compared to teacher-controlled projects.

INTRODUCTION

A great race is being run in schools, with the outcome impacting the future of students. Educators and school budgets strain to keep pace with the rapid growth and capabilities of cutting edge technology (Hirsch, 2005). Considerable gaps occur between acquiring technology and adapting it for effective instruction. Hippomenes, in Greek Mythology, runs a race against Atalanta in order to win her hand in marriage. To attract her attention, Hippomenes tosses golden apples onto her path. The Apple iPod promises to be the golden apple for educators striving to help students keep pace. Sparking student enthusiasm through imaginative educational applications of technology, the iPod's adaptive capabilities to education are extensive. Compared to other handheld devices, it is affordable and has clones that market similar capabilities. Hitting the market in 2001, many universities and

DOI: 10.4018/978-1-61520-897-5.ch008

Copyright © 2010, IGI Global. Copying or distributing in print or electronic forms without written permission of IGI Global is prohibited.

schools began examining the iPod's educational adaptability (Bomar, 2006; French, 2006; Hastings, 2005; Vess 2006).

Teachers are being trained in educational applications of new technologies with very little time spent on mastering how to use the technology. Lennex and Nettleton's (2009) research revealed that bad technology instruction from teacher education candidates can be overcome. The iLRN model, developed by Lennex & Nettleton (2009), shows the observed effects of initial student instruction provided by the teacher. The quality of the directions determines the extent to which students depend on the teacher for further feedback and technical assistance. If a teacher is *perceived* as not understanding even a small part of the technology, Lennex (2008) discovered that P-12 students are unlikely to ask for clarification of assignments or for any further assistance. Exploration and peer coaching replaced the teacher. Teachers who encouraged this interaction discovered that this scaffolding of student knowledge produced final student projects that demonstrated higher levels of critical thinking and creativity when compared to teacher controlled projects. Using the handheld technology generated final products that exceeded project parameters (See Fiugure 1: iLRN model).

This chapter will also examine current research studies on the strengths and weaknesses of handheld technology in the educational environment and examine the technology standards for teachers and students from the International Society for Technology Education (ISTE) and the National Council for the Accreditation of Teachers (NCATE). It will provide some examples of how the iPod can be used effectively in the classroom. Based on our research into the introduction and use of the iPod in educational settings, the chapter will explore a learning dynamic that occurred when using the Apple iPod as a focal point in P-16 education.

TECHNOLOGY MISCONCEPTIONS

The focus on education should not be on the technology but the teaching that is used with it. The mythology surrounding educational technology must be eradicated. The first myth that undermines the use of technology is that students are omniscient when it comes to understanding technology. Many teachers believe that by virtue of having grown up in a technologically rich society, today's students have an innate understanding of technology. This is unfortunate because there is a digital divide between students. Access to technology is not equal throughout the United States or the world. There are areas of the country where Internet access is not available or only available through limited access. Nearly three-fourths of the American population uses the Internet on a regular basis according to the Global Information Technology Report 2008-2009 (Dutta &Mia, 2009). Yet only 50% of students have access to computers in homes or schools (Reynolds & Lennex, 2009). Complicating the issue further is the gender gap in the use of technology. The average amount of time girls spend using technology is significantly less than the amount of time boys use it. This gap widens as girls enter middle and high school (Canadian Teacher's Federation, 2003; Sanford &Madill, 2006). Even though teachers are aware that disparities exist, students are taught as if, by virtue of their age, they are proficient in technology.

In an education class, the researcher asked undergraduate teacher education candidates to brainstorm ways in which an iPod might be used as a teaching tool. These handheld devices were new to the market at the time. The researcher was explaining that her plan of allowing students to borrow the device was not practical, since the very act of hooking the iPod up to another computer and downloading material would cause the stored information to disappear. During this discussion, two or three students hastened to explain that with certain precautions, one could go from an office to home personal computer (pc) without any problems. Twenty years younger than their professor, they grew up using video games and computers. They were the digital natives. While the candidates tried to talk the researcher through the steps of how to save purchased items, four other students looked at each other in disbelief. One exclaimed, "That explains it. We didn't know *why* our iPod kept erasing itself every time we used each other's computers." Although we make characterizations of technology understanding about persons born after 1983, not all are what they seem.

In the 1970's many American public schools created elite squads of students who were trained in audio-visual media repair. These students were expected to be able to jump up and fix a filmstrip projector or movie reel at a moment's notice for their teachers. The overall assumption was that the technology was too complicated for the teachers to master, and the trained students would provide those teachers with the tech support they needed. Thirty-five years later, many teachers still turn to their students when they have questions about navigating the computer or working with new technology. Teachers expect their students to know more, merely because they are students and popular literature assures them that this is so. Klecker (2004) noted pre-service teachers who used basic computing skills such as word processing and PowerPoint, spent at least one hour per week online, and conversed mainly through e-mail communications. Lennex (2007) found that prospective incoming college freshmen looked first to the Internet to gauge program value and expected teachers to advertise courses with syllabi and supporting materials. Teacher educators increasingly look to the Internet for video and picture editing, networking, and sources of research information. Very few pre-service teachers e-mail, instead preferring mobile technologies such as texting (Britten & Clausen, 2009). Digiovanni, (2009) found that almost 100% of pre-service teachers surf the Internet regularly and 60% used iPods. This is not to say all pre-service teachers, like P-12 students, are fluent with technology. Using technology for personal purposes and using it in the classroom to support achievement of students are two completely different concepts.

Teachers do their students a disservice when they have false expectations of student skill levels. Pre-assessment of technology skills will result in clearer instruction in technology use. Teachers' assumptions can negatively impact student learning by failing to provide adequate instruction on using technology advantageously. The only way to become proficient with technology is through exploration and practice.

Teachers Using Technology

School districts have struggled to absorb the cost of placing technology in classrooms. Teacher education programs routinely include technology courses for pre-service teachers, yet there are many teachers who do not integrate technology into their lessons. Dillenbourg (2008) contends that the majority of teachers are technologically literate because society has increasingly begun to incorporate tool use in all aspects of life. It is a fallacy to believe that teachers do not know how to use technology. From iPods, e-mail, texting, blogs, Internet searches, calculators, GPS units, and video games, many forms of technology have become pervasive in society. Yet there is a disconnect between society and the classroom. Although teachers' comfort levels have increased, there is not a corresponding rise in the use of technology in the classroom.

Teacher educator professional associations, such as ISTE, established standards for technology literacy among teachers and students. In 2008, the organization revised their standards for teacher performance. The National Educational Technology Standards (NETS) for teachers states five broad standards: (1) facilitate and inspire student learning and creativity, (2) design and develop digital-age learning experiences and assessments, (3) model digital-age work and learning, (4) promote and model digital citizenship and responsibility, and (5) engage in professional growth and leadership. Standard Three, model digital-age work and learning, would directly relate to objectives of teaching with handhelds. This standard states that the "teachers exhibit knowledge, skills, and work processes representative of an innovative professional in a global and digital society." Indicators for this standard further state teachers should:

a. demonstrate fluency in technology systems and the transfer of current knowledge to new technologies and situations
b. collaborate with students, peers, parents, and community members using digital tools and resources to support student success and innovation
c. communicate relevant information and ideas effectively to students, parents, and peers using a variety of digital-age media and formats
d. model and facilitate effective use of current and emerging digital tools to locate analyze, evaluate, and use information resources to support research and learning (ISTE, 2008, paragraph 3).

ISTE is a partner for the National Council for the Accreditation of Teacher Education (NCATE). In most American colleges of education, NCATE accreditation is required to recommend candidates for teaching licenses.

The concept of using technology is inherent with some digital natives (Lennex, 2007; Lennex, 2008). At the elementary level, much depends on the level of technological activity in the home as to the expectation of use in schools. The more one uses technology in the home, the more likely a child will think it should be part of a classroom (Britten, 2009). Given that popular gaming such as Wii and Nintendo DS have spilled into many classrooms as learning tools, and social networking, such as Second Life, has become an important part of economic and social application theory, handheld technology is necessarily innovative in public schools. Most classrooms have at least one computer although its use is usually restricted to the teacher. Schools may have Internet access, but students may be restricted from using it. Many schools claim they have Internet access for students but it is not readily available. Classrooms with more than 5 or 6 computers available for students are rare. Computer lab schedules may conflict with class time and library computer stations are not available for every student. Many computers in media centers are restricted to serving as old-fashioned card catalogs, causing even fewer computers to be available for student use. The amount of time students may spend on available computers is usually limited and does not invite time for exploration. Often, students are not provided with the kind of access needed for meaningful research (Poff, 2008). It should be noted, however, that only about half of all P-12 school children have access to Internet at home (Lennex & Flynn, 2009).

Are teachers ready to teach with technology? Sometimes the schools lack appropriate technology to support teacher use and application in the classroom (Lennex, 2006). According to Koehler and Mishra (2006), we must have teachers ready to engage in technology, pedagogy, and content knowledge. The nation's teaching force creates teachers who rely primarily on the stand and deliver method of isolated teaching. In this way, every teacher is an island in his or her classroom. Each of them must somehow develop unit plans for their disciplines. While some teachers are lucky to work with teams to develop unit and lesson plans to meet state or national goals, others are left to their own devices. Teachers that are prepared to use research and theory-proven methods in the classroom are more likely to succeed in providing clear instruction with technology to students (Anthony & Coghill-Behrands, 2009; Archambault & Oh-Young, 2009).

While university and college programs should graduate teachers with an abundance of technological competency, effective teachers have mastered curricular content knowledge (Lipper, 2007). With technology, teachers can go to the Internet and pull together a lesson on any topic. Type in *Lesson Plans* on the Google search engine and in.16 seconds, 19, 300,000 sites for lesson plans will pop up. How does downloading a prepared lesson plan from the Internet differ from using lesson plans that accompany text books? Pre-service teachers must be taught to evaluate all resources, software, technologies, and instructional materials to determine their appropriateness.

Many textbooks now have online resources and activities for both teachers and students. Pre-service teachers need guidance on how to effectively adapt evaluated resources. The request for extra instructional materials primarily comes from middle school and elementary teachers who are teaching curriculum in unfamiliar content areas. When teachers do not have a firm grasp of the curriculum, their ability to discern quality materials is compromised.

One way to help teachers sort through pedagogically sound materials is to establish a professional learning community. In this model, small groups of teachers learn how to use and adapt new techniques or materials, apply them to the classroom, and then discuss their shared experiences. In a professional learning community, teachers learn from both their own experiences and that of each other.

The teacher preparation programs at many universities have begun to adapt the professional learning community model and change the way in which pre-service teachers receive professional training. Professional Development School (PDS) programs provide a supportive, practical learning environment for pre-service teachers to understand pedagogy application. After learning theory at the university, the pre-service teacher spends each week several hours learning alongside an experienced teacher. This school-university partnership provides ongoing professional development for classroom teachers, pre-service teachers, and university faculty. Working together, students are able to learn, apply, and discuss their experiences. A good PDS model includes time for pre-service teachers to become part of the community of practice in the school (Wenger, 2001), as well as developing a shared experience with other pre-service teachers.

Several PDS students recently returned from their elementary classroom, exclaiming the many ways their mentoring teachers used a Smart Board. Ironically, on the same day, a mentoring teacher raved about how much she had learned about creating specialized documents and spreadsheets from a pre-service teacher. A professional learning community may provide a venue for teachers to develop practical technological skills.

Teachers may have access to their school's intranet for storing digital materials. In many parts of the United States, schools have become paperless. This technology has not been fully utilized but has great potential once its capabilities are understood by both teachers and administrators. There are still some glitches with server crashes and inadequate back-up systems that make teachers and students nervous about total dependence on the server as a repository. Cheap flash memory drives (in some cases 4 Gb for $10) are making this much easier to overcome.

Some textbook manufacturers provide online laboratories or exercises, but true digital textbooks are not yet fully embraced by modern classrooms. Wireless e-books or Kindle-based books have not been seriously considered as a replacement for traditional books. In a model classroom where textbooks are on an e-book reader, information could be kept current through regular updates. The costs could be nominal compared to a hardcover textbook.

The cost, installation, and maintenance of

technology effects utilization of technology. Districts, schools, and teachers have limited budgets. Hirsch (2005) suggests that schools should take advantage of the technological devices students already are using and, as a cost saving measure, adapt them for instructional use. Few schools have taken advantage of the *One Laptop per Child* notebook (OLPC). This handheld is very cost-effective [around $100 per unit] and is being used in third world countries to provide basic networking and computing programs. The vision of OLPC is to bring educational opportunities to all children and their teachers. Netbooks also provide cheap, efficient Internet access. The scaled-down computer laptop is highly competitive at around $250. It has less storage capacity, but wonderfully provides what most people need: Internet access. There are a number of other inexpensive laptops that consumers are looking toward in purchasing technology for their school-age children.

Teachers with strong content knowledge will usually be able to determine the best software for the goals and objectives of a unit. The use of that technology depends on the comfort level of the teacher. One important technology issue for teachers is the question of support. Has the teacher been taught to troubleshoot for minor problems? How much support does the school provide if technology fails? How much time should be devoted to creating back-up plans? If software or peripherals are adopted, who then maintains them? Using handhelds and wireless technologies is more of a boon to schools because they are easier to store and monitor. Even without adequate support, teachers are urged to use technology in their classrooms.

Project Dataseam is an initiative from the Brown Cancer Research Center in Louisville, Kentucky. The initiative is funded through the Department of Commercialization and Innovation within the Kentucky Cabinet for Economic Development and the Kentucky Department of Education. It is designed to provide educational resources to coal producing counties as part of the coal severance funding. These monies help provide school districts in those counties with low cost Macintosh-based computers. Schools must agree to pay for the training of teachers and leave the computers "on" when not in use. The Brown Cancer Center in Louisville, Kentucky, uses the computer networks at night, when schools are closed, to process data. To date, more than 6,000 processors work in the evening, when schools are closed, to analyze cancer research data for the Center.

According to a pre and post technology readiness survey conducted (N=980) of Dataseam workshop participants, 92% of teachers believed student performance was enhanced by technology use. In the post surveys, participants indicated that they would like to have more targeted content training. They would like more make-it and take-it or ready-made activities to use in their classrooms. Themes for technology professional development echo this sentiment (Koehler & Mishra, 2006; Kress & Silva, 2009). Teachers do not see themselves as having the creativity or the time available to create curriculum supportive technological instructional materials.

Collegiate level teacher educators do not prepare teacher education candidates to find information for every aspect of their content knowledge, pedagogy, and technology integration. Expert discipline knowledge does not naturally translate into technology integration competency. College instructors do not focus on instructional technology. Teachers entering into a modern classroom may have been trained in technology skills rather than specific technologies. Traditional pre-service teachers are more likely to be goal and achievement oriented.

Because technology and software are frequently upgraded and dramatically alter their capabilities every few years, teachers need to relearn technology, upgrade teaching methods, and adapt new software. As technologies evolve, teachers will find better instructional programs. For teachers to use technology as an instructional tool, professional development must be conducted

Table 1. Pre and post survey results from Dataseam workshop surveys, 2005-2008

	Strongly Disagree	Disagree	Agree	Strongly Agree	Yes	No
PRE SURVEY RESULTS						
I believe that learning with technology enhances student performance.	24	2	234	645		
I am likely to seek out opportunities for students to use technology for learning.	24	16	324	522		
I am likely to use the new Apple computers with my students.	28	51	349	459		
I am primarily here because my attendance was mandated.	309	316	188	95		
Have you had any previous Apple Macintosh training?					245	558
POST SURVEY RESULTS						
I believe that learning with technology enhances student performance.	4	3	269	637		
I am likely to seek out opportunities for students to use technology for learning.	4	6	320	587		
I am likely to use the new Apple computers with my students.	7	10	325	572		

more effectively. In many schools, successful integration of instructional technology is dependent on the social climate. Schools where teachers are encouraged to experiment with alterative teaching methods must accept that there will be a learning curve for teachers. The current driven atmosphere of student achievement through accountability testing can create a culture where teachers are afraid to use technology because it is viewed as a time-waster. Neither teachers nor students are given time to explore and become proficient with new technologies.

In some content areas, the use of technology may be tied to learning and achievement. Mathematics is one discipline where handheld technology has become an integral part of the discipline. Students and teachers use handheld devices in many forms, including graphing calculators and iPods. The iPod is relatively new. Educational uses are still being investigated. Although its technical capabilities can be matched with other devices: Camera, voice recorder, CD player, and video player, its mobility is what causes it to be an exceptional educational tool. Pre-service teachers, after tutoring students for several weeks, created a list of ways the iPod might be used to help students learn more effectively.

1. Create a picture file of famous people, events, places, etc. (Social Studies and Art)
2. Record step by step instructions for a project. Download pictures of each step so students can compare their project with the directions. (All subject areas)
3. Download pictures so that they can be shown on a television in order to enlarge it for a visually impaired child. (All subject areas)
4. Teachers and parents can keep in touch each day by using the voice recorder instead of writing notes and making phone calls. (All subject areas, especially English)
5. Record the teacher working examples for students so they can visually see the steps. Record the directions orally at the same time. (Science and Mathematics)
6. Students will record themselves reading a written piece aloud. (All subject areas)

Teachers not only must learn to use such devices as an instructional tool, they must also learn to effectively train their students to use the devices. When teachers do not fully comprehend the capabilities inherent in a device, they are reluctant to use it with their students.

Student Instruction

Teachers must have sound pedagogical practice (Gagne, 1965) regardless of the instructional tools they wish to employ. Lessons should have definable goals, objectives, and appropriate assessments for students. The types of technology teachers choose to implement must be based on the achievement of learning goals by students. Learning obstacles may arise when employing new technology and teachers must be aware of problems that may occur. Teachers must be comfortable teaching with a technology.

Often, students' misinterpretation of instruction is based on their perceptions of teacher knowledge. Educators unwittingly widen this divide by their own comments, such as, "I don't know much about how this technology works" or "Let me double check the instructions and make sure we aren't going to break something." In a more situational way, classrooms are their own social unit in which rules and behaviors are defined by circumstance. The classroom develops what Nardi and O'Day (2002) call an informational ecology; an "information ecology... [composed of] people, practices, values, and technologies." (p.49). This framework examines how people adapt and interact with technology. A teacher with strong pedagogical and content knowledge may have difficulty instructing digital natives if they perceive the teacher to be less than fluent (Koehler & Mishra, 2006).

The iLRN Model

Soviet psychologist Lev Vygotsky (1978) created a theoretical framework that suggested that tools and signage (language, number systems) mediated activities. Development, or learning, occurred through the activity that took place in a social context that influenced the learner. Leontiev extended Vygotsky's work and developed a triangular model to conceptualize human activity. In this model, the tool, the subject [the person interacting with the tool] and the object [purpose for the activity] all impact each other. (Benson, Lewler, & Whitworth, 2008; Hasan, 2001; Kuutti, 1996; Nardi, 1996; Yamagata-Lynch. 2007; Zurita & Nussbaum, 2007). At one corner of Leontiev's model,rests the purpose of the activity; the object. In another corner rests the subject; the person who handles the tool in some form, all of which are intermingled to provide an outcome.

Engstrom developed the analytical framework even further by introducing another layer of analysis over Leontiev's. His additions include a deeper examination of the activity mediated by the tools through examining the context of the activity. These new additions include consideration of the rules surrounding the activity, the roles of the participants in the activity, and the people involved in the activity (Kuutti, 1996; Nardi, 1996; Zurita & Nussbaum, 2007). The contextual factors surrounding the use of technology are very important to the learning that occurs. Vygotsky identified a crucial learning step between levels of development that he dubbed the zone of proximal development (ZPD). This zone is "the distance between the actual development as determined by independent problem solving and the level of potential development as determined through problem solving under adult guidance or in collaboration with more capable peers" (p. 86). However, unlike Piaget (Charles, 1974), who believed the individual moved to the next developmental level *after* learning occurred, Vygotsky believed that learning occurred *after* moving to the next level (Gredler, 2005).

Although Vygotsky stressed the teacher-student relationship in proximal development learning (Gredler, 2005) knowledgeable peers can provide guidance from one level to the next. Vygotsky (1978) believed that the teacher was the more influential of the two. At the most basic level, a teacher is one who imparts instruction, based on expert knowledge of the discipline being studied. However, when it comes to technology the assumption has been made by both school administrators and teachers that students are more knowledgeable; that technology is for the young. This myth is still being passed from school to school. Just as playing an instrument or learning a new skill takes time and practice, so too, does learning to use technology with ease. Teachers must learn to not only use technology, but to adapt it to meet instructional needs.

Applicable Activity Learning Models

Within a single grade level classroom, children exhibit a great deal of variation in what they learn. Through observation and data collection, teachers regularly adjust the curriculum and teaching strategies to be most effective for their students (Dillenbourg, 2008). Making adjustments for students is part of the culture building process for the classroom. Together, teachers and students create a language for learning that is unique to their classroom. Shared activities and experiences also help build a unique and nurturing learning environment. This construction of a classroom culture creates a learning climate that provides opportunities for students to learn from each other as well as the teacher. The teacher's role in allowing this to occur is crucial to ensuring that learning is occurring at several levels. For example, the researcher's fifth grade students were asked to create a PowerPoint presentation on the Civil War. The researcher had little experience with this technology. Students were provided with minimal technical instruction, and were encouraged to develop technology skills by imitating and learning from each other. On presentation day, the Power Points whistled, flashed, and sang. Mastery of the learning necessary for the manipulation of technology was impressive. The time these students spent exploring and sharing in the computer lab allowed them to develop valuable technological skills.

Teachers who assign projects or problems with rigid criteria, will find that final projects will have a cookie cutter quality to them. Jonessen (2002; 2000) suggests that projects or problems must be ill-defined or ill-structured for student learning to occur. Teachers using Janesson's ill-structured approach expect student work to be more creative. It is the difference between an art project in which everyone glues down the same five shapes to make the same picture and another in which students create their own shapes and pictures. The teacher must create a classroom climate where students feel free to take risks. While the teacher may create or shape the environment, peer interaction has an even stronger effect on student learning and creativity. Student imitation of more capable peers often leads to projects that far exceed the instructor's criteria. The interaction between students and the teacher's ability to create an accepting learning environment directly affects the creativity and learning of students.

In the researcher's first year of teaching, she created *Share Day*; a monthly project designed to help students break down research projects into small, easily managed sections. Each month, fifth grade students were asked to create a project based on a different aspect of a country they were assigned to research. The teacher deliberately assigned projects that went from being highly structured in September to being more flexible and open-ended by the end of the year. The initial success of Share Day led her to continue refining and assigning the projects for several years. Jonassen's (1999) problem based learning model provides students with a problem that is not clearly defined so students will learn through their experiences. The instructor scaffolds lessons to provide the learners with the information they need at the appropriate time. The students construct learning through their own problem solving. The teacher collected some interesting data that suggested ways in which creativity was transmitted from student to student. If at least three projects in the first two assignments were presented to the class with any sign of creativity [a flag made of tissue paper flowers or a puffy paint map with jewels marking important towns], an exponential growth of creativity in student projects was charted during the succeeding months. Not only did gifted and average students develop their creative skills, but special education students also improved as a result of the collective experience. By the end of the year, many special education students earned a reputation for their creativity. On the other hand, if the first few assigned projects did not extend beyond the teacher's parameters, the students never developed their creativity. Without peer examples, the spark did not emerge throughout the year. Open-ended projects and teacher encouragement were not enough to off set lack of positive peer examples.

Vygotsky (1978) believed that collective activity would be beneficial for children who struggled with learning and that appeared to be the case in the teacher's classroom. The differences in student products from year to year appeared to be directly linked to students' imitations of their peers. The teacher approached the projects with the same suggestions and ideas each year. The variable was the number of students in the classroom willing to take risks with the assignment. If a peer did not emerge in the class to lead the way, the students never seemed to develop projects that were more than adequate for the assignment. The difference in the caliber of the projects was the difference between a student draping a desk with a string of colored Christmas lights, slapping a metal colander on his head, and blasting off through time to share the historical events in Germany compared to the student who read aloud a report taken from an encyclopedia. It appeared that there had to be a creative peer at the next level of development in order for movement to occur. The iLRN model (See Fiugure 1) demonstrates how teacher *and* peer interaction may have an effect on student learning.

According to Bielaczyc and Collins (1999), when teachers use learning communities in the classroom, student learning occurs as a result of shared knowledge. Through working in small groups, students will contribute their varied background knowledge to solving the task and the result is improved understanding by each member. An important aspect of Bielaczyc and Collin's theory of collaborative learning is the teacher's role in the purposeful development of the community. Instructors design problems that require students to work together and share information. Rather than individual learning being the focal point, lessons are designed for group instruction.

While B.F. Skinner's theory of behaviorism might attribute changes in student output to the effect of shaping through the application of the appropriate stimuli (Gredler, 2005), the results seem to be more indicative of imitation and the development of classroom culture. Whether or not creativity may be taught, certainly the freedom for creative exploration can be taught and imitated. While each year a random sampling of students per grade level might indicate that students were at the same development level, their levels of potential development, as evidenced by the products they produced, would show wide variations in mental age. In the classroom it was not the teacher-student interaction that created the leaps, but the student-student-teacher interactions. The teacher must create a classroom culture where student exchanges are encouraged. Vess (2006) wrote, "When applications are based on solid learning theory and designed with appropriate outcomes in mind, they can transform the educational experience for students, build communities of learners, promote more active engagement or materials, and achieve the (essential) learning outcomes" (p. 479). Teachers must analyze the goal and purpose for using technology as an instructional tool. Both Jonnessen and Bielaczc and Collins have developed instructional design models that offer a framework for student learning within a social context, but with each, the teacher orchestrates (Dillenbourg, 2002) the educational experience. The instructor is in control and tweaks the environment to enhance learning

Individuals respond within their limited perceptions to the needs of their cultural environment. The cultural norm for schools is that students behave in different patterns when responding to the teacher and to each other. Benedict (1934) speaks of the individual contributing to the whole cultural product in such a way that the culture is differentially enhanced. If everyone behaved as society norms and mores dictated, then culture would not change. Dramatic changes occur in classrooms as a result of charismatic individuals determining the priorities and products of the teacher's lesson objectives. Malinowski (1944) states that "changes in behavior, and thus in cultural functioning, occur as a result of derivation of unique needs" (p. 38).

As societies change and the collective begins to use new technological products, a greater need to incorporate norms and mores governing the behaviors and teaching of the products occurs. Organization regarding these norms and mores within culture governs the extent to which teacher educators prepare teacher education candidates to use the technology products in future classrooms. Malinowski (1944) believes that a cultural need becomes a "limiting' factor within a group" (p. 90). The way(s) in which that need is met is determined by the socially acceptable parameters of the given situation. In the case of schools, students are supposed to look to their teacher for organization and guidance with lessons. The teacher (Gagne, 1965) leads the classroom with an organized thought toward objectives and assessments to meet curricular goals. If the teacher has a clear content lead, but an unclear technological lead, what then happens to her audience of students? The researchers discovered students, armed with their own cultural norms and mores regarding technology, began to lead themselves toward classroom learning (Collins, 2004; Kress & Silva 2009).

The iLRN model was developed based on the interactions of students, in grades P-12, in reaction to handheld technology based learning. Students used a variety of handhelds [i.e. iPods, laptops, graphing calculator] in learning situations. Teachers gave instructions regarding content and products for daily lessons. However, the students began to develop behaviors inconsistent with teacher directions. Student leaders emerged from the random, heterogeneous groupings. This leadership did not appear dependent on social standing. Through the analysis of digital tapes, students can clearly be seen to fixate on the actions and words of student leaders. This fixation is called "entrainment." Collins (2004) describes entrainment as "an emotional energy that excites a social situation to the point of synchronous thought and action" (p. 49). Students develop their own sense of place within the group context. Some are leaders only in this situation, while others may have a charismatic presence that causes followers to perform actions related to the group. As Durkheim (2003), Foucault (1994), and Goffman (1963) have described with representation of self and interaction ritual (IR), one may represent an ideal only within a group at a given moment.

Collins (2004) has identified markers within IR that indicate charismatic leading. These markers include pitch of voice, synchronization of movement, alternating speech, and even laughing. If one likes the other member(s) of conversation, the results will occur at split second timing. For example, students might receive new information and simulations through the handheld technology but the actual socialization of repetitive use occurs with cultural interaction among peers. Ritual interaction (Collins, 2004) occurs "when focus on an artifact or verbalization occurs among two or more people" (p. 48). This focus is communicated within the social grouping and group participants are recognized.

The iLRN Model in Practice with Handhelds

The iPod is an example of an available handheld technology whose capabilities are not fully understood by students or teachers. The Apple iPod

Figure 1. The iLRN model

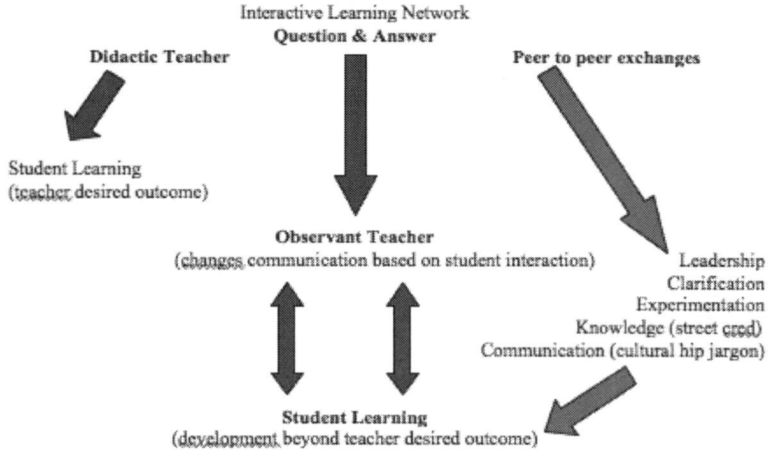

hit the market in 2001. Over the last few years it has quickly evolved to include many features. It is a small handheld device that provides a portable platform for recording sound, music, data, and visuals. Early attempts to use the iPod as a classroom technology were focused on specific course assignments. Read (2005) wrote that iPods were used as a recording device for interviews. It was also used as a platform to download music to put in the library on reserve for a music class (Stephens, 2005). Another use for the iPod was to gather audio book downloads for students to listen to in their spare time. The iPod provides an easy way for students to listen to audio books. The teacher might download one story at a time or several chapters of a textbook on the iPod. Students may listen to the iPod as they read along with the story. The playback rate can be adjusted to match student speed. (Bomar, 2006).

When teacher education candidates use an iPod as a part of their instruction with P-12 students, they may not be providing accurate instructional information of the device. The iLRN model, developed by Lennex and Nettleton (2009), demonstrates teacher and student interactions. The model revealed that poor technology instruction from teacher education candidates could be overcome within the classroom environment. In this model, the teacher provides initial student instruction. The quality of the directions determines the extent to which students depend on the teacher for further feedback and technical assistance. If a teacher is *perceived* as not understanding even a small part of the technology, Lennex (2008) discovered that P-12 students are unlikely to ask for clarification of assignments or for any further assistance. Exploration and peer coaching replaced the teacher. Teachers who encouraged this interaction discovered that this scaffolding of student knowledge produced final student projects that demonstrated higher levels of critical thinking and creativity when compared to teacher controlled projects. Using the handheld technology generated final products that exceeded project parameters. When the teacher discouraged peer interactions or exploration of the handheld device, final outcomes were sterile and limited to fulfilling the teacher's request. The iLRN model demonstrates the influence of peer social context on Vygotsky's zone of proximal development, The ZPD is the knowledge to be gained through interaction with teachers, peers, and others (Bransford & Cocking, 2000). In the case of learning with handheld technology, this is exclusively among peers. The following case studies demonstrate teacher education candidates (TEC) and student interactions among P-12 populations.

In Case 1 (see Table 2: Art instruction case study), the TEC introduced handheld technology to fourth graders. The students were supposed to take still pictures with a smart stik and digital video camera. The purpose was to create still images for an interpretation of *Jack and Beanstalk*. The interaction between the teacher and students indicated that the teacher did not know how to operate the camera beyond basic functions. Quickly there was a problem with the technology.

The TEC in this case study did not appear to be comfortable with technology, yet produced through the use of an online service, a stop-motion video from a combination of the student's smart stiks. Students were successful in creating pictures not because of the teacher's instruction, but rather through the iLRN model.

Case 2 (see Table 3: Elementary school case study) presents children in grades one through five being introduced to iPods in a non-classroom situation. Groups consisted of homerooms which cycled among various booths every ten to fifteen minutes. In this interaction, the groups of children were given two video iPods (vPod) which contained, in a videos folder, a video produced by the school principal. One audio iPod classic was also used for music only. While the children were quite interested in the workings of the iPods, the teachers were constantly taking the devices from children. The teachers admitted to the researcher that they were afraid the children would break the vPods. The teachers stated "they were not familiar with iPods," and "the kids did not use technology regularly." The teachers were also obviously trepidatious about letting the children have experiential learning with iPods.

Handheld technology is a tool to help education occur (Koehler & Mishra, 2006). Teachers and students need to become technically competent on devices in order to use them most effectively. The steps of development and the study of the capabilities of the technology are important. Developing a unit of study where the technology becomes a tool instead of the centerpiece relies on the teacher thoroughly understanding the technology. Once the teacher becomes comfortable with the technology, then it can be harnessed for use in the classroom. Of course, not all students want to jump into using technology. Some students prefer to watch while others want their hands on the technology. Peer interaction can lead the way for learning.

CONCLUSION

Students demonstrate good use of technology through sheer curiosity. Teachers are leaders in the classroom (Gagne, 1965), but their leadership must be based on understanding what direction they are leading their students. In studies with iPods, students in grades one through eight often attempt to use technology in non-familiar ways. If a teacher is present, students will sometimes ask about particular functions or how to achieve certain products.

Lowther, Ross, and Morrison (2003) conducted a study to examine the use of laptops in the classroom. Teachers involved in the pilot study received over fifty hours of specialized training and were relatively comfortable with computers. Classroom students leased laptops for $50.00 per month. In the control groups, the classrooms had five to six computers and the teachers did not receive training. After a year, the students using the laptops were more comfortable using computers and their writing scores improved. The teachers were all positive about the experience. In the control groups, students enjoyed computer use but their writing scores had not increased as much as the laptop group. The non-laptop teachers wanted more computers in their classroom in order to provide students with a better computer/student ratio (Lowther, Ross, & Morrison, 2003). The more time people spend interacting with

Table 2. Art instruction case study

Minutes into lesson	Observed Behavior	Interpretation
Before lesson	The TEC did not set up the digital video cameras in preparation for students to use with smart stiks.	TEC either did not pre-plan or does not know how to set up the cameras.
2:00	The lesson began and many hands go up as questions are asked. In front of the class, the TEC explained to the Videographer (V) that the class was working on plot and asked V to set up the cameras.	Students might see TEC as not knowing how to set up the video cameras or as unprepared
6:30	Students begin taking pictures of scenes and place scene materials.	
11:20	Student B attempts to use camera but the smart stik is full. V is approached by the TEC and asked what to do, " I do not know how to erase card images." The videotape is turned off until 13:09 to accommodate erasing card images on all cameras.	Student perception of TEC as incompetent with technology is reinforced.
13:09	Student B's Group: B does most of the clay manipulation	After smart stiks were cleared, it appeared to researcher that TEC had competence of the technology. However, the teacher does not manifest confidence beyond basic functions of the technology. Clearly taking pictures was the objective, but students were teaching each other more than they were asking questions of the teacher.
14:00	B joins another group. Girl, W, is carefully pushing photo button.	
14:44	W explains to R. "You've got to hit photo... yeah that's right... you just took a picture." W is looking into the view screen as he affirms a picture is taken. B gets up to look at camera and screen. B tells R, "No, wait." B holds R's right elbow. W continues to explain procedure. R looks uncertain about what is happening. S pays no attention to discussion and continues working with clay models.	In both instances, students were peer teaching. One student acts as the leader while others seek their advice before continuing with the activity. At no time is the TEC asked by this group or affirmation or continuation of either the technology or the clay manipulation.
14:54	Group 2: Girl, Q, kneels on top of table so she can reach the camera buttons. She asks the TEC circulating through the room about how to take the picture. TEC touches button with eraser, saying, "You just push the button for a picture."	Student asks TEC for technology information. TEC gives instruction on how to take a picture with the video camera. For one minute, students in this group ask TEC about both technology and clay manipulation.
14:55	Q uses her pencil to touch the button and asks, "Like that?" TEC responds, "Yeah, now take the picture." TEC reminds the group she wants everyone to get a chance to take a picture. TEC leaves the group.	
15:20	Boy, Z, takes a picture, climbs on to table, and then smiles at result.	
15:48	Boy, X, changes scene and stands, then leans to take picture. Smiles at result.	
16:14	Girl, E, walks up to box with her arms folded and forgets to change scene. Classmates remind her. She starts to take picture. Girl, F, looking through the view screen, looks at it and says, "Yeah, take that, it's good." E takes the pictures and smiles broadly.	The students have been peer teaching on the technology and clay manipulation. The students appear to be rapidly changing strategies to acquire the best photos.
16:36	Girl G looks at screen and smiles, "That's good." G takes picture and giggles, then smiles broadly as she leaves the camera.	

continued on following page

Table 2. continued

Minutes into lesson	Observed Behavior	Interpretation
16:59	Z is back on the table, trying to look at view screen. He uses his left hand cupped above the screen to cut the glare. Another student, J, tries to stop him from looking at camera.	Z does not touch the view screen to move it to decrease the glare. It appears to be an attempt by J to keep Z from harming their photos, or the camera. Students appeared to be taking well-being responsibility for the technology equipment.
17:19	F tells the others to change the claymation action and then she takes a picture.	
17:57	Back to Group 1: The group and TEC are checking out their pictures. B makes an "ooh" sound and widens eyes.	B is clearly pleased with progress. She has moved among three groups in this session.
18:49	Girl, M, asks TEC how to do something with images on smart stik. TEC puts fingers to mouth, eyes droopy and says, "I don't know how to do that, I'm sorry." TEC moves to another group at table.	No instruction given to girl by TEC. TEC is reinforcing her inability to work with the technology. In this case, TEC appeared to know how to manipulate but chose not to teach students. Student cannot proceed with desired photo manipulation.

Table 3. Elementary school case study

Minutes into taping	Observed Behavior	Interpretation
45:58	Boy 1 gains control of vPod after discussing with Boy 2. They both share ear buds.	
46:06	Teacher is holding vPod for Boy 3. Presenter tells teacher, "Oh they can hold it." Teacher asks, "Are you sure?" Presenter replies, "Yes. They're pretty sturdy… just don't put them in the washing machine." Presenter smiles broadly. Boy 3 does not manipulate controls but watches the video, as do two other classmates.	Teacher is afraid technology will be broken.
46:30	Boy 1 hands vPod to Boy 4.	
46:36	Boy 4 takes out ear bud. Boy 2 offers an earbud to Boy 3.	
47:10	Teacher takes vPod away from the Boys 2, 3, & 4. Teacher is blinking heavily, holding lips tightly, and grasping vPod until knuckles whitened.	Teacher is tense and worried about the technology breaking. Students have not been provided with any chance to manipulate or explore the technology and its capabilities.
47:52	Teacher hands the presenter a vPod. Immediately seven hands go up and children say "I haven't seen it."	Teacher would like to omit the worry of technology breaking or responsibility of technology. Presenter has assured her of technology sturdiness but teacher appeared to be nervous.
47:55	Teacher leaves the group.	Teacher left group without saying anything to students or presenter. She returned within a few seconds to take the group elsewhere.
48:00	A child said, "it's [the vPod] off." Presenter tells children to, "Push the big round button in middle…it will usually take you right back to where you were."	The students rarely asked for assistance in using the vPods. Unless forced to restrain themselves, students plunged forward and attempted to use the devices. They are an intuitive device that facilitates student learning.

a technology in this case computers, the more comfortable and proficient they will be with the technology (Lowther & Morrison, 1998). The difference in teacher training is significant, because it provides another variable that quite possibly may have impacted this research. The fact that the laptop teachers received intensive training before students began their year using laptops seriously impacted their teaching strategies and their lesson design. "Properly designed podcasts may become another effective tool for students using them in a particular way" (French, 2006, p. 58).

FUTURE DIRECTIONS

The learning theories developed using video iPods (i.e. iPod classics) in education could be expanded to all handheld technologies. It is safe to say that portable technology is the future of schools. Standard technology is too expensive, is too bulky and is not functional for the thin client needs of today's students. The memory capacity and speed of many traditional desktops or even laptops is far below that of available mobile technology. As educators we should strive to provide the best educational supports for the curriculum. Like Atalanta, focusing on the golden apples, educators can bring focus to the curriculum with handheld technologies, like the iPod. The iTouch is the latest classroom friendly version of the iPod. Although the iTouch is Internet capable, most schools have restricted or password protected access to the Internet. Several hours of video and text information can be stored onto the iTouch to be used in classroom interactions.

Teacher training should include not only information on basic uses of instructional technology, but also the means by which to allow students to work well in conjunction with the technology. Teacher educators must undertake technology competence. While content knowledge gives curriculum a good foundation, teacher support of curriculum through technology products is often quite basic. The training omits much on the varied uses of the software.

Teacher education must change to meet the needs of our future learners. College classes and the way in which they are delivered must also change. By the end of the last century, technology courses were viewed as obsolete. The "teach how to use an overhead" courses became absorbed or eliminated. Teacher education courses should follow a PDS model in that teacher education candidates at all levels are regularly included in classroom instruction in order to teach technology use and support. This inclusion, when properly supervised and guided, will lead to greater confidence in classroom management and innovation. TEC's should have scaffolded field experiences beginning from teacher education program entrance. The nature of constructive learning should also include basic technological skills and their application in the classroom. Technology is a support to curriculum. In a PDS, the TEC would be working continuously in a classroom and would become more familiar with the school's technology capabilities. The TEC would also have more feedback from mentors on their use of technology to support curriculum. The guidance of mentors should include analysis of assessment both with and without technology supports. A Teacher Productivity Assessment (TPA) or similar method of analyzing a unit's goals, methods, individual and collective student needs, and overall performance should be included for each semester of PDS field experience.

REFERENCES

Anthony, R., & Coghill-Behrends, W. (2009). Teachers of the future: Report on a national survey. In C. Crawford et al. (Eds.), *Proceedings of Society for Information Technology and Teacher Education International Conference 2009* (pp. 1696-1697). Chesapeake, VA: AACE.

Archambault, L., & Oh-Young, C. (2009). Putting the T in PCK: exploring the nature of the TPCK framework among K-12 online educators. In C. Crawford et al. (Eds.), *Proceedings of Society for Information Technology and Teacher Education International Conference 2009* (pp. 4008-4014). Chesapeake, VA: AACE.

Benedict, R. (1934). *Patterns of culture*. Boston: Houghton Mifflin Company.

Benson, A., Lewler, C., & Whitworth, A. (2008). Rules, roles, and tools: Activity theory and the comparative study of e-learning. *British Journal of Educational Technology, 39*(3), 456–467. doi:10.1111/j.1467-8535.2008.00838.x

Bielaczyc, K., & Collins, A. (1999). Learning communities in classrooms: A reconceptualization of educational practice. In Reigeluth, C. M. (Ed.), *Instructional-design theories and models: A new paradigm of instructional theory* (2nd ed., pp. 269–292). Mahwah, NJ: Lawrence Erlbaum Associates.

Bomar, L. (2006). iPods as Reading Tools. *Principal, 85*(5), 52–53.

Bransford, J., Brown, A., & Cocking, R. (2000). *How People Learn: Brain, Mind, and Experience & school*. Washington, DC: National Academy Press.

Britten, J., & Clausen, J. (2009). Using what they bring with them. In C. Crawford et al. (Eds.), *Proceedings of Society for Information Technology and Teacher Education International Conference 2009* (pp. 1744-1747). Chesapeake, VA: AACE.

Britten, J., Estridge, M., Volmer, K., & Clausen, J. (2009). The digital natives are speaking. In C. Crawford et al. (Eds.), *Proceedings of Society for Information Technology and Teacher Education International Conference 2009* (pp. 1741-1743). Chesapeake, VA: AACE.

Canadian Teacher's Federation. (2003). *Kids take on media: Summary of finding*. Retrieved January 15, 2007, from www.ctf-ee.ca/en/projects/MERP/summaryfindingd.pdf

Charles, C. M. (1974). *Teacher's petite Piaget*. Belmont, CA: David S. Lake Publishers.

Collins, R. (2004). *Interaction Ritual Chains*. Princeton, NJ: Princeton University Press.

Digiovanni, L., Schwartz, S., & Greer, C. (2009). I think, iPod(cast), I learn: using digital media and podcasting in teacher education. In C. Crawford et al. (Eds.), *Proceedings of Society for Information Technology and Teacher Education International Conference 2009* (pp. 1812-1819). Chesapeake, VA: AACE.

Dillenbourg, P. (2008). Integrating technologies into educational ecosystems. *Distance Education, 29*(2), 127–140. doi:10.1080/01587910802154939

Durkheim, E., & Emirbrayer, M. (2003). *Sociologist of modernity*. San Francisco: Wiley-Blackwell.

Dutta, S., & Mia, I. (2009). *The global information technology report 2008-2009*. Retrieved April 1, 2009, from http://www.insead.edu/v1/gitr/wef/main/fullreport/index.html

Foucault, M. (1994). *The Order of Things: An Archaeology of the Human Sciences*. New York: Vintage Books.

French, D. (2006). iPods: informative or invasive? *Journal of College Science Teaching, 36*(1), 58–59.

Gagne, R. (1985). *The Conditions of Learning and the Theory of Instruction* (4th ed.). New York: Holt, Rinehart, and Winston.

Goffman, E. (1963). *Stigma: notes on the management of spoiled identity*. New York: Prentice Hall.

Gredler, M. E. (2005). *Learning and instruction - theory into practice*. Upper Saddle River, NJ: Pearson Education, Inc.

Hasan, H. (2001). An overview of techniques for applying activity theory to information systems. In H. Hasan, E. Gould, & P. Larkin (Eds.), Information systems and activity theory: Vol. 2, Theory and practice (pp. 2-33). New South Wales, Australia: Wollongong University Press.

Hastings, N., & Tracey, M. (2005). Does media affect learning? Where are we now? *TechTrends*, *49*(2), 28–30. doi:10.1007/BF02773968

Hirsch, J. (2005). Applying Students' Own Devices in the Classroom. [from Education Full Text database.]. *School Administrator*, *62*(10), 8. Retrieved February 27, 2007.

ISTE. (2008). *International Society for Technology Education teacher standards*. Retrieved April 10, 2009, from http://www.iste.org/Content/NavigationMenu/NETS/ForTeachers/2008Standards/NETS_ or_Teachers_2008.htm

Jonassen, D. (2000). Instructional design model for well-structured and ill-structured problem solving learning outcomes. *Educational Technology Research and Development*, *45*(1), 65–95. doi:10.1007/BF02299613

Jonassen, D. H. (1999). Designing constructivist learning environments. In Reigeluth, C. M. (Ed.), *Instructional Theories and Models: A New Paradigm of Instructional Theory* (2nd ed., pp. 215–239). Mahwah, NJ: Lawrence Erlbaum Associates.

Jonassen, D. H. (2002). Integration of problem solving into instructional design. In Reiser, R. A., & Dempsey, J. V. (Eds.), *Instructional Design and Technology* (pp. 107–122). Upper Saddle River, NJ: Merrill Prentice Hall.

Klecker, B., Lennex L., & Lackner, K. (2004). *Evaluating the integration of technology in a teacher preparation program*. (ERIC Document Reproduction Service No. ED 481667).

Koehler, M., & Mishra, P. (2006). Introducing tpck. In AACTE committee on innovation and technology (Eds.), Handbook of technological pedagogical content knowledge (tpck) for educators (pp. 3-31). London: Routledge Press.

Kress, T., & Silva, K. (2009). Using digital video for professional development and leadership: understanding and initiating teacher learning communities, In C. Crawford et al. (Eds.), *Proceedings of Society for Information Technology and Teacher Education International Conference 2009* (pp. 2841-2847). Chesapeake, VA: AACE.

Kuutti, K. (1996). Activity theory as a potential framework for human-computer interaction research. In

Lennex, L. (2006). Is this on the test? Technology integration perception in teacher education classes. In C. Crawford et al. (Eds.), *Proceedings of Society for Information Technology and Teacher Education International Conference 2006* (pp. 1695-1700). Chesapeake, VA: AACE.

Lennex, L. (2007). The faculty Web page: contrivance or continuation? *TechTrends*, *51*(5), 32–37. doi:10.1007/s11528-007-0067-z

Lennex, L. (2008). Digital natives and the use of video iPods: a Lewis and Clark expedition. In C. Crawford et al. (Eds.), *Proceedings of Society for Information Technology and Teacher Education International Conference 2008* (pp. 4913-4915). Chesapeake, VA: AACE.

Lennex, L., & Flynn, H. (2009). Wisely using cyberspace: needs analysis of P-12 teacher Web pages. In C. Crawford et al. (Eds.), *Proceedings of Society for Information Technology and Teacher Education International Conference 2009* (pp. 3473-3480). Chesapeake, VA: AACE.

Lennex, L., & Nettleton, K. (2009). *Ipods & the iLRN theory: A new vision for classroom Connections*. Unpublished raw data.

Lipper, D., & Sagehorn, E. (2007). How to hire tech-savvy teachers. Interactive educator, (Winter), 28-32.

Lowther, D., & Morrison, G. (1998). The NTeQ model: a framework for technology integration. [from Education Full Text database.]. *TechTrends*, *43*, 33–38. Retrieved April 9, 2009. doi:10.1007/BF02818173

Lowther, D., Ross, S., & Morrison, G. (2003). When Each One Has One: The Influences on Teaching Strategies and Student Achievement of Using Laptops in the Classroom. [from Education Full Text database.]. *Educational Technology Research and Development*, *51*(3), 23–44. Retrieved April 9, 2009. doi:10.1007/BF02504551

Malinowski, B. (1944). *A scientific theory of culture and other essays*. Chapel Hill, NC: University of North Carolina Press.

Nardi, B. (Ed.), *Context and consciousness: Activity theory and human-computer interaction* (pp. 17–44). Cambridge, MA: MIT Press.

Nardi, B. A. (1996). Activity theory and human-computer interaction. In Nardi, B. A. (Ed.), *Context and Consciousness* (pp. 7–16). Cambridge, MA: The MIT Press.

Nardi, B. A., & O'Day, V. L. (1999). *Information ecologies: Using technology with heart*. Cambridge, MA: The MIT Press.

One Laptop per Child (OLPC). (n.d.). Retrieved April 2, 2009, from http://www.laptop.org/en/?gclid=CPi7w_y72pkCFQ9JagodgnhNXw

Poff, J. (2008 December). Don't void our voices. *Edutopia*, 10.

Read, B. (2005). Duke U. Assess iPod Experiment and Finds It Worked--in Some Courses. [from Education Full Text database.]. *The Chronicle of Higher Education*, *51*(43), A28. Retrieved February 27, 2007.

Reynolds, A., & Lennex, L. (in press). Can you read this? 508 compliance among Kentucky schools?

Sanford, K., & Madill, L. (2006). Resistance through video games: It's a boy thing. *Canadian Journal of Education*, *29*(1), 287–306.

Stephens, M. (2005). The iPod Experiments. [from Education Full Text database.]. *Library Journal Net Connect*, *22*, 24–25. Retrieved February 27, 2007.

Tech Trends.

Vess, D. (2006). History to go: why I teach with iPods. *The History Teacher*, *39*(4), 479–492.

Vygotsky, L. S. (1978). *Mind in society: The development of higher psychological processes* (Cole, M., John-Steiner, V., Scribner, S., & Souberman, E., Eds.). Cambridge, MA: Harvard University Press.

Wenger, E. (1999). *Communities of practice: Learning, meaning, and identity*. New York: Cambridge University Press.

Yamagata-Lynch, L. (2007). Confronting analytical dilemmas for understanding complex human interactions in design based research from a cultural-historical activity theory (CHAT) framework. *Journal of the Learning Sciences*, *16*(4), 451–484.

Zurita, G., & Nussbaum, M. (2007). A conceptual framework based on activity theory for mobile CSCL. *British Journal of Educational Technology*, *38*(2), 211–235. doi:10.1111/j.1467-8535.2006.00580.x

ADDITIONAL READING

Bomar, L. (2006). iPods as Reading Tools. *Principal*, *85*(5), 52–53.

Carlson, S. (2004). Duke U. Will Give iPod Music Players to All Freshmen. [from Education Full Text database.]. *The Chronicle of Higher Education*, *50*(47), A21. Retrieved February 22, 2007.

Carlson, S. (2004). With This Enrollment, a Toy Surprise. [from Education Full Text database.]. *The Chronicle of Higher Education*, *51*(4), A29–A30. Retrieved February 27, 2007.

Carlson, S. (2005). The Net Generation in the Classroom. *The Chronicle of Higher Education*, *52*(7), 34–37.

Erlauer-Myrah, L. (2006). Applying Brain-Friendly Instructional Practices. *School Administrator*, *63*(11), 16–18.

French, D. (2006). iPods: Informative or invasive? *Journal of College Science Teaching*, 36(1), 58-59. Retrieved February27, 2007, from Education Full Text database.

Gee, J. P. (2003). *What video games have to teach us about learning and literacy*. New York: Palgrave Macmillan.

Goodyear, P., & Ellis, R. A. (2008). University students' approach to learning: Rethinking the place of technology. *Distance Education*, *29*(2), 141–152. doi:10.1080/01587910802154947

Grose, T. (2004). Duke Sings a New Tune. [from Education Full Text database.]. *ASEE Prism*, *14*(3), 14. Retrieved February 27, 2007.

Gurian, M., Henley, P., & Trueman, T. (2001). *Boys and Girls Learn Differently!*San Francisco, CA: Jossey-Bass.

Gurian, M., & Stevens, K. (2006). How Boys Learn. *Educational Horizons*, *84*(2), 87–93.

Gussin, L. (1995). Constructive lessons: building and playing simulation games. *C. D. Rom Professional*, *8*(5), 40–50.

Hastings, J. (2005). Cool Tools. [from Education Full Text database.]. *School Library Journal*, *51*(9), 42–45. Retrieved February 27, 2007.

Hayes, E. (2005). Women, video gaming, and learning: beyond stereotypes. *TechTrends*, *49*(5), 23–28. doi:10.1007/BF02763686

Katehi, L. & Ross, M. (2007). Technology and culture: Exploring the creative instinct through cultural interpretation. *Journal of Engineering of Education*, 96(2), 89-60. Retrieved April 1, 2009 from Education Full Text Database.

Lai, C. W., & Wu, C. C. (2006). Using handhelds in a jigsaw cooperative learning environment. *Journal of Computer Assisted Learning*, *22*, 284–297. doi:10.1111/j.1365-2729.2006.00176.x

NCATE. (2009). National Council for the Accreditation of Teacher Education. Retrieved April 10, 2009, from http://www.ncate.org.

Park, B. (2006). The Science of Learning Meets the Art of Teaching. *Education Canada*, *46*(4), 63–66.

Passig, D., & Levin, H. (2000). Gender preferences for multimedia interfaces. *Journal of Computer Assisted Learning*, *16*, 64–71. doi:10.1046/j.1365-2729.2000.00116.x

Read, B. (2005). Duke U. Assess iPod Experiment and Finds It Worked--in Some Courses. [from Education Full Text database.]. *The Chronicle of Higher Education*, *51*(43), A28. Retrieved February 27, 2007.

Read, B. (2005). Duke Will Scale Back Its iPod Giveaway to Students. [from Education Full Text database]. *The Chronicle of Higher Education*, *51*(32), A30. Retrieved February 27, 2007.

Read, B. (2005). Seriously, iPods Are Educational. [from Education Full Text database.]. *The Chronicle of Higher Education*, *51*(28), A30–A32. Retrieved February 27, 2007.

Read, B. (2006). Duke Stops Giving Students Free iPods but Will Continue Using Them in Classes. [from Education Full Text database.]. *The Chronicle of Higher Education*, *52*(36), A39. Retrieved February 27, 2007.

Roach, R. (2004). Incoming Duke Freshmen Receive Apple iPods. [from Education Full Text database.]. *Black Issues in Higher Education*, *21*(20), 46. Retrieved February 27, 2007.

Sanford, K., & Madill, L. (2006). Resistance through video games: It's a boy thing. *Canadian Journal of Education*, *29*(1), 287–306.

Siu, K. W. M., & Lam, M. S. (2005). Early childhood technology education: A socio-cultural perspective. *Early Childhood Education Journal*, *33*(6), 353–358. doi:10.1007/s10643-005-0003-9

Stephens, M. (2005). The iPod Experiments. *Library Journal (1976)* [from Education Full Text database.]. *Net Connect*, *22*, 24–25. Retrieved February 27, 2007.

Summerville, J., & Reid-Griffen, A. (2008). Technology integration and instructional design. *TechTrends*, *53*(5), 45–51.

Sweedyk, E., & de Lael, M. (2005). Women, games, and women's games. *Phi Kappa Phi Forum*, *85*(2), 25–28.

Underwood, J. D. M. (2007). Rethinking the digital divide: Impacts on student-tutor relationships. *European Journal of Education*, *42*(2), 213–222. doi:10.1111/j.1465-3435.2007.00298.x

Section 3
Social and Affective Issues

Chapter 9
Technology to Enhance the Affective Learning Outcomes of Teacher Trainees

Nor Aziah Alias
Universiti Teknologi MARA, Malaysia

Nor Aiza Alias
Kepong Secondary School, Malaysia

ABSTRACT

This chapter focuses on the utilization of technology to enhance the learning outcomes of pre-service teachers in the context of post secondary four year teacher education program provided by higher education institutions. A brief description of technology in teacher education precedes the discussion on the learning outcomes with a specific focus on the affective outcomes. Several guiding principles for enhancing the affective learning outcomes of pre-service teachers are furnished prior to describing a technology supported immersive learning approach to elicit such outcomes. The chapter concludes with a Malaysian immersive learning example that utilises the internet technology and collaboration with practitioners in schools.

INTRODUCTION

Technology is certainly not a panacea to all educational problems but it has become indispensable to educators in schools and higher education institutions. This is especially true for computer and internet technologies. At the very least, the word processor aids the preparation and management of class instruction. This chapter focuses on how technology can be employed to enhance the affective outcomes of teacher trainees in teacher education. We specifically opt to deliberate on affective learning outcomes due to the challenges of educating teachers who are not only expected to have the knowledge, skills and affective attributes but to impart all three components to the students they are teaching. Teaching also takes place in an ill-structured, dynamic setting; it draws on various knowledge and directs at diverse groups of students whose characteristics and dispositions differ from one another. It is an overwhelming task and rather a difficult one to measure the outcomes of graduates of teacher education who are poised to "*teach more by what they are than by what they say*". We refer to

DOI: 10.4018/978-1-61520-897-5.ch009

Copyright © 2010, IGI Global. Copying or distributing in print or electronic forms without written permission of IGI Global is prohibited.

pre-service teachers and teacher trainees as those who are undergoing teacher education programs and have yet to graduate. We seek to limit the discussion in this chapter to the four year teacher education program normally conducted by higher education institutions (HEIs) in countries such as United States and Malaysia. Such university based programs have been scrutinized and challenged on its effectiveness to produce educators (Russell & Wineburg, 2007). There ought to be a re-examination of the outcomes of such programs especially amidst the competition with other alternative pathways to teaching licensure. Moreover, the higher education environments are invariably different from those in the schools. Education in higher education tends to differ from the real life contexts. HEIs play the role of furnishing educational theories and classroom models. More often than not, delineation of theories and practice occur as practices in schools are imagined, visualized and simulated. Some instructors may not even have the experience of teaching in schools. There is a need to minimize the demarcation between the pre-service teachers' understanding and what is in store in the real school setting. To do so, we call for the use of the increasingly affordable and ubiquitous technology to support learning in all the learning domains, at all levels and via different modes.

TECHNOLOGY AND TEACHER EDUCATION

There is no denying that technology has advanced by leaps and bounds over the years. What was the awe of the 70s are now almost obsolete or have taken different forms in terms of production or delivery. An example would be the video. The analog era saw video production as tedious and time consuming but now children are able to produce videos of acceptable quality using hand held digital camera or mobile phones and editing them via simple video editing software. Computers evolve from being unique to being ubiquitous. The high tech wonders of the 80s which included the monitor with the flickering green text and other peripherals that essentially required a room to be housed in are now installed in lightweight tablet PCs or I Pods. Technology not only converges; it is more durable and affordable. We no longer see technology as the gadgets for the rich. In fact, people are fast becoming consumers of technology. We are also witnessing a diminishing affluence divide due to the all pervading technology. The emergence of the World Wide Web and the internet transform lives as the internet serves as a communicator, infotainer and service provider. People express themselves, work and learn on the move; with the internet, they connect and interact. Educators cannot deny the significance of the internet in the teaching-learning process since students are now "born and bred in the web era"

In this chapter, we will loosely refer to technology as the tool and techniques for learning and for the delivery of instruction. Hence, it may range from media such as videos and information and communication systems to process (soft) technologies. Table 1 illustrates some of the available hard and soft technology including hardware, categorized accordingly with reference to Sun Associates (2001). In terms of technology use, Davis (1997) also classifies them into the following areas: (1) enhancement of productivity, (2) technology literacy, (3) technology assisted learning, and (4) technology tools for learning (mind tools, etc).

Betrus and Molenda (2002) provide an informative account of how technology in teacher education has evolved since the 1920s. They reflected on how educational media was substantially affected by the emergence of computer technologies of the 1980s. The internet has also brought colossal changes to teacher education providers. Tomei (2003) classifies technology in a progressive utility level from the use of technology for literacy (understanding), for collaboration, decision-making, infusion (learning with technol-

Table 1. Categories of technology

<table>
<tr><td colspan="3">Hard technology</td></tr>
<tr><td rowspan="2">Hardware
• Audio Recorder
• Digital Still Camera
• Document Camera
• Laptop
• Tablet PC
• Overhead Projector
• Portable LCD Projector
• TV with DVD
• Interactive board
Handheld devices
• Camcorder
• Cell phones
• iPODs
• PDA
• MP3
Assistive technology (devices)</td><td>Application technology and Productivity Tools
• Word Processing
• Spreadsheet
• Databases
• Desktop Publishing
• Multimedia and presentation tool (graphics, sound, pictures, animation)
• Movie maker
• Podcasts
• Authoring tool
• Data collection and analysis
• Organization and brainstorming</td><td>Communication technology
Web ware
• Emails
• Web 2.0
• Webinars
• Wikis
• Blogs, weblogs,
• Community/ usergroups - facebook, friendster
Wireless and mobile
• Wi Fi
• GPS
• GPRS
• SMS, MMS</td></tr>
<tr><td>*Exploratory and integrated technology
• Simulation tool
• Virtual Reality
• Gaming
• Intelligent Tutor
• Integrated learning systems
• Learning management system</td><td>Resource technology
• Repositories
• E-book
• Online Library, encyclopedia
• Services – editing, search engines
• Web Video - Youtube</td></tr>
<tr><td colspan="3">Soft technology /Process technology - Based learning (project, problem, work, resource, brain-based</td></tr>
</table>

* Exploratory technology combines some content with a particular delivery strategy to encourage students to explore a subject and construct their own knowledge (Sun Associates, 2001)

ogy), integration (teaching with technology) and the study of technology itself. How research on technology in teacher education has transformed is also a fact not to be dismissed. These research that span decades have proliferated from a dominantly positivistic paradigm to interpretivism and critical theory (Willis, Thompson and Sadera, 1999). The typical systematic quantitative research has also made way for a more emergent and practice-oriented designs such as action, developmental and design based research. Educational researchers in the field of teacher education nonetheless display a common understanding that technology can only be maximized into practice if its integration into the classroom is appropriately managed.

In teacher education as in other higher education programs, technology has consistently been integrated into the teaching and learning process in many different ways and for various purposes (Brush et al, 2003; Hsiang, 1999; Thomas, Larson, Clift & Levin, 1996). The current literature on technology in teacher education is basically divided into several categories which are (1) the provision of technology as a subject in teacher education programs (basically for literacy), (2) the integration of specific technology in teacher education programs to ensure its use by the graduates when they enter their profession as teachers and (3) the issues surrounding pre service teachers and in service teachers with regard to their use of technology in the classrooms. Murray and Zemba-Saul (2008) for instance, look at how providers of university based teacher education programs use modern digital tools to prepare teacher trainees. They specifically zoom on the use of laptops and found that teachers would use this tool on a one to one initiative to transform teaching. Internet technology has also been harnessed to enhance networking such as Pratt's (2008) multipoint e-conferencing between English teacher education students on school placements, their host teachers and their university tutors. The use of blogs and e-portfolio to scaffold reflective practice such as that studied by Hughes and Purnell (2008) is another technology integration topic that has incited much interest. So is technology to support constructivist teaching as addressed by Bednar and Charles (1999) and Hull and Saxon (2009).

Cooper and Bull (1997) earlier found that teacher educators who are comfortable with technology will graduate technological leaders for schools that hire them. Either by offering technology as a subject or by embedding it in other subjects or activities, teacher education graduates must grasp the knowledge and skills that will allow them to successfully integrate technology into their teaching. However, Fulton, Glenn and Valdez (2004) contended that many teacher candidates do not come away with those skills. What is being taught in teacher education programs may significantly differ from what is practiced by teachers in the actual classrooms. This is supported by Cleaves and Toplist (2008) who discovered that pre-service teachers hardly use technology to enhance the teaching of conceptual knowledge; they were utilizing it only for presentations. In addition, Harshbarger (1995) and Winters (2004) again found that many pre-service teachers did not recognize the need for certain technology in their teaching until they had become in-service teachers and by then, they were not sure what to and how to do it. It is not however, the intent of this chapter to dwell on technology integration issues in general. Having stated all of the above, we would like to direct the reader to the questions once posed by Wellington (1995):

1. Should technology be used mainly to introduce teachers to the technology they will meet in their future teaching?
2. Should it play a part in the 'delivery' of teacher education?
3. Can it be used to 'do teacher education differently'?
4. Can it be utilized to re-structure teacher education programs?

We find his questions still relevant in the current discourse on technology. The area of technology in teacher education is indeed an immense and intricate one. In the light of student centered education, we propose another question to compliment Wellington's:

5. How can technology be utilized to support the different outcomes in teacher education?

The main thrust of this chapter is hence, the utilization of technology to support the learning outcomes of teacher trainees in higher education, in this case the affective learning outcomes.

A discussion on outcomes is incomplete without acknowledging Benjamin Bloom who in 1956 pioneered the study of learning outcomes with his three learning domains of cognitive (knowledge), affective (attitudes) and psychomotor (skills). Until now, his taxonomies of outcomes in each domain are still referred to. Ewell (1985) states that a distinction between cognitive and affective outcomes is a distinction between gains in knowledge and changes in attitudes or values. The affective domain (from the Latin affectus, meaning "feelings") includes a host of constructs, such as attitudes, values, beliefs, opinions, interests, and motivation. Krathwohl's affective domain taxonomy is perhaps the best known of any of the affective taxonomies (Huitt, 2001).

The taxonomy is ordered according to the principle of internalization, characterization being the highest level. The five levels are explained below.

1. Receiving refers to the student's willingness to attend to particular phenomena of stimuli (classroom activities, textbook, music, etc.)
2. Responding refers to active participation on the part of the student. At this level he or she not only attends to a particular phenomenon but also reacts to it in some way.
3. Valuing is concerned with the worth or value a student attaches to a particular object, phenomenon, or behavior. This ranges in

degree from the simpler acceptance of a value (desires to improve group skills) to the more complex level of commitment (assumes responsibility for the effective functioning of the group).

4. Organization is concerned with bringing together different values, resolving conflicts between them, and beginning the building of an internally consistent value system.
5. Characterization by a value or value set. The individual has a value system that has controlled his or her behavior for a sufficiently long time for him or her to develop a characteristic "life-style." Thus the behavior is pervasive, consistent, and predictable

Other than Krathwohl, Martin and Reigeluth (1999) put forward another conceptual model of the affective domain. They acknowledge the complexity of the affective domain and propose six dimensions of affective development as depicted in Table 2.

We will refer to both Krathwohl's and Martin and Reigeluth's work when we synthesize the teacher education outcomes to be presented next. For the purpose of our discussion, affective learning outcomes are behaviours that indicate beliefs, feelings and attitudes. These are demonstrated behaviors indicating attitudes of awareness, attention, concern, and responsibility, ability to listen and respond in interactions with others, and ability to demonstrate those attitudinal characteristics, disposition or values which are appropriate to the field of study. It is also related to students' values, perceptions, goals and interests

LEARNING OUTCOMES OF PRE-SERVICE TEACHERS

For decades, educational indicators have been based on a combination of input, process and output. Gauging an educational system output simply means looking at the graduates and their level of attainment. Since graduation rates do not tell us everything about the quality of graduates, there is a need to stress on learning outcomes. Educators must consider not only the particular skills and facts they want students to retain, but what kinds of things they want students to be able to do, and what kind of traits and abilities they will need to lead a rewarding, successful lives after graduation (McNeir, 1993). For instance, in teacher education, we need to establish the attributes of the teacher that we aspire to develop at the end of the program so they are physically, cognitively and emotionally ready to go to schools and teach. The Malaysian Standards for Education program

Table 2. Definitions of the dimensions of affective development

Term	Definition
Moral development	Building codes of behaviour and rationales and following them, including developing pro social attitudes, often in relation to caring, justice, equality etc.
Social Development	Building skills and attitudes for initiating and establishing interactions and maintaining relationship with others.
Spiritual development	Cultivating an awareness and appreciation of one's soul and its connection with other souls, with God and with all His creation
Emotional development	Understand one's own and others' feeling and affective evaluations, learning to manage those feelings, and wanting to do so
Aesthetic development	Acquiring an appreciation for beauty and style, including the ability to recognize and create it, commonly linked to music and art, but also includes the aesthetics of ideas
Motivational development	Cultivating interests and desire to cultivate interests, based on the joy or utility they provide, including both vocational and avocational pursuits.

for instance, espouses characteristics and "must have elements" in the teachers who graduated from such programs. Teachers are expected to

1. Be multi skilled to face globalization and the borderless world.
2. Be resourceful in recognizing and making use of existing and new market segments.
3. Possess research skills in the prospect of the teacher being a researcher in the new environment of the teaching profession.
4. Be familiar with new concepts of education and training such as student centered learning, e-learning, outcome based student assessment, recognition of prior learning and international standards in education.
5. Be aware of the new trends in education such as quality assurance, accreditation and academic load/credit that are based on learning outcomes.
6. Take into consideration the diversity and heterogeneity of the student population in planning their educational approaches and understanding that students are the products of traditional and smart schools and some are adult learners, part-time or full-time.
7. Collaborate with prospective employers to obtain feedback when designing educational programs. These employers could also provide training places for the graduates. (Malaysian Ministry of Education, 2003)

Another example is the superb details spelled out by the Vanuatu Ministry of Education (2006) where teachers are expected to have key attributes in four categories. The categories are

1. Professionalism which includes professional values, professional knowledge and disposition and continuous professional development
2. Content of teaching which deals with what is taught. It includes subject matter, attitudes and values, learning processes, and skills. It includes things that are transmitted both explicitly and implicitly and takes into account language skills across the curriculum, content presentation in an integrated way and incorporation of cultural values
3. Practice of teaching which is what a teacher does and how it is done. This encompasses planning and evaluation, management and instruction, communication and consideration of individual needs, abilities/disabilities and aspirations.
4. Interaction within the school and with families and the community which highlights the need for teachers to engage meaningfully with other stakeholders in education

With the expectation to produce competent teachers running high, education programs are designed to incorporate not only the content knowledge but also pedagogical knowledge (PK), pedagogical content knowledge (PCK), technological knowledge (TK), generic and soft skills, and values and attitudes that include the love of knowledge and continuing professional development. Of late, technological pedagogical content knowledge or TPACK has also been introduced as another facet of knowledge required to ensure effective and efficient technology integration by the teacher. As explained by Mishra and Koehler (2006), TPACK involves an understanding of the complexity of relationships among students, teachers, content, technologies, and practices. It is about the capability of the teacher to combine the content knowledge (subject matter that is to be taught), technological knowledge and pedagogical knowledge (theories, practices, processes, strategies, procedures, and methods of teaching and learning). Mishra and Koehler (2006) espouse TPACK as the connections and interactions between the three types of knowledge. We foresee TPACK to gain grounds in future teacher education discourse and research as technology continues to expand and transform the way students live and learn.

In teacher education, instruction and learning go beyond the psychomotor and the cognition. For a program to be effective, it has to be enquiry based and related to real life practices. Pre-service teachers need to see the relevance of theories in authentic school setting and to be able to apply what has been professed in lecture and discussion sessions in the university lecture halls. Teacher trainees also need to be aware of current local and global scenarios. Peacock (2000) asserts that one of the challenges for teacher educators in the current information society is to prepare pre-service educators to teach and develop thinking skills and inquiry in the educational environment to ensure that teachers become good thinkers, by *experiencing* what good thinkers do.

A glean of current literature and excerpts from speeches and writings of eminent educationist direct us to a myriad of affective attributes needed in a teacher education graduate. Teachers are expected to have the professional knowledge, values and disposition and the ability to plan, manage and instruct. Most of these are tied to fostering motivation, interest and awareness. The critical attributes according to Thomas Friedman, a Pullitzer prize winner are the desire and the ability to teach much more than the curriculum and a special mix of intellect, care, and authority that a teacher possesses that earns that teacher the respect of the students. A Malaysian educationist, Abdul Rahim Abdul Majid espouses similar teacher characteristics that include competence in the subject taught, fairness in perception, speech and action and concern for the welfare of the pupils. Cochran-Smith (2000) proposes that the outcomes of teacher education should be associated with "what teachers can do with what they know". It is also in agreement with Lampert and Ball (1999) who suggest that knowing teaching means understanding in such a way that one is prepared to perform (or practice) in a given situation for which one cannot fully prepare in advance. They emphasize how teacher candidates should know what they need to know rather than focusing on simply what they need to know. We see this as a progression of awareness and responsiveness to the workplace or school and educational issues. In lieu of the multifaceted nature of teacher education, we propose the broad outcomes of teacher education to encompass the components in the following Table 3.

Our concern is the learning affective outcomes of teacher education. We agree with Kikin-Gil (2006) that the affective is effective and giving attention to affective learning is an effective venue to produce good teachers. We also believe that good teaching requires wisdom and teacher trainees can only attain such level if they subject themselves to more than just opening their senses and minds. They also need to open their hearts and to feel. And in order to feel, they must experience. We also acknowledge the complexity of dimensions and levels in achieving these outcomes. Empathy for instance, may be developed through the different levels as shown in Table 4.

It is indeed, a challenge to scrutinize each affective outcome in teacher education. And it is not within the scope of this chapter to detail out each outcome. We seek to proceed with a general idea of affective learning outcome and focus on how technology may be roped in to support the interpersonal, intrapersonal and perceptual affective outcomes of pre-service teachers. In terms of indicators, measures of educational outcomes are fundamentally cognitive achievements and skills. Affective characteristics are not easily measured but efforts are underway to identify the various levels of feelings and attitudes learners develop after each lesson or learning experience.

TECHNOLOGY TO ENHANCE THE AFFECTIVE LEARNING OUTCOMES OF TEACHER TRAINEES

There are countless means to support the affective learning outcomes in teacher education. Service learning as reported by Angelova

Table 3. Outcomes of teacher education

Cognitive (Knowledge)	Content knowledge	Subject matter Educational theories Pedagogical knowledge Pedagogical content knowledge
Psychomotor (Skills)	Practical skills related to teaching	Teaching Methodologies Technological Technological pedagogical Technological pedagogical content knowledge
	Generic/ soft skills – skills that transverse	Scientific and Problem Solving Information Management Life Long Learning: Leadership Communication Teamwork
Affective (Feelings, beliefs, attitude)	Interpersonal	Social skills, empathy, building interactions
	Intrapersonal	Moral, spiritual, emotional and motivational
	Perceptual/ insight	Understanding the occupation of a teacher; awareness of current educational scenario and the multidimensionality of teaching

(Adapted from Alias & Alias,2009)

(2009) and Jenkins (2008), journaling (Bolin, Khramtsova, & Saarnio, 2005), involvement in reading circles (Zeegers, 2008) and role plays (Magenheim, 2003) are among the few. What we do within the four walls of the classroom may also be appropriate to initiate affective learning outcomes. The avenues to do so have multiplied over the years due to the technological advances. However, technology must be tackled with caution. Reports on limited use of technology and ineffective preparation of teacher trainees to use technology are still prevalent (Moursund & Bielefeldt, 1999; Brush & Appelman, 2007). Technology employment in teacher education must be accomplished in a manner that they are linked to the principles upon which the design of the learning experience is built upon. Affective learning outcome that involves beliefs, feelings and attitudes calls for realistic, relevant, and stimulating instruction that elicit purposeful emotional involvement (Simonson & Maushak, 2001). On this note, we put forward five guiding principles for enhancing teacher trainees' affective learning outcomes.

Table 4. Levels and indicators of empathy

Outcome	Level	Indicator
Empathy	Receiving	The student listens and gains awareness of the matter or problem faced by others
	Responding	The student ask questions and perceives the feelings of others regarding the matter
	Valuing	The student accepts and values the significance of the matter to others
	Organization	The student consolidates her/his feelings and understands the bigger picture of the matter
	Characterization	The student feels what others feel – he/she projects compassion and comprehension of the matter

(Adapted from Alias & Alias,, 2009)

- **Guiding Principle 1:** Knowledge of practice and practice of knowledge in real setting
- **Guiding Principle 2:** Early engagement in future workplace environment
- **Guiding Principle 3:** Corroboration and reflective collaboration with practitioners
- **Guiding Principle 4:** Learning in context; rich task in authentic environment
- **Guiding Principle 5:** Continuous interaction and progression of knowledge of the workplace/ school and school culture

Based on these principles, we are advocating a technology supported immersive learning as one of the strategies for enhancing affective learning outcomes. Our main tactic is *early immersion* in the school environment. Teacher trainees should be given the opportunity to self- assess their knowledge and compare their perceptions with reality early in the teacher education process. This means not waiting until the last stage of the program before sending them to schools. Then again, this does not necessarily mean that the teacher trainees will be physically stationed in schools. They only need to be in touch with the schools, to interact with practitioners, to understand the current situations and to apply the theories in order for them to have an insight into the profession and to value what they learn in class. This is where both hard and soft technology and TPACK comes in. In the ensuing discussion, we will exploit both the soft technology that is the immersive learning approach and the hard technology to support it. Within Koehler and Mishra's TPACK framework, we are operating on the technological and the pedagogical knowledge (refer Figure 1).

Figure 1. Relationship between content, pedagogical and technological knowledge

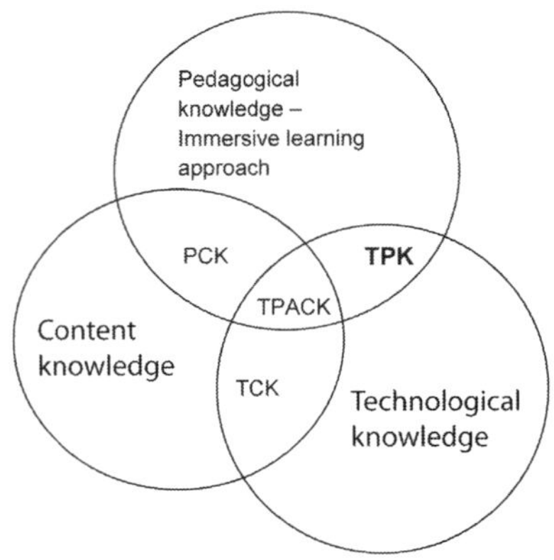

An Immersive Learning Approach to Support Affective Outcomes

In education, the use of the clause immersive learning has been rigorously associated with language learning where the learner speaks only the intended language to be learned. Content immersion is more prevalent in this language learning while cultural immersion referring to the experience of the person immersed in the culture and norms of a community is essential in ethnographic studies. Another growing area that is drawing much attention is the design and development of immersive simulations in virtual environments.

We are proposing immersive learning as a process where learning is promoted by the learner experiencing as closely as possible the minutiae of the real environment. We see immersion as a form of engagement, be it individually or in a collective mode. This may include engagement in terms of emotions or in the physical nature of the real setting. To be immersed is basically to be in and a part of the environment rather than in a detached mode. Learning within community settings is immersive. Learning by sharing thick, rich experience is also immersive. Hence, for a teacher trainee, immersive learning is about experiencing, absorbing and understanding the nuances of the multicultural and multifaceted nature of teaching, managing the classroom and interacting with pupils and parents. Immersive learning should not be limited to a "touch and go" whereby immersion ends when the student leaves after the period of school stay. Rather, it should be a continuous interaction and progression of knowledge of the workplace/ school and school culture.

An example of an immersive learning project is the Integration Program for Malaysian Pre service Teachers to be organized in the rural areas of East Malaysia. Teacher trainees from all over the country will be stationed in remote areas schools where even the basic amenities are unavailable. They will be assisting the school teachers while absorbing the culture and learning the ways of indigenous students who they may someday teach. It is an excellent immersion platform. This initiative however, incurs quite a hefty sum of money and involves only a few students from the different universities.

Clausen and Mallaby (2008) provide another account where instructors at a college initiated partnerships with the local school district and others within the university community to provide immersive contexts for student learning. The student teams explore four specific "Spaces" in order to understand how the community affects children, families, and school personnel. These spaces provide teacher education students with complex contexts to explore, investigate, and ultimately understand. Other examples include the use of virtual reality and 3D immersive worlds (Mio, 2006; Cheney, Matzen, Sanders, Bronack, Riedl, & Tashner, 2008).

How does immersive learning support affective outcomes? By being immersed in a particular environment, the learner develops an understanding of its intricacies. Immersive experiences promote learning beyond the lectures and discussion in the classrooms. They allow students to join forces on interdisciplinary projects with instructors and communities outside their higher education institutions and may extend throughout the country or the world. Through immersive learning, students are engaged in an active learning process that is connected to the real life scenarios. By being engaged in their future workplace environment, immersive learning allows teacher trainees to know what is currently practiced and to actually practice what they know in theory. They learn to collaborate with school teachers who will also corroborate on what the trainees' need to know when they start out in the teaching world. Learning becomes contextual as they perform rich task in authentic environments. An illustration of how affective learning outcomes can be achieved through immersive learning is depicted in Table 5. We contend that the higher the degree of immersion, the higher the level of affective learning outcomes achieved.

A gradual and consistent immersion through various modes is warranted to ensure practicality and effectiveness. Teacher trainees cannot be in schools all the time. Technology hence, comes into play. Immersive learning may not be tied to complex technologies; simple, accessible technology could be adequate to aid such learning. There are various technologies to engage the teacher trainees in an authentic school setting without incurring too high a cost. An ongoing asynchronous conversation with a school teacher will suffice to incite interest in current developments in schools. The central aim is for the teacher trainees to experience as closely as possible the minutiae of the real classroom and school environment. Malaysian teacher trainees watching the American movie "Freedom Writers" may be moved at that instance but the difference in culture and educational system may not be relevant enough to raise further awareness. A simple picture of Malaysian rural school children can perhaps be more apt to rouse the emotions and stimulate consciousness of Malaysian teacher trainees. Immersive learning should persist throughout their study. Short burst experiences that are sporadic may not be effectual to sustain the affective outcomes.

To aid further discussion, we provide a continuum of the technology tools in teacher education based on its complexity and accessibility in Figure 2. We refer to simple technology as ones that are easily accessible and require least programming. In this case, computer simulation refers to the utilization of simulation software and tool.

Table 5. Achievement of affective learning outcomes through immersive learning

Affective components	Learning outcomes	Example of immersive activity or task	What can be achieved through immersive learning
Interpersonal	Empathy	Trainees read school teacher teacher's reflection and ponder Trainees watch videos of scenarios and events that take place in real classrooms Trainees observe school counsellors in session	Trainees raise their level of awareness and understanding of the school, students and current educational scenario
	Social skills, building interactions	Trainees ask for input from school teachers on matters pertaining to lesson plans and classroom management Trainees and school teachers co-identify researchable issues and conduct action research	Trainees develop the necessary etiquette and attitude to address a fellow teacher. Trainees collaborate and teachers corroborate on matters pertaining to teaching and managing real classrooms
Intrapersonal	Moral and spiritual	Trainees work on an authentic disciplinary case Trainees go for externship in multiracial and multicultural setting Trainees work with underprivileged school kids Trainees pay visits to areas stricken with poverty	Trainees judge and challenge their own values when faced with alternative ones Trainees develop a heightened awareness of their functions in relation to others
	Emotional and motivational	Trainees identify and provide service to a "foster school" Trainees set up weekend or online tutorial sessions to help school kids Trainees volunteer as "big sister/big brother" to school kids	Trainees feel the joy and become involved with school children Trainees become keen and interested when rewarded with authentic experience
Perceptual/ insight	Understanding profession, awareness current scenario and the multidimensionality of teaching	Trainees develop instructional materials based on needs analysis conducted in a school Trainees shadow school teachers Trainees teach in schools during teaching practicum	Trainees understand the barriers and challenges in the profession they are venturing into; trainees have a foresight of what is in store

(Adapted from Alias & Alias,, 2009)

How one can utilize technology to support affective learning outcomes through immersive learning depends on the degree of immersion itself. Table 6 suggests some of the technology that can be employed to support the different levels of immersion. The degree of immersion is based on how close one is experiencing the details of the real environment. We acknowledge the fact that the degree of immersion does depend on the duration even though there is no indication of the time dimension in the table.

Figure 3 further explicates the examples of activities and the level of technology required to support immersion. Low immersion tends to occur when the interaction is limited to one between the trainee and materials rather than people and place. Nonetheless, a simple video clip may bring reality into the trainee's realm and elicit feelings that are synonymous to experiencing the real thing. This is supported by Abell, *et al.* (1996 as cited in Kumar and Altshuld, 2002) who stated, "video allows pre-service teachers to enter a classroom virtual world and witness events as they occur" (p. 138).

A Case of Immersive Learning at a Malaysian University

In this section, we will describe a Malaysian case of how technology is employed to support affective learning outcomes through immersive learning. The case was a pilot study of a simple technology supported environment developed for a group of teacher trainees who were in their third year of study. What spurred our motivation were the concerns voiced by the trainees themselves, their teaching practicum supervisors and the receiving schools on the lack of congruence between what is being taught in university lectures, what the trainees bring with them to school and what is in store for them in schools. We took into consideration the constraints of time and place. Firstly, we utilized an online forum that allowed those who

Figure 2. Technology continuum

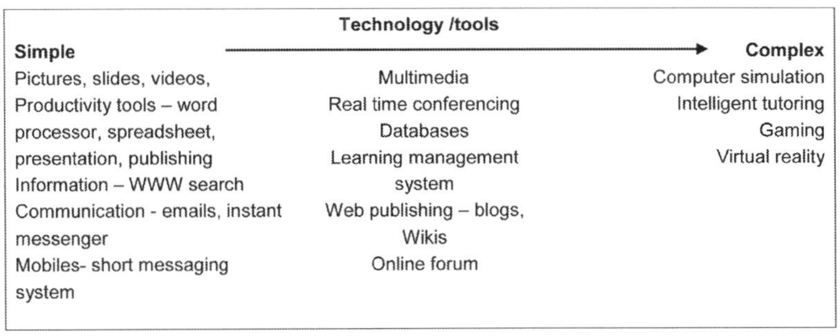

Table 6. Technology and degree of immersion

		Immersion		
		Low	**Medium**	**High**
Technology	Simple	Pictures, audio files video clips	Web messaging (emails, instant messenger) Wireless messaging – SMS	-
	Moderate	Blogs Streaming video Podcasting	Wikis Web community (facebook, etc) Online forum/usergroups	Real time conferencing
	Complex	-	Computer simulation	Virtual reality

Figure 3. Immersive activities and technology required

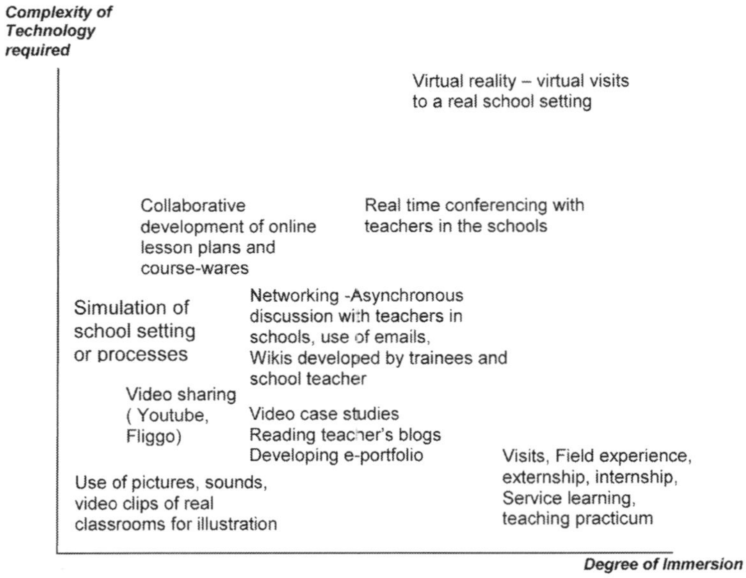

access it to respond and contribute to an issue in hand. We invited school teachers to share their experience and concerns while teacher trainees in the university logged in to read and respond to the issues raised. The trainees received first hand information without being in schools. The school teachers were able to portray the real world and describe authentic problems while letting out their concerns and having their voices heard. We permitted venting out emotions and display of both positive and negative thoughts. Secondly, we utilized the input from the teachers to allow the students to explore researchable issues on Malaysian education. Students identified areas of research and provided relevant research questions based on the teachers' narratives. Thirdly, we provided transcriptions of the teachers' reflections as data for an exercise in qualitative data analysis.

In one instance, the teacher wrote about the size of classes in her school:

On average, each class in my school has 44 students except Form Six classes. Believe it or not, our two Remove classes have enrolments of 60 and 61 respectively! How can a teacher be expected to teach effectively with so many students in class? Class control is obviously difficult, if not impossible, and students are easily distracted by their peers. ....A very enthusiastic teacher might try to memorize the names of his/ her students a.s.a.p., but I doubt that it can be accomplished within 2 months. With 5 or 6 classes to teach, a teacher actually has approximately 250 names to remember! As for me, I'm trying hard to cope but I do wish we have fewer students in each class so that I can concentrate on teaching and nurturing these young minds without leaving out any of them. Is that too much to ask?

The students responded, reflected on their own experience, expressed their astonishments, put forward what they felt, agreed and disagreed, gave ideas and recommendations on top of suggesting possible research that could be conducted. We categorized the responses from students and found evidences of the different levels of affective learning outcomes. Below are some examples from each category.

... a class can accommodate up to 98 students? Wow, I never knew that classes in Malaysian schools can be so big. (empathy/ receiving).

......to be honest, that is one of the reasons that make me sooo scared to be a teacher later on.. having a big number of students..with different backgrounds??, and with different attitudes ?? kids nowadays, u know... (emotional/responding)

... I still remember when I was in my primary school, there were 40-45 students in my class. Our teacher could not pay attention to all of us.

... it hurts when the teacher doesn't even notice our existence. (emotional/responding).

The teacher trainees also discussed effective classroom management, the value of interactions in big classes, positive thinking and risk taking. Many proposed the use of technology. The school teacher initially felt that there was a discrepancy between what the students know and what was actually happening in a real school. She contended that most of the students were very idealistic when responding to the issue. They lacked empathy and did not comprehend the multifaceted nature of teaching in schools. They were not familiar with the administrative red tapes, the diversity of the students and the constraints faced by teachers in terms of infrastructure and technology integration. Some perceived teachers to be prone to complaining all the time. These confirmed our concern about the teacher trainees' ability to apply what they learned in real situations. A prevalent aspect was the trainees' assumptions that human behaviours were generally predictable and theories would work anywhere. Nonetheless, the trainees projected a better understanding of the profession and empathy as the interaction continued between their peers and the school teachers throughout the semester.

One of the students wrote:

I agree with _______(friend's name)'s suggestions which were to improve the facilities and increase number of teachers, HOWEVER, as we all can see, the writer is only a teacher, She cannot build the facilities, and she cannot increase the number of teacher, it's all the administration's job. So, it will be hard for her and of course for us, to change this situation. We may make a complaint or suggestion, but let's be realistic here, even though there are changes, it will take some time..

Another responded:

Frankly speaking, through my own thought, teaching an 'over-loaded' class is not an easy thing to be handled. We might easily lose our patience while dealing with the naughty students and the noise which is usually beyond of our control. We as future teachers have to look at the other things (we have to do) other than the teaching itself...... We will not be teaching the students alone but we will be connected with other tasks as well such as marking students' work (tests, homework, exam papers etc) accomplishing administrative work (preparing test, preparing project proposal) so on and so forth. I want to make it simple; a 'heavy-work' load of being a teacher is waiting for us

During the qualitative exercise, the students were able to discern the different themes in a teacher's explication of her experience in teaching both rural and urban schools in Malaysia. They came to realize the uniqueness, the disparity and the similarities of experience in teaching in the schools. Despite the lesser degree of immersion, the sharing space proves to be useful in enhancing the trainees' affective learning outcomes. In the process of getting knowledge of current practice and practicing their knowledge in an authentic setting, they reflect on their own conceptions, values and on their future career. A student described her new found awareness:

It (the sharing of experience) gives us the idea of how it is actually to become a teacher.. and somehow I think that the experience has provided us with the evidence that (the) teaching profession can no longer be the last resort. I get annoyed with those who underestimated teachers.. I agree with the kind of authentic exposure (we had).

The web technology required to bring in the authentic data and experience to the teacher trainees' sphere is non complicated and available to both parties. Contributing to the forum is second nature to the students. The practice is context driven, brings in cultural aspect, builds on experience and knowledge the contributors bring to the sharing space, exposes common misconceptions and creates connections between classroom learning and issues in the real world. The teacher trainees gain insight, display heightened awareness, question their existing knowledge and also develop effective questioning and communication skills. The sharing process is collaborative and corroborative as well as students confirm with the practitioners what they know in theory and what can be applied in schools.

Future Recommendations

The case presented provides a sneak peek into how immersion can be initiated through the use of a simple online forum. Future initiatives should explore more complex technology to provide immersive experience to pre-service teachers. A virtual world where they can interact with virtual characters in school, conduct a teaching session with virtual students and gain feedback from automated supervisors on lesson plans and assessment would be a fascinating immersive environment. Real time synchronous conferencing should also be considered to bring forth genuine experiences. Alternately, less complex video case studies may bridge theory and practice and induce reflection among the pre-service teachers.

CONCLUSION

The chapter illustrated our ideas on how immersive learning may bring about affective learning outcomes. We hope the discussion in the chapter will instigate further discourse on these outcomes and how they can be buoyed by technology supported immersive learning experiences. We demonstrate the use of simple technology to scaffold and support intrapersonal and interpersonal dialogues that are paramount to generating affective outcomes as expounded by Cleveland-Innes and Ally (2007). Further integration of multiple technologies are recommended to generate the self processes necessary to initiate what Cleveland- Innes and Ally termed as 'learning to feel". The education profession needs teachers who are passionate and who teach with their hearts. In order to develop such teachers, teacher educators must render more than just the dissemination of knowledge and skills. The affective domain must be duly addressed.

REFERENCES

Alias, N. A., & Alias, N. A. (2009). Improving the affective learning outcomes of trainees in teacher education: An immersive approach. In Nygaard, C., & Holtham, C. (Eds.), *Improving Students Learning Outcomes in Higher Education.* Copenhagen: Copenhagen Business School Press.

Angelova, M. (2001, December 22). Impact of service learning on the cognitive and affective development of pre-service teachers. *The Free Library*. Retrieved April 7, 2009, from http://www.thefreelibrary.com/Academic+Exchange+Quarterly/2001/December/22-p568

Bednar, A., & Charles, M. (1999). A constructivist approach for introducing pre-service teachers to educational technology: Online and classroom education. In J. Price et al. (Eds.), *Proceedings of Society for Information Technology and Teacher Education International Conference 1999* (pp. 1796-1801). Chesapeake, VA: AACE

Betrus, A. K., & Molenda, M. (2002). Historical evolution of instructional technology in teacher education programs. *TechTrends*, *46*(5), 18–21. doi:10.1007/BF02818303

Bolin, A., Khramtsova, I., & Saarnio, D. (2005). Using student journals to stimulate authentic learning: Balancing Bloom's cognitive and affective domains. *Teaching of Psychology*, *32*(3), 154–159. doi:10.1207/s15328023top3203_3

Brush, T., & Appelman, R. (2003). Transforming the Pre-service Teacher Education Technology Curriculum at Indiana University: An Integrative Approach. In C. Crawford et al. (Eds.), *Proceedings of Society for Information Technology and Teacher Education International Conference 2003* (pp. 1613-1619). Chesapeake, VA: AACE

Brush, T., Glazewski, K., Rutowski, K., Berg, K., Stromfors, C., & Hernandez Van-Nest, M. (2003). Integrating technology in a field based teacher training program: The PT3@ASU Project. *ETR&D*, *51*(1), 57–72. doi:10.1007/BF02504518

Cheney, A., Matzen, N., Sanders, R., Bronack, S., Riedl, R., & Tashner, J. (2008). Social constructivism in a 3D immersive world. In K. McFerrin et al. (Eds.), *Proceedings of Society for Information Technology and Teacher Education International Conference 2008* (pp. 2922-2929). Chesapeake, VA: AACE.

Clausen, J., & Mallaby, M. (2008). Immersive learning and effective technology integration: Educational foundations redefined. In K. McFerrin et al. (Eds.), *Proceedings of Society for Information Technology and Teacher Education International Conference 2008* (pp. 1987-1991). Chesapeake, VA: AACE

Cleaves, A., & Toplis, R. (2008). Pre-service science teachers and ICT: Communities of practice? *Research in Science & Technological Education*, *26*(2), 203–213. doi:10.1080/02635140802037344

Cleveland-Innes, M., & Mohamed Ally (2007). Learning to feel: Education, affective outcomes and the use of online teaching and learning. *EURODL 2007, 2*. Retrieved December 12, 2008 from http://www.eurodl.org/materials/contrib/2007/Cleveland_Ally.htm

Cochran-Smith, M. (2000). *The outcomes question in teacher education.* AERA Vice Presidential Address for Division K (Teaching and Teacher Education), AERA Annual Meeting, April 2000. Retrieved 15 November, 2008 from http://www2.bc.edu/~cochrans/default.html

Cooper, J. M., & Bull, G. L. (1997). Technology and teacher education: Past practice and recommended direction. *Action in Teacher Education*, *19*(2), 97–106.

Davis, J. E. (1997). *Categories of technology use in education.* Retrieved December 18, 2008, from http://www.quasar.ualberta.ca/edpy485/edtech/category.htm#category

Ewell, P. T. (1985). *Assessing educational outcomes. New Directions for Institutional Research, 47.* San Francisco, CA: Jossey-Bass.

Fulton, K., Glenn, A. D., & Valdez, G. (2004). Teacher education and technology planning guide. Naperville, IL: Learning Point Associates. (ERIC document Reproduction Service No. ED489530).

Harschbarger, R. J. (1995). Training pre-service and in service teachers in the use of technology. In *Electronic Proceedings of the Eighth Annual International Conference on Technology in Collegiate Mathematics*, Houston, Texas, November 16-19, 1995. Retrieved January 10, 2009 from http://archives.math.utk.edu/ICTCM/i/08/C085.html

Hsiang, M. Y. (1999). *Technology assisted reflection: A study of pre-service teacher education in middle school Language Arts and Social Studies and secondary school English and Social Studies.* Unpublished Dissertation, North Carolina State University.

Hughes, J., & Purnell, E. (2008). Blogging for beginners? Using blogs and eportfolios in teacher education. In *Proceedings of the 6th International Conference on Networked Learning* (pp. 144-152).

Huitt, W. (2001, April). Krathwol et al.'s taxonomy of the affective domain. In *Educational Psychology Interactive*. Valdosta, GA: Valdosta State University. Retrieved October 4, 2008, from http://chiron.valdosta.edu/whuitt/col/affsys/affdom.html

Hull, D. M., & Saxon, T. F. (2009). Negotiation of meaning and co-construction of knowledge: An analysis of experimental analysis of asynchronous online instruction. *Computers & Education, 52*, 624–639. doi:10.1016/j.compedu.2008.11.005

Jenkins, S. (2008) *The impact of in-class service-learning on cognitive and affective learning outcomes*. Paper presented at the 2008 Annual Meeting of the American Political Science Association in Boston, MA. Kikin- Gil, R. (2006). Affective is effective: How information appliances can mediate relationships within communities and increase one's social effectiveness. *Personal and Ubiquitous Computing, 10*(2006), 77-83.

Kumar, D. D., & Altshuld, J. W. (2002). Complimentary approaches to evaluating technology in science teacher education. In Kumar, D. D., & Altshuld, J. W. (Eds.), *Evaluation of Science and Technology Education at the dawn of the new millennium* (pp. 165–185). New York: Kluwer Academics. doi:10.1007/0-306-47560-X_7

Lampert, M., & Ball, D. (1999). Aligning teacher education with contemporary K-12 reform visions. In Darling-Hammond, L., & Sykes, G. (Eds.), *Teaching as the learning professions: Handbook of policy and practice* (pp. 33–53). San Francisco, CA: Jossey Bass.

Magenheim, J. (2003). Social, affective and normative aspects of learning in ICT-enriched learning environments: collaborative exploration of societal aspects of ICT. In. *Proceedings of the Conferences in Research and Practice in Information Technology Series, 23*, 85–88.

Martin, B. L., & Reigeluth, C. M. (1999). Affective education and the affective domain: Implications for instructional-design theories and models. In Reigeluth, C. M. (Ed.), *Instructional-design theories and models: A new paradigm of instructional theory* (*Vol. 2*, pp. 485–509). London: Lawrence Erlbaum Associates.

McNeir, G. (1993). Outcome Based Education: Tool for restructuring. *Oregon School Study Council (OSSC). Bulletin, 36*(8).

Mio, A. (2006). Effect of experience in immersive vr on application image. In C. Crawford et al. (Eds.), *Proceedings of Society for Information Technology and Teacher Education International Conference 2006* (pp. 1385-1392). Chesapeake, VA: AACE

Mishra, P., & Koehler, M. J. (2006). Technological Pedagogical Content Knowledge: A Framework for Teacher Knowledge. *Teachers College Record, 108*(6), 1017–1054. doi:10.1111/j.1467-9620.2006.00684.x

Moursund, D., & Bielefeldt, T. (1999). Will new teachers be prepared to teach in a digital age? A national survey on information technology in teacher education. Santa Monica, CA: Miliken Exchange on Education Technology (ERIC Document Reproduction Service No. ED 428 072).

Murray, O., & Zembal-Saul, C. (2008). Educate at Penn State: Preparing beginning teachers with powerful digital tools. *Journal of Computing in Higher Education, 20*, 48–58. doi:10.1007/s12528-008-9000-5

Peacock, L. (2000). Thinking skills to creatively enhance information competence. *Academic Exchange Quarterly, 4*(3).

Pratt, N. (2008). Multipoint e-conferencing with initial teacher training students in England: Pitfalls and potential. *Teaching and Teacher Education, 24*, 1476–1486. doi:10.1016/j.tate.2008.02.018

Russell, A., & Wineburg, M. (2007). Towards a national framework for evidence of effectiveness of teacher education programs. *Perspectives.* Policy Papers published by the American Association of State Colleges and Universities.

Simonson, M., & Maushak, N. (2001). Instructional technology and attitude change. In Jonassen, D. (Ed.), *Handbook of research for educational communications and technology* (pp. 984–1016). Mahwah, NJ: Lawrence Erlbaum Associates.

Sun Associates. (2001). *Evaluating technology integration.* Retrieved January 11, 2009, from http://www.sun-associates.com/resources/categories.html#anchor237232

Thomas, L., Larson, A., Clift, R. T., & Levin, J. (1996). Integrating technology in teacher education programs: Lessons from the teaching tele-apprenticeships project. *Action in Teacher Education, 17*(4), 1–8.

Tomei, L. A. (2003). *The taxonomy for the technology domain.* Retrieved June 24, 2009, from http://academics.rmu.edu/~tomei/taxonomy/

Wellington, J. J. (1995). The role of new technology in teacher-education - A case-study of hypertext in a PGCE Course. *Journal of Education for Teaching, 21*(1), 37–50. doi:10.1080/02607479550038734

Willis, J., Thompson, A., & Sadera, W. (1999). Research on technology and teacher education: Current status and future directions. *ETR&D, 47*(4), 29–45. doi:10.1007/BF02299596

Winters, R. (2004). Differentiated tech use: under what conditions, for what purposes? In C. Crawford et al. (Eds.), *Proceedings of Society for Information Technology and Teacher Education International Conference 2004* (pp. 2750-2754). Chesapeake, VA: AACE

Zeegers, M. (2008). Beyond cognition: Affective learning and undergraduate education student engagement in learning. In ECER 2008, Göteborg, Sweden 10-12 September, 2008.

Chapter 10
From Online Role-Play to Written Argumentation:
Using Blended Learning in Lessons on Social Issues

Kati Vapalahti
University of Jyväskylä, Finland

Miika Marttunen
University of Jyväskylä, Finland

Leena Laurinen
University of Jyväskylä, Finland

ABSTRACT

This chapter reports on a teaching experiment conducted during a blended learning course in social work in a Finnish university of applied sciences (polytechnic). The aim was to investigate how students' multidimensional understanding of social problems could be fostered. As argumentative methods, the study used writing tasks, online role-play, and drama work. The data consisted of essays written by 65 students (experimental group 29; controls 36) in each of three phases, plus online discussions. The essays were based on 1) the students' personal experiences, 2) general facts, and 3) a fictional case taken from the online role-play. Varying the focus of the writing task affected students' standpoints on the effects of adolescents' intoxicant use on their well-being. Moreover, the use of argumentative methods applied in the blended learning environment both broadened and deepened the students' argumentation, helping them to understand the diverse nature of an ill-structured problem.

INTRODUCTION

According to the Pisa study (OECD, 2006), Finnish schools have shown good learning results. Nevertheless, social problems such as bullying are common in Finnish schools (National Institute for Health and Welfare, 2008). Thus, it is important to develop suitable methods for teaching problem-solving skills related to social issues.

As well as teachers, there are various professionals working on social issues in Finnish schools. Youth educators and social workers, for example,

DOI: 10.4018/978-1-61520-897-5.ch010

Copyright © 2010, IGI Global. Copying or distributing in print or electronic forms without written permission of IGI Global is prohibited.

often co-operate with teachers on issues that are of social, educational and mental concern to adolescents. Social pedagogical work of this kind (see Hämäläinen, 2003; Blatchford, Kutnick, Baires, & Galton, 2003) has many similarities with the work of guidance counselors (see Peavy, 1997, pp. 19–25; Borgen & Hiebert, 2006). The aim in social pedagogies is like the aim of guidance counselors, namely to help students to manage in their lives, both at present and in the future.

Also school teachers encounter a variety of social problems in their work. The ability to understand social questions from different viewpoints (e.g. those of a client and relevant stakeholders) is thus essential. Moreover, working with adolescents often requires engagement in critical debate. In the present study, we developed methods that we considered suitable for the education of professionals in the youth education field. It should be noted that even if they were planned for future social workers and youth counselors, the methods presented here can be applied in teacher education, and at elementary and high school level. The methods were applied in a teaching experiment in which online and face-to-face learning environments were integrated.

BACKGROUND

Argumentation in the Study of Social Issues

Argumentation can be characterized as verbal, social, and rational interaction, aimed at justifying or disproving a given standpoint. When one is studying social issues, argumentation can be seen to have a two-fold character: it is learning *to* debate, i.e. learning argumentation skills in order to develop critical thinking and problem-solving skills, and also learning *from* debate, i.e. learning content through an argumentative debate (see Andriessen, Baker, & Suthers, 2003; von Aufschnaiter, Erduran, Osborne, & Simon, 2008). Learning *to* debate is valuable when, for example, teachers discuss intoxicant issues with young people. On the other hand, learning *from* debate may help students to achieve a deeper understanding of social problems (see Andriessen, Baker, & Suthers, 2003).

Logical structures are important, since they embody the characteristics of good argumentation, that is, argumentation that includes at least a claim and grounds (see Toulmin, 1958). In informal reasoning, evidence for a claim is generated and evaluated in cases where information is unclear or problems are ill-structured (Means & Voss, 1996). In everyday argumentation, in addition to knowledge, people also utilize values when making decisions (Kolstø, 2006). Professionals working with adolescents often have to deal with ill-structured problems. The solutions to these are frequently unpredictable, and contain many alternatives (Jonassen, 1997). This means that logical models of argumentation alone are not enough; indeed, they may be unsuitable in a good deal of informal everyday reasoning.

Supporting Multidimensional Thinking by Argumentation

Collaborative argumentation is a means to deepen independent critical thinking and multidimensional understanding. It requires elaboration, reasoning and reflection as well as social and collaborative skills (Andriessen, Baker, & Suthers, 2003). In collaborative learning through argumentation, participants try to solve a conflict by debate in order to construct knowledge and to understand different viewpoints (Andriessen, 2002, pp. 443–444). Laurinen and Marttunen (2007) define collaborative argumentation as a learning situation in which learners seek together to understand the core issues of a topic, by co-examining different standpoints, arguments, and counter-arguments. Developed argumentation requires counter-arguments (von Aufschnaiter, Erduran, Osborne, & Simon, 2008; Kuhn, 1991; Osborne, Erduran, & Simon, 2004). The critical evaluation of alternative standpoints is a step towards critical thinking and an understanding of the reasons underlying complex social problems (see Kuhn, 1991).

The results of a recent cross-cultural study among secondary school students have suggested that more practice is needed in argumentation, in particular, in students' analytical and critical reading (Marttunen, Laurinen, Litosseliti, & Lund, 2005). In an earlier study, Felton and Kuhn (2001) found that even when adolescents were engaged in a dialogue, their argumentative strategies were weak. The challenges that face students in their argumentation in learning contexts have also been examined by other researchers (Andriessen, Baker, & Suthers, 2003; van Bruggen, Kirschner, & Jochems, 2002; Weinberger, Stegmann, Fischer, & Mandl, 2007). Kuhn (1991), for example, found that when people were asked to generate their own theories on given social problems, the theories often included naive epistemological understanding, and were presented without alternatives.

In order to stimulate argumentative discussion, inspiring tasks are needed. Such tasks may include the challenge of ill-structured problems (Veerman & Treasure-Jones, 1999), role-play (Simonneaux, 2001), questioning (Veerman, Andriessen, & Kanselaar, 2002), dialogue tools (Hirsch, Saeedi, Cornillon, & Litosseliti, 2004), and diagrams (Lund, Molinari, Séjourné, & Baker, 2007). Moreover, Osborne, Erduran, and Simon (2004) emphasize the importance of a sense of social context, and the provision of suitable instruction as means to facilitate argumentation. More recently, a study on computer-supported collaborative argumentation has been conducted (Fischer, Kollar, Haake, & Mandl, 2007).

Stimulating Argumentation in Computer-Assisted Learning Environments

Because triggering argumentative interaction is challenging, teachers need tools for designing effective learning environments. Argumentation may be supported, for example, with instructional scripts (see Kollar, Fischer, & Slotta, 2007; Weinberger, Stegmann, Fischer, & Mandl, 2007). The aim of the instructional script is to increase prospective interaction and to foster collaborative learning in online, face-to-face or integrated environments (Dillenbourg & Jermann, 2007).

Instructional scripts may be divided into macro- and micro-scripts. Macro-scripts are pedagogical models for the sequencing of group activities by using e.g. roles (Dillenbourg & Tchounikine, 2007; Dillenbourg & Hong, 2008). According to Häkkinen and Mäkitalo-Siegl (2007), the aim of macro-scripts is indirectly to create an environment for effective interaction. Macro-scripts may consist of individual activities (e.g. personal tasks), collaborative activities (e.g. small group interaction), and collective activities (e.g. class-wide discussions) (Dillenbourg & Tchounikine, 2007). One example of an argumentative macro-script is an "ArgueGraph" (see Dillenbourg & Jermann, 2007). The "ArgueGraph" consists of four phases, which are 1) multiple-choice questionnaires on a topic (individual activity) followed by graphs that indicate students' answers in questionnaires, for further discussion and pair formulation; 2) questionnaires for answering in pairs (collaborative activity); 3) a face-to-face session for merging students' arguments into a theory of the topic (collective activity); and 4) the individual writing of a synthesis of arguments related to the theoretical framework (individual activity).

Micro-scripts, for their part, are direct instructional prompts that guide specific activities such as counting numbers together or answering a single question. Students are expected to internalize the micro-scripts progressively so that they can apply them automatically (Dillenbourg & Hong, 2008). Micro- and macro-scripts often overlap during long courses.

The use of instructional scripts presents many challenges. According to Hesse (2007), instructional scripts may even lead to unwanted results. As an alternative to using instructional scripts to help learners advance in a learning situation, Hesse prefers scripts based on the learners' awareness of group interaction, learning situation, and history of actions taken. Häkkinen and Mäkitalo-Siegl (2007) consider that the use of scripts may present challenges when computer-supported scripts are integrated into class work. Moreover, they are concerned that many teachers have weak pedagogical skills in the use of scripts. Macro-scripts do not seem automatically to produce high-level collaboration; different groups seem to need different kinds of scripting (Hämäläinen, 2008, p. 69).

Dillenbourg, Järvelä, and Fisher (2009) claim that the effectiveness of particular media has been overestimated; they refer especially to the use of asynchronous (non-real time, in contrast to face-to-face or chat discussions) online communication tools in isolation. As an alternative to a one-sided use of media tools they recommend the use of integrated macro-scripts. There, the online and face-to-face environments complement each other across multiple social levels (e.g. individual, collaborative, and collective), multiple contexts (e.g. classroom, home) and multiple media (e.g. with or without computers, videos, or mobile phones). Teachers in these kinds of learning environments are required to orchestrate different forms of coordination (Dillenbourg, Järvelä, & Fisher, 2009).

The integrated macro-scripts have features similar to those of *blended learning*. Garrison and Vaughan (2008, p.5) define blended learning as a combination of the best features of oral face-to-face communication and written distance-learning communication, applied in a thoughtful and coherent way (see also Osguthorpe & Graham, 2003). In an earlier study, Garrison and Kanuka (2004) saw blended learning as a potentially a good method, capable of bringing about meaningful and effective learning. Nevertheless, they also emphasized the challenges it presents in the planning phase. The challenges are related to merging the distinct approaches and properties of face-to-face and online learning (Garrison & Vaughan, 2008, p. 11). This suggests a need for further research if we wish to learn more about applying multiple learning environments in an appropriate way.

Multiple learning environments are topic currently receiving attention in formal and non-formal learning, not only in schools but also in working life. Social and youth work is traditionally based on face-to-face communication, but in recent years online environments have also been utilized. Thus, teaching based on blended learning would appear to have strong potential in the study of social issues.

The present study deals with integrated macro-scripts aimed at triggering argumentation. The teaching experiment as a whole consists of an integrated macro-script, including such activities as writing on adolescents' use of intoxicants from different perspectives (individual activity), online role-play (collaborative activity), and drama work (collaborative and collective activities). All these activities within the macro-script also include micro-scripts for guiding learners in a stricter way. In the writing tasks, the students were given suggestions by the teacher for the kinds of issues to be discussed (i.e. physical, psychological, and social issues). Moreover, both the online role-play discussions and the drama work were prompted by role descriptions. Blended learning, in turn, was organized in this study by integrating online role-play and face-to-face drama work.

AIM OF THE STUDY AND RESEARCH QUESTIONS

While argumentation has been found to have benefits for learning (e.g. Andriessen, 2002; Dillenbourg, Järvelä, & Fisher, 2009; Weinberger, Stegmann, Fischer, & Mandl, 2007) and for developing critical thinking (Kuhn, 1999), it has not been systematically exploited in the study of social issues in higher education. Consequently, the aim of this study was to promote multidimensional thinking on ill-structured social problems among students of social work, within a blended learning environment. Argumentation skills were practiced by means of various argumentative methods in a course on intoxicant work. All the students (experimental group and controls) wrote a short essay in each of three phases within the experiment. The experimental group participated in lectures and practiced argumentation in role-play, followed by drama work. The control group only wrote the essays.

The research questions were as follows: 1) Would varying the focus of the writing tasks stimulate students' argumentation in their three successive essays? 2) Would the quality of argumentation in the essays of the experimental and the control groups differ? 3) How actively did students participate in an asynchronous (non-real time) role-play? 4) Would argumentative blended learning arrangements (online role-play followed by drama work) affect the breath and depth of students' argumentation in their essays?

METHOD

Participants and Data Collection

The experiment was carried out in a Finnish university of applied sciences (polytechnic). The first stage which lasted one month, was conducted in the spring of 2007, on an experimental group of students (n=29, aged 21–29) from a degree program in social work. The students in the control condition (n=36, aged 19–51), also from the social work program simply wrote essays in the fall of 2008.

All the participants (experimental and controls) wrote three essays on adolescents' use of intoxicants, one in each of three different phases. The focus of the task was different in the different essays. In the first essay, the students (with absences, 25 in the experimental group, 36 in the control group) were asked to describe *their own use of intoxicants when under age, and its effects on their own well-being* (physical, psychological, and social). In the second essay the students (23 experimental, 33 control) were asked to discuss *adolescents' use of intoxicants in general, and how it affects their well-being.* In the third essay all the students (27 experimental, 31 control) wrote about *a fictional young girl's use of intoxicants as presented in an online role-play case, and its effects on her well-being.* The experimental students did this after having engaged in online role-play discussion and drama work. In total, the essay data consisted of 175 essays: 75 by the experimental group, and 100 by the control group.

In addition, the data included students' asynchronous online role-play discussions (215 messages altogether) via Moodle. The students were divided into four discussion groups, each with 7–8 members. They were asked to contribute discussions at least once a day over a five-day period.

Teaching Experiment and Blended Learning Arrangements

Figure 1 shows the design of the study. The whole teaching experiment, which included writing tasks, lectures, online role-play and drama work, is defined as an integrated macro-script in this study. The blended learning, in turn, covers online role-play discussion (phase 5), small-group drama (phase 6), and class-wide drama (phase 7). The experimental group participated in eight phases and the control group in three phases of the teaching experiment.

The pedagogical purpose of phase 1 was to activate students' thinking on the topic. The lectures on intoxicant work (Phase 2) dealt with both adolescents' use of intoxicants and general content related to intoxicant work. The aim behind the essay on adolescents' use of intoxicants in general (Phase 3) was to consolidate knowledge gained from the lectures. The lecture on collaborative argumentation (Phase 4) prepared the students for their subsequent asynchronous role-play discussion (Phase 5), followed by drama work (Phases 6 and 7). Before the role-play the students

Figure 1. Teaching experiment and the design of the study

Phase of the experiment	Activity	Task	Condition	
			Experimental (n=29)	Control (n=36)
1	First essay (15 min).	Writing on one's own use of intoxicants when under age, and its effects on one's own well-being.	X	X
2	Lectures (20 x 45 min).	Participating in lectures on intoxicant work.	X	
3	Second essay (15 min).	Writing on the effects of adolescents' use of intoxicants on their well-being in general.	X	X
4	Lectures (4 x 45 min).	Participating in lectures on collaborative argumentation.	X	
5	Online asynchronous role-play (5 days).	Engaging in online role-play at least once a day.	X	
6	Small group drama work (45 min).	Participating in small group drama work face-to-face.	X	
7	Class-wide drama work (45 min).	Presenting drama presentations class-wide and engaging in discussions after the presentations.	X	
8	Third essay (15 min).	Writing on the effects of a fictional young girl's use of intoxicants (presented in the phase 5 online role-play) on her well-being.	X	X

Note: X=participation in the activity; blended learning covers the phases 5, 6, and 7.

were given instructions and roles for their online discussion. Knowledge gained from the lectures was assumed to be utilized by the students in their online role-play and drama work.

During the asynchronous role-play discussion (Phase 5) the students engaged in a debate on the problem of a fictional young girl's use of intoxicants. Thus, the students discussed the problematic use of intoxicants by adolescents, with reference to the case of a young girl and her immediate surroundings. The discussion was based on students' real-life experiences and knowledge of the topic. The students' task was to find solutions to the problem. Four discussion groups, with either seven or eight members in each group, were set up randomly. Three of the group members were given the role of proponents ("brother," "classmate" and "principal of the school") while three were given the role of opponents ("father," "mother" and "classmate") of a proposition. The proponents were in favor of the proposition that adolescents should be allowed to organize for themselves events of a type where alcohol use is common, while the opponents took the opposite view. The perspective of the young girl ("Liisa") was not defined, and the students who took that role defined it for themselves. In addition, one group had the role of a health nurse; his/her task was to act as an expert on health issues arising in the discussion. The students were also given short descriptions of their roles. The asynchronous online role-play was intended to increase students' multidimensional understanding of adolescents' use of intoxicants.

In the drama work the students continued with the case discussed during the online role-play. During the small-group drama work (phase 6), the students' groups remained the same as they had been during the online role-play. Each group was given a different drama task (see below), intended to deepen their online role-play discussion. In this phase the students, as well as preparing their drama presentations, also collected arguments for and against the topic they were discussing. In phase 7, after the small-group work, the students presented their dramas to the whole class. The drama methods were based on forum-theatre techniques (see Boal, 1992), such as image-theatre techniques, improvisation, and role-work. Whole-class discussions followed the drama presentations.

The drama tasks given to the groups were based on the solutions that they had arrived at during their online role-play discussions. The first group was asked to present a performance to the whole class about the future of the characters in the online role-play and to discuss with the audience whether the representation was realistic or not. The second group was asked to debate in front of the whole class, taking the roles they had been given in the online role-play, on the theme *adolescents' use of alcohol should be better controlled in the future.* The third group was asked to present to the whole class a fictional meeting in which they acted out in the roles that they had been given. Their aim was to promote understanding of the topic *adolescents' organization of a free-time event*, which had also been their topic in the online role-play discussion. The fourth group was asked to discuss the topic *alcohol should be forbidden at student events* in front of the whole class, taking their fictional roles. As a final element, the methods that were used were reflected on by the whole class. Finally, the aim of the writing about a fictional young girl's use of intoxicants as presented in an online role-play case was to activate students' thinking on adolescents' intoxicant use from one person's viewpoint.

Analysis of the Students' Essays and Online Role-Play Discussions

The essays were analyzed by categorizing standpoints and arguments according to Toulmin's (1958) argumentation model. The model contains the following components: a claim, data, a warrant, a backing, a rebuttal, and a qualifier. In previous studies many researchers have simplified the components of the model to a claim, data and warrants (Kolstø, 2006); to a claim, data, and reasons (Kollar, Fischer, & Slotta, 2007); or to a claim and grounds (Marttunen & Laurinen, 2001; Weinberger, Stegmann, Fischer, & Mandl, 2007). In the present study, standpoints (claims), arguments (data, warrants, and backings) in support of the standpoint, and counter-arguments (rebuttals) were identified in the students' essays.

Standpoints were grouped into four categories according to the students' views on the effects of the use of intoxicants on adolescents' well-being: 1) no effects, 2) positive effects, 3) negative effects, and 4) both positive and negative effects. *Arguments* were classified as *primary*, *secondary*, and *tertiary* arguments. Primary arguments supported the standpoint directly, secondary arguments deepened the primary arguments, and tertiary arguments, in turn, deepened the secondary arguments. *Counter-arguments* questioned either the standpoint or arguments at different levels. An example of the analysis is presented through the following extract from one essay:

---use of alcohol harmed Liisa's [the girl in the online role-play case] well-being [standpoint, negative effect]. ---Her school work was going badly [primary argument], because she was often drank, and was even drunk at school [secondary argument]. She could not be responsive to learning and interaction at school because of her use of alcohol [tertiary argument]. However, drinking will only really harm her if she does it regularly [counter-argument] (student no. 7, third essay).

The students' online discussions were analyzed by counting how many messages each student sent via Moodle during the prescribed five-day period. The number of messages gave a rough measurement of students' motivation to participate in online discussion.

Statistical Analysis

The numbers of standpoints, arguments, and counter-arguments in the essays were counted. The association between the numbers of various standpoints and the students' essays written in the three phases were tested with Fisher's exact test for both the experimental and the control conditions. In order to obtain a more detailed picture of the expected and observed counts of the standpoints, standardized residuals were used. The residuals were adjusted to follow a normal distribution (adjusted standardized residuals, see Bewick, Cheek, & Ball, 2004, p. 47).

The data proved limited in meeting the assumptions of parametric techniques: the size of the data was quite small and the values of the dependent variables were not normally distributed (see Bland, 1988, pp. 216, 238). Thus, non-parametric tests (Kruskal-Wallis and Mann-Whitney tests) were used to compare the results between the essays written in the different phases, and between the experimental and control conditions. The Kruskal-Wallis test was used to test the differences in the means of the number of arguments and counter-arguments between the students' three essays (see Gall, Borg, & Gall, 1996, p. 403). Two-by-two comparisons were made with the Mann-Whitney test between the different essays, and between the experimental and control conditions (see Bland, 1988, pp. 217–224).

The inter-rater reliability of the analysis was examined by having two researchers classify 12% (9 out of 75) of the essays by the experimental group. The agreement percentages for the raters were 67% for standpoints, 82% for arguments, and 69% for counter-arguments.

RESULTS

Standpoints Taken in the Essays by the Experimental and Control Groups

Fisher's exact test indicated that there was an association between the numbers of different

Figure 2. Associations between the different standpoints and the students' essays in different phases in the experimental and control groups

Group	Standpoint	Phase of writing													
		First essay				Second essay				Third essay				Total	
		f	%	*ASR*	*p*	*f*	%	*ASR*	*p*	*f*	%	*ASR*	*p*	*f*	%
Experimental	No effects	13	**54.2**	**5.0**	***	1	4.3	-2.3	*	1	3.7	-2.7	**	15	20.3
	Positive effects	3	12.5	1.9	ns.	0	0.0	-1.4	ns.	1	3.7	-0.5	ns.	4	5.4
	Negative effects	4	16.7	-3.3	**	17	**73.9**	**3.4**	**	12	44.4	0.0	ns.	33	44.6
	Both positive and negative effects	4	16.7	-1.7	ns.	5	21.7	-1.0	ns.	13	**48.1**	**2.6**	**	22	29.7
	Total	24	100.0			23	100.0			27	100.0			74	100.0
Control	No effects	22	**64.7**	**6.1**	***	1	3.2	-3.6	***	3	9.7	-2.7	**	26	27.1
	Positive effects	3	8.8	1.7	ns.	1	3.2	-0.3	ns.	0	0	-1.4	ns.	4	4.2
	Negative effects	5	14.7	-4.4	***	22	**71.0**	**3.6**	***	16	51.6	0.9	ns.	43	44.8
	Both positive and negative effects	4	11.8	-2.1	*	7	22.6	-0.2	ns.	12	**38.7**	**2.3**	*	23	24.0
	Total	34	100.0			31	100.0			31	100.0			96	100.0

Note: ASR=adjusted standardised residuals; ***=$p<.001$; **=$p<.01$; *=$p<.05$; ns. =non-significant

standpoints and the three successive essays, both in the experimental (Z=33.231, p<.001) and in the control (Z=46.336, p<.001) groups. Figure 2 shows the percentages and adjusted standardized residuals for the different standpoints in both groups.

When writing about their own use of intoxicants when under age (first essay), the students typically, in both groups, reported that their own use of intoxicants did not affect their well-being (54%, ASR=5.0, p<.001, in the experimental group; and 65%, ASR=6.1, p<.001, in the control group). When the focus was on adolescents' use of intoxicants in general (second essay), the negative effects of intoxicants were emphasized in both groups: 74% of the students (ASR=3.4, p<.01) in the experimental group and 71% of the students (ASR=3.6, p<.001) in the control group took the view that adolescents' use of intoxicants had only negative effects on their well-being. When the focus was on a young girl's use of intoxicants (third essay) 48% (ASR=2.6, p<.01) of the students in the experimental group and 39% (ASR=2.3, p<.05) of the controls stressed both positive and negative effects.

Number of Arguments in the Students' Essays

Figure 3 shows that the mean number of arguments in total was highest in the second essays and lowest in the first essays, in both the experimental group (means 7.9 and 3.3) and the control group (means 6.5 and 2.6). When the three essays were compared for the occurrence of different levels of arguments, primary arguments were the most frequent and tertiary arguments the most infrequent in all cases. The Kruskal-Wallis test indicated that both the numbers of arguments at each level (primary, secondary, tertiary) and the total number of arguments differed between the three different essays in both groups.

The results of the two-by-two comparisons performed for the different levels of argument between the different essays are depicted in Figures 1–4.

Arguments in Total

On average, the students put forward more arguments in total in their second and third essays than in their first essays (Figure 4). However, when the means for the second and third essays were compared, the differences proved statistical significance only in the control condition (6.5 vs. 4.9, U=358.50, p<.05). The differences between means for the first and the second essays, and for the first and the third essays, were significant for both the experimental group and the control group (values from U=104.50, p<.001 to U=209.00, p<.001).

Figure 3. Numbers of arguments in the students' three successive essays (Kruskal-Wallis test)

Group	Level of argument	Phase of writing									Kruskal-Wallis test		
		First essay			Second essay			Third essay					
		f	*M*	*SD*	*f*	*M*	*SD*	*f*	*M*	*SD*	χ^2	*p*	*df*
Experimental	Primary	58	2.3	1.7	105	4.6	2.4	96	3.6	1.7	15.74	***	2
	Secondary	21	0.8	1.0	55	2.4	1.8	66	2.4	1.6	19.75	***	2
	Tertiary	6	0.2	0.7	21	0.9	1.2	19	0.7	0.9	6.81	*	2
	Total	85	3.3	3.4	181	7.9	5.4	181	6.7	2.9	19.69	***	2
Control	Primary	69	1.9	1.1	114	3.5	1.7	79	2.6	1.1	18.88	***	2
	Secondary	20	0.6	0.7	72	2.2	1.7	53	1.7	1.1	25.03	***	2
	Tertiary	4	0.1	0.4	25	0.8	0.9	19	0.6	0.8	15.46	***	2
	Total	93	2.6	2.2	211	6.5	4.3	151	4.9	3.0	29.85	***	2

Note: ***=p<.001; **=p<.01; *=p<.05; ns. =non-significant

When the means for arguments in total in the different essays were compared between the experimental and the control group, the difference was significant only in the students' third essay (means 6.7 vs. 4.9, U=262.00, p<.01).

Primary Arguments

The mean number of primary arguments (Figure 5) was highest in the students' second essay (M_{exp}=4.6, M_{cont}=3.5) and lowest in their first essay (M_{exp}=2.3, M_{cont}=1.9). All the differences between the essays were significant under both conditions (values from U=122.50, p<.001 to U=261.50, p<.001).

When the experimental and control groups were compared on the mean number of primary arguments, the difference was significant in the second essay (means 4.6 vs. 3.5, U=259.00, p<.05) and the third essay (means 3.6 vs. 2.6, U=273.50, p<.001).

Secondary and Tertiary Arguments

Under both experimental and control conditions the students used the highest number of secondary arguments (M_{exp}=2.4, M_{cont}=2.2) and tertiary arguments (M_{exp}=0.9, M_{cont}=0.8) in their second essays (Figures 3 and 4). The differences between the first and second essay, and between the first and third essay were significant under both conditions (values from U=113.00, p<.001 to U=368.00, p<.01).

Figure 6 shows that the students in the experimental group used more secondary arguments in their third essay than the controls (means 2.4 vs. 1.7, U=302.50, p<.05). However, when the means for the number of tertiary arguments were compared between the experimental and control groups (Figure 7) the differences were quite small (ns.).

Counter-Arguments

On average, the students produced only a few counter-arguments in their essays, and the majority did not produce any counter-arguments at all.

Figure 4. Total number of arguments in the students' three essays

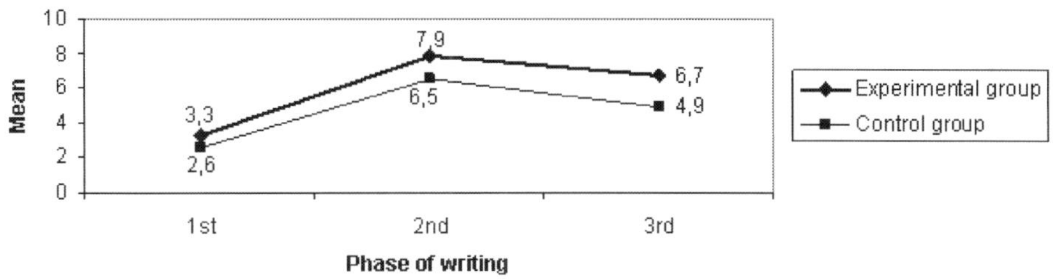

Figure 5. Number of primary arguments in the students' essays

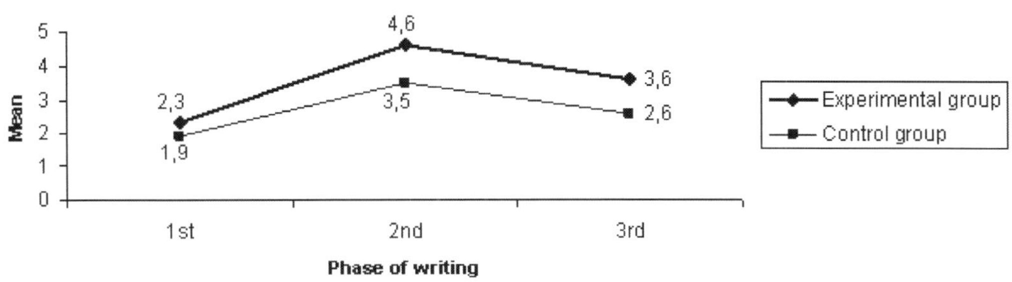

Figure 6. Number of secondary arguments in the students' essays

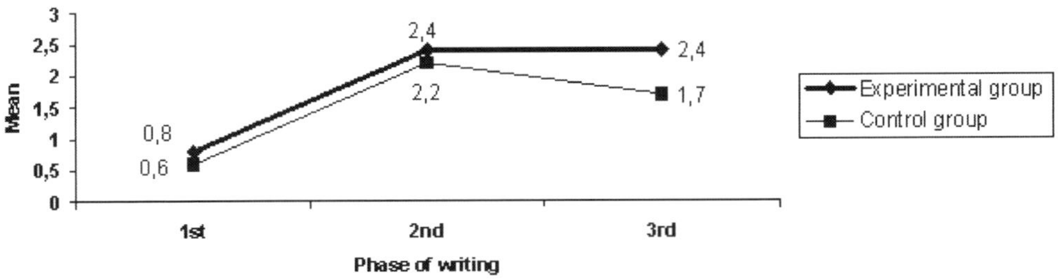

Figure 7. Number of tertiary arguments in the students' essays

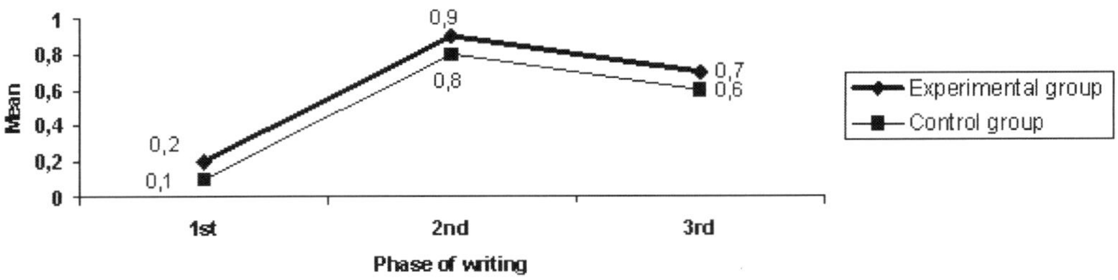

In the experimental group, counter-arguments were completely absent in 76% of the students' first essay, 65% of second essay and 70% of third essay. The corresponding figures for the control group were 64%, 61%, and 84%. The results showed no significant differences either between the different essays or between the experimental and control conditions.

Students' Level of Participation in the Online Role-Play

The students were asked to contribute to the role-play discussion via Moodle at least once a day over a five-day period. Most of the students participated in the discussion more actively than was required: in all, 72.4% participated more often than the required five times, and 20.7% of the students engaged in the discussion 10–13 times. Only 17.2% of the students participated in the discussion exactly the five times required and 10.3% less than five times. Nevertheless, all the students contributed to the online role-play at least three times. The messages sent by the students were typically extensive. The following text extract depicts the nature of the online role-play discussion. The extract comes from the first part of the problem-solving of one group (group 4):

Classmate "Mara": I didn't mean that the party should be stopped. I just would wish it would have some program other than drinking?! Because not all of us youngsters actually want to get drunk? Not even tipsy!!

Classmate "Pirjo": I would still stress that nobody is forced to take alcohol at the party, and not everyone actually does. And in my opinion no-one is left out just because they don't drink. Actually, people often worry more about those who drink too much, and when it starts to seem like they can't control themselves or calm down, we ask them to leave the party. At least when I've been present, the party has never been any kind of boozing party. It's been the sort of civilized occasion where people have behaved appropriately.

Classmate "Mara": You're quite right, no-one is forced to drink, but most of them actually do drink ... And because of that, those who don't drink feel uncomfortable or weird because they're a minority, because you always hear comments like, "Why aren't you drinking" and "Are you some kind of wimp." Of course not from everyone, but there are some partygoers who think that you can't have fun without alcohol... Although I definitely don't think that way myself.

Mother "Laura": I completely agree with what my husband said. It's amazing that other parents and school staff haven't intervened in the matter. That kind of thing wouldn't have happened in the place we lived in before. Don't the members of staff take any responsibility for the matter, since this is a blot on the reputation of the whole school, and doesn't this kind of carrying-on bother other parents?!?

"Liisa": Hey, mother and father, stop all this fussing around! If you're going to make a song and dance about this I'll never have any friends here! Everybody will get angry with me if you now prevent the organizing of this party for future! Let it go now, I've learned my lesson and I won't get plastered like that again ... please, trust me, okay...

Principal of the school "Riitta": Liisa, take it easy. It's important to discuss this issue! I think that we can get a reasonable solution to this situation. Laura and Keijo [father], I fully understand your worry when you've just have moved here. The situation must really upset you right now, but I can tell you that these events have been organized for decades, and we've never previously had things getting out of hand like this. The friendship party is an event organized by the eighth-graders themselves – not by the school. We've seen it as something that has a positive effect on the pupils' interaction. The pupils have been enthusiastic about the event, and it has played a part in influencing the young people and giving them more autonomy. Adults haven't had to intervene in the event, but of course they'll have to intervene in the future, if the situation doesn't stay within proper bounds otherwise. The idea wasn't that the party would need alcohol to develop a good group spirit. Youngsters and parents, how would you set out developing the party? In my opinion, there's no reason to stop the party just because of one case – and in so doing complicate the good relations between pupils and teachers, or change the enthusiasm of the youngsters into feelings of bitterness towards us.

DISCUSSION

General Conclusion

The purpose of this study was to develop argumentative teaching methods (integrated macro-scripts constituted by writing tasks involving different foci, online role-play discussion, and drama work) within a blended learning environment, with a view to stimulating students' argumentation. The students' argumentation was compared between three essays written in three different phases, and between an experimental group and a control group. Overall, the results suggest that the argumentative methods used here promoted students' argumentation and their ability to understand adolescents' use of intoxicants from multidimensional viewpoints.

First of all, practicing argumentation in the blended learning environment seemed to both broaden and deepen students' argumentation on the topic. Compared with the control group, the students in the experimental group used more arguments *in total* and also more primary arguments and secondary arguments in their third essays (written after the online role-play and drama work). The number of primary arguments can be taken to indicate the *breadth* of the argumentation, and the number of secondary and tertiary arguments the *depth* of the argumentation.

Compared with the control group, the students in the experimental group also used more *primary* arguments in their second essays, i.e. after the lectures on intoxicant work. Thus, the lectures alone seemed to have a broadening effect on students' argumentation. However, there seemed to be a particularly beneficial effect – a *deepening* effect – later, when the lectures were merged with the practice of argumentation that occurred in the blended learning environment. This is evidenced by the clear difference between the experimental group and the control group in the use of secondary arguments in the third essay.

Under both conditions, the total number of arguments increased from the first essay to the second essay, but decreased from the second essay to the third essay. The decrease in the number of arguments may be due to the more challenging nature of the task assigned in the third essay as compared to the second one. However, this decrease was statistically significant only in the control group.

The online role-play discussion forum seemed to be inspiring for the students. Although they were asked to contribute to the online discussions at least once a day during the five-day period, the majority of them (72%) contributed more often than required. Indeed, one fifth of the students sent messages twice as often as required, or even more frequently.

Kuhn (1991) emphasizes the value of counter-arguments when envisioning alternatives with respect to one's own standpoint. The consideration of alternatives, according to Kuhn, enables individuals to make valid and evidence-based claims regarding social issues. However, the production of counter-arguments in written texts seems to be difficult for students. Most of the students in the present study used no counter-arguments in their essays. In the first essay, the reason for this may be that when the students wrote about their personal use of intoxicants, their standpoint was, of course, supported by arguments, but not questioned through the use of counter-arguments. In the third essay, the lack of counter-arguments may be due to the fact that the most frequent line of argument was that the young girl's use of intoxicants, as it emerged in the online role-play, had both positive and negative effects on her well-being. In itself, this indicates the controversial nature of the issue in question. The second essay contained the largest number counter-arguments, although the number was small.

The results also showed that students' standpoints on the effects of adolescents' use of intoxicants on their well-being was affected by varying the focus of the writing task. When the students in the experimental group wrote about their own use of intoxicants when under age, slightly more than a half (54%) of them saw this as having no effect on their well-being. The high frequency of that standpoint may be explained by the fact that 72% of the students described their own use of intoxicants when under age as either non-existent or moderate. When the students wrote on adolescents' use of intoxicants in general, the majority in the experimental group (74%) saw this as having only negative effects on young people's well-being. This result may reflect public opinion. People often discuss social problems on a general level, solely on the basis of the information received from the media. This means that different situations related to the use of intoxicants and individual motives are often excluded from consideration. For example, in their study of middle-age and elderly people (N=246) Minnebo and Eggermont (2007) found a correlation between television exposure (television being perhaps the primary source of information on young people) and a negative perception of young people's substance use. In addition to wholly negative effects, many students (48%) of the experimental group in the present study saw both positive and negative effects in the young girl's use of alcohol as portrayed in the online role-play. The positive effects mentioned were mostly of a social nature.

The different writing tasks that the students were given on adolescents' use of intoxicants encouraged them to put forward a variety of standpoints. The standpoints that the students produced in the different tasks may illustrate a possible real-life situation in intoxicant work in which people often do not see any problems in their own use of intoxicants, but do so with regard to other people. The implication may be that argumentative writing tasks are potentially valuable in achieving a multidimensional understanding on social issues. For professionals working with adolescents, it is essential to understand different viewpoints even if there is no need to concur with them.

The writing tasks were closely integrated with the teaching experiment. The first writing task aimed at activating students to think about intoxicant use through reflecting upon their own prior experiences, the second one was related to the lectures on intoxicant work, and the third writing task involved a blended learning environment (online role-play discussion and drama work). The merging of writing assignments with the other learning environments may have the clearest advantages for domain-content learning (Tynjälä, 2001).

Blended Learning in Teacher Education

Multiple learning environments appear to be of particular benefit in deepening people's understanding of a topic. In addition to solely teacher-led knowledge-sharing during lectures, students have to elaborate the topic in a more extensive way, and from different viewpoints. During the online discussions and the drama work on adolescents' use of intoxicants, the students in the present study utilized both their own experiences and the information acquired in the lectures. The asynchronous online discussion forum provided students with an equal opportunity for debate, encouraging especially students who were not normally very active in face-to-face situations (see Cheung & Hew, 2004). The use of an asynchronous online format also made it possible for students to reread the written arguments that had been presented during the online role-play discussion. Since the discussion lasted five days, the students had plenty of opportunity to reflect on and deepen their ideas on the topic. The drama work that was based on the role-play discussions provided the students with a further opportunity to enter more deeply into interaction and discussion.

The teaching experiment presented here may be applied as an example in cases where intention is to have extended learning environments involving the integration of online and face-to-face learning. For teachers, it is important to have skills for designing large and multiple learning environments as an alternative to single teaching sessions. By combining multiple learning environments, the teachers have better possibilities to provide meaningful and effective learning experiences for students. This view is supported by Garrison and Kanuka (2004), who stress the value of blended learning environments in facilitating critical thinking and higher-order learning.

The theme (adolescents' use of intoxicants), the case (a fictional young girl's use of intoxicants), and the tasks (writing tasks, online role-play discussion, and drama work) of the present study can be applied in various learning contexts, and with students from different fields and of different ages. Moreover, the form of the integrated macro-script presented above can be copied or slightly modified and applied to different themes – such as youth criminality or truancy – with appropriate changes. Nevertheless, as Dillenbourg, Järvelä, and Fisher (2009) point out, it is important to remember that computer-assisted learning is not a recipe for producing learning at the method level; it applies more to the design level, in supporting the conditions for effective group interaction, such as explanation, argumentation, and mutual regulation.

The problematic nature of the case that the students had to solve during the blended learning (online role-play followed by drama work) was perhaps one reason why the argumentation produced in the third essay was deeper in the experimental group than in the control group. The use of cases in teacher education has been found to be beneficial to learning, among both pre-service and in-service teachers (Levin, 1995). According to Levin, students and novice teachers, in particular, may achieve more elaborated understandings of the issues in the case. In addition, they may become aware of the need for critical reflection on their own thoughts. The problems that teachers encounter in their work are ill-structured in nature, and they should thus be practiced during teachers' professional education (Cheung & Hew, 2004). As far as in-service teachers are concerned, a case-based learning environment may be of particular benefit in fostering their reflective skills and meta-cognitive thinking.

FUTURE RESEARCH DIRECTIONS

While the current study contributes to the understanding of integrated macro-scripts and blended learning in stimulating argumentation, caution is needed in generalizing the results, since they are heavily context and group dependent. However, this is also the case with many other pedagogical macro-script studies (see e.g. Hämäläinen, 2008). There is, in any case, clearly a need for further research on the effectiveness of the integration of online and face-to-face learning. The aspects to be investigated would include particularly various social and contextual effects on learning (see Häkkinen, & Mäkitalo-Siegl, 2007), the themes that can profitably be discussed online and face-to-face, and the various learning environments and methods that can be blended.

The results of the present study suggest that argumentative methods in the blended learning environment have benefits for the study of social issues in higher education, because they seemed to trigger students to put forward multifaceted standpoints and engage in deep argumentation. In future research, one might wish to look more closely at the various ways in which students can learn to transfer the information taught in lectures to their practical problem-solving – something that in the present study was done through online discussions followed by drama work, and through essay writing.

Finally, it can be suggested that this study represents an attempt to merge theoretical studies with the requirements of professional practice. This would seem to be an essential procedure in higher education, but it is one that has not so far been adequately implemented, either in higher education (Tynjälä, 2001) or in teacher education (Korthagen, 2001).

REFERENCES

Andriessen, J. (2002). Arguing to learn. In Sawyer, R. K. (Ed.), *Cambridge handbook of learning science* (pp. 443–444). Cambridge, UK: Cambridge University Press.

Andriessen, J., Baker, M., & Suthers, D. (2003). Argumentation, computer support, and the educational context of confronting cognitions. In Andriessen, J., Baker, M., & Suthers, D. (Eds.), *Arguing to learn. Confronting cognitions in computer supported collaborative learning environments* (pp. 3–25). Dordrecht, The Netherlands: Kluwer.

Bewick, V., Cheek, L., & Ball, J. (2004). Statistics review 8: Qualitative data–tests of association. *Critical Care (London, England)*, *8*(1), 46–53. doi:10.1186/cc2428

Bland, M. (1988). *An introduction to medical statistics*. Oxford, UK: Oxford University press.

Blatchford, P., Kutnick, P., Baires, E., & Galton, M. (2003). Toward a social pedagogy of classroom group work. *International Journal of Educational Research*, *39*(1–2), 153–172. doi:10.1016/S0883-0355(03)00078-8

Boal, A. (1992). *Games for actors and non-actors* (Jackson, A., Trans.). London: Routledge.

Borgen, W., & Hiebert, B. (2006). Career guidance and counseling for youth: What adolescents and young adults are telling us? *International Journal for the Advancement of Counseling*, *28*(4), 389–400. doi:10.1007/s10447-006-9022-5

Cheung, W. S., & Hew, K. F. (2004). Evaluating the extent of ill-structured problem-solving process among pre-service teachers in an asynchronous online discussions and reflection log learning environment. *Journal of Educational Computing Research*, *30*(3), 197–227. doi:10.2190/9JTN-10T3-WTXH-P6HN

Dillenbourg, P., & Hong, F. (2008). The mechanics of CSCL macro-scripts. *International Journal of Computer-Supported Collaborative Learning*, *3*(1), 5–23. doi:10.1007/s11412-007-9033-1

Dillenbourg, P., Järvelä, S., & Fisher, F. (2009). The evolution of research on computer-supported collaborative learning: From design to orchestration. In Balacheff, N., Ludvigsen, S., de Jong, T., Lazonder, T. A., & Barnes, S. (Eds.), *Technology enhanced learning: Principles and products* (pp. 3–19). Amsterdam: Springer.

Dillenbourg, P., & Jermann, P. (2007). Designing integrative scripts. In Fischer, F., Kollar, I., Mandl, H., & Haage, J. M. (Eds.), *Scripting computer-supported collaborative learning. Cognitive, computational, and educational perspectives* (pp. 275–301). New York: Springer. doi:10.1007/978-0-387-36949-5_16

Dillenbourg, P., & Tchounikine, P. (2007). Flexibility in macro-scripts for computer-supported collaborative learning. *Journal of Computer Assisted Learning*, *23*(1), 1–11. doi:10.1111/j.1365-2729.2007.00191.x

Felton, M., & Kuhn, D. (2001). The Development of Argumentative Discourse Skill. *Discourse Processes*, *32*(2–3), 135–153. doi:10.1207/S15326950DP3202&3_03

Fischer, F., Kollar, I., Haake, J. M., & Mandl, H. (2007). Perspectives on collaboration scripts. In Fischer, F., Kollar, I., Mandl, H., & Haage, J. M. (Eds.), *Scripting computer-supported collaborative learning. Cognitive, computational and educational perspectives* (pp. 1–10). New York: Springer. doi:10.1007/978-0-387-36949-5_1

Gall, M. D., Borg, W. R., & Gall, J. P. (1996). *Educational research. An introduction* (6th ed.). New York: Longman.

Garrison, D. R., & Kanuka, H. (2004). Blended learning: Uncovering its transformative potential in higher education. *The Internet and Higher Education*, *7*(2), 95–105. doi:10.1016/j.iheduc.2004.02.001

Garrison, D. R., & Vaughan, N. D. (2008). *Blended learning in higher education. Framework, principles, and guidelines*. San Francisco: Jossey-Bass.

Häkkinen, P., & Mäkitalo-Siegl, K. (2007). Educational perspectives on scripting CSCL. In Fischer, F., Kollar, I., Mandl, H., & Haage, J. M. (Eds.), *Scripting computer-supported collaborative learning. Cognitive, computational and educational perspectives* (pp. 263–271). New York: Springer. doi:10.1007/978-0-387-36949-5_15

Hämäläinen, J. (2003). The concept of social pedagogy in the field of social work. *Journal of Social Work*, *3*(1), 69–81. doi:10.1177/1468017303003001005

Hämäläinen, R. (2008). *Pedagogical scripts to facilitate computer-supported collaborative learning*. Jyväskylä, Finland: University of Jyväskylä, Finnish Institute for Educational Research.

Hesse, H. (2007). Being told to do something or just being aware of something? An alternative approach to scripting in CSCL. In Fischer, F., Kollar, I., Mandl, H., & Haage, J. M. (Eds.), *Scripting computer-supported collaborative learning. Cognitive, computational and educational perspectives* (pp. 91–98). New York: Springer. doi:10.1007/978-0-387-36949-5_6

Hirsch, L., Saeedi, M., Cornillon, J., & Litosseliti, L. (2004). A structured dialogue tool for argumentative learning. *Journal of Computer Assisted Learning, 20*(1), 72–80. doi:10.1111/j.1365-2729.2004.00068.x

Jonassen, D. H. (1997). Instructional design models for well-structured and ill-structured problem-solving learning outcomes. *Educational Technology Research and Development, 45*(1), 1043–1629. doi:10.1007/BF02299613

Kollar, I., Fischer, F., & Slotta, J. (2007). Internal and external scripts in computer-supported collaborative inquiry learning. *Learning and Instruction, 17*(6), 708–721. doi:10.1016/j.learninstruc.2007.09.021

Kolstø, S. D. (2006). Patterns in students' argumentation controlled with a risk-focused socio-scientific issue. *International Journal of Science Education, 28*(14), 1689–1716. doi:10.1080/09500690600560878

Korthagen, F. A. J. (2001). *Linking practice and theory: the pedagogy of realistic teacher education.* Paper presented at the Annual Meeting of the American Educational Research Association, Seattle, April 2001.

Kuhn, D. (1991). *The skills of argument.* Cambridge, UK: Cambridge University Press.

Kuhn, D. (1999). A developmental model of critical thinking. *Educational Research, 28*(2), 16–25.

Laurinen, L., & Marttunen, M. (2007). Written arguments and collaborative speech acts in practicing the argumentative power of language though chat debates. *Computers and Composition, 24*(3), 230–246. doi:10.1016/j.compcom.2007.05.002

Levin, B. B. (1995). Using the case method in teacher education: The role of discussion and experience in teachers' thinking about cases. *Teaching and Teacher Education, 11*(1), 63–79. doi:10.1016/0742-051X(94)00013-V

Lund, K., Molinari, G., Séjourné, A., & Baker, M. (2007). How do argumentation diagrams compare when student pairs use them as a means to debate or as a tool for representing debate? *International Journal of Computer-Supported Collaborative Learning, 2*(2–3), 273–295. doi:10.1007/s11412-007-9019-z

Marttunen, M., & Laurinen, L. (2001). Learning of argumentation skills in networked and face-to-face environments. *Instructional Science, 29*(2), 127–153. doi:10.1023/A:1003931514884

Marttunen, M., Laurinen, L., Litosseliti, L., & Lund, K. (2005). Argumentation skills as prerequisites for collaborative learning among Finnish, French and English secondary school students. *Educational Research and Evaluation, 11*(4), 365–384. doi:10.1080/13803610500110588

Means, M. L., & Voss, J. F. (1996). Who reasons well? Two studies of informal reasoning among children of different grade, ability, and knowledge level. *Cognition and Instruction, 14*(2), 139–178. doi:10.1207/s1532690xci1402_1

Minnebo, J., & Eggermont, S. (2007). Watching the young use illicit drugs: Direct experience, exposure to television and the stereotyping of adolescents' use substance use. *Young, 15*(2), 129–144. doi:10.1177/110330880701500202

National Institute for Health and Welfare. (2008). *School Health Promotion Study.* Retrieved February 1, 2009, from http://info.stakes.fi/kouluterveys/tulokset/koko2008pk.pdf.

OECD. (2006). *Science competencies for tomorrow's world. Analysis. Volume 1. Programme for International Student Assessment (PISA).* Organization for Economic Co-operation and Development. Retrieved November 28, 2008, from http://www.oecd.org/dataoecd/30/17/39703267.pdf

Osborne, J., Erduran, S., & Simon, S. (2004). Enhancing the quality of argumentation in school science. *Journal of Research in Science Teaching*, *41*(10), 994–1020. doi:10.1002/tea.20035

Osguthorpe, R. T., & Graham, C. R. (2003). Blended learning environments: definitions and directions. *The entity from which ERIC acquires the content, including journal, organization, and conference names, or by means of online submission from the author. Quarterly Review of Distance Education*, *4*(3), 227–233.

Peavy, V. (2003). *Sociodynamic counseling. A constructivist perspective*. Victoria, Canada: Trafford.

Simonneaux, L. (2001). Role-play or debate to promote students' argumentation or justification on an issue in animal transgenesis. *International Journal of Science Education*, *23*(9), 903–927. doi:10.1080/09500690010016076

Toulmin, S. (1958). *The uses of argument*. Cambridge, UK: Cambridge University Press.

Tynjälä, P. (2001). Writing, learning and the development of expertise in higher education. In G. Rijlaarsdarn, P. Tynjälä, L. Mason, & K. Lonka (Volume Eds.), Studies in writing. Writing as a learning tool: integrating theory and practice (Vol. 7, pp. 37–56). Dordrecht, Netherlands: Kluwer.

van Bruggen, J. M., Kirschner, P. A., & Jochems, W. (2002). External representation of argumentation in CSCL and the management of cognitive load. *Learning and Instruction*, *12*(1), 121–138. doi:10.1016/S0959-4752(01)00019-6

Veerman, A., Andriessen, J., & Kanselaar, G. (2002). Collaborative argumentation in academic education. *Instructional Science*, *30*(3), 155–186. doi:10.1023/A:1015100631027

Veerman, A., & Treasure-Jones, T. (1999). Software for problem solving through collaborative argumentation. In Andriessen, J., & Coirier, P. (Eds.), *Foundations of argumentative text processing* (pp. 203–229). Amsterdam: Amsterdam University Press.

von Aufschnaiter, C., Erduran, S., Osborne, J., & Simon, S. (2008). Arguing to learn and learning to argue: case studies of how students' argumentation relates to their scientific knowledge. *Journal of Research in Science Teaching*, *45*(1), 101–131. doi:10.1002/tea.20213

Weinberger, A., Stegmann, K., Fischer, F., & Mandl, H. (2007). Scripting argumentative knowledge construction in computer-supported learning environments. In Fischer, F., Kollar, I., Mandl, H., & Haage, J. M. (Eds.), *Scripting computer-supported collaborative learning. Cognitive, computational and educational perspectives* (pp. 191–211). New York: Springer. doi:10.1007/978-0-387-36949-5_12

ADDITIONAL READING

Chinn, C. A. (2006). Learning to argue. In O'Donnell, A. M., Hmelo-Silver, C. E., & Erkens, G. (Eds.), *Collaborative learning, reasoning, and technology* (pp. 355–383). London: Erlbaum.

Clark, B. C., & Sampson, V. D. (2007). Personally-seeded discussions to scaffold online argumentation. *International Journal of Science Education*, *29*(3), 253–277. doi:10.1080/09500690600560944

Clark, D. B., Sampson, V. D., Weinberger, A., & Erkens, G. (2007). Analytic framework for assessing dialogic argumentation in online learning environments. *Educational Psychology Review*, *19*(3), 343–374. doi:10.1007/s10648-007-9050-7

Craig, R. T., & Tracy, K. (2005). "The issue" in argumentation practice and theory. In F. H. van Eemeren, & P. Houtlosser (Eds.), Argumentation in practice (pp. 11–28). Amsterdam: John Benjamins.

Dillenbourg, P. (2002). Over-scripting CSCL: the risk of blending collaborative learning with instructional design. In P. A. Kirschner (Ed.), Three words of CSCL. Can we support CSCL? (pp. 61–91). Heeren, Nederland: Open University of Nederland.

Erduran, S., Simon, S., & Osborne, J. (2004). TAPping into argumentation: Developments in the application of Toulmin's argument pattern for studying science discourse. *Science Education*, *88*(6), 915–933. doi:10.1002/sce.20012

Erkens, G., Prangsma, M., & Jasper, J. (2006). Planning and Coordinating Activities in Collaborative Learning. In O'Donnell, A. M., Hmelo-Silver, C. E., & Erkens, G. (Eds.), *Collaborative learning, reasoning, and technology* (pp. 233–263). London: Erlbaum.

Hämäläinen, R. (2008). Designing and evaluating collaboration in a virtual game environment for vocational learning. *Computers & Education*, *50*(1), 98–109. doi:10.1016/j.compedu.2006.04.001

Hämäläinen, R., Oksanen, K., & Häkkinen, P. (2008). Designing and analyzing collaboration in a scripted game for vocational education. *Computers in Human Behavior*, *24*(6), 2496–2506. doi:10.1016/j.chb.2008.03.010

Järvelä, S., Häkkinen, P., Arvaja, M., & Leinonen, P. (2004). Instructional support in CSCL. In Strijbos, J.-W., Kirschner, P. A., & Martens, R. L. (Eds.), *What we know about CSCL: and implementing it in higher education* (pp. 115–139). Dordrecht, The Netherlands: Kluwer. doi:10.1007/1-4020-7921-4_5

Kobbe, L., Weinberger, A., Dillenbourg, P., Harrer, A., Hämäläinen, R., Häkkinen, P., & Fischer, F. (2007). Specifying computer-supported collaboration scripts. *International Journal of Computer-Supported Collaborative Learning*, *2*(2–3), 211–224. doi:10.1007/s11412-007-9014-4

Kollar, I., Fischer, F., & Hesse, F. W. (2006). Collaboration scripts – a conceptual analysis. *Educational Psychology Review*, *18*(2), 159–185. doi:10.1007/s10648-006-9007-2

Koschmann, T. (2003). CSCL, Argumentation, and Deweyan Inquiry: Argumentation *is* learning. In Andriessen, J., Baker, M., & Suthers, D. (Eds.), *Arguing to learn. Confronting cognitions in computer supported collaborative learning environments* (pp. 261–269). Dordrecht, The Netherlands: Kluwer.

Newmann, F. M. (1991). Higher order thinking in the teaching of social studies: Connections between theory and practice. In Voss, J. F., Perkins, D. N., & Segal, J. W. (Eds.), *Informal reasoning and education* (pp. 381–400). Mahwah, NJ: Erlbaum.

Oulton, C., Dillon, J., & Grace, M. M. (2004). Reconceptualising the teaching the controversial issues. *International Journal of Science Education*, *26*(4), 411–423. doi:10.1080/0950069032000072746

Quignard, M. (2005). A collaborative model of argumentation in dyadic problem-solving interactions. In van Eemeren, F. H., & Houtlosser, P. (Eds.), *Argumentation in practice* (pp. 69–85). Amsterdam: John Benjamins.

Sampson, V., & Clark, D. B. (2008). Assessment of the ways students generate arguments in science education: current perspectives and recommendations for future directions. *Science Education*, *92*(3), 447–472. doi:10.1002/sce.20276

Schwarz, B. (2003). Collective reading of multiple texts in argumentative activities. *International Journal of Educational Research*, *39*(1–2), 133–151. doi:10.1016/S0883-0355(03)00077-6

Stahl, G. (2007). Scripting group cognition. In Fischer, F., Kollar, I., Mandl, H., & Haage, J. M. (Eds.), *Scripting computer-supported collaborative learning. Cognitive, computational and educational perspectives* (pp. 327–335). New York: Springer. doi:10.1007/978-0-387-36949-5_18

Suthers, D. D. (2007). Roles of computational scripts. In Fischer, F., Kollar, I., Mandl, H., & Haage, J. M. (Eds.), *Scripting computer-supported collaborative learning. Cognitive, computational and educational perspectives* (pp. 177–187). New York: Springer. doi:10.1007/978-0-387-36949-5_11

van Eemeren, F. H., & Grootendorst, R. (2003). *A systematic theory of argumentation. The pragma-dialectical approach*. Cambridge, UK: Cambridge University Press. doi:10.1017/CBO9780511616389

van Eemeren, F. H., Grootendorst, R., & Kruiger, T. (1987). *Handbook of Argumentation Theory. A critical survey of classical backgrounds and modern studies*. Dordrecht, The Netherlands: Foris.

Waghid, Y. (2005). Action as an educational virtue: toward a different understanding of democratic citizenship education. *Educational Theory*, *55*(3), 323–342.

Weinberger, A., Stegmann, K., & Fisher, F. (2007). Knowledge convergence in collaborative learning: Concepts and assessment. *Learning and Instruction*, *17*(4), 416–426. doi:10.1016/j.learninstruc.2007.03.007

Wiley, J., & Bailey, J. (2006). Effects of collaboration and argumentation on learning from web pages. In O'Donnell, A. M., Hmelo-Silver, C. E., & Erkens, G. (Eds.), *Collaborative learning, reasoning, and technology* (pp. 297–321). London: Erlbaum.

Chapter 11
Women and Technology, Upon Reflection:
Linking Global Women's Issues to the Digital Gender Divide in Urban Social Studies Education

Judith Cramer
Columbia University, USA

Margaret Smith Crocco
Columbia University, USA

ABSTRACT

Two collaborating urban university educators document their evolving understanding of the ways in which technology, gender and social studies intersect to challenge traditional assumptions in teacher education. The "male" culture of computing, notoriously unfriendly to girls in schools, is part of a well-documented digital gender gap. Though teacher preparation curricula often make little reference to gender, most American education students are female, and are taught by females in a profession often referred to (derogatively) as "feminized." Through their efforts to infuse technology in a course on global women's issues, and in the surrounding pre-service master's degree program, the authors learned to see the role of digital technology in new ways. Joining the subject of female empowerment worldwide to issues of technology access, use, and culture in schools, they used research on the digital gender divide to expand technology's role in their curriculum from mere method to essential course content.

INTRODUCTION

What makes software good for education?

- It costs less than a hundred dollars.
- You can learn it in less than half an hour. And
- (pause here for effect) it delivers a lot of bang for the buck.

With this definition of digital excellence, we welcomed our students to a new Technology Seminar at Teachers College, Columbia University, at the beginning of the 21st century. Like most teacher educators, when we began our collaborative work on

DOI: 10.4018/978-1-61520-897-5.ch011

Copyright © 2010, IGI Global. Copying or distributing in print or electronic forms without written permission of IGI Global is prohibited.

technology infusion we regarded digital technology simply as a tool to support course content, the (intellectual) "bang." Early on in the process, we discovered that "less is more," especially when it comes to preparing student teachers for under-resourced urban schools.

Eight years later, we see digital technology both as content and tool in social studies education. Our experience infusing technology into a pre-service social studies program has changed our perspective. Reflecting on our work now, we see that at its heart has been finding ways to infuse technology into social studies curricula that pay attention to the digital divide of gender. The strategies we have developed for technology integration reflect our evolving understanding of several complexities:

- The relative silence on the subject of gender in teacher education, despite the fact that gender issues exist in education generally and in social studies education particularly;[1]
- The challenges and opportunities afforded by the effort to infuse technology, itself a gendered subject, into a course focused on gender issues; and
- The dynamic state of digital technology, manifested recently in the shift from desktop to cloud computing, and the proliferation of social networking sites.

We offer this chapter to provide useful models and adaptable examples to teacher educators who may be confronting the same complexities or paradoxes. We want to share a few of the curriculum projects we devised for our students, and, with reflection, were able to improve. At each stage of our work we sought student input and critique, through class discussion, journal entries, individual and group interviews and end-of-course surveys. Our own reflective practice took the form of writing, which often incorporated students' responses to various technology initiatives. The discipline of writing, and especially writing collaboratively, proved a goad to intellectual clarity, rigorous assessment, and, eventually, to contextualizing our work through research at the intersection of technology, gender and social studies.

Throughout this chapter we cite our experiences and the reflections on these experiences that took the form of published articles, in order to indicate how reflection helped us improve our practice. In addition, we describe in detail the evolution of our approach to technology infusion in one course designed for pre-service students: Women of the World: Issues in Teaching. While changes in technology afforded new possibilities, at the same time, our own understanding of the relationship of digital technology to women's empowerment became more sophisticated. Our original philosophy of "less is more" remains in place, and remains appropriate to the range of situations our graduates encounter in their student teaching placements, where technology equipment, support, and internet access may all be problematic. However, we now know how to use our simple tools in more profound ways. We still use the concept-mapping software *Inspiration*, for example, the first digital tool we adopted, but instead of relying on it for a whole project, now we integrate it with online learning activities such as (a) building an archive of sites on *delicious.com* for (b) creating a *WebQuest* about women.

Ultimately we came to understand, through our encounters with a series of digital divides, based not just on the factors of race, class and economics in our city, but on gender in the socially constructed "male" world of computing, and on pedagogic hierarchies in the disciplinary subcultures of schooling, how technology not only could be, but should be, more than mere tool. Our predominantly female graduates would likely encounter mandated curriculum (and textbooks) that give women in history and women's social issues little attention, if any, as well as a school computer culture notoriously unfriendly to girls. Yet, by looking at technology from the perspective of a course on the world's women, they could also see it "as one of the most powerful tools available... to interrupt the inheritance of patriarchy" (Crocco & Cramer, 2005, p. 41). Reflection combined with action produced ways to address the digital divide of gender and to empower young women (and young men) to use gender—reflectively—in their own teaching careers.

Women of the World: Issues in Teaching provided an intellectual platform in which to test ideas for overcoming the gender divide in technology. This elective course, offered once a year in a master's degree program in social studies, regularly enrolls between 15 and 30 master's students, about 75% of whom are female. Since its subject is gender issues, and its students are primarily female, the course offered a suitable environment to try to add value to the study of women by using technology tools that could be mastered without detracting from the main focus of the course — content from history, anthropology, and sociology illuminating the history and status of women and girls worldwide.

For readers unfamiliar with the evolving problem of digital divides, perhaps a brief word of explanation is in order. Although researchers have documented amelioration of some digital divides related to race, class, age, and income, one that has persisted is the divide between girls and boys regarding technology use. Even today in the United States, women are under-represented in computer science and engineering, for example, with women numbering fewer than one in five among doctoral students in these disciplines (OECD, 2009, p. 14). In fact, as a field, computer science has seen a regressive trend in women's participation, when measured by the number of college majors and advanced degrees (Sanders, 2005). Research on technology use summarized in several chapters of the *Handbook of Gender Equity* (Klein, 2007) and elsewhere over the last fifteen years (Brunner, 2003; Hanson, 1997; Sanders 2005) shows that girls have been less likely than boys to be frequent users of many technologies, especially video games. While recent studies of teenagers and Web 2.0 technologies, such as those undertaken by the Pew Internet & American Life Project (Lenhart & Madden, 2003, 2005, 2007; Rainie & Hitlin, 2005), indicate that these patterns of technology use may be evolving, it still remains true that, in general, girls have a lower sense of self-efficacy regarding technology use than boys (Brown, S., Boyer, M., Mayall, H., Johnson, P., Ming, L., Butler, M., 2003).

As two female teacher educators preparing a cohort of primarily female graduate students for entrance to a predominately female profession, we assumed that our pre-service teacher program might provide an interesting ecology in which to explore the intersection of gender, technology, and social studies. In this chapter, we document our consideration of and evolving strategies for infusing technology into a master's certification program in the teaching of social studies that posits the importance of gender to that process. We hope the insights we offer here, distilled by ongoing reflection on our practice, may be of use to other teacher educators.

THE SOCIAL STUDIES PROGRAM: EARLY EFFORTS

In this section, we describe our early efforts to shape a technology approach for the pre-service master's level social studies program at Teachers College (TC). We began our work together under a PT3 grant-funded initiative to integrate technology in teacher preparation programs across the College. For three years (2000–2003) our goal was to ensure that our students would leave the program knowing how to choose simple, inexpensive yet effective tools, such as *Inspiration* and *Timeliner*, to add value to their social studies teaching. The history of this work, which brought us face to face with digital divides related to race, class, and gender, is presented in an essay in the *Journal of Computing in Teacher Education* (Crocco & Cramer, 2004).

One of these divides was the very great disparity between TC's technology infusion ideal and the reality awaiting student teachers in the urban schools where most of them did their student teaching and worked after graduation. We anticipated part of this divide: scarcity of equipment. What we did not anticipate, however, was our students' reports of the disinterest their cooperating teachers expressed about using technology. While it would be easy to attribute this attitude to the lack of equipment, we learned from our research into subject cultures (see Goodson & Mangan, 1995; Means, Penuel & Padilla, 2001) that unlike teachers in other school subjects, history and social studies teachers have been among the most reluctant to bring computers into their classrooms.

We recognized the need during the grant experience to investigate our students' attitudes about and skills in using technology, including facility with standard tools such as email and educational applications such as concept-mapping software. We reproduce here a screen shot of the results of a 2003 inquiry into our students' technological expertise. As is apparent, at least for most of the "digital natives" (Prensky, 2001) who comprised our class, student proficiency related mainly to conventional uses of technology like word processing, rather than to educational software such as *Inspiration.*

As our efforts at introducing technology into the pre-service program unfolded, we were forcefully reminded by our students that technology must be embedded in meaningful content to win their interest. Having come to TC after five years as a middle and secondary school technology specialist, during which she had created content-based technology projects across the curriculum (Scharf & Cramer, 2002), Cramer knew this. Likewise, Crocco, who had written on the value of a constructivist approach in teacher education (Crocco, 2001), should have predicted that a mandated Tech Seminar, with a narrow focus on computer applications, would likely provoke student resistance. Later, reading reports of other PT3 grant institutions posted on the U.S. Department of Education Web site, we learned that many had made the same early mistake. At TC, students articulated dissatisfaction with the Tech Seminar on several grounds: its "one size fits all" format did not take account of the fact that some entering students knew a lot and some knew nothing (see Figure 1). In crowded computer labs at the College, large classes of students had to double up, with experienced learners helping beginners. Apart from this, they argued, the Tech Seminar was a waste of time, anyway, because the New York City schools they were assigned to provided little equipment and even less encouragement for them to try applying what they learned; besides, there were other pressures on their time, such as preparing high school students for state exams.

Reflecting back on the three-year developmental process of devising the program's technology policy, we believe that we benefited from student critiques in ways we did not anticipate then. The issues students raised—access to the computers in their schools, where equipment was generally poor and scarce; the school's culture of computing, exclusionary and competitive, with math and science classes usually commandeering what lab time there was; and the disinterest in technology shown by the social studies teachers mentoring them—these remained in our minds and later informed our research-based efforts to make technology play a significant, empowering role for the (largely female) future teachers we worked with in Women of the World.

For the program-at-large, we decided on a two-pronged strategy. Under the PT 3 grant, we began infusing technology in all our courses, thus partially eliminating the need for a Tech Seminar. We decided also to require students to take workshops offered by the Computing and Information Services at our institution. They could take any two workshops they wished; they simply needed to document the fact that they had taken two. This approach ameliorated previous student resistance to the one-size-fits-all format of the Tech Seminar

Figure 1. Teachers College pre-service students' self-reported technology expertise profile shows more facility with standard software programs than with educational applications. © 2003 Judith Cramer

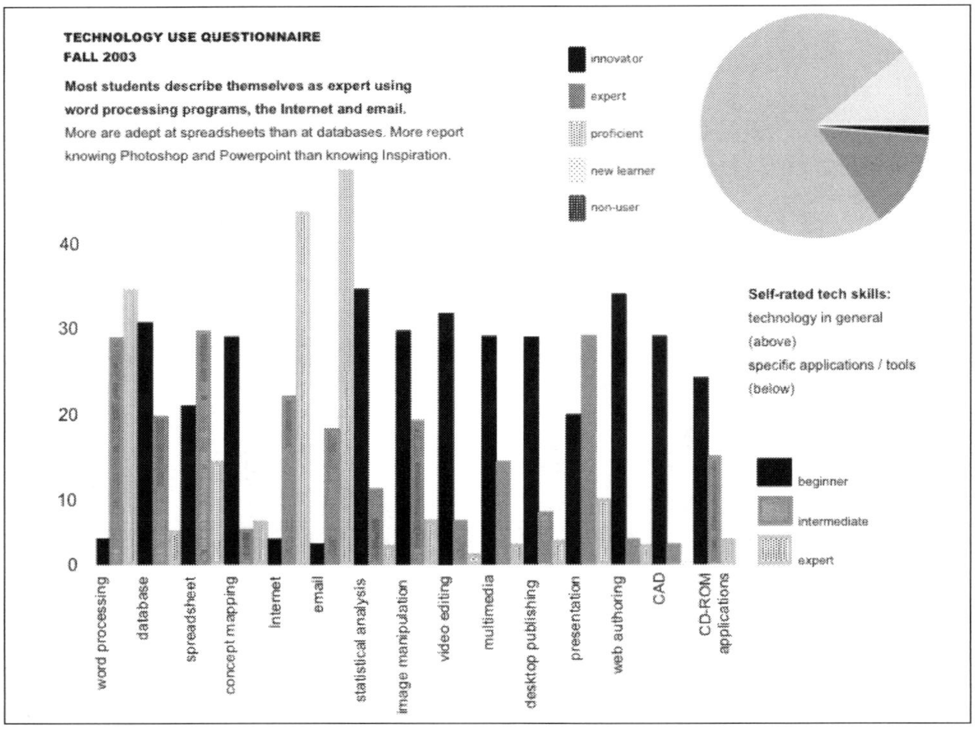

and allowed for a customized solution to enhancing student skills in technology use. We were committed to creating a technology-rich teacher preparation program that would offer our graduates a glimpse of what was possible in bringing a constructivist, student-centered approach to the use of technology in social studies classrooms (Coppola, 2005).

WOMEN OF THE WORLD: SECOND STAGE EFFORTS

Although originally we were confident that technology belonged on the methods rather than content side of our master's level certification curriculum, that is not where it stayed. As we reflected further about technology's place in the social studies, we concluded that digital tools must be examined as content as well as process, especially considering our largely female cohort from the standpoint of women's history.

From the perspective of feminist historians such as Gerda Lerner, whose works on patriarchy (1985, 1992) are core texts in Women of the World, digital technology, particularly the Internet, can be seen as a way to create the global female communication network that is necessary to interrupt patriarchy. From the perspective of our own ongoing research, at the intersection of gender, technology and social studies (see Crocco, Cramer & Meier, 2008), expert use of technology by women social studies educators can be a way to work against patriarchy and its artifact, sexism, and for gender equity, in the technology-inflected culture of schooling.

Reflecting on these connections in a presentation for the Society for Information Technology and Teacher Education (SITE), subsequently published in SITE's affiliated online journal (Crocco

& Cramer, 2005a), we offered one model for using technology to bring women's history into high school social studies classes:

We looked for digital tools that are attractive, easy to learn, inexpensive and therefore generally accessible, and adaptable to a wide variety of topics and settings. We designed projects for the students that brought digital tools into connection with significant skills dimensions in the teaching of social studies: the organization of complex data, the uncovering of misconceptions in thinking about social studies topics, the relationships between historical narrative and other forms of representation, such as literature, chronology and change, and cause and effect...[W]e also brought a set of strong values to this enterprise that dictated the need for these technology applications to enhance the constructivist, student-centered pedagogy we wish to foster in our teacher education program.[2] *(Crocco & Cramer 2005a, p. 42)*

To sequence our technology projects in the most effective way, we adopted ideas Gee had recently put forth in *What Video Games Have to Teach Us about Learning and Literacy* (2003). Following the lesson he drew from video games about "frontloading feedback," we moved from simple to more complex uses of technology, by a) turning to more sophisticated tools after beginning with simple ones, and b) combining tools, as described above. We also applied the notion of "pleasurable frustration" that he reported propelled his young son from level to level in video games. We tried to aim for a level of expertise just at the limit of our students' competencies, though, admittedly, this was made difficult by the diversity of their technology backgrounds (visualized through self-reported data, in Figure 1). Women of the World's technology strategies, as we had formulated them in 2004, are captured in this image of a screen from our slide presentation at SITE (Figure 2).

One measure of our approach's effectiveness was the fact that students began to innovate with technology, doing more than we asked in their assignments. As we reported in our paper, several asked to combine tools; one student decided to create a Web site to publish her work on the Internet, though that had not been mandated. Most striking, and most gratifying to us, was the connection our students, men and women alike, made between technology competence and the empowerment of women, locally as well as globally. "Teachers

Figure 2. Summary slide, "Technology use, women, and global studies in social studies teacher education," Best paper award recipient, SITE 2004. ©2004 Judith Cramer and Margaret Smith Crocco

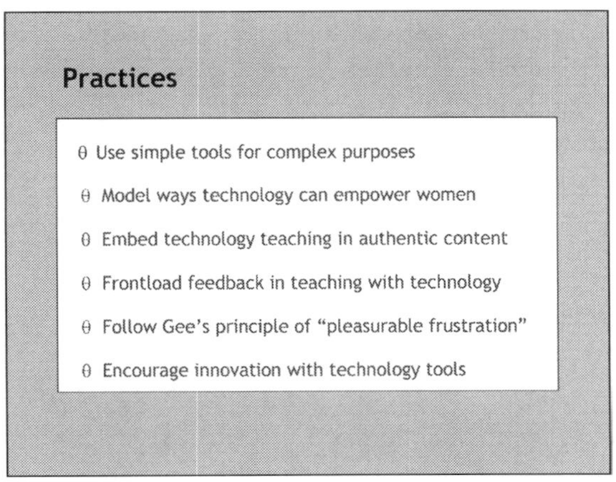

don't get enough technological instruction," wrote one respondent to our anonymous end-of-course surveys; offered another: "women need to become technologically versed."

Early Projects with Inspiration® and Timeliner®

Student surveys from cohorts of Women of the World students (2001-2003) showed *Inspiration* to be the clear favorite among technologies used in the course. One reason for this, obviously, is that the concept-mapping program conformed to our articulated definition of a superior digital tool. In this case, however,

- The specified cheap price was actually zero, when students received 30-day demo disks provided by the publisher, so they could load the software on their home computers;
- The requisite short learning time was facilitated by Cramer's in-class instruction on two useful software programs, Inspiration and Timeliner, together at the beginning of the term;
- The crucial element, or "bang," resulted from our work devising meaningful projects to connect these software tools to women's global experiences and the theme of female empowerment.

Inspiration, a digital tool originally developed for business, with a formulaic interface that could be construed as limiting, became a powerful lever for raising technology-based learning goals when connected to data sets in Joni Seager's (1997) *State of Women of the World Atlas*, a required text in the course (Crocco & Cramer, 2005a). Similarly, *Timeliner*, a program our students found even more limited in its interface and capacities than *Inspiration*, and which came in second in the popularity contest, was still the one that most students chose to use for final projects because we connected it to a popular fictional reading, *In the Time of the Butterflies*, Julia Alvarez's poetic account of the martyred Mirabal sisters in the Dominican Republic under Trujillo.

We asked students to construct two timelines around the Mirabal sisters' story: one pinpointing events as seen or told by a historian; the other visualizing the same events from the perspective of Alvarez's narrative. Deceptively simple, this project could be used to explore a complex literary idea with high school students: how a novelist expands some events or episodes and contracts others, almost like an accordion player, in order to sound a theme. Figure 3, a slide from our SITE presentation, shows a single panel taken from one of the classroom projects that resulted from this assignment. The panel displays flags of two different colors, indicating the two timelines, and primary source images, including portraits of the murdered *mariposas* (butterflies) as the Mirabal sisters were called. Most dual timelines created by students on *In the Time of the Butterflies* comprised 20–30 panels in *Timeliner*.

Inspiration® and Timeliner,® Upon Further Reflection

We continue to rely on the ideas of concept mapping and timelining, while recognizing that particular software programs used by educators, even very good ones, like *Hyperstudio*, may go in and out of the marketplace without warning. *Inspiration* piloted a new online version in spring 2008, which at first blush appears to be better than Web-based conceptual mapping tools made available by *Mindmeister* (www.mindmeister.com) and *Gliffy* (www.gliffy.com), for instance. Our students have used *Timeliner* successfully with their oral history projects, to situate individual lives in historical contexts. Some students have constructed oral history timelines with *Inspiration*. Of the two, *Inspiration* has proved the most useful to us as teachers. Among its many classroom uses are: brainstorming, debunking myths, project

Figure 3. Slide from SITE presentation created to illustrate timeline projects based on Julia Alvarez' novel "In the Time of the Butterflies." © 2004 Margaret Smith Crocco and Judith Cramer

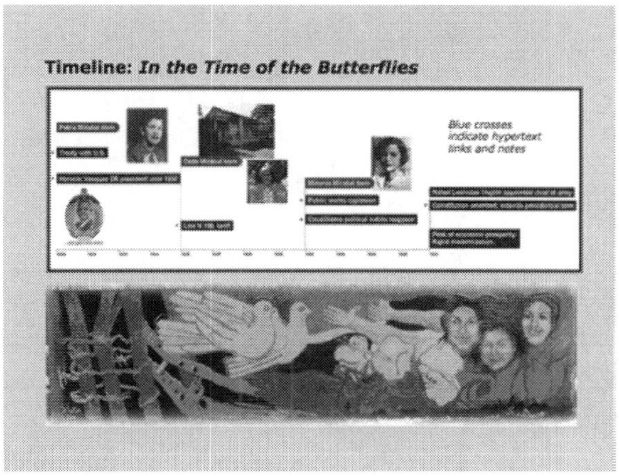

planning, and conceptualizing where doing so requires visualization (e.g., "backwards design").

Introducing WebQuests into Women of the World

Our first round of reflections on our work in Women of the World pushed us in contrasting directions. In response to persistent student complaints about the gap between College technology ideals and City schools' technology realities, we developed a requirement we called "scalability" in curriculum design with technology. A retrenchment made to help students cope with an apparently intractable digital divide, scalability meant that students must be able to show how the technology-based projects they created for high school students could work in a one-computer classroom, not just in the full lab situation they found at TC. At the same time, on the basis of our students' willingness to innovate with technology, we moved in the other direction, to push the digital envelope. Here we set out to see if a tested but so far rather conservatively deployed technology tool, the *WebQuest*, could be marshaled to our cause.

WebQuests became a key technology in Women of the World following a controversy in the class that developed over the novel *Shabanu: Daughter of the Wind*, which was added to the reading list in 1999, following two unsuccessful attempts to find a suitable book about South Asian women. Reflecting in a later essay on the issues raised by using fiction to teach world history, Crocco (2005) noted that

> *[t]he stumbling blocks to selection of a good text were akin to those faced by social studies teachers at the K-12 level: avoiding the pitfalls of essentialism, cultural relativism, and ethnocentrism.... providing a reading experience my students would enjoy; and simply finding a book that my students could actually use in their own teaching of secondary social studies, especially in New York City's public schools...(p. 566).*

In the decade since its publication in 1989, *Shabanu* had won numerous literary awards; the book had made Suzanne Fisher Staples, its journalist author, a sought-after spokeswoman for young adult fiction. But as a Westerner, or outsider, writing about Islamic culture and society, Staples had also attracted controversy. After two Pakistani-American students at Teachers College expressed strong reservations about the novel to Crocco, referring her to several Web sites on which Islamic organizations advocated proscribing the book from US classrooms and libraries, she undertook a research project (2000–2003) designed to learn what lay behind the critical reaction to *Shabanu*.

Crocco concluded that "developing educators' and future educators' capacity to read all texts, fiction and non-fiction, as well as visual media, with a sophisticated post-colonial consciousness ought to be an important task of 21st century teacher education" (p. 578). Such a task became the basis for the first *WebQuest* constructed for Women of the World (see: http://www.tc.edu/faculty/Crocco/webquestshabanu.htm). Previously we had included *WebQuests* in the course by selecting models for our students to imitate from *WebQuest* inventor Bernie Dodge's site (www.webquest.org). Generally students had chosen to create *WebQuests* around topics raised by other literary readings, such as the perennial course favorite, *In the Time of the Butterflies*. The *Shabanu WebQuest* allowed us to test this digital tool as a medium for addressing controversial issues, a central aim of social studies education, and one never far from the subject of gender.[3]

An article we wrote reflecting on our work for readers of *Social Education* (Crocco & Cramer, 2005b) explains why we chose to explore the *WebQuest's* possibilities for teaching about the world's women, and the process we used to help our students distinguish genuine *WebQuests*, which meet pedagogic criteria defined by Dodge, from the many "digital reports on famous females," as one student termed them, that masquerade as *WebQuests*, and occupy a chunk of Internet real estate, even on Dodge's own portal, as he is the first to point out. Though initially our students were loath to criticize material from an "official" site like Dodge's, eventually they did connect the "lite" approach of many so-called *WebQuests* "on women" with the superficial treatment of women's history in their own high school education and textbooks.

By taking the *Shabanu WebQuest* in class, students learned first-hand what makes Dodge's invention live up to his criteria for an authentic digital aid to teaching and learning. The online debate over Staples' novel, taking place on various Islamic organizations' and teacher associations' Web sites, constituted a highly specific and extremely current discussion platform, available to them only on the Web. Their quest—to determine whether we should include *Shabanu* in the curriculum or not—modeled real life controversies they would surely face in their future work. By the time the activity had concluded, students were eager to tackle *WebQuest* design themselves. They enthusiastically accepted the challenge laid out by Dodge in "Five Rules for Writing a Great WebQuest" (2001) to create their own *WebQuests* on women of the world.

We asked for a *WebQuest* on a topic of their own choosing discussed in Joni Seager's *State of Women of the World Atlas* or Chila Bulbeck's *Reorienting Western Feminisms* (1997), two important course texts. We rely on these resources, in particular, to help our students meet the dual challenges of ethnocentrism and cultural relativism as they explore such controversial global women's issues as female genital mutilation, or topics like arranged marriages and veiling, both of which figure in the plot of *Shabanu*.

Select something you would teach at the secondary level. Aim for a "backwards design" process in which you use Inspiration to map out your goals and work backwards from those goals to the design of the WebQuest. On the last day of the course, be prepared to share your work with the rest of the class. Write a 3-5 page paper to accompany the WebQuest explaining your choices. (p.145)

Subsequent reflection on this project led to the article for *Social Education* (Crocco & Cramer, 2005b), describing three student *WebQuest* projects in detail. One, investigating the gendered side of the AIDS epidemic in Africa, involves a scenario in which the Gates Foundation plans to give money to five countries; a second focusing on the gendered nature of international trafficking, culminated in a UN Conference to be held in Montreal in 2005. Team members represent five different countries that must evaluate their involvement in diverse aspects of trafficking, in order to report about the problems for their nation at the conference. The image shown here (Figure 4) represents perhaps the most controversial topic chosen: how gender is determined, or, in the words of this *WebQuest's* author, "What do you think makes a man a 'man' and a woman a 'woman'?" (Zapanta, 2006, p. 10). In order to investigate "the connection between gender role and the cultural concept of the person" (p. 10), students assume the status of cultural anthropologists who study several cultures that present more than two genders.

Although a recent *New York Times* article about the *muxe* of Mexico (Lacey, 2008) testifies to general interest in this subject, admittedly, as we cautioned in our essay, not all the examples created by our cohort of graduate students are suitable for secondary school classrooms. But they make a convincing case that authentic *WebQuests* can be crafted around difficult subjects.

WebQuests for Women of the World, Upon Further Reflection

A frequent criticism of the *WebQuest* design is that it is too teacher-centered. Cramer, who has taught TC's professional development workshops on *WebQuests* for a number of years, has heard career teachers voice this objection repeatedly. Our pre-service students also wondered: If teachers formulate the inquiry questions, select all the Web sites, design the team structures and create the assessment rubrics, how is it possible to think of *WebQuests* as constructivist or student-centered?

The "take then make" method we used with *WebQuests* in Women of the World suggested a way to meet this criticism. Students in primary grades might "take" a *WebQuest*, to become familiar with the form's structure and aims. In upper elementary or middle school, students might begin to take ownership of *WebQuests* by contributing to some aspect of their design. The assessment rubric, for instance, is one element students could "make." Or they can brainstorm the essential question(s) using *Inspiration*, and search for the Web sites that all teams visit to acquire preliminary understandings. High school students, especially those who have had these experiences, might become curriculum creators by making *WebQuests* from scratch.

Now Web 2.0 tools like the social book marking site *delicious* (www.delicious.com) offer students a way to maximize their computer time and to keep track of their sources, particularly if they are working on their *WebQuests* collaboratively, at home or from multiple school computers. All students enrolled in Women of the World 2008 opened accounts on *delicious* at the beginning of the term to use in various assignments. *Delicious* has direct applicability to *WebQuest* creation but many other uses as well. Dodge also now maintains a helpful new interactive feature on his site, the WebQuest Garden, which is both a template for creating a *WebQuest*, complete with prompts, and a hosting service, free for 30 days and only $20 for two years. It is so easy to create a *WebQuest* on the Garden that the novice will be delighted.

What is most exciting about the *WebQuest* for our purposes in Women of the World is the opportunity it provides for students to dig deeply into subject matter related to women's lives around the world and with this material to create learning opportunities for their own students that pose questions (rather than simply providing answers) about critical contemporary issues dealing with gender. This is to say that the issues posed affect women and men, their lives, communities, and intertwined futures refracted through the prism of social justice. Bringing technology into the

Figure 4. Title page of a WebQuest on gender's meanings and social construction in diverse cultures, created for Women of the World: Issues in Teaching. © 2006 Jaclyn T. Zapanta. Used by Permission

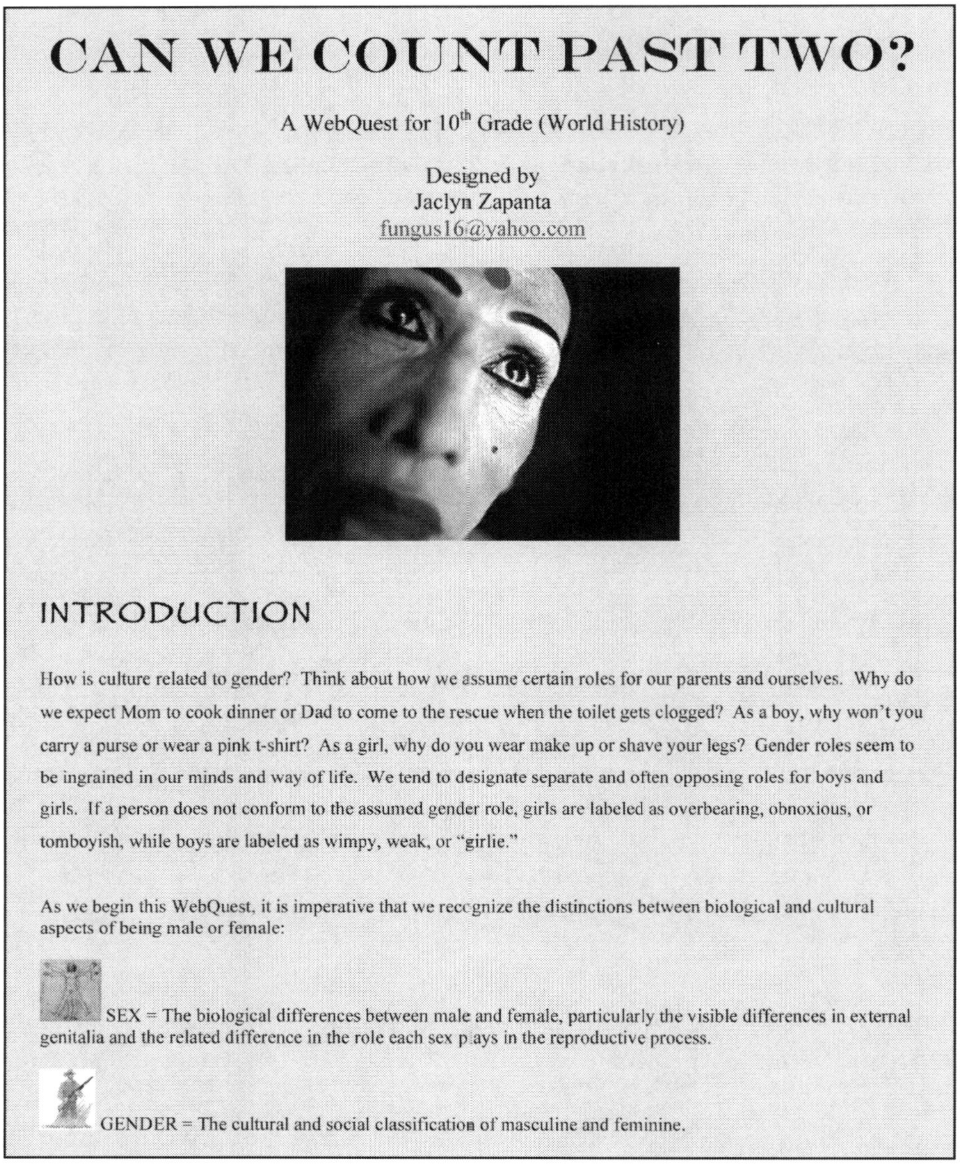

CAN WE COUNT PAST TWO?

A WebQuest for 10th Grade (World History)

Designed by
Jaclyn Zapanta
fungus16@yahoo.com

INTRODUCTION

How is culture related to gender? Think about how we assume certain roles for our parents and ourselves. Why do we expect Mom to cook dinner or Dad to come to the rescue when the toilet gets clogged? As a boy, why won't you carry a purse or wear a pink t-shirt? As a girl, why do you wear make up or shave your legs? Gender roles seem to be ingrained in our minds and way of life. We tend to designate separate and often opposing roles for boys and girls. If a person does not conform to the assumed gender role, girls are labeled as overbearing, obnoxious, or tomboyish, while boys are labeled as wimpy, weak, or "girlie."

As we begin this WebQuest, it is imperative that we recognize the distinctions between biological and cultural aspects of being male or female:

SEX = The biological differences between male and female, particularly the visible differences in external genitalia and the related difference in the role each sex plays in the reproductive process.

GENDER = The cultural and social classification of masculine and feminine.

classroom in this way can be seen as a 21st century disruption of the age-old problem of patriarchy.

Women of the World: Future Directions

For a course on citizen media, Cramer had developed digital photojournalism projects with the social networking site *Flickr* and the intriguing low-cost software, *Comic Life*. In 2008 we decided to introduce these tools into Women of the World. The 2008 course focused on the topic of women's representation/self-representation. To start the process of reflection, we invited students to take photos with digital cameras on location in New York City and post them to the

Flickr group "Tell a Story in 5 Frames." Their assignment was to create a five-frame essay on the theme of contemporary women's experiences. "Fashion Over Function," a witty photo essay by a male member of the class documenting contemporary women's obsession with shoes, garnered plaudits from the *Flickr* group's members (see: http://www.flickr.com/groups/visualstory/discuss/ 72157606080910709/). Students could then choose to create a *WebQuest* on the theme of female representation or to use *Comic Life* to develop a short graphic novel representing an aspect of contemporary women's lives, from their photo shoot or oral history project.

Although we have had only one semester's worth of experience trying these new approaches, they have yielded some fascinating work. We reproduce here three pages from a *Comic Life* project based on a student's oral history with her grandmother (Figure 5). The multimodal graphic novel format allowed the student to construct a story that combined her own photography, including a picture of herself with her grandmother; pictures from her grandmother's scrapbook, such as the evocative cover image; researched historic images from online archives; and verbatim quotations from her interview in the form of speech balloons. Together these three pages, selected from nineteen created by this student, suggest the possibilities of rich invention that a new generation of simple yet powerful tools like *Comic Life* and *Flickr* can bring to teacher education classrooms, and by extension to schools. Engaged in the creative act of representing women through images and multi-level texts (Saraceni, 2003; McCloud, 1993, 2000), our students in Women of the World 2008 had a first-hand experience of the choices authoring agents make in attempting to portray the complex realities of contemporary women's lives.

What has become clear over our years of working with software and computers in the Women of the World class is the degree to which we have moved from seeing these merely as tools to understanding them more broadly as content for the course. As we demonstrate these approaches in our classroom, we are—self-consciously yet proudly—aware of the fact that we are two middle-aged women, true "digital immigrants" (Prensky, 2001), who stand before a class of (mostly) young women demonstrating the affordances of such tools in teaching social studies. Because two women use these tools to facilitate consideration of women as historical and anthropological subjects, in yet another sense the tools become part of the

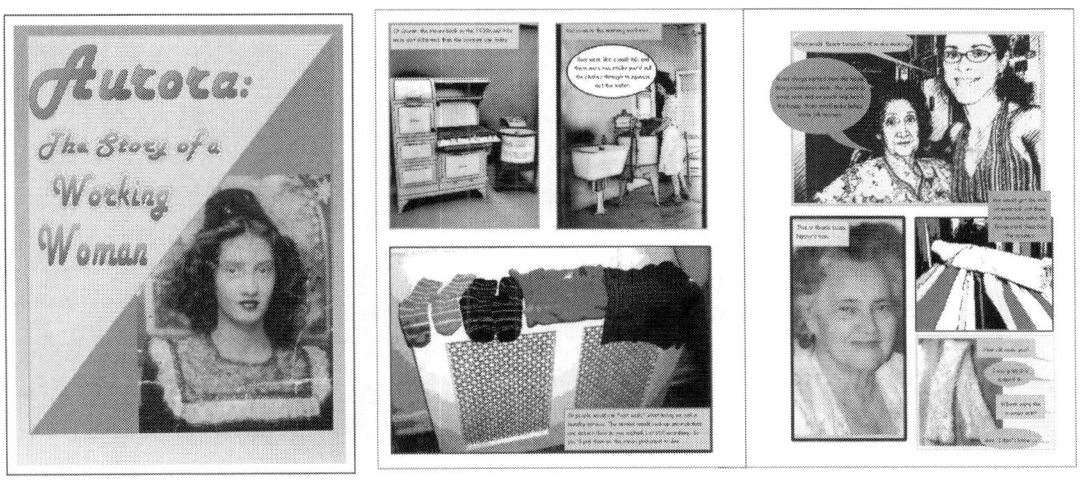

Figure 5. Cover and spread excerpted from 18-page graphic novel created from an oral history project by a student in Women of the World: Issues in Teaching. © 2008 Wendy M. Cortes. Used with permission

classroom content, helping women investigate women's lives, including their engagement with digital media, in new and exciting ways. We hope that by modeling the use of technology to teach about women's lives, we enable our students—future teachers for the most part—to carry both the technology and the attention to gender into their own classrooms.

CONCLUSION

The efforts at improving the place of technology in social studies teacher education described here raised a number of questions for us about the place of gender in our field. These questions motivated us to collaborate with another colleague on a survey of twenty years of research at the intersection of technology, gender, and the social studies (Crocco, Cramer & Meier, 2008). Unfortunately our survey confirmed what we had suspected: how little attention social studies researchers on technology have paid to gender. But outside the social studies field, much research has been done on this topic. The research clearly shows that access to computers is no longer a problem for most women. It also demonstrates that although women typically use computers for different purposes than men, they do use computers as much as men when they are interested in what can be done with digital media, especially to facilitate interpersonal communication. Unfortunately, however, to some extent, women still exhibit lower levels of self-efficacy than men in using computers.[4]

Recent work by researchers at the Pew Internet & American Life Project (Lenhart & Madden, 2003, 2005, 2007; Rainie & Hitlin, 2005) and The MacArthur Foundation (Jenkins et al, 2006; Muziko et al., 2008) provide demographic data suggesting that young women are comfortable in the *Facebook* culture, one that is markedly different from the old computer culture, with its isolating tendencies. Indeed, women's interest in and facility with digital environments focused on social networking may allow them to surpass men in their engagement with some forms of computing, especially those which depend on collaboration and communication—abilities that studies have long shown to be female strengths (Clegg, 2001). In our review essay we suggest redefining gender from a gap to be eliminated to a difference to be explored (Crocco, Cramer & Meier, p. 130). Further, we believe that the Web's new "participatory culture" (Jenkins et al., 2006) is a promising area for research, especially in social studies. Here girls not only hold their own but often excel. Our experience with Women of the World offers the social studies field a glimpse of what is possible when gender becomes a key course interest. We invite other teacher educators and researchers to look into it in their domains too.

REFERENCES

Alvarez, J. (1995). *In the time of the butterflies*. New York: Plume.

Blackwell, P., Applegate, J., Earley, P., & Tarule, J. (2000). *Education reform and teacher education: the missing discourse of gender*. Washington, DC: American Association of Colleges for Teacher Education.

Brown, S., Boyer, M., Mayall, H., Johnson, P., Ming, L., & Butler, M. (2003). The GlobalEd Project: Gender differences in a problem-based learning environment of international negotiations. *Instructional Science*, *31*(4–5), 255–276. doi:10.1023/A:1024677708501

Brunner, C. (2003 April). Approaching technology. *Women's Educational Equity Act Resource Center Digest*, 1-16. Retrieved November 7, 2007, from http://www.edc.org/WomensEquity

Bulbeck, C. (1997). *Reorienting western feminisms*. Cambridge, UK: Cambridge University Press. doi:10.1017/CBO9780511552151

Clegg, S. (2001). Theorising the machine: Gender, education, and computing. *Gender and Education*, *13*(3), 307–324. doi:10.1080/09540250120063580

Coppola, E. (2005). *Powering up: Support for constructivist teaching with technology*. Paper presented in Philadelphia, PA at the National Educational Computing Conference. Retrieved from http://www.iste.org/Content/NavigationMenu/Research/ NECC_Research_Paper_Archives/NECC_2005/Coppola-Eileen-NECC05.pdf

Cortes, W. (2008). Comic Life. Oral history presentation, New York.

Crocco, M., & Cramer, J. (2004). A virtual hall of mirrors? Confronting the digital divide in urban social studies teacher education. *Journal of Computing in Teacher Education*, *20*(4), 133–137.

Crocco, M., & Cramer, J. (2005). Technology use, women, and global studies in social studies teacher education. *Contemporary Issues in Technology & Teacher Education*, *5*(1), 38–49.

Crocco, M. S. (2001). Leveraging constructivist learning in the social studies classroom: A response to Mason, Berson, Diem, Hicks, Lee, and Dralle. *Contemporary Issues in Technology and Teacher Education, 1*(3), 386-394. Retrieved April 7, 2009, from http://www.citejournal.org/vol1/iss3/currentissues/socialstudies/article2.ht

Crocco, M. S. (2005). Teaching *Shabanu*: The challenges of using world literature in the social studies classroom. *Journal of Curriculum Studies*, *37*(5), 561–582. doi:10.1080/0022027042000310692

Crocco, M. S., & Cramer, J. (2005). Women, WebQuests, and controversial issues in the social studies. *Social Education*, *69*(3), 143–148.

Crocco, M. S., Cramer, J., & Meier, E. (2008). (Never) Mind the gap! Gender equity in social studies research on technology in the twenty-first century. *Multicultural Education & Technology Journal*, *2*(1), 19–36. doi:10.1108/17504970810867133

Doolittle, P., & Hicks, D. (2003). Constructivism as a theoretical foundation for use of technology in social studies. *Theory and Research in Social Education*, *3*(1), 72–105.

Evans, R. W., & Saxe, D. W. (Eds.). (1996). *Handbook for teaching controversial issues: NCSS bulletin 93*. Washington, DC: NCSS.

Gee, J. P. (2003). *What video games have to teach us about learning and literacy*. New York: Palgrave Macmillan.

Goodson, I. V., & Mangan, J. M. (1995). School cultures and the introduction of classroom computers. *British Educational Research Journal*, *21*(5), 613–628. doi:10.1080/0141192950210505

Hanson, K. (1997). *Gender, discourse, and technology*. Center for Equity and Diversity Working Paper No. 5. Retrieved June 9, 2009, from http://www.eric.ed.gov/ERICWebPortal/custom/portlets/recordDetails/ detailmini.jsp?_nfpb=true&_&ERICExtSearch_SearchValue_0=ED418913&ERICExtSearch_SearchType_0=no&accno=ED418913

Hargittai, E., & Shafer, S. (2006). Differences in actual and perceived online skills: The role of gender. *Social Science Quarterly*, *87*(2), 432–448. doi:10.1111/j.1540-6237.2006.00389.x

Jenkins, H., Clinton, K., Purushotma, R., Robison, A. J., & Weigel, M. (2006). Confronting the challenges of participatory culture: media education for the 21st century. *The MacArthur Report: Building the Field of Digital Media and Learning*. Retrieved February 7, 2008, from http://digitallearning.macfound.org/site/c.enJLKQNlFiG/b.2029291/k.97E5/ Occasional_Papers.htm

Klein, S. (Ed.). (2007). *Handbook of gender equity* (2nd ed.). New York: Lawrence Erlbaum.

Lacey, M. (December 7, 2008). A lifestyle distinct: The muxe of Mexico. *The New York Times, Week in Review*, 4.

Lenhart, A. (2003). The ever-shifting Internet population: A new look at Internet access and the digital divide. *Pew Internet & American Life Project*. Retrieved November 7, 2007, from http://www.pewinternet.org/report_display.asp?r=88

Lenhart, A., & Madden, M. (2005). Teen content creators and consumers. *Pew Internet & American Life Project*. Retrieved November 7, 2007, from http://www.pewinternet.org/PPF/r/166/report_display.asp

Lenhart, A., & Madden, M. (2007). Social networking websites and teens: An overview. *Pew Internet & American Life Project*. Retrieved November 7, 2007, from http://www.pewinternet.org/PPF/r/198/report_display.asp

Lerner, G. (1985). *The creation of patriarchy*. New York: Oxford University Press.

Lerner, G. (1992). *The creation of feminist consciousness*. New York: Oxford University Press.

Mason, C., Berson, M., & Diem, R. Hicks, Lee, J., & Dralle, T. (2000). Guidelines for using technology to prepare social studies teachers. *Contemporary Issues in Technology and Teacher Education, 1*(3), 386-394. Retrieved April 7, 2009, from http://www.citejournal.org/vol1/iss1/currentissues/socialstudies/article1.htm

McCloud, S. (1993). *Understanding comics*. Northampton, MA: Kitchen Sink Press.

McCloud, S. (2000). *Re-inventing comics*. Northampton, MA: Kitchen Sink Press.

Means, B., Penuel, W. R., & Padilla, C. (2001). *The connected school: Technology and learning in high school*. San Francisco: Jossey-Bass.

Mizuko, I., Horst, H., & Bittanti, M. boyd, D., Herr-Stephenson, B., Lange, P. G., Pascoe, C. J., & Robinson, L. (2008). Living and Learning with New Media: Summary of Findings from the Digital Youth Project. *The MacArthur Report: Building the Field of Digital Media and Learning*. Retrieved March 28, 2009, from http://digitallearning.macfound.org/site/c.enJLKQNlFiG/b.2029291/k.97E5/ Occasional_Papers.htm

OECD. (2009). *Equally prepared for life? How 15 year old boys and girls perform in schools*. Retrieved June 20, 2009, from http://www.oecd.org/

Oliver, D. W., & Shaver, J. P. (1966). *Teaching public issues in the high school*. Boston: Houghton Mifflin Company.

Prensky, M. (2001). Digital natives, digital immigrants. *On the Horizon, 9*(5), 1-6. Retrieved April 8, 2009, from http://www.marcprensky,com/writing/Prensky-DigitalNatives, DigitalImmigrants-Part1.pdf

Rainie, L., & Hitlin, P. (2005). The Internet at school. *Pew Internet & American Life Project*. Retrieved November 7, 2007, from http://www.pewinternet.org/PPF/r/163/report_display.asp

Sanders, J. (2002). Something is missing from teacher education: attention to two genders. *Phi Delta Kappan, 84*(3), 241-44. Retrieved November 2002, from http://www.pdkintl.org/kappan/k0211san.htm

Sanders, J. (2005). *Gender and technology in education: A research review*. Retrieved November 7, 2007, from http://www.josanders.com/pdf/gendertech0705.pdf

Saraceni, M. (2003). *The language of comics*. London: Routledge.

Scharf, E., & Cramer, J. (2002). Desktop poetry project. *Learning and Leading with Technology, 29*(6), 28–31, 50–51.

Seager, J. (1997). *State of women of the world atlas* (2nd ed.). New York: Penguin.

Volman, M., & von Eck, E. (2001). Gender equity and information technology in education: The second decade. *Review of Educational Research, 71*(4), 614–634. doi:10.3102/00346543071004613

Whitley, B. (1997). Gender differences in computer-related attitudes and behavior: A meta-analysis. *Computers in Human Behavior, 13*(1), 1–22. doi:10.1016/S0747-5632(96)00026-X

Zapanta, J. T. (2004). *Can we count past two?* Zittleman, K., & Sadker, D. (2002). Gender bias in teacher education texts. *Journal of Teacher Education, 53*(1), 168–180.

FURTHER READING

Boyd, D. (2007). Why youth (heart) social network sites: The role of networked publics in teenage social life. In Buckingham, D. (Ed.), *MacArthur Foundation Series on digital learning, youth, identity, and digital media* (pp. 1–26). Cambridge, MA: MIT Press.

Brooks, J., & Brooks, M. (1993). *In search of understanding: The case for constructivist classrooms*. Alexandria, VA: Association for the Study of Curriculum Development.

Brunetti, I. (Ed.). (2006). *An anthology of graphic fiction, cartoons and true stories*. New Haven, CT: Yale University Press.

Carlin, J., Karasik, P., & Walker, B. (Eds.). (2005). *Masters of American comics*. New Haven, CT: Yale University Press.

Crocco, M. S. (2005). Women and the social studies: The long rise and rapid fall of feminist activity in the National Council for the Social Studies. In Woyshner, C., Watras, J., & Crocco, M. (Eds.), *Social education in the twentieth century: Curriculum and context for citizenship* (pp. 142–159). New York: Peter Lang.

Crocco, M. S. (2006). Gender and social education: What's the problem? In Ross, E. W. (Ed.), *Social studies: Purposes, problems and possibilities* (3rd ed., pp. 171–197). Albany, NY: State University of New York Press.

Cuban, L. (2003). *Oversold and underused*. Cambridge, MA: Harvard University Press.

Donovan, J. D., Bransford, J. W., & Pellegrino, S. (2005). *How people learn: Bridging research and practice*. Washington, DC: National Academy for Education.

Eisner, W. (1985). *Comics and sequential art*. Tamarac, FL: Poorhouse Press.

Gertler, N. (Ed.). (2002). *Panel one: comic book scripts by top writers*. Thousand Oaks, CA: About Comics.

Giles, R. (2006). *How to use Flickr: The digital photography revolution*. Boston, MA: Thomson.

Gravett, P. (2005). *Graphic novels: Everything you need to know*. New York: Collins Design.

Horrigan, J., & Murray, K. (2006). Home broadband adoption in rural America. *Pew Internet & American Life Project*. Retrieved November 7, 2007, from http://www.pewinternet.org/PPF/r/176/report_display.asp

Horrigan, J., & Smith, A. (2007). Home broadband adoption 2007. *Pew Internet & American Life Project*. Retrieved November 7, 2007, from http://www.pewinternet.org/PPF/r/217/report_display.asp

International Society for Technology in Education. (2007). *National education technology standards for students: The next generation*. Retrieved November 7, 2007, from http://www.iste.org/inhouse/nets/cnets/students/pdf/NETS_for_Students_2007.pdf

Kroski, E. (2005). The hive mind: Folksonomies and user-based tagging. *Infotangle*. Retrieved April 5, 2009, from http://infotangle.blogsome.com/2005/12/07/the-hive-mind-folksonomies- and-user-based-tagging/

Marlow, C., Naaman, M., Boyd, D., & Davis, M. (2006). *Position paper, tagging, taxonomy, Flickr, article, to Read.* Paper presented at Collaborative Web Tagging Workshop at WWW 2006. Edinburgh, Scotland, May 22. Retrieved April 9, 2009, from http://www.danah.org/papers/

Marri, A. R. (2007). Working with blinders on: A critical race theory content analysis of research on technology and social studies education. *Multicultural Education & Technology Journal*, *1*(3), 144–161. doi:10.1108/17504970710822359

Mason, C., McGlinn, M. M., & Siko, K. L. (2005). Twenty years of technology: A retrospective view of *Social Education*'s technology themed issues. *Social Education*, *69*(44), 155–161.

Ohler, J. B. (2007). *Digital storytelling in the classroom: New media pathways to literacy, learning, and creativity*. Thousand Oaks, CA: Corwin Press.

Richardson, W. (2006). *Blogs, wikis, podcasts and other powerful Web tools for classrooms*. Thousand Oaks, CA: Corwin Press.

Rosenzweig, R. (2006). Can history be open source: Wikipedia and the future of the past. *The Journal of American History*, *93*(1), 117–146.

Sabin, R. (1996). *Comics, comix, & graphic novels: a history of comic art*. New York: Phaiden.

Shirky, C. (2005). Ontology is overrated: Categories, links, and tags. *Clay Shirky's Writings About the Internet: Economics & Culture, Media & Community*. Retrieved from http://shirky.com/writings/ontology_overrated.html

Shirky, C. (2008). *Here comes everybody: The power of organizing without organizations*. New York: Penguin Press.

Thornton, S. (2005). *Teaching social studies that matters*. New York: Teachers College Press.

Weiner, S. (2003). *The rise of the graphic novel: faster than a speeding bullet*. New York: Nantier Beall Minoustchine.

Weiner, S. (2006). *The 101 best graphic novels*. New York: Nantier, Beall & Minoustchine.

Wright, B. (2001). *Comic book nation: The transformation of youth culture in America*. Baltimore: Johns Hopkins University Press.

ENDNOTES

1. For a discussion of the lack of attention to gender in teacher education, see: Blackwell et al. (2000); Crocco & Cramer (2005); Sanders (2002, 2006); Zittleman & Sadker (2002).
2. For a discussion of why constructivism is an appropriate underlying philosophy for technology integration in the social studies, see: Crocco (2001); Doolittle & Hicks (2003); Mason, et al. (2000).
3. On teaching controversial issues, see the NCSS Handbook on Teaching Controversial Issues edited by Evans & Saxe (1996), and

the classic work on Teaching Public Issues by Oliver & Shaver (1966).

4 For a discussion of the term self-efficacy, as it applies to women and technology, see: Brown, et al. (2003); Hargittai & Shaffer (2006); Sanders (2005); Volman & Eck (2001); Whitley (1997).

Section 4
Subject-Specific Teacher Education

Chapter 12

Preparing Qualified Elementary School Teachers:

Connecting Mathematics and Science by Integrating Data Collection Technology into Methods Courses

Irina Lyublinskaya[1]
College of Staten Island / CUNY, USA

Nelly Tournaki
College of Staten Island / CUNY, USA

ABSTRACT

This chapter describes a process for the implementation of data collection technology that the authors introduced into the science and mathematics methods courses for preservice elementary-school teachers in a public, urban college. The curriculum of the methods courses was developed to include inquiry-based lab activities that utilize probeware and various data collection interfaces. The lesson plans and the reflections that the authors collected from the 124 preservice teachers over three semesters show that the courses not only exposed them to a variety of data collection instruments, but also changed their attitudes and confidence levels about using such technology in the classroom. The results of this project suggest that preservice teachers perceive data collection technology as a tool for the clear demonstration of otherwise hard to teach science and mathematics concepts to their students. After using data collection technology in their method courses, preservice teachers were able to create their own inquiry-based activities, in which their students were involved in collecting real time data, generating hypotheses, analyzing data, and drawing conclusions. The data collected from the preservice teachers also showed that they needed more experience and practice to better understand the benefits of this type of technology for their future students as well as for their own learning.

DOI: 10.4018/978-1-61520-897-5.ch012

Copyright © 2010, IGI Global. Copying or distributing in print or electronic forms without written permission of IGI Global is prohibited.

INTRODUCTION

Our technology-based society is advancing at such a rapid pace that universities are struggling to prepare students with the technology skills they need for today. Millions of dollars are being poured into the purchase of technological equipment for today's classrooms, but the hardware is worthless if school faculty members are unfamiliar with its function and educational application (Association for the Advancement of Computing in Education, 2003). Over the last two decades, many government agencies have set up relevant curriculum standards to direct the implementation of educational technology, including the International Society for Technology in Education (2008). Further, non-government organizations such as the Society for Information Technology and Teacher Education (http://site.aace.org/), founded in 1990, promote research and practice in the use of technology in teacher education.

There is, however, an ongoing debate regarding how teacher education programs can most effectively prepare teachers to use technology in their teaching. Kay (2006) recently completed a meta-analysis of sixty-eight refereed journal articles that suggested various strategies on how to incorporate technology into preservice teacher education. The following ten strategies for the incorporation of technology emerged from his review: 1) Delivering a single technology course; 2) Offering mini-workshops; 3) Integrating technology in all courses; 4) Modeling how to use technology (i.e. faculty using technology in their own teaching practice); 5) Using multimedia (i.e. technology case studies, online courses, electronic portfolios); 6) Collaboration (i.e. establishing partnerships among universities, colleges and K to 12 schools to create technology-rich learning experiences); 7) Mentor teachers (i.e. continuous professional development); 8) Practicing technology in the field (i.e. actively support the production and delivery of technology-based lessons by preservice teachers); 9) Focusing on education faculty (i.e. faculty development); and 10) Improving access to software, hardware and/or support (i.e. laptop programs).

Teacher Knowledge as it Relates to Technology

Though research about teachers has examined the complex and ill-defined concept of *teacher knowledge* (Carter, 1990; Cochran-Smith & Lytle, 1999; Fenstermacher, 1994; Munby, Russell, & Martin, 2001), only recently have education researchers started to examine teacher knowledge as it relates to technology. Knowledge is essential because teachers use it to determine their actions in the classroom. Thus, it is strategic to identify the relevant knowledge base that teachers draw upon and develop when they learn to teach with technology. It is widely accepted in the education community that teacher knowledge has three components– Content Knowledge, Pedagogical Knowledge, and Pedagogical Content Knowledge (Grossman, 1988; Shulman, 1987). When teachers integrate technology with their professional knowledge they yield four types of knowledge related specifically to technology (Hughes, 2000, 2005; Hughes & Scharber, 2008): Technology Knowledge (TK), Technology Pedagogical Knowledge (TPK), Technology Content Knowledge (TCK) and Technological Pedagogical And Content Knowledge (TPACK). TPACK describes that body of knowledge that teachers need for teaching with and about technology in their assigned subject areas and grade levels. TPACK is depicted as knowledge that relies on the interconnection and intersection of content, pedagogy (teaching and student learning), and technology (Margerum-Leys and Marx, 2002; Mishra, and Koehler, 2006; Niess, 2005; Pierson, 2001; Zhao, 2003). Based on research both with preservice (Niess, 2005) and in-service (Niess, Suharwoto, Lee, & Sadri, 2006) mathematics teachers, Niess further clarified these central components of TPACK as the knowledge and beliefs that a teacher demonstrates that are consistent with:

1. An overarching conception about the purposes for incorporating technology in teaching.
   - This conception is what the teacher knows and believes about the nature of the subject matter, what he or she thinks it is important for students to learn, and how technology supports that learning. These foundations of the teacher's knowledge and beliefs about teaching with technology serve as a basis for his or her decisions about classroom instruction (objective, strategies, assignments, curriculum and text, and evaluation of student learning).
2. Knowledge of students' understandings, thinking, and learning with technology.
   - In this area, the teacher relies on and operates from his or her knowledge about how students learn with technologies and believes that technologies are useful in learning appropriate subject matter.
3. Knowledge of curriculum and curricular materials that integrate technology into learning and teaching.
   - With respect to the curriculum, teachers discuss the topics and ideas in a technology-enhanced environment, how student learning activities are organized, scaffolded, structured, and assessed, and how best to implement a variety of technologies that are available for teaching particular topics.
4. Knowledge of instructional strategies and representations for teaching and learning with technologies.
   - With respect to teaching and learning, the teacher adapts technologies in different ways to meet specific instructional goals and the needs of the range of learners in the class.

Others (Deier, 2001; Dun, Feldman, & Rearick, 2000; Margerum-Leys & Marx, 2002; Mishra & Koehler, 2006) have distinguished fairly similar categories of technology knowledge.

BACKGROUND

Teaching for Understanding through the Use of Technology: An Overview of our Mathematics and Science Methods Courses

In mathematics and science classroom, the teacher's goal is not merely the pursuit of more precise quantifiable data, but also illumination of mathematical and scientific principles and processes in a manner that promotes broad student understanding. This goal is not strongly dependent on cutting-edge technology. In fact, student understanding can be hindered by complicated processes and equipment. Thus, it is the teacher's responsibility to balance the competing goals of instructing students in the basic principles of mathematics and science in a way simple enough to promote student understanding and representing the processes of science and scientific research in a manner that is true to the discipline. In this Chapter, we describe how the inclusion of probeware and data collection interfaces, in the activities designed for our mathematics and science methods courses for preservice teachers, provides authentic "real-world" reflection of scientific research while facilitating student understanding. The activities follow the constructivist approach and the preservice teachers are exposed to the process of Backward Design in which they 1. Identify desired results that their students should achieve, 2. Determine acceptable evidence, and 3. Plan learning experiences and instructions (Wiggins & McTighe, 2005).

More specifically, we describe inquiry-based lab activities that we developed and implemented in both our mathematics and science methods classes, with 124 preservice elementary school teachers, over three semesters. These activities address core National Science Education Standards and National Council of Teachers of Mathematics (NCTM) standards for mathematics. The average age of the participants was 25.5 years, with 91% of the group in their 20s, 6% in their 30s, and 3% over 40; 91.6% were females and 2.4% were males, which is typical of elementary education teachers; 85.5% were Caucasian, 3.2% African American, 5.6% Hispanic, and 5.6% Asian.

The activities exposed the preservice teachers to a variety of data collection instruments that can be used in the elementary science classroom as well as helped them to refresh science and mathematics concepts they had learned in their content courses. We utilized Vernier probeware and data collection interfaces, such as Go!Link® interface, used with computers, EasyLink® interface, used with TI-84 graphing calculators, and LabQuest®, a stand-alone interface (see Figure 1).

The unique feature of the activities is the natural connection they make between a science topic and a mathematics concept, which in turn allows the teacher to integrate science and mathematics learning in the elementary classroom. Each activity was completed by the preservice teachers in a classroom setting modeling collaborative group work that they, in turn, would be expected to facilitate, as an inquiry-based science or math activity, with their future students. Each activity was followed by discussions of common student misconceptions, the place of the activity in the science and mathematics curriculum, lesson planning, alternative assessment options, issues of classroom management, and other pedagogical topics. As part of the course requirements preservice teachers developed their own inquiry-based activities that incorporated data collection technology. Finally, the chapter includes an analysis of qualitative data, such as pre-service teachers' reflections and their developed activities. Finally, the impact of integrating data collection technology into mathematics and science methods courses on preservice teachers' attitudes and confidence towards using this technology in their future teaching is discussed.

INTEGRATION OF DATA COLLECTION TECHNOLOGY IN METHODS COURSES

Challenges of Technology Integration in Teacher Education

Research clearly indicates that in order to use technology effectively as a tool to help students it takes a great deal of education and experience (Coley, Cradler, & Engel, 1997; ISTE, 1999; Milken Family Foundation, 2001; NCATE, 1997; Thomas & Cooper, 2000; U.S. Department of Education, 2000). In spite of this challenge, tech-

Figure 1. Vernier data collection Technology (© 2009, Vernier software and technology. Used with permission)

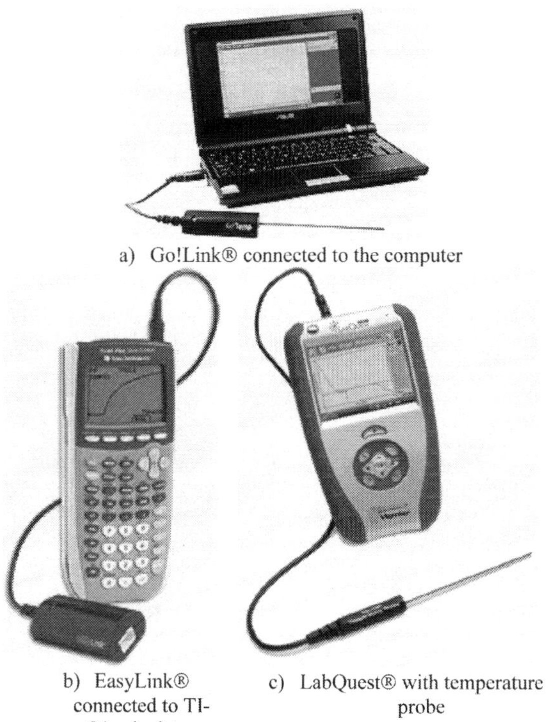

a) Go!Link® connected to the computer

b) EasyLink® connected to TI-84 calculator

c) LabQuest® with temperature probe

nology does not permeate the typical preservice teacher's education experience. There are several reasons for the insufficiency of technology integration in teacher education programs, including, first, there are environmental factors such as support, sharing of resources, and training; second, personal social cognitive factors like faculty attitudes, anxiety, self-efficacy, willingness to make a time commitment and face the risks involved with using technology, competency, beliefs and perceptions of the technology's relevance, and lack of knowledge (Dusick, 1998; Snider, 2002); third, there is resistance of cooperating teachers to the institutionalization of educational technology (Medcalf-Davenport, 1999; Strudel & Wetzel, 1999); and fourth, because technology changes so quickly, "recommended best practices are a constantly moving target" (Cooper & Bull, 1997, p. 97). Nevertheless, it is crucial for preservice educators to be flexible and "evaluate the use of technology as a process of change" (Snider, p. 231). Despite the challenges, new technologies are becoming easier to use and less costly, so that they can be more easily integrated in both college classrooms and in elementary and secondary education classrooms. Instructional data collection technology is an example of technology that has such qualities.

Instructional Data Collection Technology

As we all know, a lot happens in the world of technology in a short period of time. Handheld devices, just a few years ago, were widely considered to be organizers with limited memory and low-resolution grayscale screens. Today, educators are using handhelds for word-processing, Internet browsing, PowerPoint, grading, scheduling, attendance, lesson-planning, e-mailing, and data collection. There are literally thousands of software applications for handheld devices (Curtis, 2005). Further, probeware and interfaces have been developed for various devices such as computers, handhelds, and graphing calculators as well as for stand-alone data analysis tools. More specifically, science probeware is a hands-on data acquisition tool which allows for real-time data collection, storage, and analysis. With more than 50 types of probes available on the market today, students can collect a variety of data. For example, a Temperature Probe is a digital thermometer that can be connected to a computer. The computer stores and displays the temperature readings obtained by the probe. As a result, probeware gives students immediate feedback on their data in the form of statistical and/or graphical analysis. In addition, probeware has the ability to provide accurate, quantitative data for variables that historically have not been measurable in school laboratories (Marcum-Dietrich & Ford, 2002).

Given their relatively low cost, handhelds are becoming an increasingly compelling choice of technology for K-12 classrooms because they enable a transition from the occasional, supplemental use of classroom computers and school computer labs to the frequent, integral use of portable computational devices (Soloway, Norris, Blumenfeld, Fishman, Krajcik, & Marx, 2001; Tinker & Krajcik, 2001). Research indicates that teachers and students respond favorably to handheld devices, which have the potential to affect learning positively across curricular topics and instructional activities. Teachers have indicated that students are more motivated, spend more time using technology, collaborate and communicate more, and in general benefit when they are given a portable and readily accessible tool (Vahey & Crawford, 2002). Students, in turn, have found handhelds easy to use, fun, and a useful for learning (van't Hooft, Diaz, & Swan, 2004). Further, researchers argue that classrooms with handheld computers differ fundamentally from those that have desktop computers in that users of handhelds interact with other computing devices as well as with each other at the same time (Cole & Stanton, 2003; Danesh, Inkpen, Lau, Shu, & Booth, 2001; Mandryk, Inkpen, Bilezkjian, Klemmer, & Landay, 2001; Roth, 2002). Overall, then handheld computers have the potential to support both personalized and collaborative learning. Roschelle and Pea (2002), for example, highlight three ways in which handheld devices have been used to increase learning collaboratively - classroom response systems, participatory simulations, and collaborative data gathering and suggest there are many more such uses (Danesh et al., 2001; Mandryk et al., 2001; Roschelle, 2003). Finally, because of their small size, handheld computers support learning outside the classroom, any time or on any day of the week (Bannasch, 1999; Inkpen, 2001; Sharples, 2002; Solo-way et al., 2001; Staudt & Hsi, 1999; Tinker, 1997).

Data Collection Technology in the Methods Classrooms

Data collection probes can be used in all classrooms since this technology creates an inquiry-based learning environment, in which students are involved in collecting real time data, generating hypotheses, analyzing data, and drawing conclusions (Lyublinskaya, 2003a & b). The activities that a teacher creates based on these probes are student-centered, which increases understanding of the concepts and methods of science and mathematics (Cortes-Figueroa & Moore, 1999; Niess, 2001, Stager, 2000). In fact, science methods courses have the obligation to prepare preservice techers on how to use calculator-based data collection technology in their classroom teaching so that their future students will benefit from these technologies (Stokes, Jenkins, Huhnke, Grey, & Manning, 2000).

In the abundance of literature on educational technology, only three studies have investigated the integration of data collection technologies in methods courses in teacher education programs; each one examined science methods classes. Lyublinskaya and Zhou (2008) conducted a quasi-experimental study in the science methods course they taught, and reported that more exposure to technology influences preservice teachers' perspectives and attitudes toward graphing calculator-based technologies, but not necessarily their confidence. Confidence and perspective are somewhat independent of each other. Gado, Ferguson, & Van't Hooft (2006) infused handheld technology-based inquiry activities into a science methods course and reported a substantial impact on preservice teachers' attitudes, self-efficacy, and conceptual understanding related to integrating technology into their future classes, increasing their understanding of the interconnectedness between science and technology. As shown in their study, Handheld Based Laboratory (HBL) can be used to motivate students and improve student understanding of science and mathematics concepts, and numerical abilities. "The use of handheld-based science activities decreased teacher-directed instructional strategies and increased student involvement in inquiry activities. As a result, they [preservice teachers] perceived that their future classroom students would benefit "tremendously" from the use of handheld computers during science investigations, promoting the notion of autonomy, allowing children to develop self-regulation and control of the learning process, helping students gain knowledge beyond what could have been attained using a textbook or a traditional laboratory investigation (p. 527)." Finally, Heflich, Dixon and Davis (2001) integrated probe ware in a science methods course and in in-service professional development and reported that teachers indicated that their perceptions of how science should be taught changed by the end of the project.

Solutions and Recommendations

We know that real-life applications, especially visual and hands-on demonstrations, enhance students' learning of essential material, meet the needs of students with different learning styles, and create additional motivation for learning a discipline. The use of experiments, demonstrations, computer simulations, and inquiry-based activities allows students to create visual images and practical understanding of science and mathematics concepts and relationships. The use of hands-on activities within the content of science and mathematics provides additional opportunities for teachers and their students to make connections and to master standards-based concepts and skills. Such technology assists us in meeting the expectations of preparing our students for the challenges of the 21st century.

Recognizing the paucity of research in the area of the use of probeware in methods courses, at the same time acknowledging its advantages in education in general, we recognized the need to include data collection technology, specifically, handheld based technology, as both learning and teaching tools in the science and mathematics methods courses we teach in a public college in New York City. Thus, over three semesters we have developed a set of inquiry-based lab activities that integrate science, mathematics, and data-collection technology for elementary education preservice teachers (Lyublinskaya, 2009). These activities aim at 1. Developing a sense of confidence in teaching science and mathematics in our preservice teachers. 2. Increasing their interest in subject areas and instructional technology. 3. Impacting their perspectives and attitudes towards using data collection technology in their future classes.

Preservice teachers in these science and mathematics courses spent nine weeks at the college in face-to-face classroom instruction and six weeks at local elementary schools for teaching practice. Each class met for 180 minutes weekly per subject for the first 9 weeks. One lab activity per week was conducted by the preservice teachers during the last hour of each session, giving them an opportunity to explore and analyze a total of about 15 activities each semester. The activities included: Freeze! The Number Line Game (distance, decimals on the number line); Stack'em Up! Adding Decimals (batteries, adding signed decimals); Switcherro! Commutative Property of Addition (batteries, decimals); Groupies! Associative Property of Addition (batteries, decimals); Electric Circuits for Multiplication and Division (series and parallel circuits, decimals); I See the Light! Fraction of Reflection (light reflection and absorption, colors, percents, fractions, decimal conversion); Cold, Warm, Hot! Comparing Decimals (temperature and heat, ordering decimals); Mix'em Up! Comparing Decimals Game (energy transfer, thermal equilibrium, mean value); Same Temperature – Different Scales. What Is the Pattern? (unit conversions, patterns); The Hottest Girl? The Coolest Boy? The Warmest Class! (temperature, measures of central tendency); Hold Everything (insulation, heat transfer, decimals); What a Drag (friction, measurements); Ocean Floor Mapping (maps, graphs); Batty about Science (bats, motion, distance, graphs); Lift the Load (simple machines, lever, proportion, ratio) (Lyublinskaya, 2009). Several examples of developed activities are analyzed below.

Working in small collaborative groups, preservice teachers completed a number of experiments and analyzed data. They also discussed conceptual questions that were raised in each lab activity. On average each activity took 30-40 minutes to complete. Whole class discussions facilitated by the professor followed each of these 'students' perspective' experiences. The pedagogical issues of using these activities in the elementary classroom were addressed in these discussions. Specifically, discussions focused on developing student-centered inquiry-based learning experiences for the children, facilitating children's learning of subject specific concepts and skills through the activities, connecting mathematical and scientific concepts in a hands-on technology based approach, and addressing the most common misconceptions children have. In addition, these classroom discussions considered the place of these activities in lesson and unit planning and in a standards-based curriculum, the role of performance based assessment, classroom management issues, and other pedagogical topics.

In order to assess preservice teachers' Content Knowledge, Pedagogical Content Knowledge, and Technological Pedagogical Content Knowledge, we required them to develop their own inquiry-based science/math activities that incorporated the data collection technology used in these courses. During the last six weeks of the semester, they had a choice to implement their own developed activities or activities used in the course in their elementary school classrooms with small groups of students in grades 2 – 4. Sample lesson plans developed and taught by the preservice teachers are discussed below.

Sample Activities and Classroom Practice

Activity 1. Freeze! The Number Line Game

The main objective of this activity is for students to learn to predict the location of positive decimal numbers on the number line and verify that prediction experimentally with a motion detector. To achieve the objective students use the Vernier Go!Motion® detector, LoggerLite® software, and a computer to construct a physical number line on the floor and to explore the locations of the positive decimal numbers on it by standing at different locations on the number line and observing the distance readings of the motion detector. The activity meets one of the NSES standards for physical science: *develop an understanding that the position of an object can be described by locating it relative to another object or to the background* (NCSESA & NRC, 1996) and one of the NCTM standards: *compare and order decimals and find their approximate locations on a number line* (NCTM, 2000). In the first part of the activity preservice teachers constructed their own number line on the floor. In order to do that, the instructor first put a 6-m long masking tape on the floor to represent the number line. The zero mark of the number line was drawn directly underneath the motion detector. The Go!Motion detector, which was connected to the computer whose screen was projected on the large screen for the whole class to see. The instructor then called a preservice teacher to stand in front of the motion detector and move slowly back and forth until the motion detector showed a distance of 1 m. (see Figure 2).

The position of the preservice teacher on the masking tape was marked as 1. The same procedure was followed with another preservice teacher in order to locate a position on the number line where the motion detector showed a distance of 2 meters; that position was marked on the masking tape as 2. This was continued until the tape was marked with integer numbers up to 6. While conducting this activity in class, the computer screen was projected onto the Smart Board, so that all of the preservice teachers could see the distance measurements and participate in the construction of the number line. The interaction resulted in the preservice teachers giving their classmates suggestions on how to move (forward or backwards) in order to find locations of integers on the number line. The construction of the real number line on the floor helped them understand that positive numbers get larger as they move away from the motion detector (that is, farther from the zero mark). It also helped them make connections between the location of the number on the number line and the distance between the zero mark and the number. Since a motion detector is very sensitive and measures distance with a 0.1 mm precision, the distance measurements are affected by even a slight body movement. Thus, the distance measurements change slightly even for a person who is standing still. The preservice teachers were instructed to round measurements to the tenth place in order to find the positions of integers on the masking tape. Although these changes were in the thousandths of a meter, the preservice teachers had a hard time understanding that, within the errors of measurement, the distance was constant and that the measurement could be

Figure 2. Experimental setup for the Number Line Game (Adapted from 33. Graphing Motion. Middle School Science with Vernier. © 2009, Vernier software and technology. used with permission)

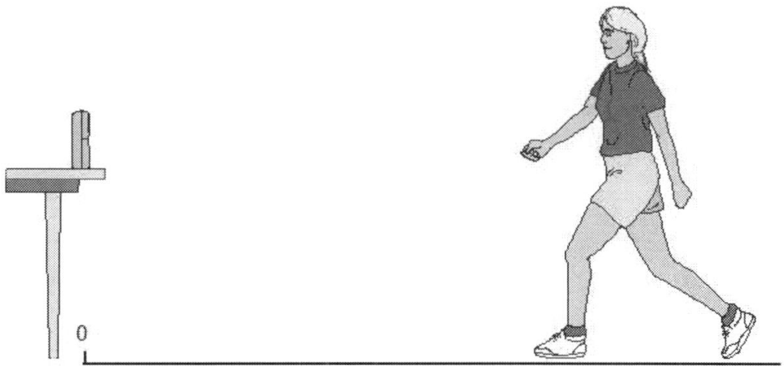

rounded. For example, when the first preservice teacher was standing 1 m away from the motion detector, the measurements were fluctuating between 0.995 m and 1.027 m. Rounding to the tenth led to the same distance of 1.0 m; however, the class needed help from the instructor to come to this understanding. These kinds of errors in measurements and the idea of equal measurements within the errors are conceptually hard science ideas for elementary school students, and it was also hard for preservice teachers. This activity helped them make the connection between the process of rounding experimental distances and errors of measurements.

In the second part of the activity the instructor gave the preservice teachers several decimals between 0 and 6. Before experimenting, they were asked to predict the locations of these decimals on the number line drawn in their worksheets and to explain the reasons for their predictions. The preservice teachers were also asked to compare each given decimal to the nearest integers on both sides and use symbols < (less than) and > (greater than) to record their comparisons. In order to verify their predictions, the preservice teachers were asked to find the location of each number that they were given on the number line on the floor. The instructor then called several volunteers to stand at the positions that they had predicted. The instructor asked one preservice teacher at a time to stand in front of the motion detector, let the class observe the readings, and, if needed, help the preservice teachers to adjust his/her position.

In the third grade classroom, in which the preservice teachers conducted this lesson in small groups, they decided to ask 3 or 4 students to stand at the positions they predicted for different decimals given to them simultaneously. The motion detector showed the distance to the student who stood closest to the motion detector (the smallest number). After this number location was verified, the student sat on the floor to allow the motion detector to measure the distance to the 2nd student, and so on. This reinforced the concept that larger decimals are located at a larger distance from the zero mark. In addition, students were asked to check the integers to their left and to their right in order to verify their comparisons. For example, a student standing at location 1.6 noticed that his number is between 1.0 and 2.0. This observation led to a class discussion on how to compare 1.6 to 1.0 and 1.6 to 2.0, to a discussion of place value, and to a discussion of distance measurements on the number line. To stretch their thinking, the children were asked the following questions:

1. Order these numbers: 2.7, 3.3, and 1.5. Can you compare them?

2. How much bigger is 2.7 than 1.5? ___. What is the distance between 1.5 and 2.7? ____
3. How much smaller is 1.5 than 3.3? ___. What is the distance between 1.5 and 3.3? ___
4. Did you notice any patterns as you answered these questions? Record your observations.

The majority of the students independently made the connection between distance from zero to a given number and the magnitude of a number; however, only about half of the students answered questions 2 – 4 above, which compared different decimals to each other. Nevertheless, after the preservice teachers let students measure distance directly on the floor, many of the students connected the result of subtraction and distance between two decimals.

The experience provided by this activity helped the third graders learn that moving towards the motion detector reduces the distance and thus makes the displayed number smaller. At the same time, moving away from the detector increases the distance, and thus the number gets larger. When predicting the position of the decimal on the number line, students moved in a direction to correct their initial prediction and to find the correct location for a given decimal. In addition, they were able to compare their positions and the numbers those positions represented and to draw conclusions about how their decimals related to the closest larger and smaller integers. Answering extension questions helped children to generalize their experimental observations and make connections between the relative locations of decimals on a number line and the distances between these decimals.

Activity 2. Mix'Em Up! Comparing Decimals and Exploring the Average

This activity was a follow up to another activity in which the preservice teachers used containers with water at different temperatures to learn about heat and temperature in science, and to learn about ordering decimal numbers in mathematics. In the preceding activity the objective in science was to understand heat as energy of the transfer process; the objective in mathematics was to understand place value and how to compare numbers by comparing digits in corresponding places. The activity uses EasyTemp® probe and a graphing calculator (see Figure 3).

The *Mix 'Em Up!* activity provided preservice teachers with the opportunity to learn about thermal equilibrium and direction of heat transfer, to compare decimals "experimentally", and to see how students can discover the meaning of the arithmetic average in a scientific experiment. This activity meets one of the NSES standards: *develop students' understanding of heat; heat can be produced in many ways, such as burning, rubbing, or mixing one substance with another. Heat can move from one object to another by conduction* (NCSESA & NRC, 1996), and one of the NCTM standards: *compare and order decimals, measures of central tendency* (NCTM, 2000). The activity is designed as a game, in which

Figure 3. Measuring temperature with temperature probe. (© 2009, Vernier software and technology. Used with permission)

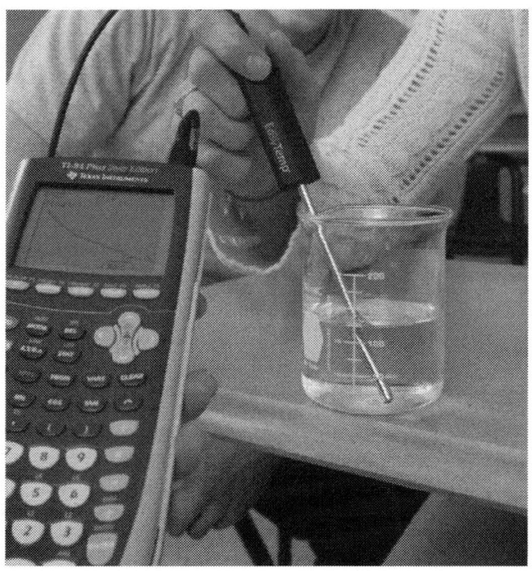

each student works with a partner. Each pair is given three containers, labeled A, B, and C. The containers are filled with the same amounts of water at different temperatures. The students are also given an empty container labeled "Mixture". One child in each pair turns away, while the other takes equal amounts of water from each container, mixes water from only two containers in the "Mixture" container, and discards the water from the 3rd container. The objective of the game is to find out which two containers were used for the mixture. To accomplish that, students have to measure the temperature of the water in each container then, compare the temperature of the water in the mixture to the temperatures of the water in containers A, B, and C. Then, the students switch roles. To add a competitive component to the game, the students use a timer to determine who was faster in finding out from which containers water was used.

Below are the two most common approaches that preservice teachers used in this activity:

1. One preservice teacher measured the temperature of water in all four containers and placed the values on the number line. Then, she measured the distance from point M (the temperature of the mixture) to each point representing the temperatures for containers A, B, and C. The two equal distances indicated which containers had been used to create the mixture.
2. Another preservice teacher suggested that the temperature of the mixture should be an average of two of the temperatures of the water in containers A, B, and C. She found the averages of all of the possible combinations of containers and determined which average was the closest to the experimental value in the 'Mixture" container.

When this activity was used with 4th grade students they started by measuring the temperatures of the water and ordering the numbers representing the temperature values. They checked their ordering by touching the water with their fingers to determine in which container water felt colder or warmer (see Figure 4).

Based on their sense of touch some students had to correct the order of decimals before they proceeded to the next step. Students then chose different approaches to solve the problem. For example, some used the number line approach, very similar to one used by the preservice teachers. They put all four temperatures on the number line and then eyeballed the point "right in between" two different temperatures, until they found which of these mid-points was the closest to the experimental temperature of the mixture. Another group used subtraction to compare the differences between different temperatures. None of the students used the formula for the arithmetic average to solve the problem. This provided the preservice teacher with the opportunity to facilitate

Figure 4. Checking order of temperatures by touch. (Adapted from 2. Why Thermometers? Elementary Science with Vernier. © 2009, Vernier software and technology. Used with permission)

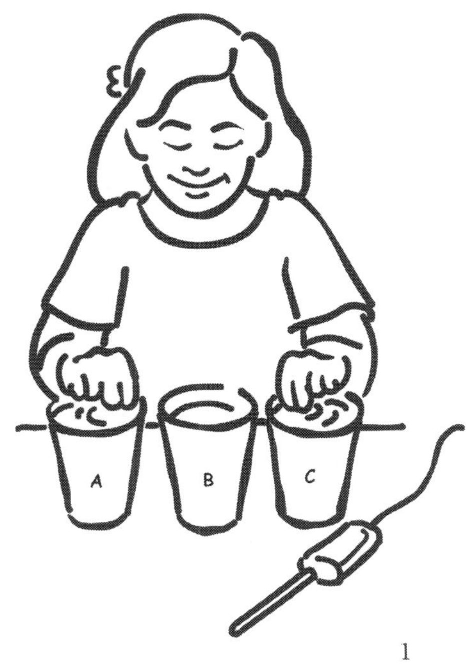

students' discovery of the fact that the average of two numbers lies exactly between those two numbers on the number line.

Activity 3. Stack'Em Up, Switcheroo, and Groupies! Commutative and Associative Properties of Addition

In this lab activity the preservice teachers used AA batteries and a Vernier differential voltage probe connected to the LabQuest® to measure the voltage across stacked batteries. The objective for science was to understand the properties of alkaline batteries and polarity; and the mathematics focus was on arithmetic operations with signed numbers and properties of addition. This activity meets the following NSES standards: *Electricity in circuits can produce light, heat, sound, and magnetic effects; electrical circuits require a complete loop through which an electrical current can pass; electrical circuits provide a means of transferring electrical energy when heat, light, sound, and chemical changes are produced.* It also meets the following NCTM standards: *Understand the meaning and effects of arithmetic operations with decimals; discover the commutative property of addition; discover the associative property of addition.*

The activity has three parts. In Part 1, students explore properties of batteries as they are stacked together and extend that to the idea of adding signed numbers. In Parts 2 and 3, students discover the commutative and associative properties of addition respectively as they measure the voltage of batteries stacked in different orders or combined in different groups. Only positive decimals were used when the preservice teachers taught this activity to elementary school students. Three AA batteries, marked A, B, and C, were given to each group of students. The students were asked to place each battery in the groove of a rule, align the negative end of the battery with the zero mark

Figure 5. Using voltage sensor with batteries. (Adapted from 33. Stacked Batteries. Elementary Science with Vernier. © 2009, Vernier software and technology. Used with permission)

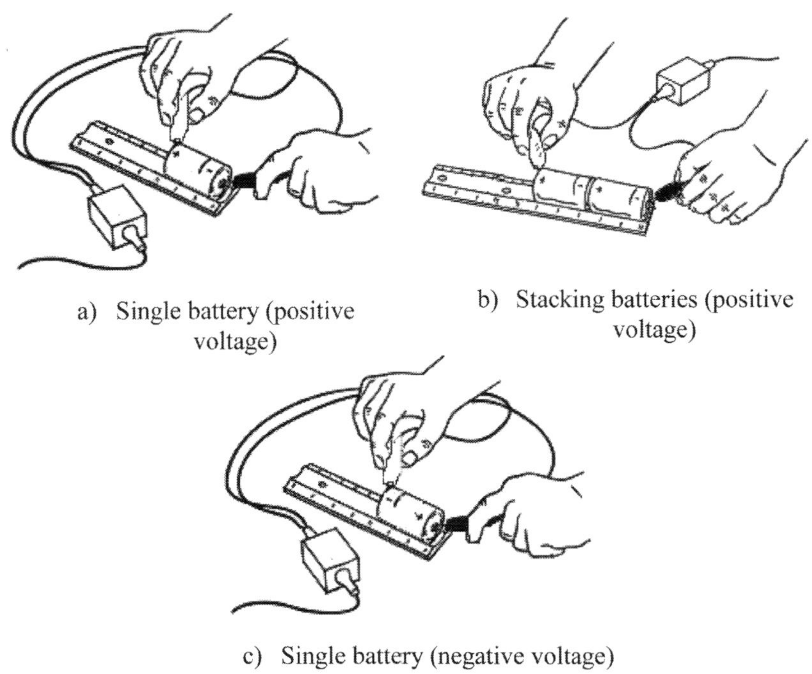

on the rule, and measure the voltage of each battery (See Figure 5a).

Due to the fact that some batteries were used and some were brand new, the voltages of the batteries differed. The voltage values of the three batteries in each group were represented by the letters A, B, and C, in correspondence to the letter designation of the batteries. Students were then instructed to keep the orientation of each battery constant. Then they were given addition number sequences (shown below) and asked to use the numbers that represented their voltage measurements in order to complete these number sequences:

$A+C=\_+\_=\_$

$B+C=\_+\_=\_$

$A+B+C=\_+\_+\_=\_$

Students then were asked to describe the strategies they used to complete the number sequences.

In order to verify their computations, the students used a voltage probe that was connected to the LabQuest. The students stacked the batteries according to the number sequence and checked their results (Figure 5b). This exercise helped the students verify their skills in adding positive numbers and also provided them with the opportunity to practice measurements using the voltage probe.

In part 2 students explored the voltage of two batteries that were joined together in different order. They were asked to write a number sequence for each case (see Figure 6).

Based on their observations, the students filled in the table above and were expected to generalize their findings and complete the following mathematical statement $A+B \square B+A$ with the correct symbol <, =, or >. Since the voltage measurements for both orders of stacking the batteries came up to be the same, the students had no problems coming up with the commutative property of addition $A+B = B+A$.

In part 3 students completed a similar activity to discover the associative property of addition. In this part of the experiment the students were asked to combine three batteries in as many different ways as they could think of while keeping the orientation of each battery the same. In order to help them, the lab worksheet asked students to measure the voltage of each individual battery first then, stack two batteries and measure the voltage of each "double" battery. They were then asked to write the number sequence for each method that they used to create a triple battery and use parentheses to indicate how they combined the batteries in each method. The voltage probe was used to determine the voltage of the "total battery" in each method. Figure 7 shows the cumulative results from the 4th grade groups that completed this activity. (The cases in which the students switched the order of the batteries are not included.):

Here, the individual voltage measurements were A = 1.45 V, B = 1.57 V, C = 1.23 V, AB = 3.02 V, BC = 2.8 V.

Figure 6. Discovery of commutative properties of addition

Stacking Order	Measured Voltage	Number Sequence
[- A +][- B +]	V	
[- B +][- A +]	V	

Figure 7. Exploring associative properties of addition

Method	Number Sequence	Measured Voltage
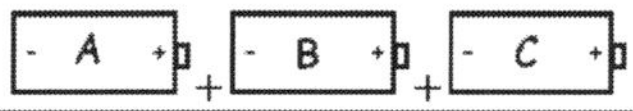	A + B + C	4.25 V
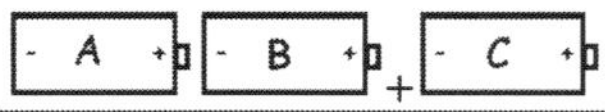	(A + B) + C	4.25 V
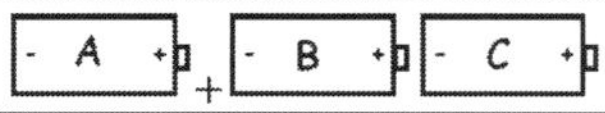	A + (B + C)	4.25 V

Both the 4th grade students and the preservice teachers were able to discover the commutative and associative properties of addition when using positive decimals. At both levels some had difficulty in using the voltage probe and in understanding where to attach the leads on the batteries in order to measure the voltage. Elementary school students had difficulty writing number sequences using parentheses to indicate how they combined the batteries. Taping combined batteries together to allow the students see the "double" or "triple" batteries, helped them make the connection between using parentheses and combining the batteries together.

If a teacher wants to differentiate instruction in order to accommodate more advanced students, the activity can include an experiment that involves negative decimals. In order to create negative decimals, the batteries are flipped, so that the positive end of each battery is placed towards the zero mark of the rule, and the ground (black) lead of the voltage sensor is attached to the positive end of the battery (Figure 5c). In this case the voltage is measured as a negative number. The following questions were used to extend students' thinking:

1. Will the commutative property hold true if you add positive and negative numbers?
2. Can you think of other arithmetic operations that will demonstrate the commutative property? Give examples.
3. Does the associative property of addition hold true for the negative numbers? Why?
4. Will the associative property hold true if you add positive and negative numbers?
5. Can you think of other arithmetic operations that demonstrate the associative property? Give examples.

Since negative decimals are not part of the elementary school curriculum, negative numbers were not used with the students. Only the preservice teachers were asked to complete the activity for the negative numbers, and it was particularly difficult for them. They had a hard time adding negative decimals and they had no understanding of operations with negatives. The experiment helped them see what happens when negative numbers are added, but due to time constraints, it was not possible to develop a true conceptual understanding of these operations with negative decimals.

Samples of Activities Developed by Preservice Teachers

Activity 1. Hibernation: 3rd grade CTT classroom

In this lesson the preservice teacher incorporated the Go!Temp® probe with a laptop computer to provide students with an opportunity to discover what happens to a person's temperature when they transition from a physical activity to complete relaxation. Here is an excerpt from the preservice teacher's lesson plan:

To begin the lesson, I will ask the students to monitor their breathing. Using an hour glass style timer, the students will monitor their respiration for one minute, counting the number of times they inhale. I will then have the students engage in a physical activity, such as jumping jacks, that will increase their heart rate, as well as their body temperature. I will utilize the Go!Temp temperature probe technology that will allow the students to accurately measure their temperature before and after the physical activity. The students will also monitor their pulse to see the difference in the pace of their heartbeat before and after the activity. They will feel their pulse, recalling prior knowledge from a music lesson that I taught them, where they learned how to monitor their pulse by placing 2 fingers on their wrist.

After the activity was completed, the preservice teacher facilitated a discussion that helped the students establish the relationship between their observations and the behavior of animals during hibernation.

Activity 2. Seasons: 4th Grade General Education Classroom

Explanations of the seasons are very challenging for students and even for adults. The majority of preservice elementary teachers have a very common misconception that seasons are caused by the changing distance between the earth and the sun during the earth's annual revolution. In this lesson the preservice teacher used the earth globe and a light probe with the TI-84 graphing calculator to find out what causes the seasons. By measuring the amount of light over time on the globe, illuminated by the light source (the sun), with the globe's axis tilted away from the sun in "winter" and toward the sun in the "spring", students discovered that the earth received less light in winter than in the summer.

The preservice teacher then facilitated discussion that helped students make connections between the amount of light and the amount of energy, and also determine reasons for this difference. Here is a quote from the preservice teacher's reflection on this lesson:

The students learned how to use the calculator connected to the light probe to take measurements of the light reflection.... The students understood and learned that the sun is not closer to earth in the summer or that it is (not) further away from earth in winter. They understood that the earth's axis is on a tilt and that the northern and southern hemispheres receive different amounts of light at the same time. The students were able to observe and record the difference in light intensity on the two hemispheres.

Since the distance between the light source and the earth globe was kept the same, students were able to determine that the tilt of the earth's axis causes the light to be direct (in the summer) or indirect (in the winter) and it is the tilt along with the rotation of the earth around the sun, rather than the earth's distance from the sun, that causes the seasons.

In both of these activities the main focus of the lesson was science. However, both preservice candidates incorporated mathematics skills and concepts, such as measurements, comparing and ordering numbers, and working with decimals, into the lessons. The use of data collection technology provided the preservice teachers with the opportunity for designing inquiry-based activities that helped their students to learn challenging science concepts.

Results and Discussion

In the previous sections of the chapter we described in detail some of the activities that preservice teachers were exposed to and created while attending their methods course in mathematics and science. In addition, in the beginning of each of the three semesters, preservice teachers were asked to reflect on their a) knowledge about technology and b) attitudes/confidence toward educational technology. Upon completion of the course they were again asked to reflect on their experience and describe changes in their knowledge and attitudes/ confidence towards data collection technology used in class.

a) Technology Knowledge (TK) and Technological Pedagogical And Content Knowledge (TPACK) self-assessment: In the initial reflections 67.3% of the preservice teachers who responded (N = 110) stated that they had TK necessary for teaching, 19.1% stated that they had some knowledge, and 13.6% stated that they did not have TK. However, only 33.3% of this group mentioned calculators or emerging technologies, such as SmartBoards, IPods, PDA, digital cameras, etc. The rest of them referred to computer technology and software or used generic terms when talking about educational technology. 42% of this group stated that they learned the technology skills on their own and 41% learned in various formal education settings. Others learned technology at their job or received informal training from friends, colleagues, or family members.

When asked about TPACK, 45.7% of preservice teachers stated that they had such knowledge, 38.1% wrote that they had some knowledge, and 16.2% did not have any TPACK based on self-assessment. However, only 46.4% of preservice teachers identified TPACK correctly, while the majority of them were describing mainly technology skills when describing their TPACK.

The preservice teachers tended to perceive data collection technology as important and interesting to their own learning and productivity; however, they perceived these technologies as more important and more interesting to their future students. In other words, the preservice teachers tended to consider data collection technology more important as a teaching tool than a tool for their own learning. This result is consistent with the emphasis of the course curriculum, which was to teach the preservice teachers how to use technology as an instructional tool in specific subject areas not to teach new content knowledge.

I was aware of data collection technology in the classroom. However, when I attended elementary school, technology was not as high tech. For example, we never measured the ocean floor. This activity did change the way I perceive the use of technology in the elementary classroom, because I did not realize how sophisticated and exciting a science lesson can be.

When I wrote my first reflection for this course it was based on my opinion of technology as a whole. I really thought that using a calculator too much in a classroom would interfere with the child's ability to build the skills necessary to perform mathematical operations. However, after the experiments that we performed in class today, I think differently. I enjoyed participating in the activities and using the technology involved. I was actually stunned to see how a calculator can measure the temperature of different things so quickly and accurately.

On average, 10% of the group incorporated some form of data collection technology during practice student teaching of their own lesson plans. Although still low, this is an important increase because in the past there was complete lack of technology incorporation in lessons developed by preservice teachers since use of data collection technology was not incorporated into the methods courses. This finding supports the literature that indicates that one of the strategies that leads to practice of technology in the field is the integration of technology in the teacher preparation courses (Kay, 2006).

b) Attitudes/Confidence toward educational technology: in the beginning of each semester the preservice teachers were asked about their attitudes towards the use of technology in the elementary classroom. Analysis of received responses (N = 110) showed that 19.1% of the preservice teachers were concerned about students becoming dependent on technology and not learning basic skills, 15.3% stated that technology could have a positive role in elementary school, but was not necessary, and 5.5% suggested that technology should not be used with young students. The majority of the preservice teachers considered the use of educational technology as necessary in elementary schools (58.2%); however, this was mostly a reference to the use of computers and the Internet.

After completing the course, 62.5% stated that they will definitely use data collection technology in teaching, while 38.5% stated that they would use it if they have more practice. Analysis of reflections on attitudes towards using data collection technology in teaching a specific subject matter indicated that 33.3% changed their attitudes towards using this type of technology in science. 49.1% stated that they will definitely use this technology in both science and mathematics, and in interdisciplinary teaching, while 7% responded that they will use data collection technology without stating specific subject areas. Only 10.5% of the group was not sure about using this type of technology in their future classrooms. Such findings support previous research on attitudes towards handheld devices (e.g. Gado, Ferguson, & van't Hooft, 2006) as well as attitudes towards computing technologies in mathematics (e.g., Gningue, 2003).

When asked if data collection technology can be used in inclusive classrooms to teach students with learning disabilities, 50.9% answered "definitely yes", 44.7% considered the pros and cons but were not sure, and only 4.4% considered this technology inappropriate for this group of students.

Statements in the preservice teachers' reflections indicated that overall, in all courses their confidence with the use of data collection technology improved throughout the semester.

I thought that calculator based technology was easy enough for the elementary level to grasp. It was fun and it had various steps in which the children will each have a different task and interact with each other.

Before this class I had no idea how to use a graphing calculator. I thought that people use it only for math not science. Now that I know & have been introduced to these technologies, I feel that I will be more comfortable to use them with my future students. I feel that I will be able to do more engaging lessons with my students to help them learn more.

I definitely have more technology based skills after I had this class. Every experiment we did in this class used technology ... learning the experiments using the calculator with so many functions I didn't even know could exist using such a small device. I was truly amazed. This will also help me bring these skills to my classroom as a future teacher.

Various levels of exposure to data collection technology in different courses influenced the preservice teachers' attitudes toward this technology to varying degrees, but the influence was positive across the board (Lyublinskaya & Zhou, 2008). Still, after one semester of exposure about 20% of the preservice teachers did not feel confident enough to use data collection technology in their teaching.

I agree that I have a bit more technology skills, but not enough to be confident in implementing technology in a class setting.

After taking this class, I think I've more technology skills to use technology in teaching, but I'll need more time to practice with all the technology devices. It's because although we did many interesting activities with technology, I didn't have enough time to know & practice more ... graphing calculator & and the devices we can connect to graphing calculators.

About 10% of the preservice teachers enjoyed using data collection technology, but weren't sure if it was appropriate for elementary school students.

I never knew this kind of data collection technology existed to be used in a classroom. It has opened my eyes that there are a lot of different types of technology that can be used in a classroom. However, I do not know if I agree with this type of technology in an elementary school classroom. The children will probably enjoy using this type of technology because it will be new to them. I think they will also be amazed by how it works.

This perception was predominant at the beginning of the semester, but by the end of the semester, when all of the preservice teachers felt more comfortable with technology, their attitudes and perceptions towards using this technology in the classroom changed.

My first impression was that the use of this technology was too advanced for elementary school students. I now disagree with my first impression because it wasn't difficult at all. The tools may seem hard to use at first but it was simply done in a few easy steps.

This course definitely changed the way I perceived technology in the elementary classroom. When I thought of the use of technology, I thought of the things in which I was used to using. For example, smart boards, desktop computers, I-pods, etc. After conducting various experiments, I realized that I can implement technology into almost any lesson! Also, I realized, after I used such technology, that my students would be just as excited as I was.

This activity changed the way I perceive the use of technology in elementary classrooms. Before this experiment I was unaware of data collection technology. Before this experiment, when I thought of technology in the elementary school classroom, I thought of computers, calculators, S.M.A.R.T boards, scanners, printers, the internet, multimedia and spreadsheets. I was unaware of what data collection technology is and that it can give students a hands-on real life experience. It is interesting how technology can provide for students real life experience in the classroom. Students are able to learn what scientists do when they map the ocean floor and find out the depth of an object under the ocean floor by using this type of technology. From this activity, I am starting to believe that there are many useful types of technology that can be used for learning and teaching experience in elementary school classrooms.

Finally, although some of the preservice teachers had initially strong reservations concerning the use of calculators in the classroom, their experience in the course changed their perceptions.

I always thought that calculator-based technology was good but if a student relied on a calculator too much they would become lazy. Now I feel that calculator-based technology should be used a lot with kids in the classroom because I think it will help them understand the topic better.

I have never had the opportunity to utilize calculator-based technology either in the classroom teaching students or in my own learning experiences in school. As a result of using this technology with lab activities we had I feel that this technology provides students with a means to further their understanding of concepts, engages student in learning and provides valuable data/information to analyze and share. This technology is essential in the science classroom in the elementary school.

Having never used calculator-based technology before, I found these activities very interesting and enjoyable and I feel it was due to the technology used. I never thought about using such technology in the classroom until we did these activities. It strongly changed the way I thought about technology in the classroom. I feel the technology enabled more critical thinking in that students can see for themselves what was occurring in the experiments. Therefore, they can better predict what will occur and what made the actions occur. I now feel technology should be included in as many lessons as possible.

FUTURE RESEARCH DIRECTIONS

Over the last decade of practice in incorporating educational technology into teacher education programs, a new model of the methods course, one that integrates technology with traditional teaching practices, has emerged. However, there are many issues that need to be further explored: How do methods courses successfully develop preservice teachers TPACK without sacrificing the traditional curriculum goals of these courses? What efforts are needed to provide preservice teachers further opportunities to use technology during their teacher practicum? Finally, data collection technology has been used primarily in science methods courses (i.e., Lyublinskaya & Zhou, 2008; Gado, Ferguson & Van't Hooft, 2006; Heflich, Dixon, Davis, 2001); research is needed to investigate its place in other methods courses as well.

CONCLUSION

A methods course that infuses handheld technology-based inquiry activities has a substantial impact on preservice teachers' conceptual understanding related to integrating technology in their future classes, their ability to create activities that incorporate such technology as well as their attitudes towards such technologies.

Interdisciplinary activities, such as the ones we reviewed, can be used as 1) Demonstration of a concept (e.g., *Freeze! The Number Line Game*). Using an activity as a demonstration allows a teacher to talk about the concepts without necessarily using multiple sets of equipment for the students. 2) Class exercises or hands-on exploration in small groups (e.g., *Mix'Em Up!*). When activities are used as class exercises or small group explorations, students have an opportunity for teamwork and interaction with each other as well as to learn specific skills like using measuring devices. Since group work is more time consuming, since it involves a small group of students working at their own pace, some activities may be divided up into parts and completed within two or three lessons. The teacher may use one part of the activity as a class demonstration and another part as independent small group work. In teaching a particular topic, the teacher has an opportunity to introduce the activities in different places within the topic. An activity could be an exploration of a new topic that would be followed by the teacher's instructions and explanations. 3) The activities could be used as review exercises. Often activities are used at the end of studied topics when students are expected to use what they have learned for applications and problem solving.

This project has all of the components of the constructivist learning paradigm. As stated by Bates (2000), "Modern education theory is moving beyond the recall of facts, principles, or correct procedures and into the areas of creativity, problem-solving, analysis, or evaluation … Learners need the opportunity to communicate with one another as well as with their teachers. This of course includes the opportunity to question, challenge and discuss issues. " The creation of this successful constructivist environment depended on the teacher, the students and the use of technology. The teacher assumed the role of a facilitator to the students and a guide to help them achieve their learning objectives. The students were active participants in the learning process: in this student-centered learning environment, the students were involved in knowledge construction, not knowledge absorption. Finally, the use of technology offered instant feedback, was a tool for clear demonstrations of otherwise hard to teach concepts, and created an inquiry-based learning environment, in which students were involved in collecting real time data, generating hypotheses, analyzing data, and drawing conclusions as early as elementary school.

REFERENCES

Association for the Advancement of Computing in Education (AACE). 2003). *A study of preservice elementary teachers' technology skill preparedness and examples of how it can be increased.*

Bannasch, S. (1999). The electronic curator: Using a handheld computer at the Exploratorium. *Concord Consortium Newsletter*. Retrieved August 10, 2003 from http://www.concord.org/library/1999fall/electronic-curator.html

Bates, A. W. (2000). *Managing Technological Change*. San Francisco: Jossey-Bass.

Borko, H., & Putnam, R. T. (1995). Expanding a Teacher's Knowledge Base. In Guskey, T. R., & Huberman, M. (Eds.), *Professional development in education* (pp. 35–65). New York: Teachers College Press.

Borko, H., & Putnam, R. T. (1996). Learning to teach. In Berliner, D. C., & Calfee, R. C. (Eds.), *Handbook of educational psychology* (pp. 673–708). New York: Macmillan.

Bransford, J. D., & Schwartz, D. L. (1999). Rethinking transfer: A simple proposal with multiple implications. In Iran-Nejad, A., & Pearson, P. D. (Eds.), *Review of research in education* (pp. 61–100). Washington, DC: American Educational Research Association.

Carter, K. (1990). Teachers' knowledge and learning to teach. In Houston, W. R., Huberman, M., & Sikula, J. (Eds.), *Handbook of research on teacher education* (pp. 291–310). New York: MacMillan.

Cochran-Smith, M., & Lytle, S. L. (1999). Relationships of knowledge and practice: Teacher learning in communities. In A. Iran- Nejad & P. D. Pearson (Eds.), Review of research in education (Vol. 24, pp. 249-306). Washington, DC: American Educational Research Association.

Cole, H., & Stanton, D. (2003). Designing mobile technologies to support co-present collaboration. *Personal and Ubiquitous Computing*, *7*, 365–371. doi:10.1007/s00779-003-0249-4

Coley, R., Cradler, J., & Engel, P. K. (1997). Computers and classrooms: The status of technology in U.S. schools. *Educational Testing Service.* Retrieved February 2, 2006, from http://www.ets.org/Media/Research/pdf/PICCOMPCLSS.pdf

Cooper, J. M., & Bull, G. L. (1997). Technology and teacher education: Past practice and recommended directions. *Action in Teacher Education*, *19*, 97–106.

Cortes-Figueroa, J. E., & Moore, D. A. (1999). Using CBL technology and a graphing calculator to teach the kinetics of consecutive first-order reactions. *Journal of Chemical Education*, *76*(5), 635–638. doi:10.1021/ed076p635

Curtis, M. (2005). The rise of the handheld computer in schools. *Media and Methods*, *41*(6), 14.

Danesh, A., Inkpen, K., Lau, E., Shu, K., & Booth, K. (2001). Geney: Designing a collaborative activity for the Palm handheld computer. In *Proceedings of CHI, Conference on Human Factors in Computing Systems*, Seattle, WA.

Drier, H. S. (2001, March). *Beliefs, experiences, and reflections that affect the development of techno-Mathematical knowledge.* Paper presented at the SITE, Orlando, FL.

Dun, A., Feldman, A., & Rearick, M. (2000, April). *Teaching and learning with computers in schools: The development of instructional technology pedagogical content knowledge.* Paper presented at the American Educational Research Association (AERA), New Orleans, LA.

Dusick, D. M. (1998). What social cognitive factors influence faculty members' use of computers for teaching? A literature review. *Journal of Research on Computing in Education, 31*, 123–137.

Fenstermacher, G. D. (1994). The knower and the known: The nature of knowledge in research on Teaching. In Darling-Hammond (Ed.), Review of research in education (Vol. 20, pp. 3-56). Washington, DC: American Educational Research Association.

Gado, I., Ferguson, M., & Van't Hooft, M. (2006). Using handheld-computers and probeware in a Science Methods course: Preservice teachers' attitudes and self-efficacy. *Journal of Technology and Teacher Education, 14*(3), 501–529.

Gningue, S. M. (2003). The effectiveness of long term vs. short term training in selected computing technologies on middle and high school mathematics teachers' attitudes and beliefs. *Journal of Computers in Mathematics and Science Teaching, 22*(3), 207–224.

Grossman, P. L. (1988). *A study in contrast: Sources of pedagogical content knowledge for secondary English.* Unpublished Doctoral Dissertation, Stanford University, Palo Alto, CA.

Heflich, D. A., Dixon, J. K., & Davis, K. S. (2001). Taking it to the field: The authentic Integration of mathematics and technology in inquiry-based science instruction. *Journal of Computers in Mathematics and Science Teaching, 20*(1), 99–112.

Hughes, J. E. (2000). *Teaching English with technology: Exploring teacher learning and practice.* Unpublished Doctoral Dissertation, Michigan State University, East Lansing, MI.

Hughes, J. E. (2005). The role of teacher knowledge and learning experiences in forming technology-Integrated pedagogy. *Journal of Technology and Teacher Education, 13*(2), 277–302.

Hughes, J. E., & Scharber, C. (2008). Leveraging the development of English TPCK within the deictic Nature of literacy. In Technology, T. A. C. I. a. (Ed.), *Handbook of Technological Pedagogical Content Knowledge (TPCK) for Educators* (*Vol. 1*, pp. 87–106). New York: Lawrence Erlbaum.

Inkpen, K. (2001). Designing handheld technologies for kids. In *Proceedings of CHI, Conference on Human Factors in Computing Systems*, Seattle, WA.

International Society for Technology in Education. (1999). *National education technology standards*. Retrieved February 2, 2006, from http://www.iste.org/Template.cfm? Section=NETS&CONTENTID=4963&TEMPLATE=/ContentManagement/ContentDisplay.cfm

International Society for Technology in Education. (2008). *National Education Technology Standards for Teachers*. Online document. Retrieved July 16, 2008, from http://www.iste.org/Content/NavigationMenu/NETS/ForTeachers/2008Standards/NETS_for_Teachers_2008.htm

Kay, R. H. (2006). Evaluating Strategies Used to Incorporate Technology into Preservice Education: A Review of the Literature. *Journal of Research on Technology in Education, 38*(4), 383–408.

Lyublinskaya, I. (2003a). *Connecting Mathematics with Science: Experiments for Precalculus.* Emeryville, CA: Key Curriculum Press.

Lyublinskaya, I. (2003b). *Connecting Mathematics and Science: Experiments for Calculus.* Emeryville, CA: Key Curriculum Press.

Lyublinskaya, I. (2009). *Technology Activities for Elementary Mathematics and Science* (2nd ed.). Long Island, NY: Whittier Publications.

Lyublinskaya, I., & Zhou, G. (2008). Integrating Graphing Calculators and Probeware into Science Methods Courses: Impact on Preservice Elementary Teachers' Confidence and Perspectives on Technology for Learning and Teaching. *Journal of Computers in Mathematics and Science Teaching, 27*(2), 163–182.

Mandryk, R. L., Inkpen, K. M., Bilezkjian, M., Klemmer, S. R., & Landay, J. A. (2001). Supporting children's collaboration across handheld computers. In *Proceedings of CHI, Conference on Human Factors in Computing Systems*, Seattle, WA.

Marcum-Dietrich, N. I., & Ford, D. J. (2002). The place for the computer is in the laboratory: An Investigation of the effect of computer probeware on student learning. *Journal of Computers in Mathematics and Science Teaching, 21*, 361–379.

Margerum-Leys, J., & Marx, R. W. (2002). Teacher knowledge of educational technology: a case study of student/mentor teacher pairs. *Journal of Educational Computing Research, 26*(4), 427–462. doi:10.2190/JXBR-2G0G-1E4T-7T4M

Medcalf-Davenport, N. (1999). Historical and current attitudes toward uses of educational technology. In Price, J. D., Willis, J., Willis, D. A., Jost, M., & Boger-Mehall, S. (Eds.), *The information technology and teacher education annual* (pp. 1424–1428). Charlottesville, VA: Association for the Advancement of Computers in Education.

Milken Family Foundation. (2001). *Information technology underused in teacher education*. Retrieved February 2, 2006, from http://www.mff.org/edtech/article.taf? _function=detail&Content_uid1=131

Mishra, P., & Koehler, M. J. (2006). Technological Pedagogical Content Knowledge: A new framework for teacher knowledge. *Teachers College Record, 108*(6), 1017–1054. doi:10.1111/j.1467-9620.2006.00684.x

Montgomerie, T. C., & Irvine, V. (2001). Computer skill requirements for new and existing teachers: Implications for policy and practice. *Journal of Teaching and Learning, 1*(1), 43–55.

Moursund, D., & Bielefeldt, T. (1999). *Will New Teachers Be Prepared to Teach in a Digital Age? A National Survey on Information Technology in Teacher Education*. Santa Monica, CA: Milken Exchange on Education Technology.

Munby, H., Russell, T., & Martin, A. K. (2001). Teachers' knowledge and how it develops. In Richardson, V. (Ed.), *Handbook of research on teaching* (*Vol. 4*, pp. 877–904). Washington, DC: American Educational Research Association.

National Council for the Accreditation of Teacher Education. (1997). *Technology and teacher education: New standards*. Washington, DC: Author.

NCSESA & NRC. (1996). *National Science Education Standards*. Washington, DC: National Academy Press.

NCTM. (2000). *Principles and standards for school mathematics*. Reston, VA: Author.

Niess, M. (2001). A Model for Integrating Technology in Preservice Science and Mathematics Content-Specific Teacher Preparation. *School Science and Mathematics, 101*(2), 102–109. doi:10.1111/j.1949-8594.2001.tb18011.x

Niess, M. L. (2005). Preparing teachers to teach science and mathematics with technology: Developing a technology pedagogical content knowledge. *Teaching and Teacher Education, 21*(5), 509–523. doi:10.1016/j.tate.2005.03.006

Niess, M. L., Suharwoto, G., Lee, K., & Sadri, P. (2006). *Guiding Inservice Mathematics Teachers in Developing TPCK*. Paper presented at the American Education Research Association Annual Conference, San Francisco, California, April.

Pierson, M. E. (2001). Technology integration practices as function of pedagogical expertise. *Journal of Research on Computing in Education*, *33*(4), 413–429.

Roschelle, J., & Pea, R. (2002). A walk on the WILD side: How wireless handhelds may change computer-supported collaborative learning. *International Journal of Cognitive Technology*, *1*(1), 145–272. doi:10.1075/ijct.1.1.09ros

Russell, M., Bebell, D., O'Dwyer, L. M., & O'Connor, K. M. (2003). Examining Teacher Technology Use: Implications for Preservice and In-Service Teacher Preparation. *Journal of Teacher Education*, *54*(4), 297–310. doi:10.1177/0022487103255985

Sharples, M. (2000). The design of personal mobile technologies for lifelong learning. *Computers & Education*, *34*, 177–193. doi:10.1016/S0360-1315(99)00044-5

Shulman, L. (1986). Those who understand: Knowledge growth in teaching. *Educational Researcher*, *15*(2), 4–14.

Shulman, L. (1987). Knowledge and teaching: Foundations of the new reform. *Harvard Educational Review*, *57*(1), 1–22.

Snider, S. L. (2002). Exploring technology integration in a field-based teacher education program: implementation efforts and findings. *Journal of Research on Technology in Education*, *34*, 230–249.

Soloway, E., Norris, E., Blumenfeld, P., Fishman, B., Krajcik, J., & Marx, R. (2001). Log on education: Handheld devices are ready-at-hand. *Communications of the ACM*, *44*(6), 15–20. doi:10.1145/376134.376140

Stager, G. (2000). Portable probeware: Science education's next frontier. *Curriculum Administrator*, *36*(3), 32–36.

Staudt, C., & Hsi, S. (1999). *Synergy projects and pocket computers*. Concord Consortium Newsletter.

Stokes, D., Jenkins, C., Huhnke, L., Grey, G., & Manning, C. (2000). Math and Science Curriculum Revision: A Collaborative Approach to Improving Preservice Teachers' Use of Technology Knowledge and Instructional Skills. In *Proceedings of World Conference on Educational Multimedia, Hypermedia and Telecommunications 2000* (pp. 1832). Norfolk, VA: AACE.

Strudel, N., & Wetzel, K. (1999). Lessons from exemplary colleges of education: Factors affecting technology integration in preservice programs. *Educational Technology Research and Development*, *47*(4), 63–81. doi:10.1007/BF02299598

Thomas, J. A., & Cooper, S. B. (2000). Teaching technology: A new opportunity for pioneers in teacher education. *Journal of Computing in Teacher Education*, *17*(1), 13–19.

Tinker, R., & Krajcik, J. (Eds.). (2001). *Portable Technologies: Science Learning in Context*. New York: Kluwer Academic/Plenum Publishers.

U. S. Department of Education. (2000). *E-learning: Putting a world-class education at the fingertips of all children*. Washington, DC: Author.

U.S. Department of Education. (2004). *National Educational Technology Plan*. Washington, DC: Author.

Vahey, P., & Crawford, V. (2002). *Palm Education Pioneers Program: Final evaluation report*. Menlo Park, CA: SRI International.

van't Hooft, M., Diaz, S., & Swan, K. (2004). Examining the potential of handheld computers: Findings from the Ohio PEP project. *Journal of Educational Computing Research*, *30*(4), 295–312. doi:10.2190/M1W6-A94D-3NKM-KBUU

Wiggins, G., & McTighe, J. (2005). *Understanding by Design*. Alexandria, VA: Association for Supervision and Curriculum Development.

Zhao, Y. (2003). *What Teachers should Know about Technology: Perspectives and Practices*. Greenwich, CT: Information Age Publishing.

ADDITIONAL READING

Cappella, E. (2000). What Children Think About Computers. *The Future of Children: Children and Computer Technology*, *10*(2), 186–191.

Clemens, A., Moore, T., & Nelson, B. (2001). *Math Intervention SMART Project (Student Mathematical Analysis and Reasoning with Technology)*. Online paper. Retrieved July15, 2008, from http://www.smarterkids.org/research/paper10.asp

Curtis, M., Kopera, J., Norris, C., & Soloway, E. (2004). *Palm OS® handhelds in elementary classroom: Curriculum and strategies*. Eugene, OR: International Society for Technology in Education.

Dick, T. (1988, April). The Continuing Calculator Controversy. *The Arithmetic Teacher*, ▪▪▪, 37–41.

Johse, V., & Ruda, C. (2003). *Explorations: Math at Your Fingertips with the TI-10*. Dallas, TX: Texas Instruments.

Levin, G. (1985). Computers and kids: The good news, children are learning valuable lessons from machines they can't intimidate or dominate. *Psychology Today*, *8*, 50–51.

Moore, M., Carter, D., Andersen, B., & Windle, T. (2007). *Elementary Science with Vernier*. Beaverton, OR: Vernier Software and Technology.

Niess, M., Lee, J., & Kajder, S. (2007). *Guiding Learning with Technology*. Hoboken, NJ: John Wiley.

Partnership for 21st Century Skills. (2004). *Frameworks for 21st Century Learning*. Retrieved July 29, 2008, from http://www.21stcenturyskills.org/

Schielack, J. F., & Chancellor, D. (2007). *Uncovering math with manipulatives and the TI-10*. Dallas, TX: Texas Instruments.

TEEMSS. (2002). *The Final Report to the Concord Consortium and the National Science Foundation on the Technology-Enhanced Elementary and Middle School Science (TEEMSS) Project*. Retrieved July 15, 2008, from http://www.vernier.com/grants/articles/teemss.pdf

Voltz, D., & Spatka, S. (2000). *Middle school science with calculators*. Portland, OR: Vernier Software and Technology.

Wartella, E., & Jennings, N. (2000). Children and Computers: New Technology — Old Concerns. *The Future of Children: Children And Computer Technology*, *10*(2), 31–43. doi:10.2307/1602688

Wenglinsky, H. (1998). *Does it compute? The relationship between educational technology and student achievement in mathematics*. Princeton, NJ: Educational Testing Service.

KEY TERMS AND DEFINITIONS

Backwards Design: An approach to designing a curriculum or unit that begins with the end in mind and designs toward that end. Although such an approach seems logical, it is viewed as backward because many teachers begin their unit design with the means – textbooks, favored lessons – rather than deriving those from the end

– the targeted results, such as content standards or understandings.

Constructivism: A learning perspective, developed in the 1970s, which is rooted in the works of Bruner, Piaget and Vygotsky, and has its foundations in cognitive learning psychology. Constructivist learning places emphasis on the learners and propounds that learning is affected by their context, beliefs and attitudes. Learners are encouraged to find their own solutions and to build upon their prior knowledge and experience.

Emerging Technologies: some emerging technologies that are finding their ways into elementary classrooms are: handheld computing devices, such as calculators, real-time data collection technology, such as computer interfaces with data probes and sensors, interactive displays, such as Smart Boar, personal electronic devices, such as Ipods, MP3 players, PDA, and cell phones, wireless technology allowing students to stay connected as they move between home and the classroom, such as tablet PC and laptops, advanced web-based technologies, such as weblogs, e-books, wiki, online journals and discussion boards, video systems, such as PlayStation, Xbox, and Nintendo

Student-Centered Learning: A model of learning in which students are viewed as active learners and take responsibility for their own learning, determine their own needs, set their own goals, monitor their own progress and determine how to reach the desired learning outcomes in a collaborative teaching environment.

TPACK: is a framework to understand and describe the kinds of knowledge needed by a teacher for effective technology Integration. The TPACK framework argues that effective technology integration for teaching specific content or subject matter requires understanding and negotiating the relationships between these three components: Technology, Pedagogy, And Content.

ENDNOTE

1 For the project described in this chapter Professor Irina Lyublinskaya was a recipient of the 2008 National Science Teachers Association / Vernier Technology Award in the college category. Professor Lyublinskaya was recognized 2008 NSTA National Convention, which took place in Boston, MA from March 27 – March 30, 2008.

Chapter 13
Collaborative Learning in Pre-Service/In-Service Communities of Practice:
Discovering How and When to Integrate Technology in Senior High Science

Ronald J. MacDonald
University of Prince Edward Island, Canada

ABSTRACT

This chapter will describe how a research-based Community of Practice (CoP) of pre-service and in-service teachers supported teachers' reflection and learning about how and when to integrate hand-held data loggers. This study suggests that the CoP narrowed the gap between theory (in teacher education) and practice (in the school classroom). Findings will describe effective ways to use hand-held data loggers in senior high school science classes, as well as in pre-service teacher education courses. The possibilities of building even stronger connections between the traditionally theoretical world of teacher education and the real world of school are suggested.

INTRODUCTION

The theme of this book – what teacher educators think and do when adopting new technologies – is of the utmost importance in today's ever-shifting educational and technological landscape. Many teacher educators think long and hard about the potential implications of embracing new technologies. They will not institute a technology for its own sake; rather they will only embed and model new technologies if they believe they can benefit students.

Technologies have been found to enhance student achievement, promote collaboration (BECTA, 2005; Cox, Webb, Abbott, Blakeley, Beauchamp, & Rhodes, 2003; Inkpen, Ho-Ching, Kuederle, Scott, & Shoemaker, 1999) and improve student motivation (Passey, Rogers, Machell, McHugh, & Allaway, 2003). Studies also suggest that when digital technologies are used in ways that support student ownership of educational processes and products, conceptual understanding improves (Dex-

DOI: 10.4018/978-1-61520-897-5.ch013

Copyright © 2010, IGI Global. Copying or distributing in print or electronic forms without written permission of IGI Global is prohibited.

ter, Anderson, & Becker, 2000; Dwyer, Ringstaff, & Sandholtz, 1991; Hennessy, Deaney, & Ruthven, 2003). It has been reported, however, that many teachers are barely coping with the new demands of technology integration and sustainability and so do not achieve these potential benefits (Cuban, 2001; Hennessy, Ruthven, & Brindley, 2005; Tearle, 2003).

Why are technologies not integrated in sustainable ways to benefit student learning? How can teacher educators model technologies that may lead to pre-service teachers' embedding technology in ways that truly support their future students' learning?

Researchers suggest that research on particular technologies has not been sufficient to point to ways to successfully embed these technologies. They report that teachers must be involved in the process of learning about embedding technologies in schools (Hennessy et al., 2005). I suggest that not only should in-service teachers be involved in the research processes that help discover ways to effectively integrate technologies but pre-service teachers too can contribute to as well as directly benefit from becoming part of the research process. A Community of Practice (CoP) (Lave & Wenger, 1991; Wenger, McDermott, & Snyder, 2002) has shown promise as a collaborative mechanism to learn about technology integration and teaching. It is through this CoP that teachers are afforded essential opportunities to reflect on their teaching (Chalmers & Keown, 2006).

In this chapter I describe how a CoP of pre-service and in-service teachers reflected on and made decisions regarding the use of hand-held data loggers in high school science. Findings regarding the workings of the CoP and how the integration of data loggers affected student attitudes (such as self-confidence in learning science and technology usefulness) will be shown. Issues and values of the collaborative CoP model for teacher education will also be discussed.

BACKGROUND

The following section presents background on communities of practice and design-based research employed in this study.

Communities of Practice: Spaces and Places for Teacher Reflection

Collaborative learning and research can be supported through a CoP. In this community, individual teachers' needs can be addressed (Hennessy et al., 2005). Kirschner & Lai (2007), describe CoPs as "places where a process of social learning occurs between people with a common interest in a subject or a problem who collaborate over longer periods of time to share and exchange ideas, find solutions, and build knowledge" (p.128). Member of CoPs collectively decide on goals, the ways to reach these goals and methods of assessing progress (MacDonald, 2008). In previous research, CoPs have been shown to be successful as a collaborative way to address educational challenges (Bereiter, 2005; Lave & Wenger, 1991; Olitksy, 2007; Scardamalia, 2003).

Barab, Barnett, & Squire (2002) suggest that we become good teachers by, reflecting on our teaching and talking with colleagues about our reflections. The study reported in this chapter is based on this guiding principle. A CoP was designed to provide opportunities for pre-service and in-service teachers to reflect on their practice and then openly discuss these reflections. When CoPs are organized to provide the necessary time in teachers' busy lives to reflect on their teaching then lasting pedagogical change may occur (Schlager & Fusco, 2003).

An important facet of CoPs is its potential to support educational goals by giving ownership to the participants in the research. This can be done in a number of ways: by giving CoP members the opportunity to contribute to the research design and implementation and to feed back new knowledge. Importantly, CoPs involving in-service teachers (and in our context pre-service teachers too) acknowledge and value the teaching and learning of teachers' everyday lives (Niesz, 2007). The CoP must make it possible for its members to be honest and comfortable with each other (Lave & Wenger, 1991); this leads to a positive group relationship (Niesz, 2007).

Situated and distributed cognition form the theoretical base for knowledge generation in CoPs. According to Lave and Wenger (1991) such learning involves social participation in local communities, situated in a particular context, where actions are perceived to be competent by members of that local community. Technology supported, online CoPs have been researched by Laferriere, et al. (2006). Findings from their work suggest that teachers with varied backgrounds and experiences can distribute understandings by sharing with and learning from each other. Research has found that experienced teachers and pre-service teachers may be able to learn from each other when integrating technologies (Barab, MaKinster, & Scheckler, 2003). In our particular context of investigating how and when to use hand-held data loggers, a synergy may result in newfound knowledge about teaching and learning with technologies, which is possible through CoPs (Scardamalia, 2003). In this research and learning context, pre-service teachers may learn a great deal about how to teach with technology. It is within this CoP that pre-service and in-service teachers are provided the opportunity to reflect upon personal and collective values, beliefs and attitudes (Chalmers & Keown, 2006).

While it has been found that CoPs give teachers a sense of ownership of the research process, the role of teacher educators as facilitators of these communities must not be undervalued. It has been suggested that they have a strong role to play in a CoP as a researcher/instructor/facilitator. We, as researchers and teacher educators, also need to feel a sense of ownership and the responsibility to provide input (Niesz, 2007). We must not feel that we are overstepping our authority in a CoP; we have important theoretically-based practices and concepts to contribute (Wubbles, 2007). A shared understanding among in-service teachers, pre-service teachers and researchers can lead to a synthesis of instructional solutions.

The study described in this chapter investigated the use of hand-held data loggers in high school science classes. CoPs have been used in a variety of ways in science teaching with some success: increasing student active learning in science (Barab, Barnett, & Squire, 2002; Krajcik & Blumenfeld, 1994); generally supporting pre-service science teachers (Hassard & Dias, 2000); and fostering inquiry in their science teaching (Barab et al., 2003; Dreon & McDonald, 2006; Goodnough, 2004). Some effective ways to solve educational challenges and build teacher collaborations were found.

Design-Based Research

The methodology employed to investigate the CoP was design-based research. Design-based research often uses several methods which result in new instructional designs and new educational theories (Davis & Krajcik, 2005; Design-Based-Research-Collective, 2003). Initially, the researcher approaches a group of teachers who are interested in the researcher's questions and research design. The teacher participants have an essential role in providing feedback to the ongoing, iterative, process. Cycles of interventions can occur where research data provide new information for both teachers and researchers and allow collaborative instructional decisions (Sandoval & Bell, 2004). CoP meetings can be an important source of data as members discuss their progress toward research goals and re-design research and classroom instructional processes.

THE PROBLEM: CONNECTING TO THE FIELD

While teachers need to learn the skills for integrating particular technologies, teacher development should focus on involving teachers in the process of learning about technology integration (Hennessy et al., 2005). That is, *in situ* technology use is the most effective and efficient way to learn how to teach with technology. For teacher educators, this principle may be extended to help pre-service teachers to discover how and when to teach with technologies. Here lies the crucial question: How can teacher educators engage pre-service and in-service teachers in the process of learning about technology integration? Accompanying this problem is the ever-increasing pressure for teacher educators to prepare pre-service teachers to be immediately successful in real world teaching contexts. This justified pressure manifests itself in a perceived (and sometimes very real) divide between theoretical teachings in teacher education programs and the on-the-ground realities of real teaching in real schools. It is often said that teachers arrive in their first teaching post having learned a great deal of theory about teaching but not having sufficiently learned how to teach with technology.

The Hand-Held Data Logger

The particular focus of the CoP discussed in this chapter was to discover how and when to integrate hand-held data logging technology in senior high science. While research has shown that the integration of technology improves students' understanding of concepts in science (Cox, Webb, Abbott, Blakeley, Beauchamp, & Rhodes, 2003; White & Fredriksen, 1998), the frequency and manner in which technologies are used in science classrooms appears to be quite different in practice from research findings (Roth & Lee, 2006). This discrepancy may be due to problems with teacher professional development opportunities for technology integration (Hennessy et al., 2005).

Hand-held data loggers resemble large graphing calculators with their own screen and the possibility of attaching over 60 different probes (e.g., motion sensors, pH meters, and force meters). They provide an authentic opportunity for students to participate in the data collection process and are one of the most powerful new technologies to actively engage students in science (Roth & Lee, 2006). These technologies also support student inquiry – an outcome much sought after by science educators – by giving instant graphic feedback (Baggott La Velle, McFarlane, & Brawn, 2003; Zucker, Tinker, Staudt, Mansfield, & Metcalf, 2008), allowing otherwise impossible data collection (Newton, 2000) and freeing students to think about higher order interpretation and analysis (Barton, 2004; McFarlane & Sakellariou, 2002). Technologies, are still predominantly used in teacher-directed, transmission pedagogy, with the teacher at the front of the class demonstrating the devices while students watch (MacDonald & Larter, 2007; Roth & Lee, 2006).

While the potential for using hand-held data loggers for learning is great, many teachers use data loggers primarily in direct-teaching ways (Hennessy et al., 2005). The teacher demonstrates the devices while students watch (MacDonald 2008b; Roth & Lee, 2006). For the most part, data loggers presented in this way have not catalyzed an increase in student inquiry in science classrooms – one of the primary goals of science education – due to the lack of effective professional development opportunities (Seah et al., 2005). Ongoing, collaborative professional development may help teachers to integrate ICTs more effectively and increase levels of student inquiry (Hennessy et al., 2005).

In the section that follows these problems will be addressed through a description of the creation and maintenance of a CoP of pre-service and in-service teachers, with a teacher educator acting both as instructor and researcher.

THE COMMUNITY OF PRACTICE SOLUTION

One solution to the problems outlined is to incorporate current research into teacher education classes. The most contextually appropriate research might come from the teacher educators/researchers themselves. This is what I have done. In the following section, I describe the methods I used in one research project and the findings that are relevant for teacher education.

Methods

Context

The research was conducted with senior high in-service teachers and their students, along with my pre-service students. That is, I both taught these pre-service teachers science methods over two semesters and supervised their second six-week practicum placement. The intention of the CoP was to link theoretical support from the teacher education program with teachers' experience. These teachers in this school provided a nexus of experience and understandings to synergize new ways to integrate technologies as well as to more generally teach science (Figure 1). This research was conducted over 18 months (2006/2008) with 12 science teachers from three senior high schools in Eastern Canada. My senior high science methods cohort (11 students) joined this CoP for the 2008 winter term.

Research Design

Design-based research method was chosen to support the CoP, as design-based research processes are very similar to the requirements of CoP design (MacDonald, 2008). That is, at the core of each is an acknowledgement that practitioners' understandings are essential to moving a community forward. The methods involved collection of data from two sources: senior high school students completed a pre- and post-survey to uncover the effects of using data loggers in their science classrooms and labs on their attitudes toward science (described below); CoP meetings; interviews with pre-service and in-service teachers, and student focus groups were audio taped to provide qualitative data.

The student survey and focus group data helped teachers and researcher assess how these technologies might benefit high school students, and what instructional decisions might follow. Through our analysis of this data we learned about the benefits and potential problems of first introducing and then using hand-held technologies in high school science classrooms and labs. The transcripts of the audio-tapes of the CoP meetings and in-service/pre-service teacher and teacher interviews were used in the analysis of the interactions in the CoP.

Figure 1. Community of practice of pre-service and in-service teachers

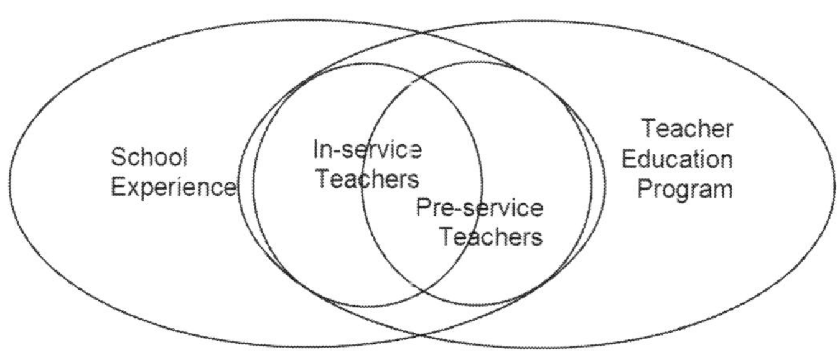

Data Sources

During CoP meetings, in-service and pre-service teachers played a significant role in setting goals, designing further CoP meetings, articulating their needs, and providing feedback about the impact of the study. There were a number of CoP activities: meetings, data logging presentations, teacher-researcher collaborative lesson planning and teaching, and an online wiki which provided for collaborative communications. Audio recording of fourteen, 60-minute interviews and eight, 60-minute focus group interviews were part of the data set. There were six classroom observations and teachers' online Wiki reflections (each teacher posted four or five times). For senior high student data, sources included four 60-minute partially structured student focus group interviews in the three study schools and a collaboratively designed student survey. (See the Analysis section for details of the data analysis.)

The student survey (the constructs, e.g., self-efficacy toward science learning, self-confidence in science ability) conducted in a pre and post design, were borrowed from a previously validated instrument by permission of the authors, the *Inquiry Science Student Assessment* (Brandon, Taum, Ayala, Young, Gray, Speitel, Nguyen, & Pottenger III, 2007). The authors found strong content-related validity evidence, through careful and thorough development process and high coefficient alphas, as well as strong concurrent validity, through positive correlations found among attitudinal scales. As well, our own factor analysis and Cronbach's alpha (>.70) procedures reconfirmed that the Likert-based survey items strongly contribute to each construct. The survey was administered at the beginning and the end of the 2008 winter semester (pre n=123, post n=97). Since in design-based research participants' concerns must be heard, when the teachers involved in the construction of the survey felt that having students use particular student identifiers would be too cumbersome, these were not included. This decision ruled out the use of dependent t-tests and resulted in independent t-test being employed. However, the same classrooms of students, with the same teachers, in the same semester took part in both the pre and post surveys.

Opportunities for Teacher Reflection

Pre-service teachers were full members of the CoP; and were given numerous opportunities to reflect on their teaching. Both pre-service and in-service teachers were asked to post reflections to an online Wiki immediately following data logger use in the classroom or lab. They were asked to reflect upon and write about three items: the curricular outcomes to be reached and what was done with the technology to help reach them; their perceptions about how the class went – what worked and what didn't; and what they would design the lesson differently the next time. These online reflections were available to all members of the CoP. Additionally, these online reflections became the items for group discussion during subsequent CoP meetings. These group discussions, as suggested by researchers such as Barab, Barnett, & Squire (2002), appear to have been the most powerful experiences to affect teachers' concepts of teaching and learning with technology.

During CoP meetings teachers were also asked to do "quick writes" – their reflections on various aspects of science teaching and learning with technology. These quick write reflections were also used as the basis for collective discussions on developing pedagogical practices.

Another specific reflection opportunity was provided to pre-service teachers. They were asked to reflect on and write about their perceptions of the theory/practice divide; the similarities and the differences they saw between educational theory and their teaching practice. Guiding questions included: What do you see in action in your placement that we have read and discussed concerning theory?; What do you want to adopt from theory that does not seem to be presently occurring in practice?; How much of a role does theory play in teaching practice? These reflections were invaluable in enabling pre-service teachers to examine their own teaching.

Analysis

Interview and focus group data were analyzed through a constant comparison method (Strauss & Corbin, 1998) to identify themes. Initial analysis built broad categories and as analysis progressed, these were subdivided into narrower categories which were coded into preliminary themes. These themes were then sub-divided into narrower themes as an in-depth analysis of the data was undertaken (Krathwohl, 1997). Constant comparison was done by two independent researchers, one working directly on the print version and the other using *NVivo* qualitative analysis software. Both methods resulted in very similar categories and themes. When researchers' categories and themes varied, the data were revisited and discussed to resolve the discrepancies. The thematic evidence presented in this chapter represents only the strongly consistent findings found throughout the data. Transcription validation was ensured through member checks and verification by second and third readers. An independent inter-rater reliability procedure was carried out to verify coding.

Correlations and independent *t*-tests formed the bulk of the statistical tests for the pre and post student survey. An example of a survey construct and its items follows:

Self-Confidence in Ability to Learn Science (1-not true at all – 6-completely true), α =.91:

- I can do almost all the work in science class if I do not give up.
- I can learn science.
- I can figure out how to do difficult work in science.
- I can master the skills taught in science class this year.
- Even if the work in science is hard, I can learn it.
- If I have enough time, I can do a good job on all my science work.

Findings and Discussion

Findings from the Pre-service and In-Service Teacher CoP

Analysis of audio-taped CoP meeting transcripts, online reflections text and interview transcripts from both pre-service and in-service teachers revealed important findings: the perceived importance of the school as a location for teacher development initiatives; the tension between curriculum content knowledge and student inquiry; and a sense that content knowledge must be delivered first. These findings are presented and discussed below. (Note: teacher quotes in this section originate from both pre-service and in-service teachers.)

Importance of the Field

Data indicated that in-service teachers relied on the school's science department for guidance and support when being introduced to new technologies and new pedagogies; this appears to ground teachers in making technology and pedagogy decisions. It was in the school, paired with support from the research-based CoP, where teachers seemed to feel most comfortable being introduced to the new technology and pedagogy. It was consistently found that in-service as well as pre-service teachers, valued learning from colleagues at their school. (Pseudonyms for teachers and schools are used.)

Greg is not teaching physics this semester but he's already come to me lots of times and I've gone to him lots of times and said, "You know this is what I'm thinking, what do you think?" ...so it's going to happen with good teachers and good schools – that's what we have.

Pre-service teachers consistently reported that they valued learning in this location as this context provided a space for in-service and pre-service knowledge and experience exchange:

I think that it's a good idea because the pre-service teachers gain from the teachers, and their knowledge, but the teachers will also be gain from the new perspectives of the pre-service teachers. So it kind of goes both ways.... and really it benefits the pre-service teachers and the teachers and aside from that it would benefit the students because they are getting better labs because of it.

Another teacher relates this consistent finding: "Maple Street School is really lucky. We have a really tight science department and we already do a lot of collaborative work together." However, at one of the schools, a physics teacher wanted to go elsewhere for support: "That's the biggest thing with me. I feel like I'm alone. And I have requested a half day to meet with a physics teacher at another school. Because we have gotten together in the past and come up with some great stuff." Teachers value their own school for support and consistently talk about this first before discussing other teacher support possibilities. Changes in teachers' work may need to be supported by colleagues in their own school before venturing beyond it.

Once teachers felt a level of comfort in their own school, they appeared ready for outside support. This was provided by the CoP in several ways: 1) *Expertise: Someone's out there.* The researcher/teacher educator, a software/hardware representative and a curriculum consultant were available in the school district. Pre-service and in-service teachers both noted that having experts support them by actually demonstrating how to use the instruments was important. One teacher's comments are representative: "Yes, I'm going to want another set of hands to help put out fires." Also, teachers often just needed to know that support was available: "I think just knowing that there is someone out there who can show up and say, "OK, let me help you out" is what is good; " 2) *Teacher reflection.* Both pre-service and in-service teachers posed challenging questions regarding the research, which revealed their own pedagogical views; 3) *Needs-based approach.* The research-based CoP appears to have been a place where teachers' needs were articulated and heard.

Balance between Curriculum Content Knowledge and Inquiry

Through audio-taped CoP meetings as well as teacher interviews a consistent theme emerged. All of the teachers expressed a tension between covering provincial curriculum goals and having students use technology to support student inquiry. At the beginning of the research, teachers expressed concerns regarding this issue:

Good science teaching is giving them enough to get them questioning and then giving them the tools to search for the answers to their own questions. But, there's a pressure, I feel. This is good science teaching, and the problem we face is that all that stuff would be great science teaching if we had the time to let them do that exploration. But we also have a constraint that they are expected to cover a certain amount of material.

Teachers consistently revealed a polarization between inquiry, where students engage in the process of doing science themselves with the hand-held data loggers and transmission models of teaching where teachers directly instruct students by delivering information. The data suggested that teachers wanted to have their students engage in student inquiry but felt transmission of information was the most efficient way to "deliver the outcomes." Teachers consistently acknowledged the value of inquiry but struggled with how this could be accomplished.

Teachers also said that student inquiry and lab work using data loggers might take too much time. After using the data loggers, however, teachers may have changed their minds. One teacher expressed this consistent finding:

The students were able to gather information quickly and graphically, which was otherwise very time-consuming before and generally avoided. Students were able to measure a force that occurs in only 0.01s time. This would be impossible to collect using older equipment. Students were engaged, were able to manipulate the new equipment very quickly, and were not at all frustrated or threatened by the new technology. No surprise there.

It was regularly found that teachers framed the issue of how and when to integrate technology by discussing the concept of balance. One particular type of balance sought was between student inquiry (aided by technology) and reaching curriculum outcomes through the transmission of information. During interviews, as teachers discussed this balance, they used their hands to portray a balance (predominantly tipped toward transmission) to represent the tension between these two pedagogies. This concept of balance was consistently represented, as evidenced by one teacher: "Good science teaching would be to find a balance between student-led inductive and deductive learning, while meeting curriculum outcomes within the time constraints of a busy school year."

As the CoP process continued many teachers began to re-examine the balance between the costs and benefits of using the data loggers in ways that fostered inquiry. As an example, the teacher quoted above who wanted to do the impulse and momentum lab in an inductive manner now appears to question the value of this method in lieu of a teacher demonstration.

There are labs that I know now that no, I'll never do this as an introductory lab, maybe as a demo in front of the class and explain what they are seeing... the momentum impulse is one you could do as a demo.

He bases this decision on the effort students put into using the data loggers versus their gains in conceptual understanding:

I don't think that it is going to work very well because of the set up time, because of all the hoops they have to jump through to set up the GLXs [data loggers], do the experiment, and read the graphs... I don't know what level of success we'll have. I think there will be a few kids that get it and the majority of the class will be like "What the hell is this?"

This teacher and others, however, still appear to recognize the learning potential of student inquiry and they want to increase their levels of student inquiry. Another teacher states:

I want to do both. I want to do the lab where you [the teacher] create your own experiment. I want to do that, I want to see how it goes. But the inquiry stuff, I guess I'm willing to do a little bit, but I'm not willing to do the whole class... not force feeding, but leading them down the right path.

Another consistently occurring aspect of balance addressed the notion that students need both teacher organized structure as well as student-led freedom of choice through science inquiry. While discussing the notion of how often he permits students to engage in inquiry, one teacher stated:

The students that are in my classroom need freedom of choice. But the kids in my classroom need structure and direction. That's the best way I can sum it up. And they are both – they're kids and they're students, and that's why I'm here. I'm just trying to figure out how I can make that balance.

Knowledge First

Teachers felt that technology integration could help after knowledge was delivered. The goal of technology was to help "perform experiments in a lab and classroom setting by the students, to reinforce concepts discussed in class," said one teacher. As the CoP developed, however, teachers began to propose that knowledge could be discovered through student inquiry (while using the data loggers), without knowledge being transmitted first. For example, one teacher conducted a lab on the concept of impulse equating to change in momentum. He first introduced this concept in the classroom, followed by proving it in the lab. After some reflection, he related that next time he will have students discover (inductively) the concept for themselves. He posted the following in the CoP online forum:

Try using the impulse and momentum lab ($Ft = mv_2 - mv_1$) immediately after Newton's Laws. Allow students to prove with the GLX [a handheld data logger] that Ft must equal mv_2-mv_1 before the concepts of impulse and momentum are even discussed. Then use this lab as a lead-in to impulse, momentum and conservation of momentum.

Findings from Student Data: Data Logger Integration

Focus group and pre/post survey data gathered from students produced a number of findings: the a caveat that curriculum content knowledge must come first; instrumentation support is essential; students prefer to use the data loggers; and a number of gender-based technology and science attitudinal differences. These findings are presented and discussed below.

Knowledge First

Students also addressed the concept of knowledge first. Two students represent a theme related to the notion that using technologies should be used to confirm knowledge already learned in the classroom. A female student stated that the use of the data logger is "a confirmation thing." She continues, "If it's something we did before, you can look at it and know what we are looking at. So if you just picked it up and measured it, motion or something, you wouldn't know what it was at all….So I think it's good that we learned to do it by hand first." This same student later concludes that "I would definitely prefer to use the GLX [data logger] because it's more interesting, but if I hadn't learned it on paper first I would have been totally lost." Males, however, consistently stated that the data logger is a useful tool, without referring to necessary teacher-provided introduction to the concepts: "I like it because it makes the lab more interesting because how else are you going to measure velocity or something without using that?"

Instrumentation Support is Necessary

Even though levels of self-confidence may vary between boys and girls, we found that both boys and girls loudly and clearly want instrumentation support. Teachers and teacher educators need to plan for both senior high students and pre-service teacher to have time to learn how to use the technology before it can be used as a learning tool. Students say they need to learn more about how to use the technology. One female student represents this consistent finding: "I'd say explain it a little more too." One male student would also appreciate more instrumentation help: "We probably have to use it hands-on for two, maybe three classes."

Student Use Preferred

One of the survey items was "Student Use Preference for Data Loggers" (as opposed to teacher use). In the pre survey, data showed that both males and females wanted to use the data loggers about the same amount, $M = 3.3$, $SD = 1.25$, $M = 3.0$, $SD = 1.24$, respectively, on a 5-point Likert scale from strong disagree (1) to strongly agree (5). In the post survey, however, females increased to a mean of 4.1 ($SD = 1.0$) compared to males ($M = 3.7$, $SD = 1.24$), which is a significant change for females, $t(57) = -3.47$, $p < .001$, $d = .93$. Females appear to want to use the technology themselves more after they used the technology in the study.

Gender Differences

Data strongly revealed that females generally prefer to be taught through teacher-directed instruction (transmission) as opposed to student inquiry: "I'd rather have written instructions telling me exactly what to do because otherwise I just feel like I'm wasting time," while males say they would rather have open-ended inquiry: "It was good that we could like try out and make our own graphs with the data logger and not just follow the instructions all the time so we could try to make our own and then someone else has to try to recreate it."

Another interesting difference emerged: when it came to students having a sense of "Technology Usefulness" (e.g., Likert item, from 1 to 5: It is important to me to do well when learning about technology.) relatively close scores between males ($M = 3.5$, $SD = 1.2$) and females ($M = 3.6$, $SD = .83$) in the pre administration were found to widen in the post administration where males increased to $M = 3.7$ ($SD = 1.23$), while females decreased to $M = 3.0$ ($SD = 1.1$), which resulted in a statistically significant difference between males and females, $t(80) = 2.53, p < 0.05, d = .57$.

Data loggers were used most frequently in Grade 11 physics. Another look at the data from only these students revealed interesting findings. All students entered their grade earned in physics. Males' grades in physics correlate with "Self-Confidence in Ability to Learn Science", $r(50) = .71$, p <.01, *Value of Science* $r(50) = .34$, $p < .05$, *Self-efficacy* $r(50) = .66, p < .05$, *Technology Anxiety* $r(45) = -0.53, p < .05$. That is, when males' grades are high so too are their scores for confidence to learn science, the perceived value of science, their self-efficacy. As males' technology anxiety decreases, their grades increase. For Grade 11 females, however, there were only two significant correlations with grades: "Self Confidence in Science Ability" $r(30) = .47$ p <.01 and "Science Anxiety" $r(30) = -.44, p < .05$. Two of these strong correlates are addressed further below. It appears that the most important influences upon grades for females are their anxiety about science and their confidence in their science ability.

As suggested above, the lower a female's science anxiety the higher their grade. Data reveal significant differences in science anxiety between males and females in both the pre and post surveys. Science anxiety stayed the same for males for pre and post at a mean of 1.7 (out of a possible high score of 6). Females post scored $M = 2.6$, $SD = 1.13$ and males scored $M = 1.7$, $SD = 0.66$ in the post survey. The post statistic represents this difference: $t(97) = 2.56$, p = 0.013, $d = .94$.

While females may develop an appreciation for the measuring and data presentation capabilities of the data logger, anxiety in using the tool was clearly evident when we talked to them. One student summed up her feelings well in a statement echoed by other females:

If you work with it every time you are in the lab, it's a lot easier when all of a sudden your partner is not there and you are working with someone else and you have to figure it out. It's like you don't really know where you are. And then there are so many different buttons to get to one spot you can confuse yourself sometimes.

Pre-service teachers also consistently found gender differences, as represented by the following interview passage:

I think you'd have to find a way to make your lessons appeal to both genders and I think generally, what I said earlier about educating the students on how to use the GLXs right from the get go would help too, maybe. It was almost like the girls were scared of them, so maybe if you were able to educate them enough then maybe they wouldn't be actually scared of the GLX or whatever. Like, they, I just remember some girls were like "Those things again!".

"Self-Confidence in Ability to Learn Science" measured a student's sense of self-efficacy for learning science (for example, "Even if the work in science is hard, I can learn it."). In the pre administration, there were no differences between gender and yet, in the post administration, females scored lower ($M = 4.70$, $SD = 1.10$, out of a high score of 6) than males ($M = 5.20$, $SD = .68$), $t(52) = 2.06$, $p < 0.045$, $d = .61$. As well, several female students indicated that their self-efficacy for learning science with the data loggers was not high. This was not found with males. This finding was elevated to a theme, "Lab confusion effects on self-efficacy." Here are three examples: "I don't think that it, even if we get a question, and we have to go find it. And I'm just left by myself to do it and usually I don't understand it." "I can get on a computer and do fine, but not something that's brand new to me." "Honestly, I don't know anything I'm doing when I'm using those data loggers. I need to know exactly what I'm practicing. Exactly what I'm doing." The majority of male students in the focus groups were more confident in their ability to use the data loggers: "When you've used them once or twice you can pretty well memorize where it's stuck. And say 'Well, I remember this from last time. I just have to do this'."

Conclusion and Implications For Teacher Education

Teacher reflection is essential to support teacher pedagogical change (Barab, Barnett, & Squire, 2002; Chalmers & Keown, 2006; Schlager & Fusco, 2003). Teacher reflection is a crucial component of CoPs. Our CoP of pre-service and in-service teachers afforded numerous opportunities for teacher reflection. Without this time to reflect upon their teaching practice they may not have truly learned from their own and others' data logger integration teaching practice. The iterative nature of the design-based research process also helped provide many cycles of reflection-informed teaching practices, assessment of teaching and the redesign of teaching practices."

The collaborative mechanism of the CoP – a blend of having pre-service teachers exposed to both theoretical understandings and teaching methods from their course work, along with on-the-ground in-service teacher support – led to important findings which have implications for teacher education. University/College courses that do not include significant influence from experienced subject teachers may be a disservice to student teachers.

Some salient conclusions from the CoP are listed below, followed by a discussion of their potential impact on teacher education courses.

Importance of the Field

Findings suggest that the first community that teachers turned to when being introduced to new technologies and new pedagogies was their school science department. This community appears to ground teachers in making technology and pedagogy decisions. It was at school where teachers seemed to feel most comfortable being introduced to the new technology and pedagogy. Changes in teachers' ways of working may need to be supported by colleagues in their own school before they venture further afield. While outside experts were welcome participants in the school at this stage, once introduced to the technology and teaching possibilities, teachers still needed to gain a degree of personal and professional comfort before meeting colleagues from other schools.

- If the school location is important to student teachers then teacher educators must acknowledge and value the possible contributions from in-service teachers. Teacher educators should find ways to link the field to the teacher education coursework.

When faced with learning a new technology and examining pedagogy, science teachers prefer the school-based CoP. They remained grounded in the best interests of their students and their school department. When they were ready, they sought outside help which also provided significant support.

- Teacher educators/researchers need to acknowledge and map out existing communities of influence in which teachers work and live. They must discover how these communities can collectively help to build a more holistic student teacher support system. This - should lead to stronger support for pedagogical change.
- To do this, teacher educators/researchers need to be significantly involved in professional development initiatives in their school districts and departments of education. By spending time and energy with committees in these bodies they will know what professional development initiatives are currently in place. They may even have the opportunity to influence future t initiatives so that they reflect a holistic network of in-service and pre-service teacher requirements.

Balance between Curriculum Content Knowledge and Inquiry

Both teachers and students appear to value the acquisition of curriculum content knowledge first before engaging in student inquiry. Pre-service and in-service teachers, however, were not comfortable with transmission as the dominant pedagogy; they also valued student inquiry (aided by technology). It has been found that these teachers engage in an economic, cost/benefit analysis to guide their pedagogical choices. They ask themselves two questions: 1. Do I teach in student-owned ways of teaching and integrating technology like inquiry, which result in a high benefit for student engagement, but cost a great deal of time and do not cover all curriculum outcomes?; or 2. Do I use transmission pedagogies which may result in lower student engagement but have a low time cost and high number of curriculum outcomes reached? These teachers want to do what is best for their students and they also want to continue to collaboratively engage in the CoP to examine their teaching beliefs and balance their pedagogical economy.

- For teacher educators, the either-or scenario posed above should be acknowledged but must also be debunked. It may not be an either-or choice, re-service teachers should be supported as their students engage in forms of technology-supported inquiry which also result in a significant number of curriculum outcomes reached.

Data Logger Integration: Implications for Teacher Education

The integration of data loggers as an element in student inquiry appears not to have improved female's self-efficacy related science beliefs or improved attitudes like science anxiety. Females appear to want hands-on learning with data loggers even more than males. There are, however, significant barriers: self-confidence in ability to learn science, high science anxiety, and a sense that technology is not useful. It was also found that females wanted data logging experiences to be teacher-guided activities. As well, females, more than males appear to value laboratory experiences with data loggers as confirmatory activities, having already learned the concepts in the teacher-directed classroom.

- Pre-service teachers need to recognize that if female students are to be afforded more opportunities to discover the possible benefits of using data loggers in science then barriers, such as lack of self-confidence and science anxiety, need to be addressed. While more research needs to find ways to address these concerns, teacher educators may need to listen to female concerns regarding data logging integration. One possible way forward is to shift the masculine ways of doing science, including decontextualized activities and mechanistic views of nature and competition (Baker, 1998), toward more authentic ways of doing science. This may provide females with the opportunity to ask societally relevant science questions and thereby gain and keep their interest (Lightbody & Durndell, 1996).

Senior high students and teachers asserted that instrumentation is essential. While the technology itself should not be the focus of learning (Hennessy et al., 2005), learning how to use the technology itself is still crucial.

- Pre-service instruction should provide sufficient time and resources for teachers to learn how to use the technology itself first, before they even contemplate using it in a teaching context. To do this, along with the teacher educator's support, technology experts could be brought into class as guest lecturers to provide technical support on how to use the technologies.

From the data, it is apparent that senior high students value ownership over how and when to integrate technology. That is, both males and females want to use data loggers themselves, rather than watch teachers use them. This finding may also apply to the context of pre-service teacher instruction.

- Student-centered instruction, in this case pre-service teacher-centered instruction, where students significantly influence how curriculum outcomes will be reached, appears to have made a difference for CoP members (including pre-service teachers). Providing this sense of ownership to pre-service teachers may yield a greater sense of responsibility to the CoP as well as to their efforts in becoming new teachers.
- Much like senior high school students' desire for student-centered learning, implications for pre-service-centered instruction are likely. That is, pre-service teachers should be given ownership of how their particular curriculum goals can be reached by permitting them to choose coursework topics and teaching methods.

Ethical Concerns and Future Research Directions

Ethical Concerns for Doing Research with Your Own Pre-service Teachers

Evaluating your own teacher education program to improve course design does not require formal ethical approval. Gathering data from pre-service teachers and then reporting findings, however, does require this step. When conducting research in this way, university and college education departments and school boards will require ethical approval. Information letters and consent forms must be included. In the research reported here, ethical approval was provided for the gathering of data from pre-service teachers at the conclusion of the science methods course. In this way, pre-service students did not feel pressure to participate in the data collection. The school principals and science department heads had indicated their support before I approached the pre-service and in-service teachers.

In future research, I will collect data from students during the course. I will ask a faculty member, unconnected to my courses, to present and collect the information letter and consent form to my pre-service teachers. To help provide pre-service teacher's with a sense of freedom to refuse to participate without harm coming to them, the interviews will be conducted in an asynchronous, chat-like, online format. This format will less likely lead to the identification of the pre-service teacher, which is important while the teacher education course is being conducted. At the end of the course in-person interviews will be conducted.

Future Research Directions: *in situ* Teacher Education

Data from the CoP research suggest that the location and the acknowledgement of experiences from in-service teachers is important. In teacher education throughout North America, there is what could be called a division of labor in the pre-service teacher education. University and colleges teach pre-service courses in their institutions and the practice teaching takes place in schools. In this model, in-service teachers have little say regarding the teaching of university courses and teacher educators have relatively little influence on what happens to pre-service teachers in their placements. With this separation of experience it is not surprising that there is a separation of theory and practice in teacher education today.

School-based professional development experiences may enhance the possibility of change in in-service teacher practice. That is, when teacher education coursework is connected to the school it may provide in-service teachers with valuable professional development experiences. They too can potentially gain from building bridges between theory and practice.

With these potential benefits to be gained for pre-service and in-service teachers it seems apparent that more research needs to be done to further investigate the benefits for teacher education and the integration of technology. With this in mind, during the academic year 2008-2009, I have attempted build stronger links to schools. Six other teacher educators/researchers from across Canada are also engaged in similar linking projects.

In my linking project I attempted to address this theory-practice divide by moving my science methods classes from the university campus to a local high school. This coursework takes place before they begin their practicum with a cooperating (supervising) in-service teacher from the school. I have asked my students to do an assignment that brings them together with in-service teachers. The teachers suggested a lab activity that the pre-service teacher initially developed. They then collaborated in the construction of this activity, taught it in the science methods course (where their in-service teacher supervisors and I provided constructive feedback) and then taught it in the in-service teacher's class. I am presently collecting data on the effectiveness of presenting a university methods class in this way. Future research projects, which value in-service supervising teachers and their schools, and that take place in a school context, could provide the data to design stronger links between schools and faculties of education and to support sustained technology integration.

REFERENCES

Baggott LaVelle, L., McFarlane, A., & Brawn, R. (2003). Knowledge transformation through ICT in science education: A case study in teacher-driven curriculum development - case study 1. *British Journal of Educational Technology*, *32*(2), 183–189. doi:10.1111/1467-8535.00319

Baker, D. (1998). Equity issues in science education. In Fraser, B., & Tobin, K. (Eds.), *International handbook of science education* (pp. 869–895). Dordrecht, Netherlands: Kluwer Academic.

Barab, S., MaKinster, J., & Scheckler, R. (2003). Designing system dualities: Characterizing a web-supported professional development community. *The Information Society*, *19*(1), 237–256. doi:10.1080/01972240309466

Barab, S., Barnett, M., & Squire, K. (2002). Developing an empirical account of a community of practice: Characterizing the essential tensions. *Journal of the Learning Sciences, 11*(4), 489–542. doi:10.1207/S15327809JLS1104_3

Barton, R. (2004). Why use computers in practical science? In Barton, R. (Ed.), *Teaching secondary science with ICT* (pp. 27–39). Maidenhead, UK: Open University Press.

BECTA. (2005). The BECTA review: Evidence on the progress of ICT in education. *ICT in Schools Research and Evaluation Series.* Retrieved September, 2005, from http://www.becta.org.uk/page_documents/research/becta_review_feb05.pdf

Bereiter, C. (2005). Design research: The way forward. *Education Canada, 46*(1), 16–19.

Brandon, P. R., Taum, A. K. H., Ayala, C. C., Young, D. B., Gray, M. E., Speitel, T. T., et al. (2007). *Phase I study of fast implementation, outcomes, and scaling up: Final report.* Retrieved June 2007, from http://www.hawaii.edu/crdg/programs/pre/scup.html

Cox, M., Webb, M., Abbott, C., Blakeley, B., Beauchamp, T., & Rhodes, V. (2003). ICT and pedagogy: A review of the research literature. *ICT in Schools Research and Evaluation Series.* Retrieved September 2005, from http://www.becta.org.uk/page_documents/research/ict_pedagogy_summary.pdf

Cuban, L. (2001). *Oversold and underused: Computers in the classroom.* Cambridge, MA: Harvard University Press.

Davis, E., & Krajcik, J. (2005). Designing educative curriculum materials to promote teacher learning. *Educational Researcher, 34*(3), 3–14. doi:10.3102/0013189X034003003

Design-Based-Research-Collective. (2003). Design-based research: An emerging paradigm for educational inquiry. *Educational Researcher, 32*(1), 5–8. doi:10.3102/0013189X032001005

Dreon, O., & McDonald, A. S. P. (2006). *Using an online community of practice to foster inquiry as pedagogy amongst student teachers.* Paper presented at the Proceedings of the 7th International Conference on Learning Sciences: International Society of the Learning Sciences, Bloomington, Indiana.

Goodnough, K. (2004). *Learning in communities of practice: The science across the curriculum project.* Retrieved June, 2006, from http://www.mun.ca/educ/faculty/mwatch/fall05/goodnough.htm

Hassard, J., & Dias, M. (2000, May). *Experiences in a constructivist community of practice: An inquiry into TEEMS: A science teacher education program.* Paper presented at the Annual Meeting of the National Association for Research in Science Teaching, New Orleans, LA.

Hennessy, S., Ruthven, K., & Brindley, S. (2005). Teacher perspectives on integrating ICT into subject teaching: Commitment, constraints, caution, and change. *Journal of Curriculum Studies, 37*(2), 155–192. doi:10.1080/0022027032000276961

Inkpen, K. M., Ho-Ching, W., Kuederle, O., Scott, S., & Shoemaker, G. (1999). *'This is fun! We're all best friends and we're all playing': Supporting children's synchronous collaboration.* Paper presented at the Computer Support for Collaborative Learning Conference '99, Stanford, U.S.

Krajcik, J. S., & Blumenfeld, P. C. (1994). A collaborative model for helping middle grade science teachers learn project-based instruction. *The Elementary School Journal, 94*(5), 483. doi:10.1086/461779

Krathwohl, D. R. (1997). *Methods of educational and social science research: An integrated approach*. New York: Addison-Wesley.

Lave, J., & Wenger, E. (1991). *Situated learning: Legitimate peripheral participation*. Cambridge, UK: Cambridge University Press.

Lightbody, P., & Durndell, A. (1996). The masculine image of careers in science and technology: Fact or fantasy? *The British Journal of Educational Psychology*, *66*, 231–246.

MacDonald, R. J. (2008). Professional development for information communication technology integration: Identifying and supporting a community of practice through design-based research. *Journal of Research on Technology in Education*, *40*(3), 429–445.

MacDonald, R. J., & Larter, A. (2007, October). A professional learning community in senior high science: Data logging and learner-centeredness. In. *Proceedings of World Conference on E-Learning in Corporate, Government, Healthcare, and Higher Education*, *2007*, 1044–1049.

McFarlane, A., & Sakellariou, S. (2002). The role of ICT in science education. *Cambridge Journal of Education*, *32*(2), 219–232. doi:10.1080/03057640220147568

Niesz, T. (2007). Why teacher networks (can) work. *Phi Delta Kappan*, *88*(8), 605–610.

Olitksy, S. (2007). Promoting student engagement in science: Interaction rituals and the pursuit of a community of practice. *Journal of Research in Science Teaching*, *44*(1), 33–56. doi:10.1002/tea.20128

Passey, D., Rogers, C., Machell, J., McHugh, G., & Allaway, D. (2003). *The motivational effect of ICT on pupils*. Retrieved September 2005, from http://www.dfes.gov.uk/research/data/uploadfiles/rr523new.pdf

Roth, W.-M., & Lee, Y.-J. (2006). Computers and cognitive development at work. *Educational Media International*, *43*(4), 331–346. doi:10.1080/09523980600926325

Sandoval, W. A., & Bell, P. (2004). Design-based research methods for studying learning in context: Introduction. *Educational Psychologist*, *39*(4), 199–201. doi:10.1207/s15326985ep3904_1

Scardamalia, M. (2003). The knowledge society network (KSN): Toward an expert society for democratizing knowledge. *Journal of Distance Education*, *17*(3), 63–66.

Schlager, M. S., & Fusco, J. (2003). Teacher professional development, technology, and communities of practice: Are we putting the cart before the horse? *The Information Society*, *19*(3), 203. doi:10.1080/01972240309464

Strauss, A., & Corbin, J. (1998). *Basics of qualitative research: Techniques and procedures for developing grounded theory* (2nd ed.). Thousand Oaks, CA: Sage.

Tearle, P. (2003). ICT implementation: What makes the difference. *British Journal of Educational Technology*, *34*(5), 567–583. doi:10.1046/j.0007-1013.2003.00351.x

Wenger, E., McDermott, R., & Snyder, W. M. (2002). *Seven principles for cultivating communities of practice*. Retrieved June, 2006, from http://hbswk.hbs.edu/item.jhtml?id=2855&t=organizations

Wubbles, T. (2007). Do we know a community of practice when we see one? *Technology, Pedagogy and Education*, *16*(2), 225–233. doi:10.1080/14759390701406851

Zucker, A. A., Tinker, R., Staudt, C., Mansfield, A., & Metcalf, S. (2008). Learning science in grades 3-8 using probeware and computers: Findings from the TEEMSS II project. *Journal of Science Education and Technology*, *17*(1), 42–48. doi:10.1007/s10956-007-9086-y

Chapter 14
Fostering Educational Technology Integration in Science Teacher Education:
Issues of Teacher Identity Development

Brenda M. Capobianco
Purdue University, USA

James D. Lehman
Purdue University, USA

ABSTRACT

This chapter describes one science teacher educator's attempts to integrate various educational technologies in an elementary science methods course, her students' responses to her attempts, and the tensions that emerged. The science teacher educator employed teacher action research as a means of systematic, reflective inquiry to examine critically how preservice elementary school science teachers think about, use, and reflect on educational technologies and how their developing professional identities intersect with adoption of these technologies. Tensions emerged from a dichotomy between what methods students perceived as "traditional" science teaching and science teaching using technology. Resulting problems of practice included: expertise in/with science and negotiating a new curriculum, control in the classroom, content coverage, and support and sense of community. The authors conclude their chapter with implications and recommendations for future research related to the significant role educational technology can play in science teacher education and science teacher identity development.

INTRODUCTION

Although technology has proliferated in recent years, it has produced relatively little change in classroom practice. In this chapter, we suggest that teacher identity plays an important role in the adoption of educational technology. In our context, an elementary science methods course, we suggest that the use of educational technology challenges traditional images of an elementary school science teacher and science instructional ideologies. We briefly describe the attempts one science teacher educator made at integrating various forms of educational technology in an elementary science

DOI: 10.4018/978-1-61520-897-5.ch014

Copyright © 2010, IGI Global. Copying or distributing in print or electronic forms without written permission of IGI Global is prohibited.

education methods course over the course of two academic semesters and among 50 preservice elementary school science teachers. The science teacher educator's primary goal was to employ teacher action research as a means of systematic, reflective inquiry to examine critically the different ways preservice elementary school science teachers think about, use, and reflect on different educational technology applications and how their developing professional identities intersect with the adoption of these educational technologies.

The research questions that guided this study included the following:

1. What attempts did the science teacher educator make to integrate educational technologies in an elementary science education methods course?
2. What were students' responses to the teacher educator's attempts to integrate educational technologies?
3. What tensions did the science teacher educator and preservice science teachers confront while learning to use educational technologies in the science classroom?
4. How did preservice science teachers' formative professional identity encourage or discourage adoption of educational technology practices?

This study draws upon two strands of literature: 1) teacher identity and 2) the use of educational technologies in preservice teacher education. We briefly describe the relevant areas of literature here before describing the particular context and methods of the study.

Teacher Identity

Teacher professional identity has emerged as an area of research, particularly within the last decade or so (Beijaard, Meijer, & Verloop, 2004; Enyedy, Goldberg, & Welsh, 2006; Leuhmann, 2007; Olitsky, 2007). Our conception of identity draws from the work of Markus and Nurius (1986) and others in which researchers explore the conception of "possible selves." Possible selves represent individuals' ideas and beliefs about who they might become, who one hopes or expects to become, as well as who one fears becoming (Dunkel & Kerpelman, 2006; Markus & Nurius, 1986). This view aligns with Helms' perspective that the self comes not just from what a person does, or his/her affiliations, but also from what a person believes, values, and wants to become (Helms, 1998). Helms argues that while much has been done, for example, on teachers' understandings of the nature of science (Brickhouse, 1990; Lederman, 2007), the ways in which science teachers obtain a sense of personal or professional identity from their subject matter are not sufficiently considered. Volkmann and Anderson (1998) have argued that the development of professional identity is a complicated process that makes preparing and mentoring teachers difficult. Affiliation and loyalty to subject matter, such as science, is critical to teachers' formation of professional identity, and to this study. We acknowledge that while affiliation to subject matter helps foster a science teacher's sense of belonging to a community, it ironically creates barriers to adopting new classroom approaches and pedagogical strategies such as the use of educational technologies. Simply put, the integration of technology in the science classroom challenges traditional images of a science teacher and science instructional ideologies (Helms, 1998; Pedretti, 2003; Pedretti, Bencze, Hewitt, Romkey, & Jivraj, 2006; Shumba, 1999). This may create a barrier to the adoption of educational technologies in science teaching and learning.

Educational Technologies in Preservice Teacher Education

Computers and allied technologies have been influencing education for more than a quarter century, and in that time we have witnessed a shift from an early emphasis on teaching programming and using computers as tutors to a greater emphasis on the use of computers as tools to enhance learning in various subjects (Wentworth & Earle, 2003). Today, computers and the Internet have achieved nearly total penetration in U.S. schools (Market Data Retrieval, 2005; National Center for Education Statistics, 2003), yet the impact of educational technology still falls short of transformative changes predicted by proponents.

Various factors contribute to what is perceived as underutilization of educational technology in the classroom. Cuban (1986, 1993) argued that the organization and culture of schools and classrooms is resistant to technology innovation. Ertmer (1999) noted that even when first-order barriers to technology integration (e.g., equipment, time, training, support) are removed, second-order barriers to integration, those that are internal to the teacher such as attitudes and beliefs, still remain. Further, technology integration is challenging because it requires teachers to understand the complex interplay of content, pedagogy, and technology to develop what has been termed technological pedagogical content knowledge (TPCK) (Koehler & Mishra, 2005). As a result, teachers continue to grapple with how best to utilize educational technologies (Dexter, Anderson, & Becker, 1999; Pederson & Yerrick, 2000).

Until relatively recently, part of the problem has been that new teachers have felt ill-prepared to utilize technology in the classroom because little attention was given to technology integration in teacher preparation. In the 1990s, several national reports raised concerns about the lack of emphasis on technology integration in teacher preparation programs (Moursand & Bielfeldt, 1999; Office of Technology Assessment, 1995; Panel on Educational Technology, 1997). These reports criticized the limited use of technology in teacher education courses, an emphasis on teaching *about* technology rather than teaching *with* technology, and lack of faculty modeling of appropriate ways to integrate technology in teaching and learning.

However, things have begun to change. Between 1999 and 2001, the U.S. Department of Education's Preparing Tomorrow's Teachers to use Technology (PT3) program funded 466 grants for nearly $400 million dollars to build the nation's capacity to prepare technology-proficient educators (Carroll, 2005). The work described in this chapter was supported by a 2000 PT3 implementation grant that had as its goals to: (a) prepare pre-service teachers to demonstrate fundamental technology competencies, using technology as a tool for teaching and learning, personal productivity, communication, and reflection on their teaching; and (b) prepare teacher education faculty to teach preservice teachers in technology-rich environments, modeling approaches that future teachers could use themselves when teaching K-12 students (Lehman, Richardson, Malewski, & Phillion, 2005). The PT3 grant provided training and technical support to faculty members who integrated technology into their practice through a year-long mentoring and support program.

In order to learn to effectively use educational technologies in K-12 classrooms, prospective teachers must see it modeled by teacher educators. This, in turn, requires that teacher educators learn to integrate the use of technology into their own practice. In the domain of science teaching, Flick and Bell (2000) suggested that science teacher educators should introduce technology in the context of science content in ways that utilize unique capabilities of the technology, address worthwhile science with appropriate pedagogy, make scientific views more accessible, and develop students' understanding of the relationship between science and technology. The case study reported herein was an attempt by one science teacher educator to meaningfully integrate technology in these ways to model for her prospective teacher effective uses of technology in the classroom.

CONTEXT OF THE STUDY AND PARTICIPANTS

This study was conducted at a large, doctoral-degree granting university of approximately 38,000 students, nearly 2,000 of which are enrolled in undergraduate teacher education programs each year. The context of the study was an undergraduate elementary science methods course generally taken by preservice elementary teachers two semesters prior to student teaching. The methods course addressed a range of topics revolving around several key themes: how children learn science, how science is taught at the elementary level, and how children's science learning is assessed. The primary goal of each course instructional unit was to help students learn more about how to engage children in scientific inquiry. Supplementing class assignments were field-based experiences in a local elementary school where students incorporated elements of inquiry by interviewing children and teaching two independent lessons using productive questions and the learning cycle.

The mode of inquiry for this study was action research. Using Carr and Kemmis's (1986) model for systematic inquiry, the first author, a science teacher educator, created an action plan, enacted her plan, made observations, and reflected on those actions. Her plan included developing and implementing lessons that incorporated the use of various educational technology applications and tools including Excel, PowerPoint, digital cameras, and lab sensors. Because action research is a spiraling process (Capobianco, Horowitz, Lincoln, & Trimarch, 2004; Carr & Kemmis, 1986; McKernan, 1988), the science teacher educator cycled through her research several times in order to clarify her starting point and refine the educational technology applications and data collection methods that she used. This took place over the course of two semesters so that the results of her action research from the first semester (Spring / N=22 students) informed the actions she took in the next semester (Fall / N=28 students). Some of these actions included modifications to her lesson plans and data collection methods.

The second author, an educational technologist, served as the science teacher educator's critical friend or consultant. In this capacity, he listened and responded to her reflections, questions, and concerns she had about teaching and learning how to use technology in the science classroom. According to Northfield and Loughran (1997), the perspective of colleagues can be very valuable and enhance the processes of self-critical inquiry (e.g., data interpretation). These conversations provided opportunities for her to highlight particular events that otherwise would have remained insignificant or invisible to her personal development as a science teacher educator.

The research methods the science teacher educator employed included maintaining a research notebook, also referred to as "journal keeping" (Cochran-Smith & Lytle, 1993; Holly, 1989), and reviewing supporting documents. The data sources consisted of daily entries in a research notebook, teacher-created student feedback forms, a modified version of the Concerns-Based Adoption Model questionnaire (Hord, Rutherford, Huling-Austin, & Hall, 1987) referred to as the Stages of Concern Inventory (SoCI), and student work (i.e., class assignments). In addition, she recorded field notes based on her own classroom observations of students' engagement with each educational technology application. Additional documents, such as lesson plans and rubrics, were reviewed.

The analysis of all qualitative data (i.e. research notebook entries, student work, open-ended responses to feedback forms, and additional documents) entailed the use of grounded theory (Strauss & Corbin, 1990). Codes and categories were generated based on subsequent reviews of all the data sources and these were later negotiated, refined and developed by the authors. Preliminary results from qualitative data were then merged with results (e.g. median scores) from the feedback forms and SoCI to identify themes and frequencies of theme occurrences. Member checks with participants were conducted to ensure validity of the claims the researchers made.

INTEGRATING TECHNOLOGY ACTIVITIES

The science teacher educator developed a series of six different class activities that incorporated the use of common productivity software, such as Excel and PowerPoint, as well as hardware including digital cameras and laboratory probeware, electronic sensors (e.g., temperature probes) interfaced to a computer (Capobianco, 2007; Capobianco & Lehman, 2006) (See Table 1). She carefully reviewed existing lesson plans for each unit and generated alternative ways of teaching the lessons using technology to support students' understanding of inquiry. For example, temperature probeware allowed students to accurately collect, organize, and communicate data related to their investigations via tables and graphs. The software accompanying the sensors provided students the opportunity to create workbooks and final drafts of their lab work which they emailed to one another at the end of the lesson. Students could critique and analyze one another's workbooks for clarity, accuracy, and the formation of logical arguments concerning the relationships between their evidence and explanations.

When designing the integration of educational technologies in each class activity, the science teacher educator paid particular attention to three key factors: 1) the unit objectives in the methods curriculum; 2) the national standards for science as inquiry that applied to each unit (see NRC, 1996, p. 121-123 for Grades K-4 and p. 143-148 for Grades 5-8); and 3) the technologies that were available and appropriate for fostering inquiry-based skills. Examples of these activities included digital journaling for young learners through the use of digital cameras; fair test investigations using temperature, pH, and cardio probeware; and PowerPoint for disseminating the results of lab investigations (see Capobianco, 2007 for more details).

Table 1. Overview of course ET applications

Unit of study in methods course curriculum	Activity	ET application	Product
1. Introduction to process skills	Determine the distribution of color in candy	Excel PowerPoint	PowerPoint presentation
2. Engaging in scientific inquiry	Design and conduct an investigation that determines the effect of SUV's on traffic	Excel Digital cameras PowerPoint	PowerPoint presentation
3. Learning to use laboratory probes	Examining the temperature of our hands (Extremity Remedy)	Lab probes	Mini-report with data table
4. Exploring children's science learning through productive questioning and journaling	Record responses to productive questions while engaging in an inquiry-based activity (e.g. Batteries & Bulbs Activity)	Digital cameras PowerPoint	PowerPoint presentation with digital photos
5. Challenging students' misconceptions	Determine the relationship between heat and temperature on making ice cream	Lab probes & software Excel	Written lab report
6. Designing a fair test investigation	Design and conduct a fair test investigation using lab probes (e.g. Cold Pack Lab)	Lab probes & software	Written lab report

WHAT THE DATA REVEALED

We begin our presentation of the results by considering students' responses to the student feedback forms and the SoCI, in an effort to determine how students thought about and used the different educational technology applications. In previous studies, we determined that methods students demonstrated relatively high and consistent levels of interest in and ability to engage in inquiry using technology (see Capobianco, 2007; Capobianco & Lehman, 2006). Students indicated relatively high interest in and perceptions of usefulness for the majority of applications. Additionally, students reported relatively high interest in integrating more than half of the educational technology applications within their own future practice. These results were encouraging,

Several trends were apparent in the pre- and post-SoCI results. On the pre-administration of the SoCI, students reported being curious about how technology can be used by science learners. Additional responses suggested that the methods students wanted practical suggestions on how to use technology for specific purposes. Students reported an overwhelming interest to know how to integrate educational technology in their respective classroom practice. Results from the post-administration of the SoCI indicated a progression from personal, task-oriented concerns to more collaborative, impact-oriented concerns. Almost 70% of the students on the post-SoCI indicated that they had some ideas and strategies about how to integrate educational technology in the science classroom effectively and productively. Interestingly, about 25% of the students reported still having personal and task-oriented concerns about using educational technology in the science classroom, which is not surprising given the fact that these students were still in the early stages of thinking about the adoption of educational technologies. Based on these results, we revisited students' reflections and responses and paid particular attention to the conflicts, tensions, and problems students reported. What follows is an overview of several of their concerns.

Problems of Practice

Despite the fact that the majority of students expressed increased confidence, comfort, and interest in the use of educational technology in science teaching as a result of their experiences in this course, there was a significant group of students who expressed decreased likelihood of integrating educational technology within their own prospective practice. Particular tensions or problems of practice consistently emerged across students' responses to open-ended responses in the feedback forms, SoCI, class discussions, and journal entries. These tensions included issues related to: 1) expertise in/with science and negotiating a new curriculum; 2) control in the classroom; 3) covering the content; and 4) support and sense of community. What follows is an overview of each of these issues.

Becoming a Science Authority and Negotiating a New Curriculum

One of the more pervasive themes to emerge concerned students' feelings that they did not know enough science to teach through inquiry using technology. On multiple occasions, students wrote comments such as, "I like using the technology but I am more concerned about knowing the science that needs to be taught," "I'm worried that I lack understanding of the science content," "The first thing I need to consider is not so much teaching science through technology, it is whether or not I really know enough science" (Journal entries, Spring & Fall, 2003). The students' concerns, like those of most novice science educators, focused on their need to know the science content and pedagogy, whereas the science teacher educator's personal concerns focused primarily on pedagogy associated with using technology. In her research notebook, she noted, "I am finding teaching this way demanding, but exciting. I find myself more mindful of their interactions with the technology, observing carefully how they use it and what questions they ask. I grapple with whether or not I know enough technology to answer their questions" (Journal entry, Spring, 2003). The educational technologist and science teacher educator quickly began to observe a pattern. They learned that the science teacher educator's anxiety for teaching inquiry through the use of technology paralleled her students' concerns for teaching science content and using technology in the science classroom. Although their anxieties did not exactly mirror one another, they did, in fact, inform the needs and concerns we have as educators. Though stressful and disconcerting at times, their collective reflections empowered the students and the science teacher educator to reveal internal processes and made them vulnerable to learning how to teach.

When the science teacher educator shared her reflections with educational technologist, he raised additional questions such as: Is it legitimate *not* to start with using technology and to focus on teaching scientific inquiry first then introduce the use of the technology? Should using technology in the science classroom be taught as a discrete enterprise or an integrated endeavor? Are there alternative solutions to integrating technology in an elementary teacher preparation program that prepares pre-service teachers to construct the technical, content, and practical knowledge necessary to teach science effectively? How can science teacher educators help their students balance content, pedagogy, and technological issues intrinsic in science teaching?

According to Pederson and Yerrick (2000), integrating technology in science content instruction is not only important but imperative. "Teacher education programs bear a large part of the responsibility to rear teachers prepared to use technology…in line with current science education visions" (Pederson & Yerrick, 2000, p. 145). They further state that science teacher educators need increased support, instruction, knowledge, and resources to aid them in this endeavor. In the project described here, the science teacher educator did receive the necessary support (including professional development, financial support for hardware/software, and technical support), made the investment, and slowly developed the novel expertise.

Underpinning the students' anxieties for teaching science were echoes of teaching science in a conventional way. Although they respected the science teacher educator's attempts to integrate educational technologies and model "expert" science teaching, problems of practice were plentiful, and resistance to educational technology surfaced. They worried that they would not have enough content knowledge or expertise to effectively plan and implement an educational technology approach, while covering required curriculum content. Embracing an educational technology perspective shifts the science teacher identity from that of expert in one particular subject area to that of affiliation and comfort with multiple disciplines. In other words, it shifts from segregation to integration (Pedretti, Bencze, Hewitt, Romkey, & Jivraj, 2006).

Maintaining Control and Establishing Autonomy

Additional student responses focused on concerns about negotiating a new curriculum and being capable of mastering this curriculum while simultaneously integrating different applications of educational technology. This was supplemented by students' persistent concern with "letting go" and allowing students to have more responsibility using technology without "losing control of the classroom" (Journal entries, Spring, 2003). Although methods students were introduced to the notion and practice of making their lessons more student-directed and open-ended when using educational technology, they frequently expressed the belief that this approach was "different" than the usual practice of science teachers and potentially problematic. As Wallace and Louden (1992) wrote, experimenting with new ways of teaching science often leads to "questioning strongly held values about content and control" (p. 513), which, in turn, we argue raise important questions about science teacher identity.

Getting through all of the Content

Integrating educational technology in the science classroom demands a science curriculum rich with inquiry-based experiences, access to the appropriate technologies, and teacher knowledge and expertise (Pederson & Yerrick, 2000). For beginning teachers, the problem of practice emerges as they begin to envision an educational technology orientation in action. On several occasions, the methods students described the integration of educational technology in the science classroom as "less content driven and more skills-based" (Feedback forms, Spring & Fall 2003), and, therefore, issues of content coverage loomed large. Additionally, students shared concerns about whether or not they could "introduce technology when I still have to get my students ready for [name of statewide test]," "I'm worried that I won't have the equipment or money to use technology in my classroom," and "It seems like using technology would take a lot of time away from my curriculum" (Journal entries, Fall 2003). Simply put, preservice teachers are concerned about covering content given the limitations imposed by high stakes testing, resources, and time. Furthermore, an elementary school teacher must be a "jack of all trades" who is required to master multiple disciplines and make sure all students are proficient across subject areas. Given these powerful forces, it is not surprising that, although educational technology has gained considerable recognition and enjoyed some successes, it has made limited strides in general classroom practice and is often marginalized in the curriculum.

Feeling a Sense of Belonging to the Science Teacher Community

Science teachers' sense of professional identity develops, in part, from their subject matter loyalty and affiliation. Affiliation to subject matter helps foster a teacher's sense of belonging to a community (Little, 1993). The methods students in this study consistently expressed concern regarding support (or lack of support) from colleagues, administrators, and/or parents as well as a lack of access to the resources necessary to enact various educational technologies in the classroom. They did not want to find themselves "outside" the community and/or without the tools necessary to become a member of the science teacher community of practice. The feeling that they might be the "only one" in the school using educational technology prompted strong responses of feeling isolated and potentially alienated. Finally, some prospective teachers wrote about disinterest or even resistance from students, and the particular problems that might pose. Again, these reactions from the methods students reinforced the idea that technology integration in elementary school science is not a "normal" pattern of practice (Wallace & Louden, 1992) or the usual experience of students in elementary school science.

CONCLUSION

In this chapter, we described how one teacher educator integrated educational technologies into her methods course. Furthermore, we described the steps we took to gather feedback from prospective teachers about how they think, use, and reflect on educational technology in the service of teaching elementary science. Our study reported on several tensions identified by preservice elementary school teachers with regard to their interest and motivation towards implementing educational technology in their prospective practice. These tensions included questions about their expertise in/with the content of science and how to negotiate a new curriculum; maintaining control in the classroom; getting through all of the content (i.e. content coverage in light of high stakes testing, etc.); and seeking out support while establishing a sense of community with other science educators. These tensions shed light on the complexities of integrating educational technology in the elementary classroom, and the problems of practice they pose for preservice teachers. We believe these tensions are due in large part to preservice teachers' emerging teacher identity. In other words, an orientation toward integrating educational technology presents a particular image of teaching in a particular content domain, in this case science, and a particular set of pedagogical challenges that are different from normal patterns of practice.

Volkmann and Anderson (1998) noted that the formation of a science teacher's professional identity is a complex process that creates difficulties for those seeking to prepare and mentor teachers. Teacher professional development programs are often compartmentalized, with prospective teachers learning about educational technology in one course and science education in another. Yet, teachers' identities form from the entirety of their experiences, which suggests it is important for teacher preparation programs to provide opportunities for the sorts of integrated experiences described in this study. These experiences can provide opportunities for dialogue about teaching, While similarities may exist between the perceptions of pre-service teachers and those of teacher educators, as in the parallels between the teacher educator's anxiety about teaching with technology and those of her students about learning science and using technology in this study, each individual forms a unique identity. So, these contexts should be used to help prospective teachers to confront and reflect upon the tensions that arise in learning how to teach.

Consideration must be given to more effectively integrating educational technology in our teacher preparation programs. Teacher educators need to address students' resistance to using educational technology, and what may be perceived as alternative or add-on practices, and help them to understand how these practices can be fundamentally productive, practical, and transformative approaches toward improving student learning. We propose cultivating, over the course of a preservice teacher's preparation program, a teacher identity that is inclusive of the norms and practices of technology and the content discipline. We propose that teacher educators consider the following recommendations for teacher education practice and implications for future research related to the significant role educational technology can play in teacher education and teacher identity development.

Informed by the tensions that emerged from the methods students' experiences, we recommend the following:

- Integrate educational technologies across teacher preparation programs so that preservice teachers see it modeled in the service of content learning and not in isolation.
- Provide space for preservice students to dialogue and reflect on the images, beliefs, and ideologies they associate with using educational technology in the classroom. By doing so, students may become more cognizant of, and conversant with, the ideologies they adopt. As a result, we hope that preservice teachers will make rational and informed choices about their prospective practice that include effective utilization of educational technology.
- Provide preservice teachers with opportunities to see examples of effective practice involving the use of educational technology in the service of teaching and learning of content. In order to consider adoption of educational technology, prospective teachers must see good examples of its use in order to envision how they might use it themselves (Ertmer, 2005).

- Provide preservice teachers with the space they need to explore their concerns, problems, and conflicts with using educational technology applications.
- Assist preservice teachers in the development of content knowledge, pedagogical content knowledge, and technological pedagogical content knowledge (TPCK) (Koehler, & Mishra, 2005) which seems critical to preservice teachers' self-efficacy and prospective practice.
- Engage preservice teachers in authentic field experiences so they can transfer what they learn in their methods class into the classroom setting.
- Employ self-critical, systematic reflective writing as a means through which preservice teachers can chronicle, highlight, and make meaning of the myriad concerns, issues, and conflicts they experience. Through ongoing reflections, preservice teachers may build not only the confidence, expertise, and comfort necessary to become effective teachers but also the professional knowledge necessary to master teaching (Abell, Bryan, & Anderson, 1998; Schon, 1987).

As we continue to explore preservice elementary science teachers' experiences with educational technology applications, other questions emerge. For example, what is the relationship between beginning teachers' beliefs about integrating educational technology in the classroom and their subsequent practice? How does a teachers' professional identity change over time? In what ways can incorporating educational technology in the elementary classroom help teachers re-shape their professional identities as practicing educators? We cannot say, with any certainty, what will happen in practice during the first years of teaching for this group of methods students. A longitudinal study would be required. However, we hope that in the context of a multi-year teacher preparation program we can encourage beginning elementary school teachers to reflect on what it means to be a teacher, challenge conventional notions of teaching and technology use, and bring educational technology into the mainstream.

REFERENCES

Abell, S., Bryan, L., & Anderson, M. (1998). Investigating preservice elementary science teacher reflective thinking using integrated media case-based instruction in elementary science teacher preparation. *Science Education*, *6*(4), 491–510. doi:10.1002/(SICI)1098-237X(199807)82:4<491::AID-SCE5>3.0.CO;2-6

Beijaard, D., Meijer, P. C., & Verloop, N. (2004). Reconsidering research on teachers' professional identity. *Teaching and Teacher Education*, *20*, 107–128. doi:10.1016/j.tate.2003.07.001

Brickhouse, N. (1990). Teachers' beliefs about the nature of science and their relationship to classroom practice. *Journal of Teacher Education*, *41*, 52–62. doi:10.1177/002248719004100307

Capobianco, B. M. (2007). A self-study of the role of technology in promoting reflection and inquiry-based science teaching. *Journal of Science Teacher Education*, *18*(2), 271–296. doi:10.1007/s10972-007-9041-z

Capobianco, B. M., Horowitz, R., Canuel-Browne, D., & Trimarchi, R. (2004). Action research for teachers: Understanding the steps for developing and implementing productive action plans. *Science Teacher (Normal, Ill.)*, *71*(3), 48–53.

Capobianco, B. M., & Lehman, J. D. (2006). Integrating technology to foster inquiry in an elementary science methods course: An action research study of one teacher educator's initiatives in a PT3 project. *Journal of Computers in Mathematics and Science Teaching*, *25*(2), 123–146.

Carr, W., & Kemmis, S. (1986). *Becoming critical: Education, knowledge, and action research.* London: Falmer Press.

Carroll, T. (2005). Forward. In Rhine, S., & Bailey, M. (Eds.), *Integrated technologies, innovative learning: Lessons from the PT3 program.* Eugene, OR: International Society for Technology in Education.

Cochran-Smith, M., & Lytle, S. L. (1993). *Inside/Outside: Teacher research and knowledge.* New York: Teachers College Press.

Cuban, L. (1986). *Teachers and machines.* New York: Teachers College Press.

Cuban, L. (1993). Computers meet classroom: Classroom wins. *Teachers College Record, 95,* 185–210.

Dexter, S. L., Anderson, R. E., & Becker, H. J. (1999). Teachers' views of computers as catalysts for changes in their teaching practice. *Journal of Research on Computing in Education, 31,* 221–238.

Dunkel, C., & Kerpelman, J. (Eds.). (2006). *Possible selves: Theory, research and applications.* New York: Nova Science Publishers, Inc.

Enyedy, N., Goldberg, & Welsh, K. (2006). Complex dilemmas of identity and practice. *Science Education, 90*(1), 68–93. doi:10.1002/sce.20096

Ertmer, P. A. (1999). Addressing first- and second-order barriers to change: Strategies for technology integration. *Educational Technology Research and Development, 47*(4), 47–61. doi:10.1007/BF02299597

Ertmer, P. A. (2005). Teacher pedagogical beliefs: The final frontier in our quest for technology integration? *Educational Technology Research and Development, 53*(4), 25–39. doi:10.1007/BF02504683

Flick, L., & Bell, R. (2000). Preparing tomorrow's science teachers to use technology: Guidelines for science educators. *Contemporary Issues in Technology & Teacher Education, 1*(1), 39–60.

Helms, J. (1998). Science and me: Subject matter and identity in secondary science teachers. *Journal of Research in Science Teaching, 35*(7), 811–834. doi:10.1002/(SICI)1098-2736(199809)35:7<811::AID-TEA9>3.0.CO;2-O

Holly, M. (1989). Reflective writing and the spirit of inquiry. *Cambridge Journal of Education, 19*(1), 71–80. doi:10.1080/0305764890190109

Hord, S. M., Rutherford, W. L., Huling-Austin, L., & Hall, G. E. (1987). *Taking charge of change.* Alexandria, VA: ASCD Publications.

Koehler, M. J., & Mishra, P. (2005). What happens when teachers design educational technology? The development of technological pedagogical content knowledge. *Journal of Educational Computing Research, 32*(2), 131–152. doi:10.2190/0EW7-01WB-BKHL-QDYV

Lederman, N. (2007). Nature of science: Past, present, and future. In Abell, S. K., & Lederman, N. G. (Eds.), *Handbook of research on science education* (pp. 831–879). Mahwah, NJ: Lawrence Erlbaum Associates.

Lehman, J. D., Richardson, J., Malewski, E., & Phillion, J. (2005). Technology connections in teacher education: Lessons from faculty development, electronic portfolios, and virtual field experiences involving distant locations. In Rhine, S., & Bailey, M. (Eds.), *Integrated technologies, innovative learning: Insights from the PT3 program* (pp. 129–141). Eugene, OR: International Society for Technology in Education.

Leuhmann, A. (2007). Identity development as a lens to science teacher preparation. *Science Education, 91*(5), 822–839. doi:10.1002/sce.20209

Little, J. W. (1993). Professional community in comprehensive high schools: The two worlds of academic and vocational teachers. In Little, J. W., & McLaughlin, M. W. (Eds.), *Teachers' work: Individuals, colleagues, and contexts*. New York: Teachers College Press.

Market Data Retrieval. (2005). The K-12 [Shelton, CT: Author.]. *Technology Review*, 2004–2005.

Markus, H., & Nurius, P. (1986, September). Possible selves. *The American Psychologist*, *41*(9), 954–969. doi:10.1037/0003-066X.41.9.954

McKernan, J. (1988). The countenance of curriculum action research: Traditional, collaborative, and emancipatory-critical conceptions. *Journal of Curriculum and Supervision*, *3*(3), 173–200.

Moursand, D., & Bielefeldt, T. (1999). *Will new teachers be prepared to teach in a digital age?* Research study by the International Society for Technology in Education, commissioned by the Milken Exchange on Educational Technology. Milken Exchange on Educational Technology. Retrieved March 16, 2009, from http://www.mff.org/pubs/ME154.pdf

National Center for Education Statistics. (2003, October). *Internet access in U.S. public schools and classrooms: 1994–2002* (Report No. NCES 2004-011). Washington, DC: U.S. Department of Education.

National Research Council. (1996). *National Science Education Standards*. Washington, DC: National Academy Press.

Northfield, J., & Loughran, J. (1997). *The nature of knowledge development in self-study practice*. A paper presented at the annual meeting of the American Educational Research Association, Chicago, IL, March 24-28, 1997.

Office of Technology Assessment. (1995, April). *Teachers and technology: Making the connection* (Report No. OTA-EHR-616). Washington, DC: U.S. Congress, Office of Technology Assessment.

Otliksy, S. (2007). Facilitating identity formation, group membership, and learning in science classrooms: What can be learned from out-of-field teaching in an urban school? *Science Education*, *91*(2), 201–221. doi:10.1002/sce.20182

Panel on Educational Technology. (1997, March). *Report to the President on the use of technology to strengthen K-12 education in the United States*. Washington, DC: President's Committee of Advisors on Science and Technology.

Pedersen, J. E., & Yerrick, R. K. (2000). Technology in science teacher education: Survey of current uses and desired knowledge among science educators. *Journal of Science Teacher Education*, *11*(2), 131–153. doi:10.1023/A:1009468808876

Pedretti, E. (2003). Teaching science, technology, society and environment (STSE) education: Preservice teachers' philosophical and pedagogical landscapes. In Zeidler, D. (Ed.), *The role of moral reasoning and socioscientific discourse in science education* (pp. 219–239). Dortecht, The Netherlands: Kluwer.

Pedretti, E., Bencze, L., Hewitt, J., Romkey, L., & Jivraj, A. (2006). Promoting issues-based STSE perspectives in science teacher education: Problems of identity and ideology. *Science and Education*, *17*, 941–960. doi:10.1007/s11191-006-9060-8

Schon, D. A. (1987). *Educating the reflective practitioner*. San Francisco: Jossey-Bass.

Shumba, O. (1999). Relationship between secondary science teachers' orientation to traditional culture and beliefs concerning science instructional ideology. *Journal of Research in Science Teaching*, *36*(3), 333–355. doi:10.1002/(SICI)1098-2736(199903)36:3<333::AID-TEA7>3.0.CO;2-Z

Strauss, A., & Corbin, J. (1990). *Basics of qualitative research: Grounded theory procedures and techniques*. Newbury Park, CA: Sage Publications.

Volkmann, M. J., & Anderson, M. A. (1998). Creating professional identity: Dilemmas and metaphors of a first-year chemistry teacher. *Science Education*, *82*(3), 293–310. doi:10.1002/(SICI)1098-237X(199806)82:3<293::AID-SCE1>3.0.CO;2-7

Wallace, J., & Louden, W. (1992). Science teaching and teachers' knowledge: Prospects for reform of elementary classrooms. *Science Education*, *76*(5), 507–521. doi:10.1002/sce.3730760505

Wentworth, N., & Earle, R. (2003). Trends in computer uses as reported in *Computers in Schools*. *Computers in the Schools*, *20*(1/2), 77–90. doi:10.1300/J025v20n01_06

Chapter 15
Pre-Service Elementary Teachers' Evaluations of Technology Tools for Mathematical Learning:
A Reflective Model

Christopher J. Johnston
George Mason University, USA

ABSTRACT

Pre-service elementary teachers are faced with numerous technology tools which can be incorporated into their mathematics lesson plans. However, these teachers may not be experienced in evaluating technology tools for mathematical learning prior to using them. This chapter presents a reflective model for mathematics teacher educators. In a three-part activity, pre-service elementary teachers identify their criteria for evaluating technology tools, evaluate several technology tools according to their own criteria, and make recommendations for or against those technology tools. As pre-service elementary teachers reflect upon the criteria they feel are essential for evaluating technology tools, they begin to identify the specific affordances and limitations of the technology tools. This chapter describes this three-part activity by placing it within the context of a model for mathematics teacher education.

INTRODUCTION

Pre-service elementary teachers have a wealth of technology tools available to them for use in mathematics instruction. However, the ways in which pre-service elementary teachers use technology depend upon their own personal beliefs and exposure to technology tools in their methods courses. Pre-service elementary teachers need to become good consumers of the technology resources available to them. This chapter offers mathematics teacher educators a framework for developing pre-service elementary teachers' skills in evaluating technology tools for mathematical learning. Research indicates that pre-service elementary teachers who evaluate technology tools and consider their unique affordances begin to focus on student learning when designing their own lessons. This chapter has been designed to assist mathematics teacher educators

DOI: 10.4018/978-1-61520-897-5.ch015

Copyright © 2010, IGI Global. Copying or distributing in print or electronic forms without written permission of IGI Global is prohibited.

who choose to incorporate reflective activities for their pre-service elementary teachers in the context of evaluating technology tools.

This chapter is the result of work done by the author with a group of pre-service elementary teachers during a required semester-long mathematics methods course. The author has developed an activity for pre-service elementary teachers in which they evaluate technology tools for mathematical learning. In the process of evaluating technology tools, pre-service elementary teachers consider their criteria for evaluation and reflect upon the specific affordances and limitations of the technology tools.

The conceptual framework guiding this chapter is displayed in Figure 1. Note that the center of the framework corresponds to one goal of mathematics teacher education, which is to develop teachers' Technology, Pedagogy, And Content Knowledge (TPACK). TPACK for mathematics is defined as: "the intersection of the knowledge of mathematics with the knowledge of technology with the knowledge of teaching and learning" (Niess, Lee, Sadri, & Suharwoto, 2006, p.1). In other words, TPACK is knowing how to teach mathematics when technology is integrated into the curriculum.

Surrounding the center of the conceptual framework are three major elements of a technology-enriched pre-service elementary math methods course, which will be discussed in this chapter: Technology Tools Available, Guidelines for Appropriate Uses of Technology in Mathematics Education, and Criteria for Evaluating Technology Tools. The author maintains that these three elements should be in place in methods coursework before pre-service elementary teachers begin creating lesson plans for mathematics which incorporate the use of technology.

Specifically, the objectives of this chapter are as follows. This chapter will:

Figure 1. Author's conceptual framework

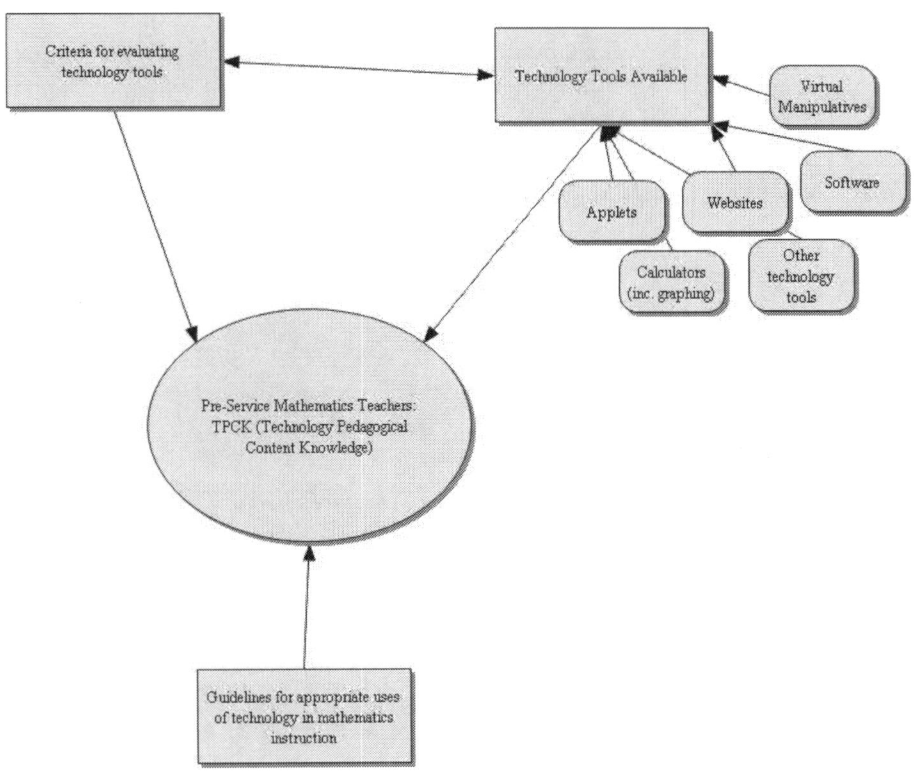

- Discuss a model of elementary mathematics methods coursework, with respect to technology, as supported by the literature;
- Identify the three critical elements of elementary mathematics methods coursework which need to be in place before pre-service elementary teachers can begin planning lessons;
- Describe, in detail, a reflective activity for use with pre-service elementary teachers in their methods coursework;
- Describe and evaluate five technology tools, which support each of the NCTM Content Standards; and
- Discuss future research directions and suggestions for other mathematics teacher educators.

BACKGROUND

Role of Technology in Mathematics Education

The National Council of Teachers of Mathematics recognizes the importance of technology in mathematics education. The Technology Principle, as set forth by the National Council of Teachers of Mathematics (2000) includes three secondary principles, which state that:

- Technology enhances mathematical learning.
- Technology supports effective mathematics teaching.
- Technology influences what mathematics is taught (p.25-26).

Similar professional organizations, including the Association of Mathematics Teacher Educators, support the appropriate use of technology in mathematics education (2006). In their position statement, they note the following desired skills of mathematics teachers upon completion of their teacher preparation programs. Teachers:

- demonstrate flexibility with high-quality and creative instructional techniques, both with and without technology, to help students explore and learn mathematics, develop mathematical thinking and communication abilities, and solve complex real-world problems;
- understand, by reflecting on how technology affords and constrains student actions and thoughts, when and how use of technology can advance learning and critical thinking, and when it can hinder the mathematical development;
- efficiently troubleshoot technology difficulties in both student and teacher use; and
- incorporate a variety of assessment techniques, including the use of technology to evaluate students' understanding of important mathematical concepts (p. 2).

This chapter specifically addresses the second bullet point of this position statement.

Pre-service elementary teachers are often introduced to various technology tools in their content and methods courses. Simply giving pre-service elementary teachers technology without considering the implications of the technology will not, in itself, increase student learning. Pre-service elementary teachers must have experiences which enable them to integrate technology into their mathematics lessons in such a way that the focus is on the mathematics, not the technology.

Technology Tools Available to Teachers

There are various classification systems in the literature. One such classification system was identified by Kurz, Middleton, and Yanik (2005), who developed a taxonomy of software within mathematics education. The taxonomy can be expanded to almost any form of technology, not just software. The five categories are:

- Review and practice tool
- General tool
- Specific tool
- Environments tool
- Communication tool

Each of these categories is explained in further detail below. While there are numerous taxonomies available in the literature, this particular taxonomy was selected for two reasons. First, it is specific to technology tools for mathematical learning. Second, it is appropriate for use by pre-service and beginning elementary teachers when classifying and exploring various technology tools in their mathematics methods coursework.

Review and practice tool. This type of software is used by students to review previously learned material; no new concepts are introduced. Students are drilled on specific skills in a particular content area, such as mathematics. Kurz, Middleton, and Yanik (2004) noted that this is a common type of technology used by mathematics teachers. This technology has been present in the classrooms for many years, so most teachers are familiar with this type of tool. Pre-service elementary teachers have, in the author's experience, traditionally used this type of tool most often, as compared to the other kinds available to them.

General tool. When the software can be used for various mathematics topics, it can be classified as general. It can be used across grade levels and for different applications. The teacher must develop the lesson to ensure that the technology is used to support the learning objectives of the lesson. Examples of this type of technology would include spreadsheets. Spreadsheets, while originally designed for business applications, have made their way into the classroom.

Specific tool. A specific tool is used to teach and/or learn one specific topic or skill. In this category, the software or technology focuses on a new concept or skill, unlike review and practice tools, which do not introduce new ideas. Examples of this type of technology include virtual manipulatives and applets, which can be used to explore new concepts or skills. Specific tools can also be classified as representations, as students learn new material through various representations (such as those afforded by virtual manipulatives.) There are two primary sources of virtual manipulatives: the National Library of Virtual Manipulatives, and Illuminations®, a project of the National Council of Teachers of Mathematics.

Environments tool. In this model, different types of learning in several subject areas are combined. Students investigate and explore in a new environment, one which is not possible in a typical classroom. Examples include online simulations, microworlds, and applications such as Star Logo®.

Communication tool. Students share information with other students, their teacher, as well as (potentially) students and teachers in other classrooms around the world. Students develop mathematical understanding as they participate in discourse. These tools may not be math specific and could potentially be used in all content areas. Examples of communication tools include chat and asynchronous discussion boards, such as those features found on Blackboard® (which is a course management tool.)

As new technologies emerge, this classification schema may need to be modified. The examples provided are not an exhaustive list; however, they give the reader a general sense of the technology tools available to teachers.

Guidelines for Appropriate Uses of Technology in Mathematics Education

Five guidelines for appropriate uses of technology were identified by Garofalo, Drier, Harper, Timmerman, and Shockey (2000) and are specific to mathematics education:

- Introduce technology in context
- Address worthwhile mathematics with appropriate pedagogy
- Take advantage of technology
- Connect mathematics topics
- Incorporate multiple representations (p. 67).

These five guidelines are explained in further detail below, and examples are given for each of the guidelines. These guidelines should be the focal point of any teacher preparation program for mathematics teachers. Other guidelines for general technology integration exist in the literature, but these are specific to mathematics education, and for that reason, they have been selected for the framework presented in this chapter.

Introduce Technology in Context

Technology should be used to support mathematical learning. Valuable classroom time should not be devoted to learning a technology tool just for the sake of using it. When planning for instruction, teachers should identify the curricular objective first, and then they should find a technology tool (if appropriate) which will support that curricular objective. For example, a pre-service teacher may have a goal for students to compare fractions. Thus, that teacher may select a fraction virtual manipulative which will allow students to explore fractions by comparing them.

Address Worthwhile Mathematics with Appropriate Pedagogy

Mathematics content should not be taught simply because technology allows it; rather, worthwhile mathematics should be taught because it meets the curricular goals and needs of the students. Further, the technology tool should support learning, not distract the student from important mathematical content. For example, a pre-service teacher may wish to use a spreadsheet to develop algebraic thinking and explore the concepts of formulas. However, if the students are so concerned with the formatting of the cells, they may miss the important mathematical content of the lesson.

Take Advantage of Technology

Technology tools offer numerous affordances, including multiple representations. For example, students traditionally view models of fractions as circular. However, technology can allow students to explore and create other fraction models. Further, technology tools allow students to explore fractions beyond twelfths typically seen in textbooks and physical manipulatives. Or students can use virtual manipulatives which allow them to rotate 2-D and 3-D objects for developing geometric thinking.

Connect Mathematics Topics

Technology can be used to help students connect mathematical ideas they have already studied. In a segmented curriculum, topics are taught in isolation with no connections to prior learning. For example, a virtual manipulative of a geoboard is useful because it can connect both geometric and measurement topics, such as area, perimeter, congruency, similarity, and other key concepts.

Incorporate Multiple Representations

Technology can be used to assist students as they make connections between verbal, graphical, numerical, and algebraic representations. Technology can both increase the number of representations available to students, as well as enhance the quality of these representations. The graphing calculator is an example of a technology tool which allows students to make connections between numeric, algebraic, and graphic representations.

Evaluation of Technology Tools for Mathematical Learning

Before pre-service elementary teachers can integrate technology into their own lesson plans, they must have opportunities to explore and evaluate technology tools for mathematical learning. In doing so, pre-service elementary teachers have the opportunity to identify the affordances and limitations of technology tools for mathematical learning.

Battey, Kafai, and Franke (2005) studied pre-service elementary teachers' criteria for evaluating and using mathematical software. They found that most pre-service elementary teachers focused on surface features, such as clear directions, rather than focusing on the content or pedagogical issues. Learning was important, but statements made by the pre-service elementary teachers indicated a concern for general learning, rather than learning important mathematical content. Finally, motivation was a key factor when selecting mathematical software. Pre-service elementary teachers were concerned about engaging and motivating software. This is not surprising, considering pre-service elementary teachers would feel more comfortable evaluating software on the basis of the engagement, motivation, and clear directions. However, as they develop their pedagogical content knowledge, it is expected that pre-service elementary teachers will look beyond these surface features and focus on deep pedagogical issues raised when using technology with their future students.

The results of this study suggest that pre-service elementary teachers consider technology and mathematical learning to be two distinct components, and that pre-service elementary teachers select software on the basis of student motivation and clear directions given by the software program. Other studies (Johnston, 2009; 2008) support this argument. By placing more emphasis on the technical features of the tools, pre-service teachers may not identify the pedagogical and conceptual affordances of technology. Pre-service teachers who view technology as a 'stand-alone" activity may use the technology to fill class time, rather than take advantage of the affordances of the technology (Battey, Kafai, & Franke, 2005.) This further supports the argument that pre-service elementary teachers need guidance when using technology in their mathematics instruction, and that teacher preparation programs need to do a better job of integrating technology into the program.

Pre-service elementary teachers must also consider the *cognitive* and *mathematical* fidelity of the technology tools they use. Zbiek, Heid, Blume, and Dick (2007) define *cognitive* fidelity of a technology tool as "the degree to which the computer's method of solution resembles a person's method of solution" (p. 1176). For example, if a pre-service teacher uses an applet to solve computation problems, then the applet should perform the task in a manner consistent with the teacher's own solution, if there is to be high cognitive fidelity. In addition, they define the *mathematical* fidelity of a technology tool as the degree to which a "technology-generated external representation" is "faithful to the underlying mathematical properties of that object" (p. 1174). In other words, if the technology tool presents or explores mathematical information, it should be consistent with mathematics as accepted by the community at large. For example, a technology tool with low mathematical fidelity may produce incorrect answers, provide misleading information, or offer errors in representations.

Why should mathematics teacher educators be so concerned about pre-service elementary teachers' evaluations of technology tools for mathematical learning? Several research studies support the belief that pre-service teachers who thoughtfully and purposefully evaluate technology tools for mathematical learning will develop lessons which benefit student learning. One case study examined two pre-service teachers (one elementary and one secondary) enrolled in a course which introduced them to various kinds of mathematical software (Kurz, Middleton, & Yanik, 2004). As these pre-service teachers began to identify the various features of the technology, they could then explain how these features could benefit student learning.

In another study, Niess (2005), found that without guidance, pre-service teachers tend to focus on their own teaching and think less about the students. Pre-service teachers need to purposefully reflect upon students' understanding, thinking, and learning as technology is integrated into a lesson plan. In this case, a guiding question for the student teachers as they planned instruction with technology was, "How will the students understand the concepts in the technology-enhanced instructional activity?" (2005, p. 521). As a result of the activities in her study, pre-service teachers focused more on student learning as a goal for mathematics instruction which is supported by technology.

Definition of Key Terms

For the purposes of this chapter, technology refers to technology tools for mathematical learning. Technology tools for mathematical learning include applets, virtual manipulatives, which are interactive, web-based visual representations of dynamic objects (Moyer, Bolyard & Spikell, 2002); specific computer-based applications such as spreadsheets, Geometer's Sketchpad®, websites, educational software, and the like. While productivity software, such as word processing and presentation tools can be used by students, they are not necessarily tools for mathematical learning.

Study Which Forms the Basis of this Chapter

This chapter discusses activities for use with pre-service elementary teachers in their mathematics methods courses. The activities were developed by the author during a research study which included 23 career-switcher pre-service elementary teachers. These pre-service elementary teachers were enrolled in a teacher licensure program, and at the time of the study, they were completing a mathematics methods course and were engaged in fieldwork at local elementary (K-6) schools. Throughout the semester, the instructor highlighted examples of good technology tools for mathematical learning, and she discussed the affordances and limitations of each. During their methods course, the pre-service elementary teachers were also required to plan and teach three lessons within their fieldwork placement sites. During the semester, the pre-service elementary teachers completed several in-class assignments with respect to technology, which are discussed in the next section.

ACTIVITIES WHICH ENCOURAGE REFLECTION BY PRE-SERVICE ELEMENTARY TEACHERS

Why Reflection?

Pre-service elementary teachers come to their methods coursework with an image of what mathematics teaching should look like, often based upon their own educational experiences. However, these educational experiences may or may not be ideal. To cite Dewey:

...quality educators and education cannot be derived from the imitation of techniques that have worked in the past, but rather teachers should be trained in analyzing and defining principles behind the techniques. In short, it is theorized that the more teacher reflectivity occurs, the better the quality of teaching (Dewey, 1933, p. 89).

Pre-service elementary teachers are sometimes conflicted between those instructional practices which are familiar to them (i.e. from their own mathematics education), and those they encounter in mathematics methods coursework.

Why, then, should pre-service elementary teachers be engaged in reflection, especially when planning for mathematics instruction supported by technology tools? Dewey (1933) notes that teachers who engage in purposeful and regular reflection consider their instructional practices in light of the reasons that support these actions, as well as the consequences which naturally follow. In short, the purpose of teacher reflection is to improve instruction. In light of this view, the author of this chapter views reflection by pre-service elementary teachers as a critical element of their teacher education program. In particular, as pre-service elementary teachers encounter technology tools for mathematical learning, they consider those elements and features of their own instruction which will most benefit student learning.

A Model of Mathematics Teacher Education

The author has described three components of mathematics methods courses which must be present before pre-service elementary teachers can begin writing lesson plans which integrate technology: introducing them to various technology tools for mathematical learning, sharing guidelines for appropriate uses of technology, and engaging pre-service elementary teachers in the evaluation of technology tools for mathematical learning. These three components are not necessarily sequential; they can occur simultaneously. Ideally, these three components of mathematics teacher education occur throughout the mathematics methods course, rather than at distinct moments in time.

Description of an Evaluation and Reflection Activity for Pre-Service Elementary Teachers

One activity which requires pre-service elementary teachers to evaluate and reflect upon technology tools for mathematical learning is described in this section. This three-part activity engages pre-service elementary teachers in the following exercises: identifying criteria for evaluating technology tools, evaluating technology tools using those self-identified criteria, and making recommendations for or against technology tools.

Prior to using technology tools in their own lesson plans, pre-service elementary teachers need experience in evaluating them. A worthwhile activity, which has been used in several methods courses, is asking pre-service elementary teachers to identify criteria which they feel are most important for evaluating technology tools. Appendix A highlights an activity sheet which can be used to serve this purpose. Note that in addition to the identification of criteria, pre-service elementary teachers are also asked to explain the rationale for each of these criteria. Why is each of these criteria important? When asked to *reflect* upon the criteria *they* would use to evaluate technology tools for mathematical learning, pre-service elementary teachers begin to consider what features of the technology tools are most important. The activity sheet requires three criteria to be identified; the instructor may increase the number (or propose no limit on the number of criteria identified) depending upon the population and goals of the methods course.

Battey, Kafai, and Franke (2005) note the criteria identified by pre-service elementary teachers when evaluating software for use in the elementary classroom. The researchers developed four theoretical categories for grouping these criteria: software features, mathematics, learning, and motivation. The pre-service elementary teachers' criteria (substantive codes), operational definitions of those codes (criteria), and theoretical categories are shown in Table 1.

Battey, Kafai, and Franke (2005) initially developed these theoretical categories, substantive codes, and operational definitions from rational number software evaluations. Specifically, teachers evaluated games. Thus, in the previous table, references to games have been replaced with references to tools. Similarly, any specific refer-

Table 1. Theoretical categories, substantive codes, and operational definitions

Codes		Operational Definitions
	Software Features	
Clarity		Clarity of directions to the user
Visual		Clear visual presentation
Technology		Ease of technology use
Purpose		Purpose of tool needs to be clear
Feedback		Feedback provided by tool for the user
	Mathematics	
General		General comments about mathematics (e.g. meets a standard [but participant does not identify a specific standard])
Specific		Specific comments about mathematics (e.g. clarity of explanation of a concept)
	Learning	
General		General comments about learning (e.g. age appropriate)
Specific		Specific comments about learning (e.g. allows for differentiation within a specific concept)
	Motivation	
Fun		Tool needs to be fun
Like		Comments on whether they like the game or not

ences to games have been removed from the list of substantive codes.

After pre-service elementary teachers have identified their criteria, the next step is to allow them to evaluate technology tools according to their own criteria. Appendix B presents an activity sheet which can be used by pre-service elementary teachers to accomplish this task. Once again, the number of technology tools does not have to be limited to three. Instructors may wish to allow their pre-service elementary teachers time to evaluate more technology tools. The technology tools can be pre-selected by the instructor, or the pre-service elementary teachers may select their own technology tools for evaluation. For each tool, pre-service elementary teachers record their criteria, use a Likert scale to evaluate the technology tool according to each of the criteria, and give reasons to support their evaluations.

Finally, pre-service elementary teachers should have the opportunity to make recommendations for or against each of the technology tools, in light of their evaluations. Appendix C presents an activity sheet which can be used by pre-service elementary teachers to accomplish this task. As they make their recommendations, either for or against each technology tool, pre-service elementary teachers reflect upon their evaluations, and they give reasons to support their recommendations.

After pre-service elementary teachers have completed this three-part activity, they are in a better position to begin integrating technology into their own lesson plans. Ideally, pre-service elementary teachers will consider the critical features of the technology tools they plan to use before implementing a lesson with students. If pre-service elementary teachers focus on the surface features of the technology tools, then the instructor should include further opportunities for pre-service elementary teachers to attend to the critical features of the technology tools: those features which promote conceptual understanding, problem solving, multiple representations, and other key pedagogical features.

DESCRIPTIONS AND EVALUATIONS OF FIVE SPECIFIC TECHNOLOGY TOOLS FOR MATHEMATICAL LEARNING

This section describes and evaluates five specific technology tools for mathematical learning. Each of the technology tools highlighted below is free and available on the Internet. No special software needs to be purchased, thereby making these technology tools accessible to all. The five technology tools were selected to highlight each of the five Content Standards of the National Council of Teachers of Mathematics (2000).

Number and Operations

A deep conceptual and procedural understanding of number sense and place value is critical to the success of all students in mathematics. Numerous resources (both physical and virtual) exist to aid students in their learning of number and operations. One such tool includes the Fractions – Adding virtual manipulative, as found on the National Library of Virtual Manipulatives website, http://nlvm.usu.edu/en/nav/frames_asid_106_g_2_t_1.html.

This tool is a useful resource because it links the algorithmic nature of adding fractions with a more conceptual understanding of how the process works. As students identify equivalent fractions, they learn the importance and need for common denominators. In addition, differentiation among students with this tool is possible because of three levels of difficulty for the types of fraction addition problems presented to the students.

Elementary students should be given other opportunities to solve problems involving fraction addition. Ultimately, they should be able to efficiently add fractions without the support of the virtual tool. However, this tool provides students with a beginning understanding of fraction addition.

Algebra

The word "algebra" often conjures up images of solving equations, variables, and graphing equations by hand. But algebra can and should begin in the primary grades, with the exploration of patterns. Young children love to find and identify patterns in the world around them. To capitalize on this curiosity, it is beneficial for students to identify patterns and extend them in a mathematical set-

Figure 2. NLVM addition of fractions tool. (© 2008 Utah State University. used with permission)

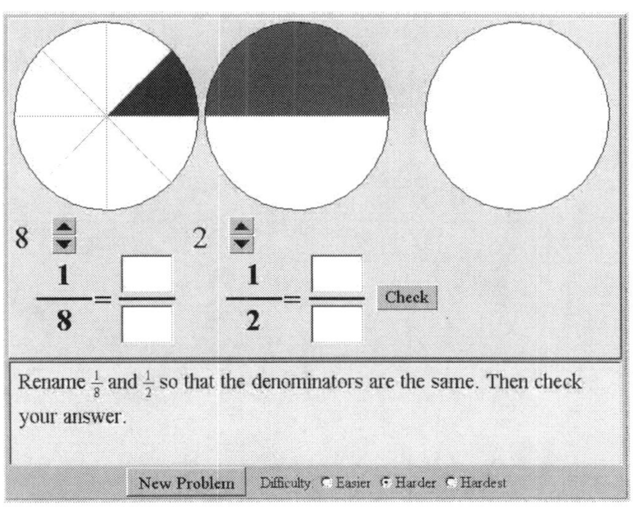

ting. One tool which allows students to do this is the Color Patterns tool, as found on the National Library of Virtual Manipulatives website, http://nlvm.usu.edu/en/nav/frames_asid_184_g_1_t_2.html.

One activity in which elementary students can be engaged is completing a color pattern. For example, a color pattern is started, and then students identify which color completes each bead in the rest of the pattern. Once they are finished, students can check their work by using one of the built-in features. If students are incorrect, they are given a message which tells them to check their work and try again. If students are correct, they are given the opportunity to go on to a new pattern.

Students should respond to questions posed by their classmates and their teachers. Such questions could include, "How did you know how to complete the pattern? Do you think there is another correct way of completing the pattern? Why or why not? How difficult was this pattern to complete? Why do you say that?"

Geometry

Examples of geometry are all around us – in nature, in architecture – almost anywhere you look, students can find examples of geometric patterns, shapes, and relationships. One example is tessellations. Students may associate tessellations with the tile work in their bathrooms, or in other places. Some students may not be familiar with tessellations. One tool which helps students explore the concept of tessellations is Shodor's tool, http://www.shodor.org/interactivate/activities/Tessellate/.

Using this tool, students can create simple tessellations from common geometric shapes, such as triangles, rectangles, and hexagons. Or, students can use the pre-selected shapes to create irregular figures, and make more complicated tessellations.

After students have had the opportunity to create their own tessellations and compare their work to other students, the teacher can lead a class discussion of tessellations in artwork, in architecture, and in other real-world settings. Other online resources are available to assist teachers as they help their students make connections to other subject areas.

Measurement

Students enjoy measuring. Teachers should take advantage of this enthusiasm for learning and provide as many measurement opportunities as possible. Geoboards offer students multiple modalities

Figure 3. NLVM color patterns tool. (© 2008 Utah State University. used with permission)

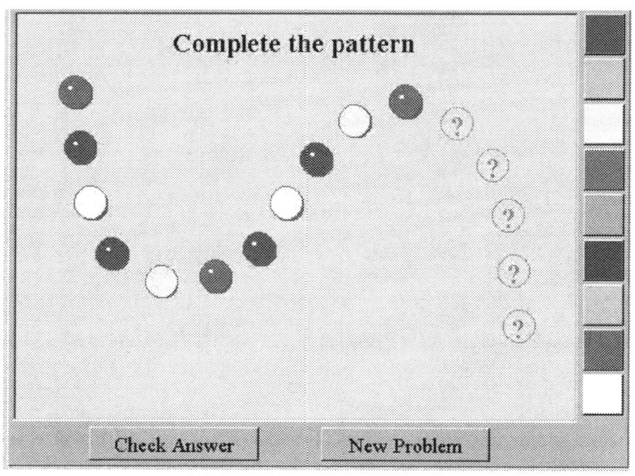

Figure 4. Shodor tessellation tool. (© 2009 Shodor. used with permission)

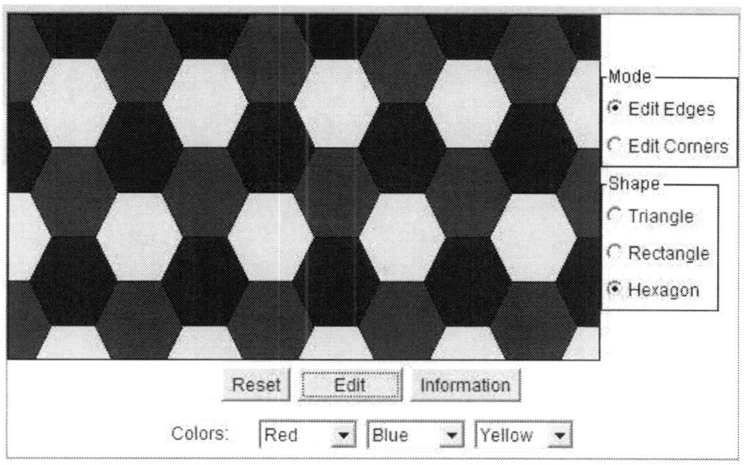

for exploring and understanding measurement. One tool available to students and teachers alike is a virtual geoboard, as found on the National Library of Virtual Manipulatives website, http://nlvm.usu.edu/en/nav/frames_asid_281_g_2_t_4.html.

Numerous activities using this tool are possible, but one worthwhile measurement activity is asking students to create three different shapes with the same perimeter, such as 12 units. Then, using the "measures" feature, students can compare the perimeter and area of each figure. The teacher may want to have students only create one type of polygon, such as a rectangle. Or the teacher may wish to have them explore creating different polygons. Another variation is stating the area (such as 20 square units), and noting what different perimeters are possible.

For an activity such as the one described above, it is important that students have dot paper to record their drawings, so they can reflect upon their work at a later date, to include a class discussion. Such

Figure 5. NLVM virtual Geoboard. (© 2008 Utah State University. used with permission)

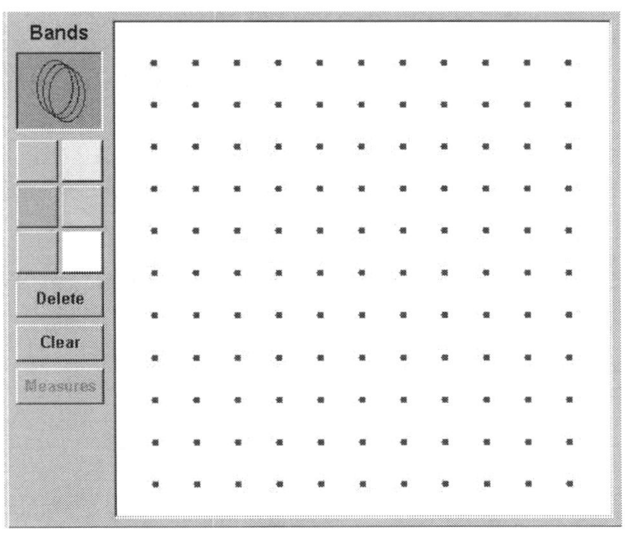

a task sheet helps students make the connection between the virtual and the written representation.

Data Analysis & Probability

Numerous data analysis tools are available on the Internet. These can be used in multiple ways. As a class, students can collect data, and then the teacher can project the graph onto an overhead screen. Or, students can create their own graphs using these tools. One such tool is a Bar Grapher, as found on the National Council of Teachers of Mathematics *Illuminations®* website, http://illuminations.nctm.org/ActivityDetail.aspx?ID=63.

Specifically, this tool allows the user to enter data he or she has collected, or for demonstration/exploratory purposes, the user can graph data which has already been programmed into the tool. In either case, students can quickly discover how to create a bar graph from a set of data.

Students can and should learn the following vocabulary of bar graphs: scale, axes, and interval. This tool, when used properly, can develop students' conceptual understanding of data analysis, specifically creating bar graphs.

FUTURE RESEARCH DIRECTIONS

The three-part activity described in this chapter has been field tested by the researcher with pre-service and in-service (beginning) elementary teachers in mathematics methods courses. Further research is needed to evaluate the effectiveness of this type of activity. In addition, research should be conducted to create and evaluate other activities which develop the mathematics Technology, Pedagogy, And Content Knowledge (TPACK) of pre-service elementary teachers. How do these kinds of activities assist pre-service elementary

Figure 6. Illuminations bar grapher. (© 2009 National Council of Teachers of Mathematics. used with permission)

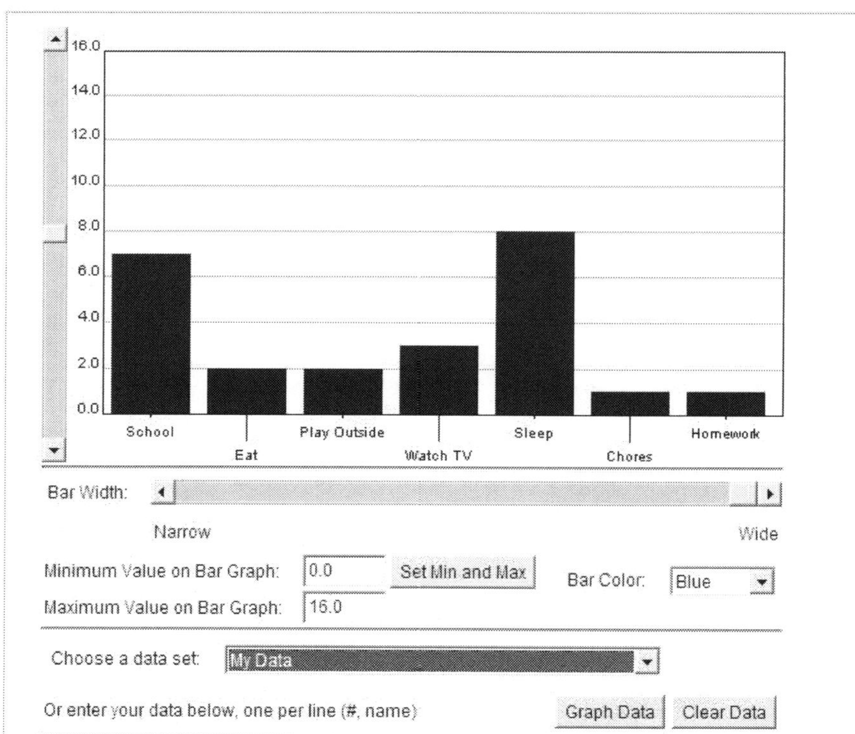

teachers as they evaluate technology tools for mathematical learning? What affordances and limitations of technology tools do pre-service elementary teachers identify? What experiences will assist pre-service elementary teachers to look beyond the surface features of technology tools so that they take full advantage of these tools? These are questions which ought to be addressed by research.

Furthermore, other populations should be studied. For example, what affordances and limitations of technology tools do experienced elementary teachers identify? Do these change over time? Another population to be considered is secondary mathematics teachers, both pre-service and in-service teachers. Are there certain criteria which secondary mathematics teachers focus? What technology tools are available at the secondary level that may not be appropriate at the elementary level? How do secondary mathematics teachers evaluate these particular tools? These are additional questions which should be addressed by researcher.

CONCLUSION

The current generation of pre-service elementary teachers, particularly those who are studying elementary education at the undergraduate level, come to mathematics methods courses with a wealth of experience in using technology, both for personal and academic purposes. However, their knowledge of technology tools for mathematical learning may be limited. This chapter has presented a model of mathematics teacher education with respect to technology, as established by the literature. The three critical components of this model include: introducing pre-service elementary teachers to various types of technology tools; modeling and discussing five guidelines for appropriate uses of technology in mathematics education; and evaluation of technology tools. This chapter has also provided the reader with a three-part reflective activity which can be used by pre-service elementary teachers in advance of lesson planning. This reflective activity requires pre-service elementary teachers to: identify their criteria for evaluating technology tools, evaluate technology tools (of their own choosing or selected by the instructor), and make recommendations for or against these technology tools. The author provided descriptions and evaluations of five technology tools, one for each of the NCTM Content Standards. Implications for mathematics teacher educators and directions for future research have been identified.

REFERENCES

Association of Mathematics Teacher Educators. (2006). *Preparing teachers to use technology to enhance the learning of mathematics: A position statement of the Association of Mathematics Teacher Educators*. Retrieved June 14, 2008, from http://www.amte.net

Battey, D., Kafai, Y., & Franke, M. (2005). Evaluation of mathematical inquiry in commercial rational number software. In Vrasidas, C., & Glass, G. (Eds.), *Preparing teachers to teach with technology* (pp. 241–256). Greenwich, CT: Information Age Publishing.

Dewey, J. (1933). *How we think: A restatement of the relation of reflective thinking to the educative process*. Boston, D. C.: Heath & Co.

Garofalo, J., Drier, H., Harper, S., Timmerman, M. A., & Shockey, T. (2000). Promoting appropriate uses of technology in mathematics teacher preparation. *Contemporary Issues in Technology and Technology Education*, *1*, 66–88.

Johnston, C. J. (2008). *Pre-service elementary teachers' criteria for evaluating technology tools for mathematics learning. Unpublished doctoral pilot study*. George Mason University.

Johnston, C. J. (2009). *Pre-service elementary teachers planning for mathematics instruction: The role and evaluation of technology tools and their influence on lesson design*. Unpublished doctoral dissertation, George Mason University.

Kurz, T., Middleton, J., & Yanik, H. B. (2004). Preservice teachers' conceptions of mathematics-based software. In. *Proceedings of the International Group for the Psychology of Mathematics Education*, *28*, 313–320.

Kurz, T. L., Middleton, J. A., & Yanik, H. B. (2005). A taxonomy of software for mathematics education. *Contemporary Issues in Technology & Teacher Education*, *5*, 123–137.

Moyer, P. S., Bolyard, J. J., & Spikell, M. A. (2002). What are virtual manipulatives? *Teaching Children Mathematics*, *8*, 372–377.

National Council of Teachers of Mathematics. (2000). *Principles and standards for school mathematics*. Reston, VA: Author.

National Council of Teachers of Mathematics. (2009). *Illuminations*. Retrieved from http://illuminations.nctm.org/

National Library of Virtual Manipulatives. (2007). Utah State University. Retrieved from http://nlvm.usu.edu/

Niess, M. L. (2005). Preparing teachers to teach science and mathematics with technology: Developing a technology pedagogical content knowledge. *Teaching and Teacher Education*, *21*, 509–523. doi:10.1016/j.tate.2005.03.006

Niess, M. L., Suharwoto, G., Lee, K., & Sadri, P. (2006, April). *Guiding inservice mathematics teachers in developing TPCK*. Paper presented at the annual meeting of the American Education Research Association, San Francisco, CA.

Shodor. (2008). Retrieved from http://www.shodor.org/home/

Zbiek, R., Heid, M. K., Blume, G. W., & Dick, T. P. (2007). Research on technology in mathematics education: A perspective of constructs. In Lester, F. K. (Ed.), *Second handbook of research on mathematics teaching and learning* (pp. 1169–1206). Reston, VA: National Council of Teachers of Mathematics.

ADDITIONAL READING

DaPonte, J. P., Oliveira, H., & Varandas, J. M. (2002). Development of pre-service mathematics teachers' professional knowledge and identity in working with information and communication technology. *Journal of Mathematics Teacher Education*, *5*, 93–115. doi:10.1023/A:1015892804607

Doerr, H. M., & Zangor, R. (2000). Creating meaning for and with the graphing calculator. *Educational Studies in Mathematics*, *41*, 143–163. doi:10.1023/A:1003905929557

Flores, A., Knaupp, J. E., Middleton, J. A., & Staley, F. A. (2002). Integration of technology, science, and mathematics in the middle grades: A teacher preparation program. *Contemporary Issues in Technology & Teacher Education*, *2*(1). Retrieved from http://www.citejournal.org/vol2/iss1/mathematics/article1.cfm.

Goos, M. (2005). A sociocultural analysis of the development of pre-service and beginning teachers' pedagogical identities as users of technology. *Journal of Mathematics Teacher Education*, *8*, 35–59. doi:10.1007/s10857-005-0457-0

Goos, M., Galbraith, P., Renshaw, P., & Geiger, V. (2000). Reshaping teacher and student roles in technology-enriched classrooms. *Mathematics Education Research Journal*, *12*, 303–320.

Goos, M., Galbraith, P., Renshaw, P., & Geiger, V. (2003). Perspectives on technology mediated learning in secondary school mathematics classrooms. *The Journal of Mathematical Behavior*, *22*(1), 73–89. doi:10.1016/S0732-3123(03)00005-1

Hazzan, O. (2000). Attitudes of prospective high school mathematics teachers towards integrating information technologies into their future teaching. In. *Proceedings of the Society for Information Technology and Teacher Education*, *11*, 1582–1587.

Hazzan, O. (2003). Prospective high school mathematics teachers' attitudes toward integrating computers in their future teaching. *Journal of Research on Technology in Education*, *35*, 213–225.

Jonassen, D. H., Carr, C., & Yueh, H. (1998). Computers as mindtools for engaging learners in critical thinking. *TechTrends*, *43*(2), 24–32. doi:10.1007/BF02818172

Kafai, Y., Franke, M., & Battey, D. (2002). Educational software reviews under investigation. *Education Communication and Information*, *2*, 163–180. doi:10.1080/1463631021000025349

Kastberg, S., & Leatham, K. (2005). Research on graphing calculators at the secondary level: Implications for mathematics teacher education. *Contemporary Issues in Technology & Teacher Education*, *5*, 25–37.

Kersaint, G. (2007). Toward technology integration in mathematics education: A technology-integration course planning assignment. *Contemporary Issues in Technology & Teacher Education*, *7*, 256–278.

Kersaint, G., Horton, B., Stohl, H., & Garofalo, J. (2003). Technology beliefs and practices of mathematics education faculty. *Journal of Technology and Teacher Education*, *11*, 567–595.

Kurz, T., & Middleton, J. A. (2006). Using a functional approach to change preservice teachers' understanding of mathematics software. *Journal of Research on Technology in Education*, *39*, 45–65.

Li, Q. (2005). Infusing technology into a mathematics methods course: Any impact? *Educational Research*, *47*, 217–233. doi:10.1080/00131880500104341

Mishra, P., & Koehler, M. J. (2006). Technological pedagogical content knowledge: A framework for teacher knowledge. *Teachers College Record*, *108*, 1017–1054. doi:10.1111/j.1467-9620.2006.00684.x

Monaghan, J. (2004). Teachers' activities in technology-based mathematics lesson. *International Journal of Computers for Mathematical Learning*, *9*, 327–357. doi:10.1007/s10758-004-3467-6

Niess, M. L. (2008). Guiding preservice teachers in developing TPCK. In Silverman, N. (Ed.), *Handbook of technological pedagogical content knowledge (TPCK) for educators* (pp. 223–250). New York: Routledge.

Niess, M. L., Ronau, R. N., Driskell, S. O., Kosheleva, O., Pugalee, D., & Weinhold, M. W. (2008). Technological pedagogical content knowledge (TPCK), Preparation of mathematics teachers for 21st century teaching and learning. In Arbaugh, F., & Taylor, P. M. (Eds.), *Inquiry into mathematics teacher education. Association of Mathematics Teacher Educators (AMTE)* (*Vol. 5*). Monograph Series.

Niess, M. L., Ronau, R. N., Shafer, K. G., Driskell, S. O., Harper, S. R., & Johnston, C. (2009). Mathematics teacher TPACK standards and development model. *Contemporary Issues in Technology & Teacher Education*, *9*(1). Retrieved from http://www.citejournal.org/vol9/iss1/mathematics/article1.cfm.

Reimer, K., & Moyer, P. S. (2005). Third-graders learn about fractions using virtual manipulatives: A case study. *Journal of Computers in Mathematics and Science Teaching*, *24*, 5–25.

Shulman, L. S. (1986). Those who understand: Knowledge growth in teaching. *Educational Researcher*, *15*(2), 4–14.

Suh, J., & Moyer, P. S. (2007). Developing students' representational fluency using virtual and physical algebra balances. *Journal of Computers in Mathematics and Science Teaching*, *26*, 155–173.

APPENDIX A

Criteria	Explanation (Rationale for Inclusion)
1. ____________	
2. ____________	
3. ____________	

Identifying Criteria

Think about the technology tools you have used in your own mathematics content and methods courses.

Below, identify your three primary criteria for selecting and using these types of technology tools in your own classroom. For each of the three criteria, explain why this is important to you.

APPENDIX B

Scoring and Evaluating Technology Tools

For each of the three technology tools you select:

- Once again, identify your three primary criteria for selecting technology tools (previous activity).
- Note the technology tool you selected. If you selected an Internet-based technology tool, be sure to include the URL.
- Rate the technology on a scale of 1 to 5 to indicate the degree to which the technology tools meets the criteria. For example, 5 means, "I strongly agree that the technology tools meets the criteria." 4 means, "I agree that the technology tools meets the criteria." 3 means, "I am not sure." 2 means, "I disagree that the technology tools meets the criteria." And 1 means, "I strongly disagree that the technology tools meets the criteria."
- Give comments which support the score you assigned to the technology tool.

A. Tool:		
Criteria	Score	Comments
1. ________________	5 4 3 2 1	
2. ________________	5 4 3 2 1	
3. ________________	5 4 3 2 1	
B. Tool:		
Criteria	Score	Comments
1. ________________	5 4 3 2 1	
2. ________________	5 4 3 2 1	
3. ________________	5 4 3 2 1	
C. Tool:		
Criteria	Score	Comments
1. ________________	5 4 3 2 1	
2. ________________	5 4 3 2 1	
3. ________________	5 4 3 2 1	

APPENDIX C

Recommendations For or Against the Technology Tools

For each of the three technology tools you selected:

- Give your recommendation for or against the technology tool, based upon your evaluation.
- Give a statement to support your recommendation, either for or against.

A. Tool:
  - Recommendation:
  - Supporting Statement:

B. Tool:
  - Recommendation:
  - Supporting Statement:

C. Tool:
  - Recommendation:
  - Supporting Statement:

Chapter 16
Reflections on a Course Designed to Encourage Technology Integration in Secondary School Mathematics

Gladis Kersaint
University of South Florida, USA

ABSTRACT

Mathematics education is used as a context to demonstrate the types of learning experiences that can be provided to preservice secondary mathematics teachers as part of a teacher education program to encourage technology integration. Specifically, the author reflects on the design, development, and implementation of a mathematics-specific technology course and considers the extent to which this course provides prospective teachers experiences to achieve the goals identified in the Mathematics TPACK (Technological Pedagogical Content Knowledge) Framework developed by the Association of Mathematics Teacher Educators. In its current form, the course addresses most of the identified guidelines; however, after reflecting on the extent to which this course might satisfy all of the indicators, the author concludes that a single course on technology integration is not sufficient. Technology integration should be considered a programmatic teacher education goal across multiple courses, both content and pedagogy.

INTRODUCTION

Ubiquitous technology has altered our views about what it means to function in today's highly connected society. In fact, extant technology has provided global access to information and has facilitated communication between and among individuals who may be in opposite ends of the world. Because new technology continues to emerge, educators have to consider and grapple with ways to take advantage of available technologies and incorporate them in educationally productive ways. In order to determine whether to use technology, educators must address important questions that include: How does one learn about available technology? How does one obtain knowledge about emergent technologies and about the best ways to integrate them effectively to support learning? What technologies should be

DOI: 10.4018/978-1-61520-897-5.ch016

Copyright © 2010, IGI Global. Copying or distributing in print or electronic forms without written permission of IGI Global is prohibited.

used? When and for what purpose should they be used? In addition to answering the aforementioned questions, those charged with preparing teachers must address additional questions that include: How do teacher educators prepare teachers to use technology effectively to support students' content development? What are design features of courses with a focus on preparing teachers to incorporate technology?

In this chapter, mathematics education is used as a context for demonstrating the types of learning experiences that can be provided to encourage preservice teachers (PSTs) to integrate technology. The chapter begins with a discussion about the various recommendations for technology use in education, in general, and in mathematics education, in particular. Then, research findings are presented to highlight affordances provided by the use of technology to support mathematics learning. The remainder of the chapter is used to reflect on the development and implementation of a mathematics-specific technology course designed to help PSTs consider their roles as instructional designers, decision-makers, and facilitators of students' learning via technology. Specifically, features of the course are highlighted to illustrate decisions made and the processes used to encourage PSTs to *learn about* and *learn to use* extant and emergent technologies to support mathematics teaching and learning. Then, the Mathematics TPACK (Technological Pedagogical Content Knowledge) Framework (AMTE, 2009) is used as a basis for reflecting on the extent to which the course meets the expectations of the mathematics education community.

RECOMMENDATIONS FOR TECHNOLOGY-USE IN EDUCATION

Teachers play a significant role in determining whether to use technology, how that technology is used, and in designing technology-enriched learning experiences for learners. Because of this, several organizations have developed standards, principles, position statements, or frameworks that encourage the use of technology to support students' learning. Addressing education broadly, the *International Society for Technology in Education* (ISTE) (2008b) released the next generation National Educational Technology Standards for Teachers (NETS•T) that encourages the use of technology to support learning and teaching of all subject matter. The NETS•T encourages teachers to use the National Educational Technology Standards for Students (NETS•S) (ISTE, 2008a) as they design, implement, and assess learning experiences to support students' learning. According to ISTE (2008b), teachers are expected to:

- *Facilitate and Inspire Student Learning and Creativity*: Teachers engage students in a variety of learning experiences that engage them in authentic problem solving.
- *Design and Develop Digital-Age Learning Experiences and Assessments*: Teachers design learning experiences that incorporate 21st Century digital tools in ways that promote student learning and are assessed in meaningful ways.
- *Model Digital-Age Learning Experiences and Assessments*: Teachers use and learn to use emergent technology to support their daily activity, the design of instruction, and communication with students, parents, and the broader community.
- *Model Digital-Age Work and Learning*: Teachers use their knowledge of current technology and emergent technology to communicate and collaborate with peers, parents, and others. In addition, they are able to use digital tools to identify and evaluate resources with potential to support students' learning.
- *Promote and Model Digital Citizenship and Responsibility*: Teachers use and teach students how to use technology in responsible ways, address the needs of a diverse

student population, and promote socially responsible interactions.

- *Engage in Professional Growth and Leadership*: Teachers function as lifelong learners of technology and of ways to use technology effectively to support teaching and learning.

In addition to the NETS•T standards that identify technological goals for all teachers, content-specific professional organizations (Association of Mathematics Teacher Educators, 2006, 2009; Australian Association of Mathematics Teachers, 2002; National Council for Social Studies, 2006;National Council of Teachers of English, 2008; National Council of Teachers of Mathematics (NCTM), 2000; National Science Teacher Association, 1999) have also produced technology statements specific to their content areas that further delineate technological expectation in their respective fields. Each of these statements acknowledges the importance of technology and encourages its use to support teaching and learning of content. Regarding mathematics, the NCTM's (2000) Technology Principle asserts that "technology is essential in teaching and learning mathematics; it influences the mathematics that is taught and enhances students' learning" (p. 24). Further, it states,

Electronic technologies—calculators and computers—are essential tools for teaching, learning, and doing mathematics. They furnish visual images of mathematical ideas, they facilitate organizing and analyzing data, and they compute efficiently and accurately. They can support investigation by students in every area of mathematics, including geometry, statistics, algebra, measurement, and number. When technological tools are available, students can focus on decision making, reflection, reasoning, and problem solving. (p. 24)

Although the Technology Principle provides an overall vision for mathematics teaching and learning, it does not provide guidelines for the use of technology. Through efforts of its technology committee, the Association of Mathematics Teacher Educators (AMTE) (2009) developed the Mathematics TPACK Framework that identifies four essential components and guidelines regarding the types of knowledge needed by mathematics teachers to design instruction that supports the learning of mathematics via digital technologies. The framework is "organized around four major areas: designing and developing technology-enhanced learning experiences; facilitating technology-integrated instruction; evaluating technology-intensive environment; and continuing to develop professional capacity in mathematics TPACK" (AMTE, no page). The final version of the framework is a result of work that occurred over a two-year period (Niess, 2008a, 2008b; Niess et al., 2009; Ronau, 2009). The Mathematics TPACK Framework's essential components and guidelines are available in Appendix A.

RESEARCH FINDINGS ABOUT TECHNOLOGY USE

Although there will continue to be a need for additional research, the education community has investigated the effect of technology usage on students' learning in general and with regards to a variety of topics (Hied & Blume, 2008; Hin & Subramaniam, 2006). Regarding mathematics, ample evidence is provided in the research literature to suggest that technology can be used effectively to enhance students' understanding of a variety of mathematics concepts (Hied & Blume, 2008), enhance students' experience in mathematics at both middle (Clements, 2000; Guerrero, Walker & Dugdale, 2004) and high school (Doerr & Zangor, 2000; Reznichenko, 2007) levels, and improve student achievement (Antonijevic, 2007; Isikal & Askar, 2005; Olkun, Altun, & Smith, 2005; Sinclair, 2004; U.S. Department of Education,

2001). When considered collectively, these studies provide support for the integration of technology in all aspects of mathematics teaching and learning.

Despite research findings that indicate the effective use of technology can enhance students' learning experiences and initiatives to increase student's access to digital technologies around the world (Organisation for Economic Co-operation and Development, 2000; Office for Standards in Education, 2002, 2004; U.S. Department of Education, 2000), studies indicate that technology is not used widely in schools, and even when they are used, there is no guarantee that they are used effectively to support instruction (Becker 2000; Cuban, 2001; Deveins, Darlow, Burdens, & Petrie, 2003; Smerdon et al, 2000). For example, just over half of the teachers in US public and private schools who had access to computers used them for classroom instruction (Smerdon et al., 2000). In addition, several reports indicate that there is an imbalance of its uses in core academic areas (Becker, 2000; Office of Standards in Education, 2002; Russell et al., 2003). Regarding mathematics, researchers have found that technology is often underused or poorly integrated in the mathematics curriculum (National Center for Education Statistics, 2001; Lawrenz, Gravely, & Ooms, 2006; Norris, Sullivan, Poirot, & Soloway, 2003; Norton, Mc Robbie, & Cooper, 2000; Office for Standards in Education, 2002).

Teachers play a critical role in determining whether and how technology will be used (Diem & Katims, 2002; Hedges et al., 2003). Studies reveal that there are a number of factors that influence teachers' technology use that include their attitudes (Coffland & Strickland, 2004; Lin, 2008; Mcalister, Dunn, & Quin, 2005); beliefs (Doerr & Zangor, 2000; Garthwait &Weller, 2005); knowledge, prior experiences, and confidence with using technology (Forgasz, 2006); and perceived usefulness of technology to support instruction (Lawrencz, Gravely, & Ooms, 2006). To meet the technological expectation of a 21st Century educational context, teacher education programs and content-specific teacher educators must assume a greater role in preparing prospective teachers to provide technology-enriched learning experiences with the potential to enhance students' content knowledge (Kersaint, Horton, Stohl, & Garofalo, 2003). Teachers must engage in professional development and teacher education programs that challenge existing views and beliefs about educational uses of technology (Lin, 2007) and prepare them to effectively use current and emergent technology (Chamblee, Slough, & Wunch, 2008).

REFLECTIONS ON THE IMPLEMENTATION OF A MATHEMATICS-SPECIFIC TECHNOLOGY COURSE

In this section, I reflect on the implementation of a mathematics-specific technology course designed to enhance PSTs knowledge about existing and emergent technology and ways to identify and design technology-enriched lessons to maximize students' mathematics learning and creativity. I begin this section by discussing key decisions made to revise the course and highlight changes that were instituted over the years. Next, I provide a brief description of course tasks and experiences provided to PSTs. Then, I describe the major course assignment that requires PSTs to work collaboratively to integrate technology in one of the mathematics courses taught at the secondary level in the United States. I conclude this section by reflecting on the extent to which this course addresses the guidelines outlined in the Mathematics TPACK Framework.

Course Development and Key Changes in Implementation over Time

When I first taught this mathematics-specific technology course, I modeled the course after the approach used by the previous instructor. The focus of the course was on teaching prospective teachers to use graphing calculator technology in the secondary mathematics classroom. Specifically, students engaged in activities that involved the use of graphing calculator technology, learned about various features of the graphing calculator, and discussed pedagogical issues related to its use. At the end of the semester, the students and I both determined that they learned a lot about mathematics and learning mathematics via technology, but they did not have sufficient understandings to support their individualized efforts to enhance mathematics learning with technology once they became teachers. In addition, more resources (e.g., technology-specific tutorials, technology-enhanced lessons) and tools (e.g., dynamic data software, web-based mathematics java applets) were becoming available. The availability of these resources suggested that it was important to prepare teachers to take advantage of them and use them appropriately to support student learning. So, I decided to revise the course.

My first step in this revision process was to place this course within the larger context of the teacher education program in which the students were enrolled. I found it important to understand the institutional context and the collective experiences provided by the range of courses to be taken by prospective mathematics teachers. With this knowledge, I would be armed with the information needed to make sound decisions regarding how this course might enhance or build upon PSTs' prior technology experiences and contribute to their overall professional development and preparation. Specifically, I was interested in determining what formal learning experiences students had with technology and the extent to which students might have experiences learning mathematics with technology. If students used technology as part of their content courses, then some assumptions could be made about PSTs' knowledge about technology and about the use of technology for learning mathematics. On the other hand, if they were not afforded opportunities to use technology while learning mathematics, then it could be assumed that the PSTs would likely have limited exposure to educational uses of technology for learning mathematics at the undergraduate level and would require additional experiences to uncover and challenge views about what it means to teach and learn mathematics with technology. These considerations were critical because there is not sufficient time in any one course to address all of the issues related to teaching and learning with technology. Understanding the teacher education context provided a basis for making decisions about time allocation and topics that would be emphasized. I used what I learned to make decisions about the nature of the course, the design and/or selection of tasks, and the extent to which information learned in the class would be supported by other courses. In addition, I explored the technological landscape of the surrounding school districts to determine the extent to which PSTs would be provided a supportive context for technology use in mathematics instruction.

During my quest for information, I learned that the majority of the PSTs entered the teacher education program having had limited or no opportunities to learn mathematics with technology at either the secondary or postsecondary level. Neighboring school districts had positive views about technology integration and had purchased technology (e.g., computers, graphing calculators, etc) to be used in the classroom, but a limited number of teachers used these tools regularly. Some of the district supervisors shared that they were excited to learn that technology integration would be part of the teacher preparation program. Apparently, they were not aware that such a course had always been part of the program. I gathered additional information from conversations with mathematics faculty members who revealed that they did not see technology as an essential component of mathematics learning, and as a result, did not incorporate it as part of their instruction. Collectively, this information 1) affirmed encouragement for technology use by school districts, 2) revealed potential areas of challenge, and specifically, potential student views regarding technology integration, and 3) revealed an area of need – PSTs needed opportunities to learn mathematics with technology. As mentioned earlier, research findings reveal that teachers' beliefs about technology and the educational uses of technology are based on their prior experiences with technology (Forgasz, 2006).

Nature of the Course

To refine the course, I continue to seek guidance from the research and practice-based literature regarding the use of technology in mathematics. For example, I considered Garafalo, Drier, Harper, Timmerman, and Shockey's (2000) description about the three ways that technology is incorporated in teacher education and used their description as a basis for revising the course. The three approaches they describe are:

1. Course Instructor as Primary User of Technology: In these cases, the teacher educator is the primary user of technology and uses it to support learning experiences (e.g., use of video cases or digital tools to demonstrate or present information).
2. Prepare Teachers to be the Primary User: In these cases, the teacher education programs prepare teachers to be the primary user of technology. Students might take a "technology for educators" course that provides them experiences with tools to support teacher productivity (e.g., record-keeping, web page production, and presentations) or requires them to develop lessons using subject-specific software.
3. Develop Teacher as Facilitator of Technology-enriched lessons: The focus is to prepare teachers to incorporate technology as part of instruction and teach them to guide their students to use technologies to explore concepts and solve problems.

I decided that aspects of all three categories were important and as a result components of each were incorporated in the course. To model technology use, I would function as a user of technology to support students' learning experiences and would incorporate technology regularly (but, not exclusively) to create a vision for the recommended type of class instruction. To prepare PSTs to be effective users of technology, I would provide information about mathematics-specific technology resources that support the presentation of mathematics during instruction (e.g., use of equation editor to write mathematically appropriate symbolism, resources available online). To encourage PSTs to be effective facilitators of technology-enriched lessons, I would provide experiences to help them learn about technology, learn to use technology, and consider how technology can be used to facilitate and enhance student learning.

Content of the Course

The mathematics-specific technology course is one of five pedagogy courses required for prospective mathematics teachers at my institution. Because of that, I had to make decisions about the content of the course. It is not a content course, so decisions about what technology to use could not be made on the basis of the mathematics topic to be addressed. For example, if teaching Geometry it would be appropriate to use dynamic geometry software to support students' learning. However, because this course is intended to be a pedagogy course, there were several things to consider that include the overall intent of the course, the mathematics content to address, technologies to integrate, and the types of experiences to provide. For example, it might be possible to design a course that provides PSTs many experiences with one technology (as this course had been implemented previously) or limited experiences with several different types of technology. There are affordances and hindrances provided by either option. In the former case, students are provided an opportunity to learn one type of technology well, which allows them time to develop confidence with that technology and focus their attention on pedagogical issues related to the use of that technology for instructional purposes. A consequence of this approach is that preservice teachers may have limited conceptions about what might be possible with other technologies. In addition, given emergent technologies, it is likely that their knowledge would be easily outdated. Using the latter approach, students might gain awareness of the variety of tools that are available, but might not gain the confidence or competence with any one tool, and as a result, may be apprehensive about the use of digital tools to support mathematics teaching and learning. After considering the pros and cons of each approach, I decided that the focus on the course would be to develop a vision for mathematics teaching and learning with technology by illustrating how various digital tools can support mathematics learning and teaching.

In order to prepare PSTs to deal with emerging technology, I decided that rather than focus on helping PSTs learn a specific technology, I would focus on helping them understand how to *learn about* and *learn to use* extant and new technologies. There are several categories of technologies available to support the teaching and learning of mathematics (see Table 1). These technologies can be used to provide opportunities for students to explore and visualize mathematics concepts, conduct mathematics experiments by making and testing conjectures, model problems, and examine patterns based on viewing multiple examples over a relatively short period of time. Over the years, the number and types of available technology continue to grow as new technologies are introduced, and others are enhanced with new features. This stresses the importance of preparing teachers to use current technology, but also preparing them to transfer current knowledge to new technologies and situations. By focusing on the range of technologies available for teaching and learning mathematics, the focus would be taken away from the a particular technology, and the emphasis would be placed on making informed decisions about the effective use of technology for supporting particular instructional tasks and purposes. In addition, this would give the PSTs opportunities to consider how technology can be incorporated regardless of the availability of a particular technology at a specific school.

The overarching goal for the course is for PSTs to leave the class feeling confident that they can be independent learners and users of technology for instructional purposes. Specifically, they would become learners of a particular aspect of technology needed to accomplish a particular instructional task and goal. This would help them understand that when using technology to support instruction, it is not necessary to know about all features of

Table 1. Examples of technologies that support mathematics teaching and learning

Category	Sample Digital Tools
Virtual Manipulatives	National Library of Virtual Manipulatives (http://nlvm.usu.edu/en/nav/vLibrary.html)
Java Applets	NCTM Illuminations (http://illuminations.nctm.org/ActivitySearch.aspx) Shodor Interactivate (http://www.shodor.org/interactivate/)
Computer Algebra Systems	TI-Nspire (http://education.ti.com/) DERIVE (http://www.chartwellyorke.com/derive.html)
Dynamic Geometry Software	Geogebra (http://www.geogebra.org/ Geometer's Sketchpad (http://www.dynamicgeometry.com/)
Dynamic Data Software	TinkerPlots (http://www.keypress.com/) Fathom (http://www.keypress.com/) Microsoft Excel

a particular technology or be able to answer all students' questions prior to using the technology. Instead, they learn that it is important to establish a learning environment that permits individual and collective problem solving with and about the technology. As part of class interactions, PSTs begin to understand that the goal is not for them to be experts about a specific technology, and that they need to investigate aspects of the digital tools that would be used to support particular instructional goals. Overall, the course provides a context for technology integration, challenging existing views about technology integration, and addressing curriculum, instruction, and assessment issues related to technology integration in mathematics learning and teaching. Decisions made about each of these areas are discussed in the paragraphs that follow.

Provide a Context for Technology Integration

Teachers have strong views about what it means to teach and learn mathematics based on their prior experiences. Because new information is filtered through pre-existing conceptions, I found it important to provide opportunities for PSTs to frame technology use within a broader perspective than their own individualized experiences with mathematics teaching and learning. To broaden their perspectives, I require PSTs to examine, reflect upon, and discuss current technology expectations for teachers and students as discussed in various standards documents, such as the ISTE (2008) NET•S and NETS•T, NCTM (2000) Technology Principle, as well as state and other local school district documents that encourage technology use in education. In some cases, teachers or district mathematics supervisors who use or encourage the use of technology regularly to support mathematics instruction are invited to talk to students in the class about what is available locally and to provide encouragement for its use. Exposing teachers to technology expectations and to individuals who support technology integration locally helps them understand that their own experiences might have been limited and that there is support for technology integration beyond this course.

Challenge Existing Conceptions about Technology

As mentioned earlier, there are a number of factors that influence teachers' decisions to use technology including their beliefs and views about teaching and learning, pedagogy, and the role of technology (Garthwait & Weller, 2005). Because of this, I deemed it important to provide PSTs experiences that uncover and reveal their views about the educational use of technology. Over the years, I have found that students who were successful learners of mathematics without technology are the most resistant to technology integration. Further, students with impoverished or limited experiences with technology tend to suggest that technology should be used to reinforce concepts learned first through pencil-paper manipulations or as a motivational tool to support class engagement, rather than as an instructional tool to support the learning of important and rigorous mathematics content (Wachira, Keengwe, & Onchwari, 2008). To address their beliefs, students are asked to read, reflect upon and discuss articles that provide information about effective uses of technology in education, in general, and in relation to mathematics education, in particular. The goal is for PSTs to have a research-based understanding of how students learn mathematics and how such learning can be influenced with the use of technology. These discussions are used to help PSTs recognize and address their views about technology and to encourage them to consider alternatives when information is provided to warrant it.

Address Curriculum, Instruction, and Assessment

Class time is used to engage PSTs in worthwhile mathematics tasks that require the use of technology to illustrate how a particular technology can be used to support mathematics learning and to support the curriculum goals espoused by the NCTM (2000) *Principal and Standards for School Mathematics*. In particular, students experience learning mathematics using various technologies (e.g., graphing calculators, computer algebra system, spreadsheets, and java applets) that, at times, uncover limitations in their own knowledge of mathematics and provide opportunities to develop or enhance their own mathematical understanding. Working independently or in groups, students complete mathematics tasks that, with some adaptation, can be used directly with secondary school students. PSTs first engage in the activities as learners who are grappling with mathematics and must provide solutions to problems or tasks that are posed. During this phase, some PSTs discover that they had limited understanding of particular mathematics topics or ideas that are clarified through exploration via technology. Then, they examine the activities as teachers to reveal their pedagogical attributes. In particular, they examine features of the mathematics tasks (e.g., questions posed, behaviors required such as the need to observe patterns, make and test conjectures, or examine visual representations) and the classroom interaction (e.g., teacher questionings, student-student and student-teacher interactions) that support the learning of mathematics. These discussions provide PSTs opportunities to consider how students' understanding and thinking develop when technology is used to support the development of conceptual understandings. In addition, PSTs consider assessment issues related to the use of the technology. They consider ways to assess students during instruction to ensure that students are learning the intended content and consider ways to assess students formally as part of course exams when technology is used regularly as part of classroom instruction.

Integrate Technology in a Course Taught at the Secondary Level

Over the years, I have adapted and continue to refine a major course assignment that provides PSTs opportunities to work in collaborative teams to integrate technology in a course taught at the secondary level. Students are provided this assignment on the first day of class and are encouraged to develop their course over time as they are learning about, learning to use, and learning to integrate technology to enhance mathematics instruction. In this section, a brief summary of this assignment is provided. A more detailed discussion about the development and implementation of this assignment is available in Kersaint (2007).

Working in collaborative groups of three or four, PSTs function as classroom teachers who are making decisions about how to integrate technology in a mathematics course (e.g., Pre-Calculus) taught at the secondary level. To complete the assignment, students consider the scope and sequence of the course for an entire school year and justify their decisions based on the appropriate use of technology. As a team, PSTs make decisions about what technology to use, when to use technology, how to use technology, and how to assess students' learning. Although each member of the team is required to develop original lessons to illustrate their individualized content, pedagogical, and technological skills, all lessons and activities included in the course integration project need not be original. In fact, PSTs are encouraged to learn about the vast amount of instructional resources available to support technology integration and to make judgments about their appropriateness based on sound criteria that they develop and justify.

PSTs are required to address the intended curriculum by examining state or national standards documents, curriculum guides provided by local school districts, textbooks and other available resources. In many cases, PSTs report that this is their first opportunity to think about the curriculum as a whole and to consider what it means to provide a year's worth of instruction. To push PSTs in their thinking, the assignment stipulates that only lessons used to introduce, develop or enhance the teaching of mathematics concepts should be included in the technology integration project. This was a purposeful decision because many PSTs initially believe that technology should only be used to reinforce understandings of content first taught using pencil-paper procedures. Technology lessons that develop students' conceptual understanding are the most challenging to develop and identify, yet they have been found to be the most likely to provide the greatest gains in students' achievement (Weglinsky, 1998). Students submit their completed assignment on a CD that includes a user-friendly navigation system that allows easy access to resources. At the end of the course, students exchange CDs with other groups, allowing them to leave the course with resources that can be used to integrate technology in courses they might teach at the secondary level.

Reflecting on the Mathematics TPACK Framework

The course described above has been implemented and refined over several years. Although tasks and activities have changed, the core features of the course have been maintained. Responses from former students and school districts provide anecdotal evidence that students are being prepared to integrate technology effectively (see Kersaint, 2007). However, I continue to reflect on its effectiveness. In the remainder of this chapter, the Mathematics TPACK Framework (see Appendix A) is used to examine and reflect on the implementation of this course, determine the extent to which the course activities and experiences address the essential components and corresponding guidelines, and discuss possible ways to address missing aspects.

Designing and Developing Digital-Age Learning Environments and Experiences

In order for teachers to develop digital learning environments and experiences, they must be provided opportunities to experience and reflect upon such experiences themselves as students. The course is designed to provide teachers such experiences. All of the guidelines related to this essential component are addressed as part of the course described above. The course activities and major course assignment provide ample opportunities for the PSTs to design, identify, locate, evaluate, and integrate mathematics tasks in the curriculum to support mathematics learning. Because they are working with peers, they have multiple opportunities to receive feedback about the developed materials as they make decisions to fulfill the course requirements. Additionally, because PSTs are asked to consider technology integration across an entire school year, they consider how students' familiarity with previously introduced technology influences the implementation of subsequent lessons. As part of the class, we discuss the need to introduce students to the technology and how to scaffold their experiences with technology. PSTs are also asked to consider how adaptations can be made with different tools to address the need to function in different school environments that may or may not have access to specific technology. Moreover, PSTs are asked to consider different ways to use technology in instruction (e.g., teacher as primary user vs. student as primary user) and incorporate technology based on the resources that are available (e.g., one computer in the class vs. access to a computer lab).

Facilitate Mathematics Instruction with Technology as an Integral Tool

The guidelines for this essential component suggest that PSTs should be provided opportunities to actually implement technology-enriched lessons in the classroom. Because the technology course does not have a field-based component, PSTs have not been required to implement lessons with students. This is clearly a shortcoming. Although students are provided tools and resources for designing and identifying lessons that incorporate technology appropriately, they are not afforded opportunities to implement these lessons or reflect on their use with actual students. This is an important component of learning to use technology for educational purposes that should be addressed. One approach for addressing this issue is to amend the course so that PSTs are provided opportunities to implement at least one lesson with a group of students. Another approach is to consider technology integration a programmatic goal and include technology-related experiences throughout the program. For example, PSTs can be asked to deliver instruction in a technology-rich environment as part of their internship experiences. If this were to occur, PSTs would have the opportunity to use technology regularly with support and feedback as they are engaged in the practice of teaching.

Assess and Evaluate Technology-Enriched Mathematics Teaching and Learning

Teachers may struggle with appropriate approaches to evaluate students' performance when technology is used regularly as part of classroom instruction. To address this, a teacher might consider implementing two sections of the exam -- one portion that involves the use of technology and a different portion in which technology is not permitted. Although this might be appropriate in some circumstances, it sends a message that the technology is not an integral part of the learning, and consequently, should not be part of the evaluation process. An alternative to this approach is to design exams in ways that allow students to use technology as needed, but that focuses on measuring students' understanding of the subject matter. In this course, Meel's (1997) article has been used as a means to help PSTs consider how to assess students. Meel describes three types of questions that may be asked when calculators are used regularly as part of mathematics instruction. They are:

- **Calculator-active items:** These items require the use of technology, because it would be difficult to obtain a solution without its usage.
- **Calculator-inactive items:** These items typically focus on the conceptual understanding of the subject matter and as a result, do not require the use of technology to determine a solution.
- **Calculator-neutral:** These items typically do not require the use of a calculator, but the calculator might be used by some students to determine a solution.

Meel also discusses how different types of exams can be developed using various combinations of these items. Attending to the purposes of assessments, PSTs discuss the various types of assessment items, and exams that might be developed to ascertain what a student knows or understands. The goal is for PSTs to learn that when developing exams the focus should not be on whether or not the technology is used, but rather, on the types of knowledge to assess and methods to measure that knowledge.

Even though assessment issues are addressed throughout the course, not all of the Mathematics TPACK indicators related to assessment and evaluation are addressed. Because the focus of this course is on the use of technology for teaching and learning mathematics, no attention has been given to the guideline that refers to "students' ethical use of technology resources in learning and communicating mathematics." My initial reaction was that this might not be relevant. However, after additional consideration, this is likely an important topic to address. All teachers need strategies for addressing issues of ethics when technology is used. For instance, mathematics teachers will likely have to address issues related to cheating on coursework, particularly given that digital tools exist that allow students to transmit information to others using wireless technologies. Also, given the vast amount of resources available online, PSTs need familiarity with copyright standards such as citing of sources of materials adapted for instructional use. Teachers who are able to recognize potential areas of difficulty and devise approaches to address them will develop confidence in their ability to manage technology implementation in a classroom setting.

Engage in Ongoing Professional Development to Enhance Technological Pedagogical Content Knowledge

As a recurring theme for the course, PSTs are asked to behave as professionals who are responsible for incorporating technology effectively to support the teaching and learning of mathematics. All assignments are expected to use standards expected of professionals. PSTs use and consider how readily available resources such as word processors, spreadsheets and PowerPoint Presentations can be used to support their productivity. For example, PSTs are introduced to equation editor, a feature of Microsoft Word, to produce mathematically appropriate symbols to communicate mathematics ideas and use screen shots to capture mathematical representations and images for use on worksheets, exams, and presentations.

This course also prepares them for professional practice by providing opportunities to work in a professional learning community to incorporate technology in a secondary-level mathematics course. They learn to work with and rely on colleagues as they complete course assignments. The major course assignment requires PSTs to reach consensus on the goals and expectations for their course, make decisions about what lessons to address and include, provide and receive feedback from each other, and work together to produce an appropriate final project. Although PSTs have opportunities to work in groups in other classes, many report that they really had to function as a team and needed the other group members to be able to complete the assignment and to produce a successful course-integration project.

Finally, because this course explores a broad range of digital tools, PSTs learn that they have not been exposed to all possible features of a particular tool or to all available technologies for teaching and learning mathematics. They begin to recognize that new tools or features will continue to emerge. Exposing PSTs to a variety of digital tools helps them understand the need and provides motivation for taking advantage of other opportunities to learn about emerging technologies. Rather than presenting the course as an end, it is presented as a means for beginning to think about what might be possible with the use of technology.

CONCLUSION

By reflecting about the implementation of a mathematics-specific technology course using the TPACK Framework, I identified areas in which the PSTs are not being well served. Specifically, I learned that it might not be possible to address all of the Mathematics TPACK guidelines in one course and that a more holistic approach might need to be taken. To provide students the range of experiences needed to support long term technology implementation, it is important to consider PSTs experiences across multiple courses in teacher education programs. Specifically, PSTs need experiences that allow them to use technology as learners of content (preferably in the context of content courses), consider and address instructional issues related to technology use, design and make appropriate judgments about technology-integrated lessons that incorporate the effective use of the technology, and implement designed lessons. If such experiences are facilitated and supported with reflection, PSTs can leave their teacher education program with the ability to design "instruction that takes full advantage of what technology has to offer, can encourage, foster, and support students construction of mathematical knowledge in a variety of ways" (AMTE, 2006).

REFERENCES

Antonijevic, R. (2007). *Usage of computers and calculators and students' achievement: Results from TIMSS 2003.* Paper presented at the International Conference on Informatics, Educational Technology and New Media in Education. ERIC Document Reproduction Services ED497737.

Association of Mathematics Teacher Educator (2009). *Mathematics TPACK Framework.*

Association of Mathematics Teacher Educators. (2006). *Preparing Teachers to Use Technology to Enhance the Learning of Mathematics.* Retrieved on February 19, 2009 from http://www.amte.net

Australian Association of Mathematics Teachers. (2002). *Standards for Excellence in Teaching Mathematics in Australian Schools.* Retrieved on February 19, 2009 from http://www.aamt.edu.au/Standards

Becker, H. J. (2000). Who's wired and who's not: Children's access to and use of computer technology. *The Future of Children: Children and Computer Technology, 10*, 44–75. doi:10.2307/1602689

Chamblee, G. E., Slough, S. W., & Wunsch, G. (2008). Measuring high school mathematics teachers' concerns about graphing calculators and change: A yearlong study. *Journal of Computers in Mathematics and Science Teaching, 27*(2), 183–194.

Clements, D. H. (2000). From exercises and tasks to problems and projects: Unique contributions of computers to innovative mathematics education. *The Journal of Mathematical Behavior, 19*, 9–47. doi:10.1016/S0732-3123(00)00036-5

Coffland, D. A., & Strickland, A. (2004). Factors related to teacher use of technology in secondary geometry instruction. *Journal of Computers in Mathematics and Science Teaching, 23*(4), 347–365.

Cuban, L. (2001). *Oversold and underused computers in the classroom.* Cambridge, MA: Harvard University Press.

Devins, D., Darlow, A., Burdens, T., & Petrie, A. (2003). *Connecting communities to the Internet: Evaluation of the Wired Up Communities programme (2000-2002).* London: Department for Education and Skills. [DFES]

Diem, R. A., & Katims, D. S. (2002). The introductioni of computers in an at-risk learning environment: A seven-year retrospectice view. *Computers in the Schools, 19*, 19–32. doi:10.1300/J025v19n01_03

Doerr, H. M., & Zangor, R. (2000). Creating meaning for and with the graphing calculator. *Educational Studies in Mathematics, 41*(2), 143–163. doi:10.1023/A:1003905929557

Forgasz, H. (2006). Factors that encourage or inhibit computer use for secondary mathematics teaching. *Journal of Computers in Mathematics and Science Teaching, 25*(1), 77–93.

Garafalo, J., Drier, H., Harper, S., Timmerman, M. A., & Shockey, T. (2000). Promoting appropriate uses of technology in mathematics teacher prepartion. *Contemporary Issues in Technology & Teacher Education, 1*(1), 66–88.

Garthwait, A., & Wellwer, H. G. (2005). A year in the life: Two seventh grade teachers implementing one-to-one computing. *Journal of Research on Technology in Education, 37*(4), 361–377.

Guerrero, S., Walker, N., & Dugale, S. (2004). Technology in support of middle grade mathematics: What have we learned? *Journal of Computers in Mathematics and Science Teaching, 23*(1), 5–20.

Hedges, L. V., Konstantopoulos, S., & Thompson, A. (2003). *NAEP validity studies: Computer use and its relation to academic achievement in mathematics, reading, and writing* (Working paper no. 2003-15). Retrieved March 12, 2009 from http://nces.ed.gov/pubsearch/pubsinfo.asp?pubid=200315

Hied, M. K., & Blume, G. W. (2008). Research on technology and the teaching and learning of mathematics: *Vol. 1. Research syntheses*. Charlotte, NC: Information Age Publishing, Inc.

Hin, L. T. W., & Subramaniam, R. (Eds.). (2009). *Handbook of research on new media literacy at the K-12 level: Issues and challenges*. Hershey, PA: IGI Global.

International Society for Technology in Education (ISTE). (2008a). *National educational technology standards (NET•S) and performance indicators for students*. Retrieved on February 20, 2009, from http://www.iste.org/

International Society for Technology in Education (ISTE). (2008b). *National educational technology standards (NET•T) and performance indicators for teachers*. Retrieved on February 20, 2009, from http://www.iste.org/

Isiksal, M., & Askar, P. (2005). The effect of spreadsheet and dynamic geometry software on the achievement and self-efficacy of 7th-grade students. *Educational Research, 47*(3), 333–350. doi:10.1080/0013188050028781 5

Kersaint, G. (2007). Toward technology integration in mathematics education: A technology-integration course planning assignment. *Contemporary Issues in Technology & Teacher Education, 7*(4), 256–278.

Kersaint, G., Horton, B., Stohl, H., & Garofalo, J. (2003). Technology beliefs and practices of mathematics education faculty. *Journal of Technology and Teacher Education, 11*(4), 567–595.

Lawrenz, F., Gravely, A., & Ooms, A. (2006). Perceived helpfulness and amount of use of technology in science and mathematics classes at different grade levels. *School Science and Mathematics, 106*, 133–137. doi:10.1111/j.1949-8594.2006.tb18170.x

Lin, C.-Y. (2008). Beliefs about using technology in the mathematics classroom. Interviews with preservice elementry teachers. *Eurasia Journal of Mathematics, Science, and Technology Education, 4*(2), 135–142.

McAlister, M., Dunn, J., & Quin, L. (2005). Student teachers' attitudes to and use of computers to teach mathematics in primary mathematics classrooms. *Technology, Pedagogy and Education, 14*(1), 77–105. doi:10.1080/14759390500200194

Meel, D. E. (1997). Calculator-available assessment: The why, what, and how. *Educational Assessment, 4*(3), 149–174. doi:10.1207/s15326977ea0403_1

National Center for Education Statistics. (2001). *The nation's report card: Mathematics 2000 (NCES Publication 2001-517)*. Washington, DC: US Department of Education.

National Council for the Social Studies. (2006). *Technology Position Statement and Guidelines*. Retrieved on February 19, 2009, from http://www.socialstudies.org/positions/technology

National Council of Teachers of English. (2008). *The NCTE Definition of 21st Century Literacies*. Retrieved on February 19, 2009, from http://www.ncte.org/positions/statements/21stcentdefinition

National Council of Teachers of Mathematics. (2000). *Principles and standards for school mathematics*. Reston, VA: Author.

National Science Teacher Association. (1999, January). *Use of Computers in Science Education*. Retrieved on February 19, 2009, from http://www.nsta.org/about/positions/computers.aspx

Neiss, M. L. (2008a). Knowledge needed for teaching with technologies – Call it TPACK. *AMTE Connection*, *17*(2), 9–10.

Neiss, M. L. (2008b). Teaching with technology: Standards for mathematics teachers. *AMTE Connection*, *18*(1), 9–10.

Niess, M. L., Ronau, R. N., Shafer, K. G., Driskell, S. O., Harper, S. R., & Johnston, C. (2009). Mathematics teacher TPACK standards and development model. *Contemporary Issues in Technology & Teacher Education*, *9*(1). Retrieved from http://www.citejournal.org/vol9/iss1/mathematics/article1.cfm.

Norris, C., Sullivan, T., Poirot, J., & Soloway, E. (2003). No access, no use, no impact: Snapshot surveys of educational technology in K-12. *Journal of Research on Technology in Education*, *36*, 15–27.

Norton, S., McRobbie, C. J., & Cooper, T. J. (2000). Exploring secondary mathematics teachers' reasons for not using computer in their teaching: Five case studies. *Journal of Research on Technology in Education*, *33*(1), 87–109.

Office for Standards in Education. (2002). *ICT in schools: Effects of government initiatives – Secondary Mathematics*. London: Author.

Office for Standards in Education. (2004). *ICT in schools: Impact of government initiatives – Secondary Mathematics*. London: Author.

Olkun, S., Altun, A., & Smith, G. (2005). Computers and 2D geometric learning of Turkish fourth and fifth graders. *British Journal of Educational Technology*, *36*(2), 317–326. doi:10.1111/j.1467-8535.2005.00460.x

Organisation for Economic Cooperation and Development. (2000). *Schooling for tomorrow: Learning to bridge the digital divide*. Paris: Author.

Reznichenko, N. (2007). *Learning mathematics with graphing calculator: A study of students' experiences*. Paper presented at the Annual Meeting of the Eastern Educational Research Association. ERIC Document Reproduction Services ED497715.

Ronau, B. (2009). Technology committee update. *AMTE Connections*, *18*(2), 12–13.

Russell, M., Bebell, D., O'Dwyer, L., & O'Connor, K. (2003). Examining teacher technology use. *Journal of Teacher Education*, *54*, 297–310. doi:10.1177/0022487103255985

Schmidt, M. E. (1999). Middle grades teacher's beliefs about calculator use: Pre-project and two-years later. *Focus on Learning Problems in Mathematics*, *21*, 18–34.

Sinclair, M. (2004). Working with accurate representations: The case of pre-constructed dynamic geometry sketches. *Journal of Computers in Mathematics and Science Teaching*, *23*(2), 191–208.

Smerdon, B., Cronen, S., Lanahan, L., Anderson, J., Iannotti, N., & Angeles, J. (2000). *Teachers' tools for the 21st Century: A report on teacher's use of technology* (NCES Publication 2000-102). Retrieved February 26, 2009 from www.nces.ed.gov/pubsearch/pubsinfor.asp?pubid=2000102

U.S. Department of Education. (2000). *E-Learning: Putting a world-class education at the fingertips of all children*. Washington, DC: U.S. Department of Education.

Wachira, P., Keengwe, J., & Onchwari, G. (2008). Mathematics preservice teachers' beliefs and conceptions of appropriate technology use. *AACE Journal*, *16*(3), 293–306.

Wenglinsky, H. (1998). *Does it compute? The relationship between educational technology and student achievement in mathematics.* Princeton, NJ: Educational Testing Service (ETS). Retrieved February 20, 2006, from ftp://ftp.ets.org/pub/res/technolog.pdf

APPENDIX

Mathematics TPACK (Technological Pedagogical Content Knowledge) Framework

AMTE believes that students at all levels, K-20, benefit from technology-enriched learning environments. Mathematics educators serve their students by considering the potential impact of a variety of forms of 21st Century digital technologies and planning accordingly.

The following framework is based on the work of Mishra and Koehler (2006). It further elaborates important considerations related to TPACK and the National Educational Technology Standards for Teachers (ISTE 2009) for those whose primary content responsibility is mathematics. It is intended to serve as a guide for mathematics educators (K-12 teachers, university faculty, teacher educators, and professional development facilitators) and researchers to plan, examine, improve, and evaluate mathematics instruction at all levels. The framework describes essential components for enhancing mathematical learning experiences via technology and is organized around four major areas: designing and developing technology-enhanced learning experiences; facilitating technology-integrated instruction; evaluating technology-intensive environments; and continuing to develop professional capacity in mathematics TPACK. Specific guidelines for each area are described below.

- **Design and develop technology-enhanced mathematics learning environments and experiences.** Educators use their knowledge of technology, pedagogy, and content to design and develop learning environments and experiences to maximize mathematics learning. They:
  a. Establish and utilize mathematical environments, tasks, experiences and resources to integrate technology tools that support learners' individual and collaborative mathematical learning and creativity;
  b. Design challenging and engaging mathematical learning experiences that utilize appropriate technologies to support the diverse needs of learners; and
  c. Identify and utilize strategies and activities that promote equitable access to and facility with technology resources.
- **Facilitate mathematics instruction with technology as an integrated tool.** Educators implement curricular plans that integrate appropriate technology to maximize mathematical learning and creativity. They:
  a. Incorporate knowledge of learner characteristics, orientation, and thinking to foster learning of mathematics with technology;
  b. Facilitate technology-enriched, mathematical experiences that foster creativity, develop conceptual understanding, and cultivate higher order thinking skills;
  c. Promote mathematical discourse between and among instructors and learners in a technology-enriched learning community;
  d. Use technology to support learner-centered strategies that address the diverse needs of all learners of mathematics; and
  e. Encourage learners to become responsible for and reflect upon their own technology-enriched mathematics learning.

- **Assess and evaluate technology-enriched mathematics teaching and learning.** Educators assess and evaluate mathematics teaching and learning using appropriate assessment tools and strategies. They:
    a. Assess learning of mathematics applying technologies when appropriate, reflect upon the assessment results, and communicate those results using a variety of tools and techniques;
    b. Assess learners' appropriate and ethical use of technology resources in learning and communicating mathematics;
    c. Use formative assessment of technology-enriched lessons and activities to evaluate mathematics learning and adjust instructional strategies accordingly;
    d. Align the technology expectations for assessment tasks and practices with that of mathematics instructional activities; and
    e. Evaluate and reflect on the effective use of existing and emerging technologies to enhance the mathematical learning of all.
- **Engage in ongoing professional development to enhance technological pedagogical content knowledge.** Educators seek, identify, and use technology to enhance their knowledge, productivity, and professional practice. They:
    a. Collaborate with others in ongoing professional activities to promote excellence in learning mathematics in technology-enriched environments;
    b. Promote social justice for access to and facility with technology in learning mathematics;
    c. Advocate, model, and promote safe, legal, and ethical use of technology for learning and exploring mathematics with learners, families and caregivers, and colleagues;
    d. Communicate and collaborate with families and caregivers, colleagues, and the larger community using appropriate technologies in order to nurture mathematical learners; and
    e. Exhibit leadership by demonstrating a research-based vision for integrating technology in teaching mathematics.

REFERENCES

International Society for Technology in Education. (2008). National Educational Technology Standards for Teachers. (http://www.iste.org/AM/Template.cfm?Section=NETS)

Mishra, P., & Koehler, M. J. (2006). Technological Pedagogical Content Knowledge: A new framework for teacher knowledge. Teachers College Record, 108(6), 1017–1054. doi:10.1111/j.1467-9620.2006.00684.x

Chapter 17
A Mathematical Problem-Solving Approach to Identify and Explore Instructional Routes Based On the Use of Computational Tools

Manuel Santos-Trigo
Center for Research and Advanced Studies, Cinvestav-IPN, Mexico

To what extent do technology developments influence teachers' instructional practices? How can teachers incorporate mathematics education research into their learning activities? What types of mathematical and didactical knowledge becomes relevant for teachers to foster students' development of conceptual understanding, and problem-solving approaches? It is argued that a community of inquiry, formed by teachers, mathematicians, and mathematics educators, becomes important to examine and analyze in-depth mathematical tasks or problems. Interaction within this community is based on fostering an inquisitive or inquiring approach to identify, to make sense, and comprehend mathematical ideas, or relations, and to solve problems. Furthermore, the use of computational tools (dynamic software and hand-held calculators) could help teachers and students explore and analyze mathematical tasks in ways that can enhance and complement paper and pencil approaches.

INTRODUCTION

Mathematical problem-solving perspectives have framed and guided the development of multiple research programs, and supported curriculum proposals in mathematics education for the last four decades (Schoenfeld, 1985; 1992; NCTM, 2000).

DOI: 10.4018/978-1-61520-897-5.ch017

Delving into the development of problem-solving research and discussing its influence in mathematics instruction requires the identification of core or fundamental issues; that is, an inquiry into problem-solving involves not only identifying themes and research directions, but also discussing the types of developments, changes and challenges that this field is facing today. What are the principles or common tenets that distinguish and unify research

Copyright © 2010, IGI Global. Copying or distributing in print or electronic forms without written permission of IGI Global is prohibited.

programs or instructional practices that are based on problem-solving approaches? To what extent have those principles evolved, been modified, or changed as a result of the development and use of computational tools? Focusing on these questions will help in characterizing and reviewing significant problem-solving developments as well as identifying key elements around the principles and possible identity of problem-solving as a domain and its corresponding academic agenda. Current themes and trends associated with problem-solving approaches document the extent to which the development of computational tools has influenced the development of research and problem-solving practices.

It is relevant to identify features associated with the characterization of problem-solving as a research and practice domain in mathematics education. Lesh & Sawojewski (2007) recognize that "the patterns that form a problem-solving identity are complex, involving varied motivational patterns, affective reactions, and cognitive and social engagement in different circumstances both within a given task and across tasks" (p. 776).

Does problem-solving in mathematics education have a common agenda, or does it have multiple themes and interpretations? Törner, Schoenfeld, & Reiss (2007) invited a group of educators who had been involved in problem-solving projects to document and discuss the influences and developments in their countries educational system. They asked them to elaborate three questions as a guide to present and structure their contributions: What are the major ideas in research? What are the main themes in curricula? And what are the relationships between research and curricula, as mediated by politics? The contributions in their publication included a variety of themes that involve the use of the terms problem and problem-solving, the study of teachers' practices, students beliefs, and cognitive and metacognitive developments, the influence of problem solving in organizing the mathematics curricula, the relation between problem-solving approaches and international assessments, e.g. Program for International Student Assessment (PISA), and the use of digital or computational tools in problem-solving activities. This multiple agenda illustrates numerous ways to utilize the construct of problem solving to investigate and promote students' construction or development of mathematics knowledge.

This chapter does not intend to review the developments in the teachers' education field and how they use problem-solving approaches (see for example, Sowder, 2007); rather, the inquiry focuses on ways in which the use of computational technology might offer a new avenue for teachers to revise, extend, and reflect on their mathematical and didactical knowledge for teaching. Thus, the focus of the chapter will be on extending a problem-solving framework proposed by Polya (1945) to include a systematic use of computational tools. To this end, a task is used to illustrate and discuss problem-solving episodes that are relevant to foster and structure the development of their students' mathematical thinking.

BACKGROUND: TEACHERS' EDUCATION AND PROBLEM SOLVING

Current reforms in mathematics curricula recognize the importance for teachers to promote their students' conceptual comprehension of mathematical content, and the development of problem-solving strategies. The National Research Council (NRC) (2001) suggests that teachers need to frame their instructional practices around five intertwined strands: conceptual understanding, procedural fluency, strategic competence, adaptive reasoning, and productive disposition. These activities are central for students to develop competencies in those strands, according to Spillane (2000, p. 144): "Reformers also propose that students develop a more sophisticated appreciation for doing mathematics including framing and solving mathematical problems, articulating conjectures, and reasoning with others about mathematics ideas: students need to appreciate mathematical activity as more than computation". It is relevant to identify and reflect on possible routes that teachers can use to develop the resources and experiences needed to understand and implement the goals associated with these reforms. Teachers to this end need to discuss mathematical tasks as they organize their lessons in a community consisting of mathematics educators, mathematicians, and themselves. Initial questions to be addressed within the community include:

1. To what extent do significant and continuous developments in mathematics education provide a framework to revise and enhance teachers' knowledge and their instructional practices?
2. What should be the role of mathematics departments and education faculties in preparing prospective and practicing teachers?
3. Or, how should the collaboration between the mathematics departments and education faculties be structured to orient and guide teachers' continuous academic development?
4. In what type of educational programs should practicing teachers participate in order to revise and extend their mathematical knowledge, and to incorporate significant research results from mathematics education into their practices?

At the outset, it is important to pinpoint the teachers' mathematical competence should go beyond the sole comprehension of only disciplinary contents; it includes what Hill et al., (2008) call mathematical knowledge for teaching and the mathematical quality of their instruction:

By "mathematical knowledge for teaching," we mean not only the mathematical knowledge common to individuals working in diverse professions, but also the subject matter knowledge that supports that teaching, for example, why and how specific mathematical procedures work, how best to define a mathematical term for a particular grade level, and the types of errors students are likely to make with particular content. By "mathematical quality of instruction" we mean a composite of several dimensions that characterize the rigor and richness of the mathematics of the lesson, including the presence or absence of mathematical errors, mathematical explanation and justification, mathematical representation, and related observables (p. 431).

The issue is how both preservice and inservice teachers develop the mathematical knowledge for teaching to exhibit consistent mathematical quality in their practices. Traditional ways to prepare high school teachers normally involve the participation of both mathematics and the education faculties. Mathematics departments offer content classes while the education faculties provide the didactic and pedagogy courses. This preparation scheme has failed to provide teacher candidates with the mathematical knowledge and sophistication needed to guide their students in the development of robust thinking. This explains why it is common to read that university instructors complain that their first-year university students lack not only fundamental mathematical knowledge (Gueudet, 2007), but also strategies and resources to solve problems that require more than the use of rules or formulae.

Many practicing teachers, for different reasons, have not learned some of the content they are now required to teach, or they have not learned it in ways that enable them to teach what is now required. ... Teachers need support if the goal of mathematical proficiency for all is to be reached. The demands this makes on teacher educators and the enterprise of teacher education are substantial, and often under-appreciated (Adler, et al., 2005, p. 361).

Davis and Simmt (2006) suggest that teachers' preparation programs should focus more on candidates' construction of mathematical ideas or relations to appreciate their connections and interpretations, and the use of various types of arguments to validate and support those relations, rather than the study of formal mathematics courses. Thus, the context to build up their mathematical knowledge should be related to the needs associated with their instructional practices, that is mathematical knowledge for teaching. "... [mathematical knowledge] needed for teaching is not a watered version of formal mathematics, but a serious and demanding area of mathematical work" (Davis & Simmt, 2006, p. 295).

Thus, teachers' mathematical knowledge for teaching can be constructed, revised, and enhanced within an interacting intellectual community that fosters an inquisitive approach to develop mathematical ideas and promotes problem-solving activities. All participants while working within this community recognize that learning mathematics is a process that takes place over time where they need to be directly engaged in sense-making activities and repeated experiences. That is, teachers need to work on mathematical tasks as members of a community that values and takes into account the participation of all members.

Learning mathematics involves long-term conceptual development, advances in abstract understanding, and improved applicability. Learning does not take place solely through learners observing some patterns in their work, even if they have generalized them explicitly. Indeed, pattern-spotting, generalizing, and reproducing patterns are merely ways in which sensate beings make sense of any succession of experiences. ... But experiences [that takes place through such engagement] might contribute to progression in understanding a particular concept (Watson & Mason, 2006, pp. 92-93).

Thus, it is central for the interactive community to promote a collaborative environment that helps examine mathematics tasks to guide or orient teachers' instructional practices. The National Research Council (1996) recognizes that inquiry plays an important role in students' learning, stating that an inquiring process involves the identification of assumptions, the critical examination of relations, and the search of explanations. Teachers and students understand and construct mathematical knowledge through an inquiring activity in which they engage in mathematical discussions, pose questions to formulate conjectures that are examined or pursued in terms of mathematical resources available, and known or discovered strategies. Under this scheme they search for different arguments to support and validate conjectures. This process demands that teachers and students alike reflect on ways to access and use their mathematical knowledge in order to make sense of situations and to solve novel problems. In 2009, the National Council of Teachers of Mathematics (NCTM) proposed that high school curricula could be structured around problem-solving activities that focus on making sense and mathematical reasoning. Thus, a key aspect in an inquiry or inquisitive approach is that it should help learners structure and organize their knowledge in terms of a web of knowledge, and skills that enables them to solve problems or learn new ideas by connecting them to what they already know.

Teachers need to interact within a community that supports and provides them with important mathematical and pedagogical elements. During the process of organizing their lessons, it is crucial for them to share and discuss their ideas openly, to understand the ideas of others in the group that could emerge while working on the tasks.

MATHEMATICAL PROBLEM SOLVING AND THE USE OF COMPUTATIONAL TOOLS

The conceptual support of a problem-solving approach relies on recognizing that teachers' development of mathematical teaching knowledge could be promoted within an intellectual community that fosters an inquiring or inquisitive approach to mathematical tasks or activities. Tasks are considered a key component in promoting students' construction of conceptual webs or networks, and developing a set of flexible strategies to be engaged in problem-solving behaviors. Gueudet (2007) stated that: "Grounding a teaching design [focusing on knowledge organization and the development of different forms of problem solving strategies] should comprise a variety of tasks, allowing development of different solutions, in order to foster a form of students' mathematical autonomy ... Working with technological devices such as dynamic geometry environments, but also computer algebra systems ... can be helpful in fostering flexibility" (p. 242). Learning mathematics and developing mathematical knowledge are processes that can be framed in terms of a set of dilemmas or problems that need to be represented, explored, and solved through the use of mathematical content or resources. Thus, a learning approach based on an inquiring process means for students to formulate questions, to identify and investigate dilemmas, to search for evidences or information, to discuss solutions, and to present or communicate the results (Santos-Trigo, 2007). It means willingness to wonder, to pose and examine questions, and to develop mathematical understanding within a community that values both collaboration and constant reflection. A mode of inquiry involves challenging the *status quo,* and it demands a continuous reconceptualization of what is learned and how knowledge is constructed. Jaworski (2006) stated that "[in a community of inquiry] participants grow into and contribute to continual reconstitution of the community through critical reflection; inquiry is developed as one of the forms of practice within the community and individual identity develops through reflective inquiry" (p. 202). Working within a community offers opportunities to search for a variety of ways to approach the tasks, as well as to identify, extend, and connect relevant mathematical concepts and problem-solving strategies that can orient teachers' instructional practices. This process also can be used as a vehicle to construct new relations or to identify new routes to reach or reconstruct classic mathematics results (Santos-Trigo, 2008). This type of teachers' interaction moreover becomes relevant to foster and develop a problem-solving approach that involves:

Seeing the mathematical content in mathematically unsophisticated questions, seeing underlying similarity of structure in apparently different problems, facility in drawing on different mathematical representations of a problem, communicating mathematics meaningfully to diverse audiences, facility in selecting and using appropriate modes of analysis ("mental", paper and pencil, or technological), and willingness to keep learning new material and techniques (Cohen, 2001, p. 986).

Finally, the use of computational tools represents an opportunity for the community to discuss mathematical tasks from perspectives where visual and computational approaches can be enhanced and naturally pursued. As a consequence, the use of the tools not only increases the opportunities for the participants to employ their experience and knowledge in order to examine the task; but also to participate in constructive discussions and to contrast the mathematical qualities of the emerging approaches to solve the tasks. The use of computational technologies offers teachers and students the opportunity to participate in activities for:

... (a) gaining insight and intuition, (b) discovering new patterns and relationships, (c) graphing to

expose mathematical principles, (d) testing and especially falsifying conjectures, (e) exploring a possible result to see whether it merits formal proof, (f) suggesting approaches for formal proof, (g) replacing lengthy hand derivations with tool computations, and (h) confirming analytically derived results (Borwein & Bailey, 2003, cited in Zbiek, Heid, & Blume, 2007, p. 1170).

Thus, common approaches based on paper and pencil environments can be enhanced widely with the use of technological tools. For instance, a dynamic software can allow the problem solvers to represent and solve problems dynamically; the controlled motion of figures (dragging) facilitates and help teachers and students recognize and explore mathematical relations within a geometrical configuration. Artigue (2010, p. 471) recognizes that "the technology itself offers now new and powerful tools for supporting and accompanying the professional development of teachers".

The use of computational tools becomes important for the community not only to identify and explore mathematical results, but also to discuss pedagogical paths associated with the construction of potential instructional routes that can be useful for teachers to guide and orient their instructional practices. Sacristan, et, al. (2010) discussed ways to use digital technologies to deal with mathematical tasks in order to promote teachers and students' development of mathematical thinking.

When teachers select or design tasks or activities to foster students' mathematical thinking development, they should be planning and visualizing what their students might do while working on the tasks. Watson & Mason (2006, p. 93) stated that "[t]o a certain extent, any lesson plan involves an implicit, if not explicit, sense of possible experiences that it is to be hoped each learner will transform into a personal learning trajectory". Problem-solving episodes emerged during the process of dealing with tasks or problematic situations. The example used to illustrate the community's work is representative of the types of tasks discussed during the problem-solving sessions held periodically. The community worked on three-hour weekly sessions during one semester. The community's members included one mathematician, two mathematics educators, three doctoral students in mathematics education, and three high school teachers; however, the unit of analysis was taken as the community itself. In general, the problems came from textbooks, research projects or studies, and tasks that involved problem formulation.

THE TASK

A square piece of paper ABCD with side l, is white on the front and blue on the back. The corner A is folded over to point A' which lies on the diagonal AC (Figure 1). Where should point A' be located on the diagonal (or how far is A' from the folding line) in order to have the total visible area, ½ blue and ½ white? (Based on Carlson & Bloom, 2005, p. 71).

A dynamic software (Cabri-Geometry) and a hand-held calculator (Voyage, 200) were used to work on this problem. The community addressed and discussed relevant mathematical features as it became involved in problem-solving activities to approach the task. Thus, the goal is not to analyze the individual approach of the participants,

Figure 1. How far should A' be from the folding line to have the total area half blue and half white?

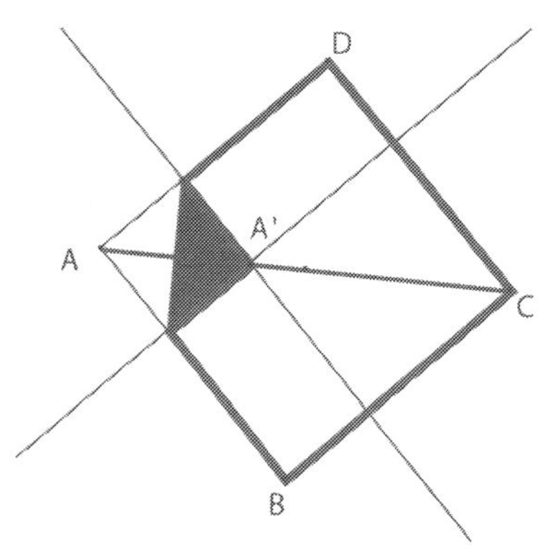

but to focus on describing behaviors that the community exhibited as a whole. The solution process is structured in episodes that distinguish key principles associated with finding solutions (Santos-Trigo & Camacho; 2009). Each episode posed and pursued set of questions during the problem-solving phases.

First Episode: An Overarching Inquisitive Principle

The core aspect in this approach is to conceptualize and examine the content of the problem (definition, theorem, etc.) in terms of questions or dilemmas that need to be explored. An overarching principle that permeates the entire problem-solving process is that teachers and students should transform the problem statement into a set of meaningful questions to be examined. Thus, the community's initial goal was to problematize the activity by identifying relevant information in the statement of the problem to explore and to make sense of the situation. Sense-making activities involve the identification and representation of mathematical objects to observe relations or patterns that are then explored. This involves quantifying and operating invariance within a mathematical system. The questions that emerged at this stage aimed at clarifying the information given in the problem statement: What are the relevant properties of a square? What does it mean to fold a vertex over to a point on the diagonal? And this also involves questions that examine figures' properties: What properties does the folding line hold? What figures are formed in blue and white colors? What happens to both areas when point A' is close to point A or close to point C? What type of triangle is formed (blue region) when point A is reflected with respect to the folding line to determine A'? How can we calculate the areas of the blue and white regions?

These and similar questions led the community to the construction of a dynamic representation of the task. This became relevant to recognize key geometric properties and relations that were later justified:

1. Triangle PA'Q is an isosceles right triangle, because a circle with centre M (the intersection point between the folding line and diagonal AC) and radius MA' passes through points A, P, A', and Q. That is, APA'Q is a square (Figure 2).
2. When point A' moves away from A the area of triangle PA'Q increases while the area of PBCDQA' decreases. The area of triangle PA'Q is visually less than the area of PBCDQA' for certain positions of A' and for other positions the opposite behavior is observed.
3. How do the areas of triangle PA'Q and the polygon PBCDQA' change when point A' is moved along diagonal AC? Is there any way to quantify and record the areas variation? Software allowed the participants to represent the area variation of both figures graphically and to identify the position of point A' where both triangle PA'Q and polygon PBCDQA' have the same area or are very close to have equal areas (Figure 3). Here, the participants observed that when point A and A' coincided, the area of the blue region was zero while the area of white region was the area of the original square.

Commentary

Two issues were stressed during this problem-solving phase: (a) the participants recognized the need of spending time to make sense of the problem statement before becoming engaged in a particular way of solving it. It was relevant for the community to clarify what the task involved and what the problem was; and that (b) they recognized that sense construction activities can be organized in terms of questioning and exploring the information embedded in the problem statement. In this process, the identification of relevant geometric properties associated with the task helped them construct a dynamic representation that was crucial to visualize a solution to the problem. This represented (Figure 3) the departure point to look for other approaches.

Second Episode: An Exploration Principle

The identification of possible routes to solve the task algebraically followed naturally from the comprehension of the problem statement. The participants recognized that the graphic approach achieved with the software provided an approximate solution to the problem. To approach this new task, they focused on ways to formally express the area behaviors. Again, the formulation of questions functioned as a key aspect to organize the activities associated with the exploration phase.

Figure 2. APA'Q is a square

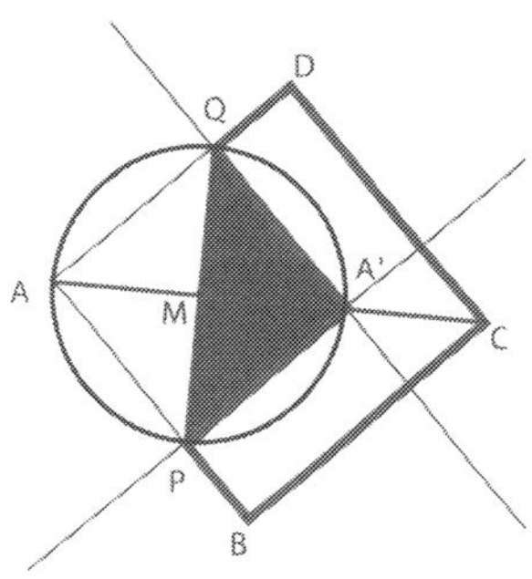

How can the area of both figures be represented algebraically? Based on figure 4, they observed that the area of square APA'Q can be expressed as x^2 and the area of square ABCD as l^2 and with this information, the triangle PA'Q and the polygon's (PBCDQ) areas are $\frac{x^2}{2}$, and l^2-x^2, respectively. Thus, they agreed that general solution could be obtained when $l^2 - x^2 = \frac{x^2}{2}$.

How is the equation ($l^2 - x^2 = \frac{x^2}{2}$) that represents the general solution related to the previous graphic solution (Figure 3)? This question led the participants to observe that in the graphic solution the value of l was 4.01 cm (side of square ABCD). They subsequently graphed both algebraic representations of the area, using a hand-held calculator to obtain the intersection point (Figure 5), represented by the coordinates of point A' where both areas are equal. That is, when the side x of triangle PA'Q is equal to 3.27415 cm the area of both regions is 5.36003 cm^2.

Figure 3. At what position of A' do triangle PA'Q, and polygon PBCDQA' have the same area?

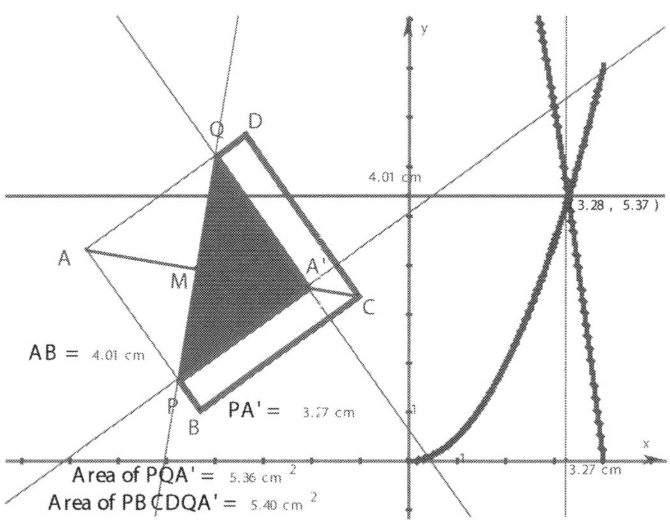

With the use of a hand-held graphing calculator, it was also possible to find the algebraic value of x in which both areas are the same. This value was obtained by solving the equation that resulted from equating the two area expressions. That is, solving $l^2 - x^2 = \frac{x^2}{2}$, leads to that $x = \frac{\sqrt{6}}{3}l$, and $x_2 = \frac{-\sqrt{6}}{3}l$ (Figure 6).

Hence, the participants observed that when the side of the square PA'QA is $x = \frac{\sqrt{6}}{3}l$, the area value of triangle PA'Q and the polygon PBCDQA' will be $\frac{6l^2}{18}$ or $\frac{l^2}{3}$. For the dynamic approach (Figure 3) the side of square ABCD is 4.01 cm and by taking this value, $x = \frac{\sqrt{6} \times 4.01}{3} = 3.2745$, and the corresponding area of both regions will be 5.36 cm^2. It was emphasized that the position

Figure 4. Representing the area of both regions (blue & white) algebraically

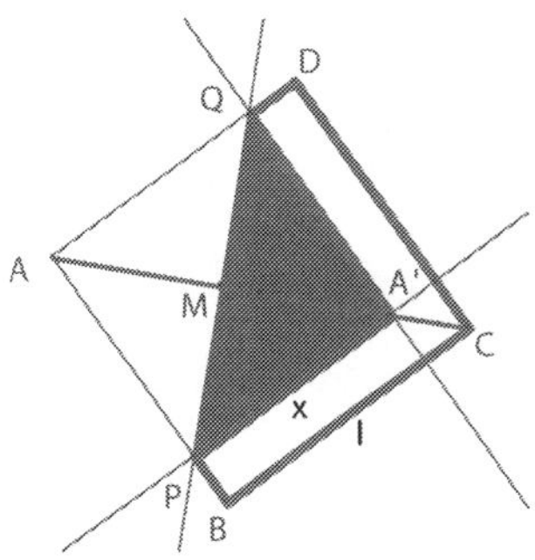

of point A' obtained through the use of dynamic software (Figure 3) was relatively close to the obtained value through the substitution of the value of 4.01 (side of the square) into the algebraic expression ($x = \frac{\sqrt{6}}{3}l$). Each tool clearly offered the participants different paths to think of the solution and, as a consequence, they used distinct strategies and resources to extend the problem's domain of analysis.

Commentary

The exploration phase focused on an algebraic representation of the area variation of the two polygons that appeared as a result of moving point A'. By denoting the side of triangle PA'Q as x, all the calculations involved while comparing both expressions could be simplified since both the blue and white areas were expressed in terms of variable x. Here, they recognized that the construction of the algebraic model of the area variation required symbolically identifying a variable to determine such model; while for the dynamic approach (Figure 3) it was only necessary to identify both polygons and the software made the corresponding calculations to graph their areas. In addition, the algebraic approach represented a general case while the dynamic approach represented a case for specific value of the side of the square.

Figure 5. Representing the graphics of both areas with the use of a hand-calculator

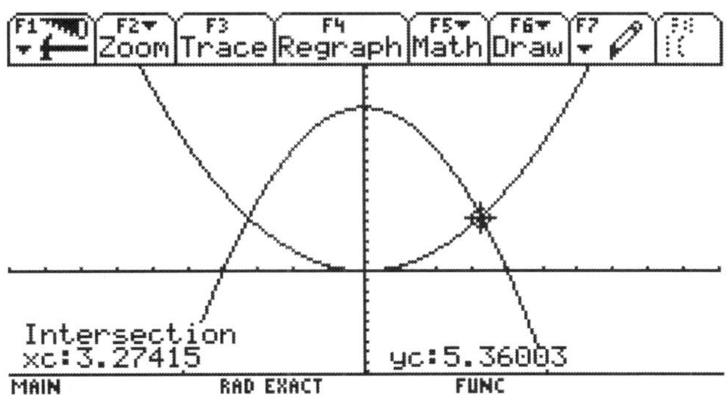

Figure 6. Solving the area equations

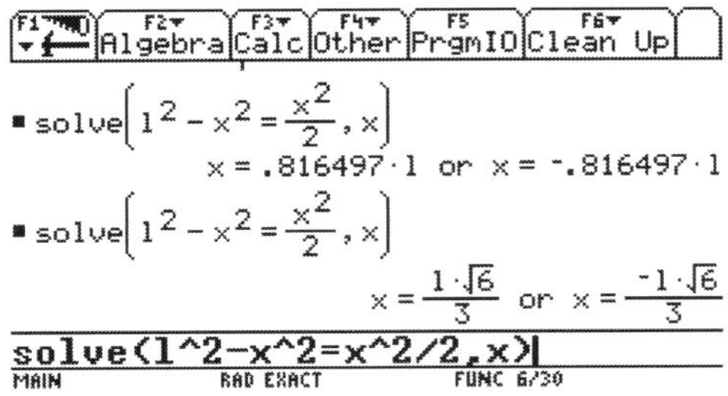

Third Episode: The Principle of Extension And Generalization

The participants asked whether the methods used to compare the area variation for the square could be extended to the case of a rectangle. They recognized that in the process of solving a problem or understanding a mathematical concept or idea it is always important to reflect on the scope of the solution or application of that concept. That is, this principle emphasizes the need for the problem solver to reflect on the range of application of the solutions methods or domain of the concept being studied.

The initial problem involved a square and at this stage, it was interesting to explore the case in which the figure was a rectangle: A piece of paper white on the front and blue on the reverse ABCD has sides a, b and $a \neq b$. As in the previous task, corner A is folded over to point A' which lies on the diagonal AC (Figure 7). Where should point A' be located on the diagonal (or how far is A' from the folding line) in order to have the total visible area, ½ blue and ½ white?

Again, the software was useful to represent and explore how the area of both polygons changed while moving point A' along segment AC. As in the previous approach, drawing the figure required the participants to think of the mathematical properties that would be relevant to represent the problem. For instance, they observed that when point A' is close to point A the blue region is a triangle; but at a certain position of A' the blue region becomes a quadrilateral (Figure 7). The construction of polygon PA'QR was based on observing that it represented a symmetric polygon of APRD with respect to line PR. That is, it holds the following properties:

Figure 7. Given a rectangle ABCE; where should point A' (on the diagonal AC) be located to have the area of PA'QR equals to the area of PBCLA'?

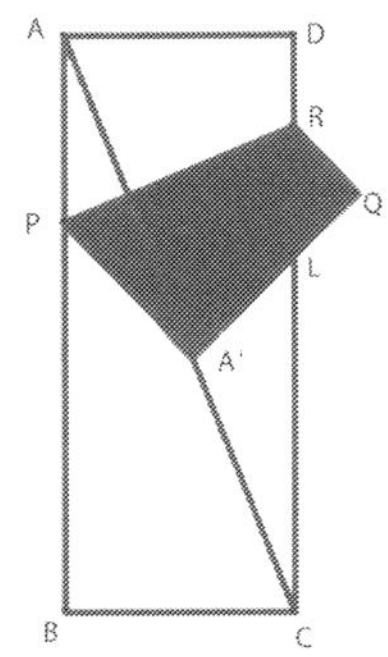

a. Point P must be on the perpendicular bisector of segment AA';
b. Angle PA'Q must be a right angle;
c. Segment A'Q needs to be the same as side AD and;
d. Angle A'QR must also be a right angle.

Again, with the help of the software it was possible to graphically examine the area changes of polygons PA'QR and PBCLA' for different positions of point A'. To determine the position of point A' in terms of the length of side BC, the participants drew a perpendicular line to side BC that passes through point A' and this perpendicular intersects side BC at point N'. Figure 8 shows that when d(B,N') was 2.88 cm, then the areas of polygons PA'QR and PBCLA' were approximately equal. The area variation could also be graphically represented, and with the use of the software the expression of the graphic representations could also be determined.

The participants observed that when point A' is moved along the segment AC, there is a posi-

Figure 8. Numeric and graphic representations of the area changes

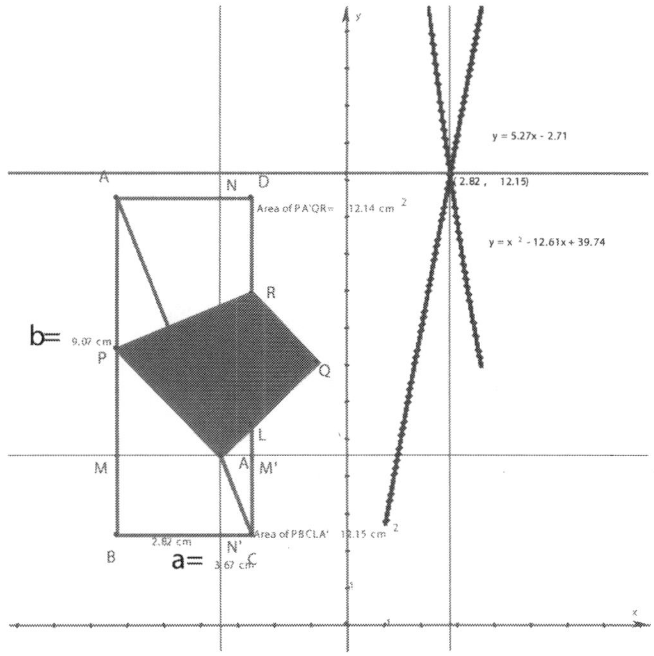

tion for A' in which the folding figure changes from a triangle to a quadrilateral. At this point the folding line (the perpendicular bisector of segment AA') will pass through vertex D (figure 7). To determine the coordinates of point A' at which the folding figure changes from a triangle to a quadrilateral, they first found the coordinates of point S which is the intersection of segment DP and diagonal AC (figure 9). In this process, the participants relied on the use a Cartesian system (an important heuristic) to find the equations of lines AC and PR. In this case they also set point B as the origin of the Cartesian system.

Then the equations were $y = \frac{a}{b}(x - a) + b$, and $y = \frac{-b}{a}x + b$ respectively. By solving these two equations they determined that the x-coordinates of point S was $\frac{a^3}{a^2 + b^2}$. Since the point S was the midpoint of AA' then the x-coordinates of point A' became $\frac{2a^3}{a^2 + b^2}$.

Figure 9. A coordinate system to determine the coordinates of point S when PD is the perpendicular bisector of segment AA'

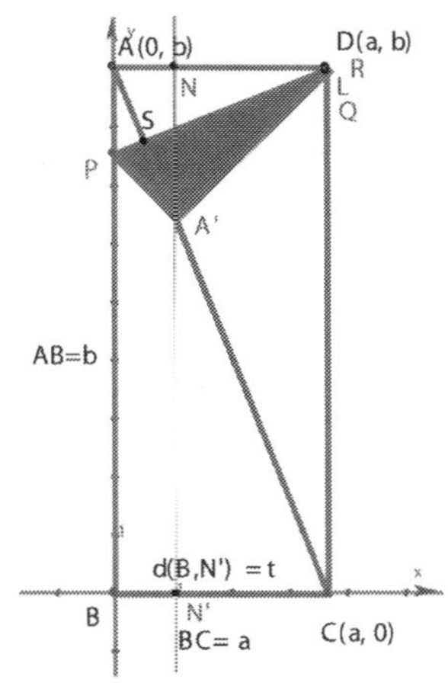

The Method's Domain

Questions emerged while working on the rectangle case: Can the method of solution be applied to all types of rectangles? Or does it always happen that the comparison of the area variation involves a quadrilateral (blue region) and a five sided polygon (white region)? The participants agreed that answering these questions is the same as answering this one: What type of relationship should sides *a* and *b* satisfy, so that the maximum area of triangle PB'D is less than the area of polygon BPA'DC? (Figure, 10).

To respond to the latter question, the participants initially found the maximum area of triangle PDA' in terms of sides *a* and *b*. They observed that the equation of line DS is $y = \frac{a}{b}(x - a) + b$, then P has coordinates $\left(0, \frac{b^2 - a^2}{b}\right)$. Therefore d(AP) $= \frac{a^2}{b}$, and the area of triangle PA'D is $\frac{a^3}{2b}$. Similarly, the area of polygon BPA'DC is $ab - \frac{a^3}{b}$. For which values of *a* and *b*, we have $ab - \frac{a^3}{b} > \frac{a^3}{2b}$? $ab - \frac{a^3}{b} > \frac{a^3}{2b}$ when $ab > \frac{3a^3}{2b}$, that is when $b^2 > \frac{3a^2}{2}$. Therefore, the expression $ab - \frac{a^3}{b} > \frac{a^3}{2b}$ holds only when $b > \sqrt{\frac{3}{2}}a$.

Figure 10. For which values of a and b the maximum area of triangle PA'D is less than the area of polygon BPA'DC?

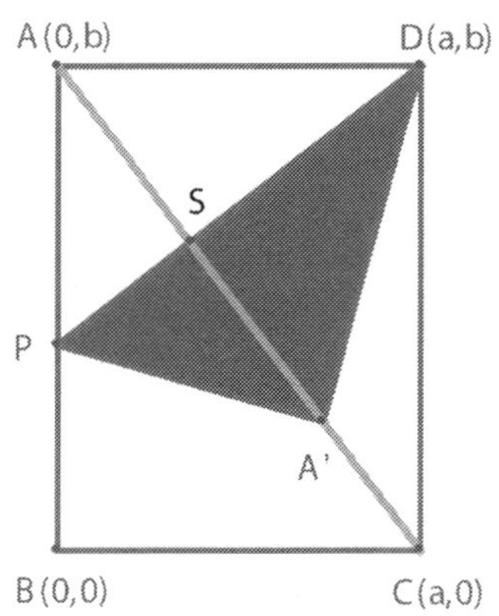

Another Connection

The dynamic representation of the problem generates other mathematical relations. For example, on figure 11 point S is the intersection point of lines PR and NN'. The participants posed the question: What is the locus of point S when point C is moved along line BC? It was observed that the locus is a parabola with focus point A and as the directrix the perpendicular line to line AB that passes through point A' (Figure 11).

Fourth Episode: Reflection Principle

Participants generally recognized that a problem-solving approach for learning mathematics involves the construction of mathematical representations of contents, situations or problems with the purpose of finding and exploring mathematical relations. In this process, any mathematical statement (problem, definition, proposition, or content) is conceptualized as a departure point for teachers, students, or problem solvers in general from which they can search for different ways to comprehend the situation or problem, and to always search for various ways of solving and extending a problem (Polya, 1945).

The community therefore had the opportunity of discussing mathematical strengths and limitations of resources, and strategies used to make sense and solve the problems. For instance, in dealing with the rectangle problem, the participants could reflect on whether the methods used to solve the square problem could be transferred and applied to this case. In addition, it was also important to reflect on the strengths provided by each tool (dynamic software or hand-held calculators) to represent and explore the problem in terms of visual, geometric, and algebraic approaches.

Participants also discussed the extent to which the set of problem-solving episodes represented an instrument that could be utilized to frame and approach other related problems. The graphic representation of area variation (Figures 3 and 5) served as a means to discuss issues that involved visually explaining optimization phenomena; while the algebraic approach represented an efficient method to analytically examine those phenomena. The general case, represented through the algebraic model, was also used to verify results obtained with the use of dynamic software; that is, the model became a tool to discuss the plausibility of the solution achieved through the use of the software.

Features of Possible Instructional Routes

The principles exhibited through these problem-solving episodes proved central to discussing possible routes to frame mathematical instruction. The community's participants asserted that there are some aspects of mathematical practices that are relevant and must be included and promoted in their instructional practices. Some of these represent practical applications of these problem-solving principles to instruction:

a. Learning activities should be structured around **an inquiring** or inquisitive approach where all the students have the opportunity to formulate and pursue question to examine, and make sense of problems or mathematical situations. For example, during the solution process of the task, it was important for the participants to initially be engaged into a scrutiny phase (through questions) to make sense of the problem statement. This phase became crucial in order to recognize relevant properties that were useful to mathematically represent the task.

b. It is an essential activity for students to **search for** diverse and multiple ways to represent and solve the task. Representing the task in different ways can offer students the opportunity to utilize distinct resources and strategies to identify and explore mathematical relations. For instance, the visual approach to the problem became relevant to identify ways in which both areas varied. The visual approach was later contrasted with the algebraic model. This model required symbolically expressing the areas.

c. **Extension and generalization** are problem solving activities that aim to evaluate the domain of the methods used to approach the tasks, and explore related connections. For example, the case of the rectangle was a natural extension to be analyzed in terms

Figure 11. What is the locus of point S when point C is moved along line BC?

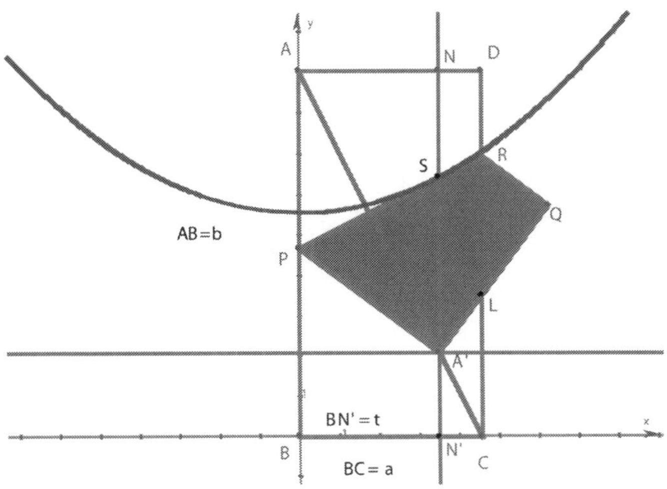

of the methods used to explore the square. It became important to examine the application range of the method used. For instance, it was necessary to find and evaluate the relation between the side of the rectangle, and the area variation of the both regions in order to identify the domain of application of the solution method.

d. **The use of computational tools** can offer students distinct routes to represent and explore mathematical relations. For example, the dynamic representation of the task becomes a powerful tool to visually examine area variation. Indeed, this dynamic approach led the participants to identify (without algebraic resources) an approximate solution. In addition, moving elements within the dynamic representation helped identify other relations or loci of particular objects; that is, dynamic representations are an opportunity for students to identify, quantify, and explore the variations in behaviors of particular elements of that configuration.

e. **In-depth study** of mathematical concepts that appear in problem-solving activities can be approached in terms of constructing a network of relations and meanings. For instance, the initial aim of identifying a point on the square's diagonal to have equal areas of the blue and white regions generated a series of questions that helped identify a web between concepts and problem solving strategies. The proper use of mathematical notation and the Cartesian system were useful strategies to simplify the problem's algebraic model. In addition, mathematical properties associated with objects (perpendicular bisector, isosceles triangles, area of square, equations solution, variation, function domain, etc.) and strategies (analyzing particular cases, looking for patterns, representing mathematical objects dynamically, etc.) were important to identify different ways to solve and extend the task.

FINAL REMARKS

Throughout this chapter I have argued that practicing, or inservice teachers, need to constantly revise both their mathematical and pedagogical knowledge for teaching. The developments in mathematics education need to be organized and structured in ways that can help teachers orient and frame their practices (Silverman & Thompson, 2008). Working on mathematical tasks within a community (formed by mathematics educators, mathematicians, and teachers), fosters the participation of its members that seems to offer the proper conditions to illustrate and practice values associated with the development or reconstruction of mathematical knowledge. In the task discussed in this paper, the use of computational tools offers teachers and students the possibility of identifying possible didactical paths to frame their instructional approaches (Simon, 2006). For example, each problem-solving episode exhibited during the solution process characterizes particular goals that involve thinking of the need for representing mathematical statements or problems in diverse ways, the need to think of various ways of approaching a task, the relevance of searching for generalizations or problem extensions, and the importance of reflecting on the extent to which the emerging methods can be adjusted and used to deal with other problems or situations. In particular, the use of computational tools offers the student the possibility of exploring the task from perspectives that include visual, graphic, numeric, and algebraic approaches. They could have the opportunity of constructing some basic mathematical results through a route that can complement those approaches based only on paper and pencil approaches.

Ways of representing and dealing with mathematical task are influenced and shaped by the use of tools (Hoyles & Lagrange, 2010). Each offers distinct opportunities for students to represent and explore the problems. Students therefore should be encouraged to use various tools, and to reflect on the strengths and limitations that each tool might offer. In summary, to make school learning experiences significant for students, teachers should reflect on potential learning routes to guide their students' development of mathematical knowledge (Sacristan, et al., 2010). That route might involve starting to construct a dynamic problem representation to identify relations or possible ways of solutions, and later to search for algebraic representations of the problem to identify and explore patterns involved in the solution process. The search for connections or extensions of the initial problem is also an important problem stage that students need to consider. Based on this information, instructors can think of and structure a plan to guide and monitor their students' development of problem solving strategies and mathematics knowledge.

ACKNOWLEDGMENT

The author acknowledges the support received from Conacyt, through projects with reference #47850 and 80359.

REFERENCES

Adler, J., Ball, D., Krainer, K., Fou-Lai, L., & Novotna, J. (2005). Reflections on an emerging field: Researching mathematics teacher education. *Educational Studies in Mathematics*, *60*, 359–381. doi:10.1007/s10649-005-5072-6

Artigue, M. (2010). The future of teaching and learning mathematics with digital technologies. In Hoyles, C., & Lagrange, J. (Eds.), *Mathematics education and technology-rethinking the terrain. The 17th ICMI Study* (pp. 463–476). New York: Springer.

Carlson, M. P., & Bloom, I. (2005). The cyclic nature of problem solving: An emergent multidimensional problem-solving framework. *Educational Studies in Mathematics*, *58*, 45–75. doi:10.1007/s10649-005-0808-x

Cohen, A. (2001). Two reactions to the mathematical education of teachers. *Notices of the AMS*, 985-991.

Davis, B., & Simmt, E. (2006). Mathematics-for-teaching: An ongoing investigation of the mathematics that teachers (need) to know. *Educational Studies in Mathematics*, *61*(3), 293–319. doi:10.1007/s10649-006-2372-4

Gueudet, G. (2007). Investigating the secondary-tertiary transition. *Educational Studies in Mathematics*, *67*, 237–254. doi:10.1007/s10649-007-9100-6

Hill, H. C., Blunk, M. L., Charalambous, C. Y., Lewis, J. M., Phelps, G. C., Sleep, L., & Ball, D. L. (2008). Mathematical knowledge for teaching and the mathematical quality of instruction: An exploratory study. *Cognition and Instruction*, *26*(4), 430–511. doi:10.1080/07370000802177235

Hoyles, C., & Lagrange, J. (2010) (Eds.). Mathematics education and technology-rethinking the terrain. The 17th ICMI Study. New York: Springer.

Jaworski, B. (2006). Theory and practice in mathematics teaching development: Critical inquiry as a mode of learning in teaching. *Journal of Mathematics Teacher Education*, *9*(2), 187–211. doi:10.1007/s10857-005-1223-z

Lesh, R., & Zawojewski, J. S. (2007). Problem solving and modeling. In F. K. Lester, Jr. (Ed.). The Second Handbook of Research on Mathematics Teaching and Learning (pp. 763-804). National Council of Teachers of Mathematics. Charlotte, NC: Information Age Publishing.

National Council of Teachers of Mathematics (NCTM). (2000). *Principles and standards for school mathematics*. Reston, VA: The Council.

National Research Council (NRC). (1996). *National science education standards*. Washington, DC: National Academic Press.

National Research Council (NRC). (2001). Adding it up: Helping children to learn mathematics. (J. Kilpatrick, J. Swafford, & B. Findell, Eds.). Mathematical Learning Study Committee, Center for Education, Division of Behavioral and Social Sciences and Education. Washington, DC: National Academic Press.

NCTM. (2009). *Focus on high school mathematics: Reasoning and sense making*. Reston, VA: The Council.

Polya, G. (1945). *How to solve it*. Princeton, NJ: Princeton University Press.

Sacristan, A. I., Calder, N., Rojano, T., Santos-Trigo, M., Friedlander, A., & Meissner, H. (2010). The influence and shaping of digital technologies on the learning –and learning trajectories- of mathematical concepts. In Hoyles, C., & Lagrange, J. (Eds.), *Mathematics education and technology-rethinking the terrain. The 17th ICMI Study* (pp. 179–226). New York: Springer.

Santos-Trigo, M. (2007). Mathematical problem solving: An evolving research and practice domain. *ZDM - The International Journal on Mathematics Education*, 523-536.

Santos-Trigo, M. (2008). On the use of technology to represent and explore mathematical objects or problems dynamically. *Mathematics and Computer Education Journal*, *42*(2), 123–139.

Santos-Trigo, M., & Camacho, M. (2009). Towards the construction of a Framework to deal with routine problems to foster mathematical inquiry. *PRIMUS: Problems, Resources, and Issues in Mathematics Undergraduate Studies Journal*, *19*(3), 260–279.

Schoenfeld, A. H. (1985). *Mathematical Problem Solving*. New York: Academic Press.

Schoenfeld, A. H. (1992). Learning to think mathematically: Problem solving, metacognition, and sense making in mathematics. In Grows, D. A. (Ed.), *Handbook of Research on Mathematics Teaching and Learning* (pp. 334–370). NY: Macmillan.

Silverman, J., & Thompson, P. W. (2008). Toward a framework for the development of mathematical knowledge for teaching. *Journal of Mathematics Teacher Education*, *11*, 499–511. doi:10.1007/s10857-008-9089-5

Simon, M. (2006). Key developmental understandings in mathematics: A direction for investigating and establishing learning goals. *Mathematical Thinking and Learning*, *8*(4), 359–371. doi:10.1207/s15327833mtl0804_1

Sowder, J. T. (2007). The mathematical education and development of teachers. In F. K. Lester, Jr. (Ed.), Second Handbook of Research on Mathematics Teaching and Learning (pp. 157-223). The National Council of Teachers of Mathematics. Charlotte, NC: Information Age Publishing.

Spillane, J. P. (2000). Cognition and policy implementation: District policy makers and the reform of mathematics education. *Cognition and Instruction*, *18*(2), 141–179. doi:10.1207/S1532690XCI1802_01

Törner, G., Schoenfeld, A. H., & Reiss, K. M. (2007). Problem solving around the World: Summing up the state of the art. *ZDM Mathematics Education*, *39*(5-6), 353. doi:10.1007/s11858-007-0053-0

Watson, A., & Mason, J. (2006). Seeing an exercise as a single mathematical object: Using variation to structure sense-making. *Mathematical Thinking and Learning*, *8*(2), 91–111. doi:10.1207/s15327833mtl0802_1

Zbiek, R. M., Heid, M. K., & Blume, G. W. (2007). Research on technology in mathematics education. In Lester, F. K. Jr., (Ed.), *Second handbook of research on mathematics teaching and learning* (pp. 1169–1207). Charlotte, NC: Information Age Publishing.

Chapter 18
Web 2.0 Tools in Social Studies Methods

Adam M. Friedman
Wake Forest University, USA

Tina L. Heafner
University of North Carolina at Charlotte, USA

ABSTRACT

This chapter presents the theory and literature behind the integration of technology, particularly the Internet, in social studies teacher education. The authors have spent significant time studying the impact of technology in the K-12 social studies environment; the results of this research are summarized in the chapter and serve as a backbone for how technology is integrated into our teaching methodology courses with the context of preparing future teachers to utilize technology as a tool to enhance content, student learning experiences, and academic achievement of their future students. Specifically, we focus on three Web 2.0 tools; blogs, wikis, and podcasts. Specific examples, vignettes, practical applications for methods instructors, and directions for the future are provided.

INTRODUCTION

The National Council for the Social Studies (NCSS) (1994) defines social studies as

...the integrated study of the social sciences and humanities to promote civic competence. Within the school program, social studies provides coordinated, systematic study drawing upon such disciplines as anthropology, archaeology, economics, geography, history, law, philosophy, political science, psychology, religion, and sociology, as well as appropriate content from the humanities, mathematics, and natural sciences. The primary purpose of social studies is to help young people develop the ability to make informed and reasoned decisions for the public good as citizens of a culturally diverse, democratic society in an interdependent world (p. 3).

On the surface, this definition gives credence to the wide variety of subject matter inherent in social studies, while simultaneously describing the purpose of teaching social studies. Upon closer scrutiny, in

DOI: 10.4018/978-1-61520-897-5.ch018

Copyright © 2010, IGI Global. Copying or distributing in print or electronic forms without written permission of IGI Global is prohibited.

order for the purpose of social studies to come to fruition, students must engage in higher-level thinking, in which they evaluate evidence, consider different perspectives, and draw their own conclusions. Accordingly, this type of discourse is precisely what is advocated in terms of student engagement by several organizations whose primary focus is on social studies education. For example, the National Center for History in the Schools calls upon students "to go beyond the facts presented in their textbooks and examine the historical record for themselves" (online) and the Center for Civic Education (1994) extols the importance of students being able to "evaluate, take, and defend positions about" a myriad of issues. Regardless of the specific social studies subject (history, political science, geography, economics), the design of instruction in which students are asked to do more than simply recall facts is imperative if the higher-level thinking goals are to be accomplished.

Various descriptions of best practices notwithstanding, social studies has a stereotypical reputation of being taught as a teacher-centered, dry subject in which a teacher, through a lecture and notes, is the disseminator of knowledge and the students are resigned to absorb it. This approach, in which students recall basic facts, and rarely if ever engage in higher-order thinking, has been described in books such as Goodlad's (1984)*A Place Called School*, and perpetuated in popular culture through movies like *Ferris Bueller's Day Off*. Oftentimes exacerbating this dilemma are end-of-course standardized examinations, which are in place in a plethora of social studies courses, and are themselves generally at a lower level of Bloom's Taxonomy (Pahl, 2003). Meier (2002) notes that these examinations can influence pedagogy, as teachers may "teach to the test" (p. 195). Further, Friedman, in his 2006 study of world history and world geography teachers, found that an end-of-course test had a negative impact on their predilection to engage students in higher-order thinking using primary source documents, as teachers in this study felt a tremendous pressure to cover all of the requisite content.

Despite the reputation of social studies and the difficulties presented by standardized examinations, the use of technology in the social studies classroom can help to bring about change in the way social studies is taught and learned. However, it is first necessary to define what is meant by technology. As Martorella (1997) notes, the definition of technology is dependent on time and place, as technology is constantly and rapidly changing. In terms of teaching and learning social studies, a class of high school students working in their school's computer lab to access the National Archives in 1989 is surely an anachronism. Twenty years later, the Internet's presence in American public schools is as commonplace as chalkboards and desks (Parsad & Jones, 2005). Friedman and Hicks (2006) note that in the past century, "'State of the art technology' has evolved from motion pictures, to radio, television, microcomputers, educational software, and static Web pages to Internet sites that foster interaction and communication between students and teachers" (p. 248). For the purpose of this chapter, we define technology as interactive computer applications, particularly the Internet and Web 2.0 software, specifically weblogs (blogs), wikis, podcasts and digital image software.

The Internet and Teaching Social Studies

In terms of teaching social studies, the transcendence of the Internet has been a development of great magnitude, as it has made resources for teachers and students (such as tens of thousands of documents and images) widely and easily available (Cohen & Rosenzweig, 2006; VanFossen & Shiveley, 2000). This in turn has the potential to transform the traditional pedagogical practices of social studies teachers, as the vast resources that are available can engage students in material. It is therefore imperative that social studies teachers be trained to teach in a manner in which they learn to incorporate technology resources into their instruction.

There is a vast literature base that advocates for the use of technology (and the Internet in particular) within social studies. Braun and Risinger (1999) refer to it in epic terms, describing it as a "truly revolutionary development" in terms of its availability of resources (p. 7). The National Council for the Social Studies (1994; 2006) has continuously supported the use of technology within social studies, and this notion has been expounded upon by various social studies researchers, for an array of reasons. Hicks and Ewing (2003) posit that the abundance of resources can foster the consideration of multiple perspectives among students while Berson (2004) describes how digital images can similarly be used.

Technology's potential for introducing new modes of instruction notwithstanding, it is imperative to note Gentry's (1995) premonition that "Applications of technology should be selected and/or continued only after determination that desirable consequences outweigh undesirable consequences" (p. 7). Echoing this, at the turn of the twenty-first century, Mason, Berson, Diem, Hicks, Lee, and Dralle (2000) authored guidelines for technology use within social studies, particularly that they "caution…against using technology for technology's sake," and prior to using technology in the social studies classroom, instructors should "Consider if the technology is allowing [students] to learn in a way that they could without the technology" (p. 107-108). In its official technology position statement six years later, the National Council for the Social Studies (2006) gave further credence to this notion, putting forth that "technology should be thought of in terms of its effect on the teaching and learning of social studies, and should be considered for use only if it will provide an improvement in one (or both) of these areas" (online). An example of this can be seen in the construct of this chapter, as the emphasis is on social studies content, with technology being used as a support mechanism.

Along these same lines, it is not necessary to teach preservice teachers how to use technology per se, as knowledge of technology itself does not necessarily translate into effective social studies instruction. Rather, it is necessary for teachers to know how to teach with it. Further, with the exception of non-traditional students returning to college to earn a teaching license, today's preservice teachers are what Prensky (2001) refers to as "digital natives," who have grown up using technology applications (p. 1).

Social studies encompasses a wide range of subjects, from history, geography, sociology, civics/government, to economics; yet each lends itself to this methodology. This chapter is not a 'how to use' guide for different technology tools; as new technology tools that are faster and have greater memory evolve, this chapter would quickly become obsolete. Rather, the thrust of this chapter is the development, discussion, and specific examples of how instruction can be designed in which technology can be used to enhance social studies content. Because teacher education programs can be thought of as a 'gateway' to teaching, this chapter will address how we use technology within social studies teacher education. This use is informed by our research of its use in the secondary social studies environment, and with the context of preparing future teachers to utilize technology as a tool to enhance content. Specifically, we focus on three Web 2.0 tools; blogs, wikis, and podcasts.

Modeling of Technology

A void exists in the literature in exploring the ways in which preservice teachers are effectively taught within their pedagogical and content training to integrate technology for teaching and learning content which engenders an intrinsic value for future implementation with learners. Despite a decade of technology instruction within teacher preparation programs and professional development training, application of technology integration in educational settings is limited and fails to significantly change content teaching and learning (Angeli & Valanides, 2009; Hew & Brush, 2007). This is especially prevalent in the field of social studies (Akengin, 2008; Bolick, Berson, Coutts, & Heinecke, 2003). Teachers continue to express lack of knowledge and skills or uncertainty in using emerging technologies with students (Hew & Brush, 2007; Koehler, Mishra, & Yahya, 2007). Research suggests that improving teacher's applications of technology is connected to their level of competency and confidence in using technologies (Angeli, 2005; Krueger, Hansen, & Smaldino, 2000; Yildirim, 2000) and their preparation in technological pedagogical content knowledge (TPCK) (Angeli & Valanides, 2009; Mishra & Koehler, 2006). Mishra and Koehler (2006) define TPCK as teachers' understanding of how to use technology explicitly to support content understanding, awareness of the interconnectedness of technology, content, and pedagogy learning outcomes, and the necessity of content-embedded technology applications. Consequently, focusing on how teacher educators are using technology to transform their teaching with technology to create new opportunities for learning content and their approach to teaching teachers to use technology in a similar manner becomes essential (Angeli & Valanides, 2009).

Questions loom as to what teacher education programs are doing to address these needs and to explore effective strategies for promoting preservice teachers' use of technology for content instruction in future classrooms. Preparation gaps exist in programmatic structures where teacher candidates are exposed to a single course on instructional technology devoid of content-specific applications (Hew & Brush, 2007). Other programmatic approaches to technology instruction provide the smorgasbord of technology where pedagogical coursework only goes as far as introducing teacher candidates to various technologies available (Hew & Brush, 2007); again, technology training is not linked to content or student understanding of content. Researchers have addressed these issues and recommend multiple experiences in using content-based technology integration throughout teacher education coursework to increase teacher candidates' technological knowledge, skills, and efficacy (Angeli, 2005; Krueger, Hansen, & Smaldino, 2000; Luke, Moore, & Sawyer, 1998; Syh-Jong, 2008; Yildirim, 2000). However, exposure alone is not enough for teacher candidates to fully understand how technology effectively teaches content and to engender a commitment to using these strategies in their future subject area instruction.

Teacher candidates "must be trained in powerful learning environments where teaching is situated in real and authentic tasks," and in ways where they "constitute a part of a larger learning and professional community for the purpose of exchanging perspectives, resolving dilemmas, and confronting uncertainty in transforming classroom practices" (Angeli & Valanides, 2009, p. 166). Thus, researchers propose that higher education faculty must model authentic and frequent applications of technology with teacher education students by providing content-based learning experiences, exposure to real applications by subject area teachers in the field, and personal opportunities to utilize technologies to teach content in clinical experiences (Angeli, 2005; Angeli & Valanides, 2009; Brush & Saye, 2009; Luke, Moore, & Sawyer, 1998; Syh-Jong, 2008). Instructional modeling of technology applications becomes the foundation from which teacher education candidates draw upon for their uses of technology reinforcing the idea that teachers model the strategies they experience in their educational training (Lever-Duffy, McDonald, & Mizell, 2005). Consequently, teacher educators need to consistently model technology as an essential and innovative instructional tool for teaching content and provide authentic learner-centered applications within content (Angeli, 2005; Angeli & Valandies, 2009; Syh-Jong, 2008).

The importance of meaningful applications of content-based technologies pushes the role of the content methods course to the forefront of technological pedagogical content knowledge (TPCK) training (American Association of Colleges for Teacher Education, 2008). It is imperative that content-specific methods instructors model effective uses of technology integration for promoting both student learning of content and teacher candidates' understanding of content pedagogy and technology-mediated learning in authentic course assignments. This view is supported by results from recent studies evaluating modeling of technology integration that suggests positive impacts on teacher candidates in terms of their pedagogical understanding of how to effectively use content-based technologies, their epistemological beliefs about technology and pedagogy, and their commitment to using technology to transform teaching and learning (Angeli & Valanides, 2009; Kim, Sachin, Westhoff, & Rezabek, 2008).

Moreover, Kim, Sachin, Westhoff, and Rezabek (2008) conducted a quantitative study of 100 preservice teachers enrolled in content methods courses to evaluate the relationship between faculty modeling of technology integration and preservice teachers' intent of using these technologies in future classrooms. Their research suggests that teacher educators learn technology-mediated pedagogy and establish beliefs about the value of technology by observing methods instructors' applications of instructional technology. Results indicate a statistically significant positive relationship between faculty technology use and preservice teachers' intent to use technology. Kim, Sachin, Westhoff, and Rezabek (2008) conclude that methods instructors "must be competent users of technology in order to influence the full development of preservice teachers who use them as role models" (p. 283). The authors propose modeling as an efficient alternative for shaping teaching behaviors when modeling of content-based technology integration is effectively used by methods instructors (Kim, Sachin, Westhoff, & Rezabek, 2008). Thus, modeling becomes a viable option for addressing ongoing debate about how to redefine teacher preparation and learning experiences to allow for content-based technology use. If teacher education candidates understand what authentic technology integration looks like in their content area and understand how to accomplish meaningful technology-mediated content instruction, they will continue to use it in schools once they start teaching (Schwarz, Myer, & Sharma, 2007).

Providing authentic and meaningful content-based learning experiences for preservice and inservice teachers are essential in helping teacher education candidates understand not only how to use advanced technologies but also the relationship between technology, content, and learning. This is especially important in social studies. Applications within social studies methods courses need to create the contextual environment to facilitate these processes and support candidates' technological pedagogical content knowledge (TPCK). Researchers suggest various discipline-specific technology applications that support the nature of content understanding and intertwine content, pedagogy, and emerging technologies (Angeli & Valanides, 2009; Akengin, 2008; Bates, 2008; Brush & Saye, 2009). Lee (2008) extends research recommendations by proposing guidelines for effectively integrating technological pedagogical content knowledge (TPCK) into a social studies context through a framework of democracy. These guidelines include ten pedagogical adaptations of the interaction among and between pedagogy, technology, and social studies content, which include:

- Locating and adapting digital resources for use in the classroom.
- Facilitating students' work in nonlinear environments.
- Working to develop critical media literacy skills among students.

- Providing students with opportunities to utilize the presentational capabilities of the Web to motivate and encourage students.
- Using the Internet to extend collaboration and communication among students.
- Extending and promoting active and authentic forms of human interaction and technology enabled social networks.
- Making use of historical source materials available through online sources.
- Promoting understandings of spatial, human, and physical systems as aided by technology.
- Expanding social experiences using technology.
- Encouraging economic literacy through the use of technology (Lee, 2008, p. 130-131).

Additionally, for teacher candidates to explore epistemological beliefs about teaching with technology and the pedagogical role technology plays in transforming social studies thinking, methods instructors need to model using advanced and emerging technologies within the social studies context and actively support reflective thinking through purposeful assignments (Akengin, 2008; Bates, 2008; Brush & Saye, 2009). Web 2.0 tools permeate everyday life and have the potential to redefine what and how we teach, learn, and prepare teachers. Ideas of how to use Web 2.0 tools in education abound (Bates, 2008; Bullen, 2008; Criswell, 2008; Hong, 2008; Groff & Haas, 2008; Yan, 2008). Further, recent data show an increased use of technology among social studies faculty (Bolick, Berson, Friedman, & Porfeli, 2007).

To counter minimal or insufficient technology applications, Brush and Saye (2009) offer strategies for effective integration of technology within social studies teacher preparation programs. They recommend providing preservice teachers with opportunities to: observe social studies teachers teaching content with technology, complete tasks in social studies methods courses that model effective technology use, explore various technology tools, and apply technological knowledge and skills in real social studies classrooms as part of their clinical experiences (Brush & Saye, 2009).

Technology in Action in the K-12 Environment

Another layer to understanding the role of technology in instructional practices is within the clinical environment; however, these experiences are limited to the technology expertise of the cooperating teacher (or practicing teacher) and there is a large degree of variability among these placements (Brush & Saye, 2009). To support teacher education candidates' knowledge and skills in integrating research-based technology for teaching social studies, we have conducted a series of technology mediated projects in secondary schools. Specifically, our studies have focused on high school students' uses of wikis in order to demonstrate their understanding of a particular topic (Friedman & Heafner, 2006, 2007, 2008; Heafner & Friedman, 2008). In each of these studies, we have utilized a quasi-experimental design, in which we have worked with two sections of the same course taught by the same teacher; one section is the control group (in which the teacher used his/her normal instructional methods) and the other has been the test group (in which students were exposed to technology resources in order to enhance their instructional experience).

Our purpose has been to test the utility of technology in supporting student learning of social studies content. In addition, the application of technology has allowed us to model effective practices for technology integration with adolescent learners; thus, bridging the divide between theory and practice. We have brought our experiences back to the methods classroom. What we have learned from our teaching, research, and uses of technology as well as our adjustments to limitations and in some cases barriers are the crux of what we extol in our methods courses in terms of technology use. From our series of studies, the overarching lessons that we have learned are the following:

1. Technology needs to be scaffolded with specific directions that encourage creativity without stifling critical thinking.
    a. This is a difficult, but not impossible, task. In other words, it is not enough to simply expose students to Internet-based resources and expect them to learn the content (Bates, 2008). Rather, it is necessary to give them material with specific, guiding questions so that students are not simply looking for a 'key word' in order to get the correct answer, but instead are guided to engage in higher order thinking (Brush & Saye, 2009; Lee, 2008).
2. Technology cannot get in the way of learning. When technology is a cumbersome tool it mitigates its potential advantage.
    a. This phenomenon was apparent in a study we undertook in which we designed a Digital Literacy Tool (DLT) that had scaffolded questions for students to consider (Friedman & Heafner, 2008). However, students were unfamiliar with this tool and by and large did not wish to use it; preferring online resources such as Wikipedia and answers.com to a much greater degree.
3. Measures of assessment must be adjusted to address the impact of technology on student learning outcomes to effectively evaluate the complexity of learning as measured in both short term and long term content retention.
    a. Similar to the above mentioned studies that focus on standardized testing, it has been our experience that it is very difficult to gauge the full extent of learning that transpires in a technology-rich environment. This is particularly the case with multiple-choice questions. For example, after comparing two sections of students on a post-test immediately following a unit of study, there was not an appreciable difference in test scores; eight months later however, not only did students in the 'test' group (those that used technology) score higher on a post-test, but interview data from students in both classes demonstrated a much greater remembrance and recollection of the unit (Heafner & Friedman, 2008).
4. 21st Century applications of technology address the limitations of traditional pedagogical practices by challenging students to think in a student-centered environment.
    a. In each of our studies, students have worked individually to create wikis that demonstrate their understanding of a particular topic. This engagement with technology reflects current literature in that many teenagers use the Internet on a daily basis (Lenhart & Madden, 2007) and do so outside of school in order to enhance their educational experience (Levin and Arafeh, 2002). For the most part, students have found this to be an enjoyable experience (Friedman & Heafner, 2007). Also, this relates to 21st century skills, as rather than memorizing information, students are engaging in higher order thinking as they create products and display them on the Internet.
5. Web 2.0 applications shift the applications of technology in learning from student as consumer to student as contributor who is actively engaged with digitally-based content.
    a. Similar to above, Web 2.0 applications allow students to become active contributors to the Internet, as opposed to recipients of information. Not only is this helpful in the sense that students are

> engaged in content, but it can simultaneously be helpful in terms of logistics. An inherent feature of Web 2.0 tools is that the information is stored on a server, thus lessening the chance that a student might lose his or her work as they might with a traditional notebook. Similarly, because there is a "sense of permanence" with these tools as data are stored, this can serve as an excellent review tool at the end of the year (Martindale & Wiley, 2005, p. 59).

The Integration of Technology in Social Studies Methods

As noted above, technology is a broad term and is constantly changing and evolving; the thrust of this chapter is on three particular Web 2.0 technologies and their use in social studies methods courses. We have found Web 2.0 software (particularly wikis) to be useful in the K-12 social studies classroom (Heafner & Friedman, 2008); therefore, as a result, we have integrated wikis as well as other Web 2.0 software (weblogs, and podcasts) into our methods courses. The remainder of this chapter will focus on the particulars of how this has been done by the authors, including specific applications, assignments, student work samples, and reflections and lessons learned. The authors are faculty at two institutions, which differ in type (public and private), as well as in terms of total enrollment and size of our teacher education program. Accordingly, the authors implement technology in a slightly different manner from one another, which it is hoped will inform the reader of how best to integrate technology into their methods courses in different contexts. Faculty member A teaches at a small, private, liberal arts university with a student enrollment of approximately 6000; accordingly, the teacher education program is small as well, with an average of 15 undergraduate and graduate secondary social studies students each year. Additionally, the campus is wireless, and each student and faculty member is issued a laptop. Faculty member B teaches in a large urban university with a student enrollment of approximately 24,000. The enrollment in teacher education programs in faculty member B's department alone exceeds the student population of the aforementioned private institution. Faculty member B teaches two to three middle and secondary social studies methods courses each semester with an approximate average yearly enrollment of over 100 middle and secondary social studies methods teacher education candidates. University technology resources are readily accessible, including wireless Internet access, to all students although no hardware resources are provided to university students.

Weblogs

Weblogs (commonly referred to as blogs) "are easily created, easily updateable Websites that allow an author (or authors) to publish instantly to the Internet from any Internet connection" (Richardson, 2006, p. 8). Blogs have increasingly been used in recent years, particularly in the political arena. For example, the website etalkinghead.com (http://directory.etalkinghead.com/) hosts a political blog directory that of this writing was a listing of 531 blogs that were organized under a broad range of political and social viewpoints. Blogs are also adaptable to educational and content goals as well as reshaping the role of users. Blogs, by nature, shift the role of users from not just consumer of information but creators of content by either posting entries on a blog or making comments on the entries posted by others. Hong (2008) offers that a blog can be "a powerful tool that enhances communication, foster critical thinking, and encourages collaborative learning, blogs have great potential in education" (p. 37).

During the first class meeting in Faculty A's course, after the syllabus has been briefly reviewed, the content of the course has been introduced, and candidates have gotten to know each other, the subsequent activity that is undertaken is for each student to create a blog for the course. There are several reasons that this is done, but the most apparent is that a blog allows students to post their thoughts about a particular topic.

On the first day of class, Faculty A asks candidates to post their educational autobiography to their blog, as well as to decide upon (and explain the reasons why) the two most important characteristics that they should possess as a social studies teacher. Faculty A has found that this allows him as well as the other students to know why each individual student has decided to embark on their career as a teacher. Other examples of blog postings are reading responses, the degree to which they will aim to have a tolerant classroom, and the degree to which they intend to integrate digital primary sources into their teaching. In terms of grading, because the topics that Faculty A asks student to post are based more on their informed opinions rather than a finished product, Faculty A typically makes this an 'all or nothing' assignment, as students receive full credit as long as they have made a post to their blog.

Simultaneous to each student making an individual comment to the class discussion, other students can comment on the original post. In many ways, this is superior to a traditional classroom discussion, as it allows (or perhaps mandates) every student to participate. Further, the use of blogs allows students to collect their thoughts and make a well-reasoned comment, as opposed to feeling on the spot in a classroom setting. Finally, as each student makes his or her post, this allows for individual interaction with the instructor who will have the time to think through a well-reasoned response; this, too, would not be possible in a traditional discussion.

The result of student blog postings is not only individualized feedback for the teacher candidate, but by reading the musings of each student throughout the semester, it is likely that this will result in the instructor understanding the perspectives of each individual candidate, ultimately forming a closer relationship with each. The use of blogs has added benefits as well, as not only will this likely translate into better in-person discussions, but the seemingly minor details of teacher education will be ameliorated through a closer instructor-student relationship, which a blog can facilitate. For example, it is often difficult to match student teacher with cooperating teachers, as a host of factors need to be weighed before these placements can be made; however, the better the instructor knows his or her students, the easier this oftentimes arduous task will be.

Blogs serve various roles within Faculty B's methods courses to scaffold teacher candidate understanding of content-based pedagogy and authentic applications with adolescent learners. Since service learning is a critical component within social studies and serves as a meaningful pedagogy for promoting civic engagement, social justice, and democratic ideals, providing learning experiences through service learning has become an important element of the methods courses that Faculty B teaches. However, exposing candidates to service learning within teacher preparation coursework alone is not enough to promote candidates wherewithal to embrace service learning as a pedagogy. Teacher candidates need structured analysis of methods and experiences to effectively understand the role of service learning as pedagogy (Anderson, Swick, & Yff, 2001; Hale, 2008). To support metacognitive analysis of service learning and professional growth, Faculty B has utilized blogs as a planning and reflective tool. Blogs provide a platform for sharing of ideas, discussion and dialogue, and facilitate rich thinking. Research suggests that for teacher candidates to employ service learning as a pedagogy they must be actively involved in the decision-making process and take ownership of implementing service projects with learners (Hale, 2008; Hart & King, 2007). In conducting service projects such as Environmental Awareness Advocacy Campaigns or Content Literacy Tutoring Programs for high poverty communities, our class blogs provided a collaborative tool for identifying community needs, brainstorming ways of addressing these needs, and designing the common service learning project to be implemented with learners. Faculty B has used blogs as a tool to support teacher candidate planning, implementation and reflection about service learning projects conducted with local urban communities. Examples of a student post and the framework for the class blog are provided.

Example of Teacher Candidate Blog Posting: "Today was the first day of our Service Learning Project. I was so excited about this activity! Last week our class decided that we wanted to paint birdhouses, plant flowers and learn about birds for our Service Project. We felt that this would be a fun, hands on activity that would get us outside and enjoying nature. We decided on the supplies we would need, the amount of time and some of the approaches we would take. We also selected our reading, Seed Folks, to introduce the idea of gardening and the environment to bring together people of diverse cultures."

To further extend contextual understanding for the application of service learning, methods course readings were structured to build candidate contextual knowledge of the urban community. These readings were supplemented by an author book talk, a walking tour to explore layers of history within the community, and a museum visit to evaluate an exhibit about community development, and the community cultural dynamics which have evolved through immigration and increased ethnic diversity. In preparation for these class experiences, teacher candidates posted questions for the author on the class blog. Subsequent to the field trip they posted pedagogical ideas for how they could use both the walking tour and museum exhibits with adolescent learners. The later use of the blog served an important purpose in helping teacher candidates think about instruction and curriculum resources. This field trip to the museum is required for all middle school students in local school systems and thus the experience served an additional purpose in helping teacher candidates consider how they too could use technology to facilitate learning. A brief excerpt of a candidate blog post follows:

".... This goes to show that hands-on experience is much better than just reading about something. I wish that all educational units could be followed by a Service Learning Project. I think they would be easy to implement into a Middle Grades setting due to the teams that the students are set up in. Hopefully I will be able to use this tactic in my own teaching."

Service learning research (Anderson, Swick, & Yff, 2001; Hale, 2008) emphasizes the importance of reflection to support future uses of this pedagogy. After the completion of service learning projects, teacher candidates debriefed and reflected on their experiences and evaluated the lessons learned for their future classrooms. These reflections and dialogue were supported through summative blog postings. Teacher candidates were encouraged to create a podcast (using Audacity) about their service learning experience and upload these to the class blog as an alternative to the written summative reflection. Candidates who selected this alternative technology tool found utility in talking rather informally about their experiences in contrast to a more formal and distant written reflection. Podcast reflections were more fluid and represented deeper, critical analysis of professional and personal growth as a result of the service learning experience. As evidenced in the following excerpt of a podcast transcript, well crafted and effectively supported service learning experiences in teacher preparation positively impact candidate understanding of students, communities, and acceptance of diversity (Anderson, Swick, & Yff, 2001; Baldwin, Buchanan, & Rudisill, 2007); while Web 2.0 tools provided the dispositional data to document candidate professional and personal growth.

Podcast Transcript: "I've never worked with students from diverse backgrounds before this class. My high school and where I tutored from was mostly your Caucasians and your southerners and whenever I found out their poverty rate was 60 percent, I was surprised. I thought that was super high. Then when I was found out that was one of the lowest in [the school system], I was shocked. Back at home it's like your poverty is in the teens, 20's maybe, but I didn't really even know, but 60 percent? That was kind of overwhelming to me.... You really wouldn't know which of those students was poverty stricken, so this experience was surprising and a good learning experience."

Reflection also is fundamental in teacher preparation and plays a significant role in candidate learning from field experiences. Another application of blogs that Faculty B has utilized in social studies methods is teacher candidate evaluation and critique of clinical experiences through weekly postings to a individually created Blog. To provide a more focused and meaningful field experience in content methods, Faculty B has established a structured clinical experience in which teacher candidates participate in a tutoring program with struggling students in middle and secondary schools. Teacher candidates, especially preservice teachers, are uncertain of their pedagogical skills, question their content knowledge, and lack confidence in their abilities to address the needs of learners. Tutoring clinical experiences serve as a safe and supportive environment for preservice teachers to hone their content knowledge and pedagogical skills. However, for this process to be successful it must be nurtured and engage preservice teachers in purposeful reflection. As a scaffolding tool, preservice teachers are guided in the diagnostic evaluation of strengths and weaknesses of learners, ongoing analysis of learner needs, strategy interventions, and self-assessment through weekly postings on their personal clinical blogs. Although access to clinical blogs is limited to class participants, clinical blogs do support a professional learning community in which preservice teachers safely share their struggles and success while interacting with peers and the instructor through collaborative dialogue to seek methods and content resources to more effectively address the needs of learners. Teacher candidates are able to utilize immediate feedback to design instruction and interventions for each weekly tutoring session.

It is worth mentioning that although teacher candidates noted within their blog postings that they "...greatly enjoyed working with an after school tutoring program" and touted that the experience as "...fun and it was not 'boring' like clinicals sometimes tend to be;" they also emphasized the value of tutoring as "....beneficial for both the student being tutored and the tutor" without focusing on the technology they were utilizing for reflection. This example of sample dialogue from student service learning clinical blog posts provides insight into the value blogs can serve to support collaborative reflection while modeling the utility of a Web 2.0 tool. Blogs became a common tool for class assignments and forum for professional exchange with the instructor and peers. It is therefore plausible to infer that the nature of technology uses camouflage teacher candidate learning about technology and technical skills development within an authentic application.

Wikis

A wiki is "a collaborative Webspace where anyone can add content and anyone can edit content that has already been published" (Richardson, 2006, p. 8). Based on a research study we have undertaken, we have written an article (Heafner & Friedman, 2008) describing the benefits and logistical hurdles of student-designed wikis in the secondary social studies environment. Wikis can be used by teachers or students in a variety of ways; the most straightforward manner being as a website that a teacher develops for their class. However, they can also be used as a one day activity or multi-day unit where students work independently or in groups to develop their own wiki to demonstrate their understanding of a particular topic, with the major advantages being that students are able to express their understanding of the topic, and subsequently being able to use their wiki as a review tool.

To fully understand history and social studies, students must learn to do history, and one example of doing history relates to analyzing primary source material. Yet, the selection and use of primary sources are perceived by teacher candidates as cumbersome and daunting, which often lead to limited application in their future classrooms. To encourage the use of primary sources and develop candidates' knowledge and skills in designing social studies instruction around primary sources, teacher candidates in Faculty B's course are assigned the task of creating a primary source wiki that includes primary sources and analysis tools to scaffold student interpretation. While content-focused assignments serve an important role in supporting candidate learning about best practices, assignments without appropriate modeling within the methods course fail to bridge the gap between theory and practice. The latter is essential to teaching candidates how to use Web 2.0 tools in authentic and meaningful ways. As a multiple-purpose model, Faculty B uses a student-created primary source kit as a wiki on Lincoln and Slavery to teach candidates how to: 1) organize primary sources in a logical sequence for intended learning outcomes, 2) scaffold student interpretation of each primary source through questioning, and 3) guide students to draw conclusions by evaluating various primary sources.

In addition to modeling primary source analysis, Faculty B also shares instructor created examples of wikis for other content topics. One such example, *It's a Matter of Perspective,* provides an important framework for discussing the potential that wikis offer in merging various types of primary sources. This example guides student thinking about the role of media in shaping American mindset and the forces which led to the rise of segregation at the onset of the 20th Century. *It's a Matter of Perspective: Music, Media, and Movies Wiki* includes the following primary sources: a popular song with racial undertones which includes a YouTube performance of the song and lyrics, a political cartoon published in a local newspaper in 1868, and YouTube excerpts from the historic and racially charged movie, *A Birth of a Nation*. Each primary source is accompanied by an analysis guide. As a class, candidates explore how the primary sources connect to Faculty B's instructional goals and the processes of selecting each source. Faculty B also models how the wiki was designed to teach teacher candidates the technology skills needed to create their own wiki.

Finally, Faculty B concludes with a discussion of the utility of student designed wikis as a strategy to promote historical thinking. Faculty B provides examples of a task description, a pathfinder (a web-based collection of primary sources), and student wikis from research conducted with secondary students (see Friedman & Heafner, Heafner & Friedman). Faculty B discusses experiences and presents data as a framework for evaluating the learning outcomes and potential implications of student uses of Web 2.0 technologies.

Faculty A purposefully waits until the methods course is about two-thirds over before wikis are introduced, and does so in a two-step manner. To describe what a wiki is, Faculty A first introduces candidates to perhaps world's most famous wiki, the commonly used online encyclopedia Wikipedia (http://wikipedia.org/) and discusses the benefits and drawbacks of its use. The use of Wikipedia is not without controversy; because of the structure of Wikipedia where anybody can log in and make edits, its use has been banned in certain academic circles (Davidson, 2007). The contention of its merits notwithstanding, Wikipedia can also be used to engage in higher-order thinking, as the 'History' tab (which is a list of every edit for a particular entry) can be analyzed in terms of the bias and perspective of the author of particular edits (Manfra, Friedman, Hammond, & Lee, 2009).

During the next class meeting, Faculty A asks candidates to create their own wiki. There are a number of sites through which they can do this, namely seedwiki.com, pbwiki.com, and wetpaint.com. Students in Faculty A's methods course are concurrently enrolled in a technology course; where among the first assignments is the development of a traditional website using Dreamweaver™. For the majority of students, this is their first experience developing a website, and as a result, they need to learn intricacies of web design, such as saving files in the correct folder and uploading to a server. While these activities are by no means overly taxing, they do tend to lead to students appreciating wikis, as there can be little argument that their use is less cumbersome and as a result their learning curve is not as steep.

In terms of an assignment, Faculty A emphasizes instructional design by which candidates can engage in higher order thinking. Candidates (because they already know how to design web sites) are very fast to catch on to the 'how-to' portion of teaching wikis, as they are usually able to create a fully functional site in less than fifteen minutes. Candidates' familiarity with web design gives Faculty A the opportunity as the instructor to emphasize content and instructional design, particularly scaffolding and differentiating questions.

In using wikis, each candidate creates a wiki that s/he can use as a particular student-centered activity as a teacher, and s/he has the option of creating it as a single-day or multi-day activity, with the idea that each student chooses a different area of study so that s/he can share his or her resources. The only requirement is that students include a combination of lower-order and higher-order objectives so that their students know 'the facts,' and are also able to apply and synthesize them.

For example, one candidate developed an activity where the task is to read three diary entries from the Battle of Gettysburg during the American Civil War, and initially answer four lower-order questions, such as what the writer was doing and her description of soldiers' experiences. These all serve as scaffolds for the higher-order portion of the assignment. In this part, students create their own diary from a Civil War battle (this too is scaffolded, as there are four battles to choose from, and hyperlinks are provided for contextual information). In so doing, they include facts from the battle, but more importantly, consider the point of view from which they will be writing. This activity serves the purpose of focusing on social studies content and is simultaneously an activity in which students would not otherwise engage, as students are creating and saving material online.

Podcasts

A podcast is "An audio broadcast that has been converted to an MP3 file or other audio file format for playback in a digital music player" (pcmag.com, 1981-2009, online). As Richardson (2006) notes, a podcast "is basically the creation and distribution of amateur radio," and similar to blogs, they have become popular in mainstream society (p. 112). A podcast can take different forms (from a conversation to a lecture on a given topic), and similar to blogs and wikis, a benefit of their use is that they allow for a permanent record of a teacher or student product.

History is the primary core discipline that comprises the overarching interdisciplinary content of the social studies. To help students learn history, students must learn to interpret primary sources using strategies and approaches of historians. Fundamental to understanding primary sources, students must learn to actively and critically read primary sources. Reading applies to the literacy strategies that historians use to make meaning of various forms of text (e.g. diaries, letters, eyewitness accounts, reports, documents, memoires, songs, etc.) and visual images (e.g. photos, political cartoons, sketches, drawings, advertisements, artifacts, etc.).

Historians first identify the facts that are in the text or images and then infer meaning based upon historical contexts such as the origin of the primary source, time period, perspective of the author, and personal or professional motives. Students lack the content knowledge and inferencing skills to effectively draw conclusions in relation to broader historical themes and big ideas; this is where the teacher provides the pedagogical interface to support student understanding. A useful strategy that Faculty B models in class to teach inferencing and primary source analysis is thinking aloud. For example, Faculty B begins reading a survivor's account of My Lai and pauses to state what would be highlighted, why Faculty B thinks this content is important, and to question the text while making connections to other social studies content. Faculty B also models how thinking about a primary source can be shifted into questions that will scaffold student interpretation of a primary source, which serves an important role in teaching students to look beyond what is right there in the text or image to infer rich and deep meaning.

Although Faculty B can apply these strategies without much effort, teacher candidates struggle with metacognition and thinking aloud as a pedagogical approach, as both require practice and authentic application with social studies content. To provide opportunities for teacher candidates to successfully utilize think aloud and hone their metacognitive skills, teacher candidates create a podcast using Audacity modeling the reading and analysis of a selected primary source for use with adolescent learners. Candidates self-critique their podcast and post the podcast and pedagogical reflection on a Blackboard discussion board for peer and instructor review.

Interviewing is another pedagogical approach that supports social studies content understanding. Interviewing and oral history are important tools of the historian for exploring perspectives of individuals who lived history, and exploration of the topographies of historical thinking is important in unraveling how a historian compares and synthesizes multiple perspectives to formulate meaning. To expose teacher candidates to interviewing and to understand the forces that shape what and how individuals remember history, candidates are assigned the task of interviewing six people of various age, gender and ethnic groups and are given an interview protocol. In preparation for the task, candidates are required to practice their interviewing skills and to consider their own thinking about history by creating a MP3 file in which they pose and answer interview questions. Candidate podcasts are shared with the Faculty B, who subsequently identifies themes which are used to initiate class discussion and collaborative analysis of candidate analysis of other interview responses. The instructor models research-based methods of categorization using the Taba Model (List, Group, Label, Conclusion) (Costa & Loveall, 2002) developed from the research of Hilda Taba (1962).

Excerpt from Methods Task Description:

What do you remember about history? Before conducting your interviews, practice your interviewing skills by creating an MP3 File using Audacity to record your responses to the interview questions. Instructor Podcast with description of the Task is provided.

While Faculty A does not encourage lecture in a social studies classroom for more than a third of any given class period, the fact remains that it is important for teacher candidates to know how to deliver an effective lecture, as a lecture is generally accepted as the fastest and most direct method of giving factual information to students. Faculty A asks discusses effective lecture and note taking strategies, particularly the components of a lecture and emphasizing the importance of asking questions. Teacher candidates then work together to compose a five-minute lecture on a topic of their choice and practice delivering it to one another. Their assignment is to choose any specific objective (i.e. 2.07, 3.06) for Ninth Grade World History on the North Carolina Standard Course of Study, and develop a 5-minute lecture on this topic. This assignment contains a clear focus on history content; however, another important feature is that it allows teacher candidates to reflect and continue to record their lecture until they are satisfied with the product that they have developed.

Assessment of Teacher Candidates

While each of the aforementioned technologies has the potential to impact the teaching of social studies methods courses, a systematic evaluation plan must be in place in order to gauge their effectiveness and impact on teacher candidate learning. We have found that the most straightforward strategy by which to do this is to include a specific grading rubric for each assignment. Within this rubric, the specific components of each technology are broken down and weighted as to their overall importance in the context of the assignment.

We have found grading rubrics to be very helpful from both the instructor as well as candidate perspective. From the instructor perspective, by determining the relative importance of different components of software, it helps us to learn the technology at a deeper level, and as a result, helps to teach it as well as answer questions about it from our class. Having specific components is also advantageous in terms of grading; because the products that students create using these technologies are quite different than traditional assignments, making grading difficult on the surface. However, having specific components of what to look for allows instructors to easily and quickly assign a grade.

From the teacher candidate perspective, rubrics are also greatly appreciated, particularly because a Web 2.0 technology assignment is oftentimes their first experience with these technologies. As a result, candidates are often not sure of our expectations, and rubrics serve the purpose of providing more certainty of what is valued as well as assessed. A clearly defined rubric allows candidates to see exactly what they need to do to be successful. The only caveat in doing this is that it will foster criterion (rather than norm) referenced grading. Modeling the use of rubrics also allows instructors to demonstrate effective assessment practices while supporting teacher candidate learning.

FUTURE RESEARCH DIRECTIONS AND CONCLUDING THOUGHTS

As noted above, the notion of technology in schools is not new, and the narrower field of technology within social studies has been prominent for over a decade. However, this chapter presents several opportunities for new research, the most apparent of which would be to scrutinize any of the three featured technology applications in one or more methods courses. Taking this a step further, the fields of social studies teacher education and instructional technology would be well informed if the participants in these methods courses were followed in the first few years of their teaching career, and the impact of these courses on these individuals as teachers, and ultimately the achievement of their students, could be measured.

Providing authentic and meaningful learning experiences for preservice and inservice teachers are essential in helping teacher education candidates understand not only how to use advanced and emerging technologies, but also the relationship between technology, pedagogy, content, and learning. The authors have shared various applications within content based methods courses that effectively create the contextual environment to facilitate these processes, and have developed methods that model our lessons learned from real-world technology integration in middle and secondary social studies classrooms. The authors have also provided examples of how we actively support reflective thinking about teaching content with technology and purposeful tasks to support social studies teachers' technological pedagogical content knowledge (TPCK). Through our continued support in professional development, research, and work in local schools, the authors are able to evaluate the utility of our methods instruction. In observing our teacher candidates that are actively seeking ways to integrate emerging technologies in the teaching of social studies, the authors are supported in their interpretation that the methods that are proposed are meaningful, authentic, and powerful applications that have the potential to transform social studies teaching and learning.

REFERENCES

Akengin, H. (2008). Opinions of prospective social studies teachers on the use of information technologies in teaching geographic subjects. *Journal of Instructional Psychology*, *35*(2), 127–139.

American Association of Colleges for Teacher Education. (2008). *Handbook of technological pedagogical content knowledge (TPCK) for educators*. New York: Routledge for the American Association of Colleges for Teacher Education.

Anderson, J. B., Swick, K., & Yff, J. (2001). *Service learning in teacher education: Enhancing the growth of new teachers, their students, and communities*. Washington, DC: American Association of College for Teacher Education.

Angeli, C. (2005). Transforming a teacher education method course through technology: Effects on preservice teachers' technology competency. *Computers & Education*, *45*, 383–398. doi:10.1016/j.compedu.2004.06.002

Angeli, C., & Valanides, N. (2009). Epistemological and mythological issues for the conceptualization, development, and assessment of ICT-TPCK: Advances in technological pedagogical content knowledge (TPCK). *Computers & Education*, *52*, 154–168. doi:10.1016/j.compedu.2008.07.006

Baldwin, S. C., Buchanan, A., & Rudisill, M. (2007). What teacher candidates learned about diversity, social justice, and themselves from service learning experiences. *Journal of Teacher Education*, *58*(4), 315–327.. doi:10.1177/0022487107305259

Bates, A. (2008). Learning to design WebQuests: An exploration in preservice social studies education. *Journal of Social Studies Research*, *32*(1), 10–21.

Berson, M. J. (2004). Digital images: Capturing America's past with the technology of today. *Social Education*, *68*(3), 214–219.

Bolick, C. M., Berson, M. J., Friedman, A. M., & Porfeli, E. J. (2007). Diffusion of technology innovation in the preservice social studies experience: Results of a national survey. *Theory and Research in Social Education*, *35*(2), 174–195.

Braun, J., & Risinger, F. (1999). *Surfing social studies*. Washington, DC: National Council for the Social Studies.

Brush, T., & Saye, J. W. (2009). Strategies for preparing preservice social studies teachers to integrate technology effectively: Models and practices. *Contemporary Issues in Technology and Teacher Education*, *9*(1). Retrieved July 7, 2009, from http://www.citejournal.org/vol9/iss1/socialstudies/article1.cfm

Bullen, A. (2008). The 'long tale': Using Web 2.0 concepts to enhance digital collections. *Computers in Libraries*, 31–35.

Center for Civic Education. (1994). *National standards for civics and government*. Retrieved January 23, 2009, from http://www.civiced.org/index.php?page=stds_toc_intro

Cohen, D. J., & Rosenzweig, R. (2006). *Digital history: A guide to gathering, preserving, and presenting the past on the Web*. Philadelphia, PA: University of Pennsylvania Press.

Costa, A., & Loveall, R. (2002). The legacy of Hilda Taba. *Journal of Curriculum and Supervision, 18*, 56–62.

Criswell, C. (2008). What Web 2.0 means for teachers. *Teaching Music, 16*(3), 1–2.

Davidson, C. (2007, March 23). We can't ignore the influence of digital technologies. *Chronicle of Higher Education, 53*(29). eTalkinghead.com. (2003-2008). *Etalkinghead's political blog directory*. Retrieved April 1, 2009, from http://directory.etalkinghead.com/

Friedman, A. M. (2006). State standards and digital primary sources: A divergence. *Contemporary Issues in Technology and Teacher Education, 6*(3). Retrieved July 6, 2009, from http://www.citejournal.org/vol6/iss3/socialstudies/article1.cfm

Friedman, A. M. (2008). Social studies teachers' use of the Internet to foster democratic citizenship. In VanFossen, P. J., & Berson, M. J. (Eds.), *The electronic republic? The impact of technology on education for citizenship* (pp. 173–195). West Lafayette, IN: Purdue University Press.

Friedman, A. M., & Heafner, T. L. (2006, March). *Student creation of social studies-specific websites to enhance historical understandings*. Roundtable presented at the annual meeting of the Society for Information Technology and Teacher Education (SITE), Orlando, FL.

Friedman, A. M., & Heafner, T. L. (2007). You think for me, so I don't have to. *Contemporary Issues in Technology and Teacher Education, 7*(3). Retrieved July 7, 2009, from http://www.citejournal.org/vol7/iss3/socialstudies/article1.cfm

Friedman, A. M., & Heafner, T. L. (2008). Finding and contextualizing resources: A digital literacy tool's impact in ninth grade world history. *Clearing House (Menasha, Wis.), 82*(2), 82–86. doi:10.3200/TCHS.82.2.82-86

Friedman, A. M., & Hicks, D. (2006). The state of the field: Technology, social studies, and teacher education. *Contemporary Issues in Technology and Teacher Education* [Online serial], *6*(2). Retrieved July 7, 2009, from http://www.citejournal.org/vol6/iss2/socialstudies/article1.cfm

Gentry, C. G. (1995). Educational technology: A question of meaning. In Anglin, G. J. (Ed.), *Instructional technology: Past, present, and future* (pp. 1–10). Englewood, CO: Libraries Unlimited, Inc.

Goodlad, J. I. (1984). *A place called school: Prospects for the future*. New York: McGraw Hill.

Groff, J., & Haas, J. (2008). Web 2.0: Today's technologies, tomorrow's learning. *Leading and Learning with Technology*, 12-15.

Hale, A. (2008). Service learning with Latino communities: Effects on preservice teachers. *Journal of Hispanic Higher Education*, *7*(1), 54–69. doi:10.1177/1538192707310511

Hart, S. M., & King, J. R. (2007). Service learning and literacy tutoring: Academic impact on preservice teachers. *Teaching and Teacher Education*, *23*(4), 323–338. doi:10.1016/j.tate.2006.12.004

Heafner, T. L., & Friedman, A. M. (2008). Wikis and constructivism in social studies: Fostering a deeper understanding. *Computers in the Schools*, *25*(3-4), 288–302. doi:10.1080/07380560802371003

Hew, K., & Brush, T. (2007). Integrating technology into K-12 teaching and learning: Current knowledge gaps and recommendations for future research. *Educational Technology Research and Development*, *55*(3), 223–252. doi:10.1007/s11423-006-9022-5

Hicks, D., & Ewing, E. T. (2003). Bringing the world into the classroom with online global newspapers. *Social Education*, *67*(3), 134–139.

Hong, W. (2008). Exploring educational use of blogs in U.S. education. *U.S.-China Education Review, 5*(10), 47, 34-38.

Kim, K., Sachin, J., Westhoff, G., & Rezabek, L. (2008). A quantitative exploration of preservice teachers' intent to use computer-based technology. *Journal of Instructional Psychology*, *35*(3), 275–287.

Krueger, K., Hansen, L., & Smaldino, S. (2000). Preservice teacher technology competencies: A model for preparing teachers of tomorrow to use technology. *TechTrends*, *44*(3), 47–50. doi:10.1007/BF02778227

Lee, J. K. (2008). Toward democracy: Social studies and TPCK. In the AACTE Committee on Innovation and Technology (Ed.), Handbook of technological pedagogical content knowledge (TPCK) for educators (pp. 129-144). New York: Routledge.

Lenhart, A., & Madden, M. (2007). *Social networking sites and teens: An overview*. Washington, DC: Pew Internet and American Life Project. Retrieved February 9, 2007, from http://www.pewinternet.org/pdfs/PIP_SNS_Data_Memo_Jan_2007.pdf

Lever-Duffy, J., McDonald, J. B., & Mizell, A. P. (2005). *Teaching and learning with technology* (2nd ed.). Boston, MA: Pearson Education, Inc.

Levin, D., & Arafeh, S. (2002). *The digital disconnect: The widening gap between Internet-savvy students and their schools*. Washington, DC: Pew Internet & American Life Project. Retrieved March 14, 2007, from http://www.pewinternet.org/pdfs/PIP_Schools_Internet_Report.pdf

Luke, N., Moore, J. L., & Sawyer, S. B. (1998). *Authentic approaches to encourage technology-using teachers*. Paper presented at the Society for Information Technology & Teacher Education International Conference, Washington, DC. ERIC Document #ED421083.

Manfra, M. M., Friedman, A. M., Hammond, T. C., & Lee, J. K. (2009, March). *Peering behind the curtain: Digital history, historiography, and secondary social studies methods*. Presentation at the annual meeting of the Society for Information Technology and Teacher Education (SITE), Charleston, SC.

Martindale, T., & Wiley, D. A. (2005). Using weblogs in scholarship and teaching. *Techtrends Linking Research and Practice to Improve Learning*, *49*(2), 55–61.

Martorella, P. H. (1997). Technology and social studies: Which way to the sleeping giant? *Theory and Research in Social Education*, *25*(4), 511–514.

Mason, C., Berson, M., Diem, R., Hicks, D., Lee, J., & Dralle, T. (2000). Guidelines for using technology to prepare social studies teachers. *Contemporary Issues in Technology and Teacher Education, 1*(1). Retrieved July 7, 2009, from http://www.citejournal.org/vol1/iss1/currentissues/socialstudies/article1.htm

Meier, D. (2002). Standardization versus standards. *Phi Delta Kappan*, *84*(3), 190–198.

Mishra, P., & Koehler, M. J. (2006). Technological pedagogical content knowledge: A framework for teacher knowledge. *Teachers College Record*, *108*(6), 1017–1054. doi:10.1111/j.1467-9620.2006.00684.x

National Center for History in the Schools. (2005). *Overview of standards in historical thinking*. Retrieved January 23, 2009, from http://nchs.ucla.edu/standards/thinking5-12.html

National Council for the Social Studies. (1994). *Expectations for excellence: Curriculum standards for social studies*. Washington, DC: National Council for Social Studies.

National Council for the Social Studies. (2006). *Technology position statement and guidelines.* Retrieved on February 11, 2009, from http://www.socialstudies.org/positions/technology

Pahl, R. H. (2003). *A*ssessment traps in K-12 social studies. *Social Studies, 94*(5), 212–215. doi:10.1080/00377990309600209

Parsad, B., & Jones, J. (2005). *Internet access in U.S. public schools and classrooms: 1994-2003. (NCES 2005-015). U.S. Department of Education.* Washington, DC: National Center for Education Statistics.

Partnership for 21st Century Skills. (2007). *Building 21st century skills.* Retrieved on February 17, 2009, from http://www.21stcenturyskills.org/route21/index.php?option=com_content&view=article&id=5&Itemid=2

Partnership for 21st Century Skills. (2009). *Framework for 21st century learning.* Retrieved on February 17, 2009, from http://www.21stcenturyskills.org/documents/framework_flyer_updated_jan_09_final-1.pdf

Pcmag.com. (2009). *Definition of podcast.* Retrieved on April 1, 2009 from http://www.pcmag.com/encyclopedia_term/0,2542,t=podcast&i=49433,00.asp#

Richardson, W. (2006). *Blogs, wikis, podcasts, and other powerful web tools for the classroom.* Thousand Oaks, CA: Corwin Press.

Schwarz, C. V., Meyer, J., & Sharma, A. (2007). Technology, pedagogy, and epistemology: Opportunities and challenges of using computer modeling and simulation tools in elementary science methods. *Journal of Science Teacher Education, 18*, 243–269. doi:10.1007/s10972-007-9039-6

Syh-Jong, J. (2008). Innovations in science teacher education: Effects of integration technology and team-teaching strategies. *Computers & Education, 41*, 646–659.

Taba, H. (1962). *Curriculum Development: Theory and Practice.* New York: Harcourt Brace and World.

VanFossen, P. (1999). An analysis of the use of the Internet and World Wide Web by secondary social studies teachers in Indiana. *The International Journal of Social Education, 14*(2), 87–109.

VanFossen, P. J. (2006). The electronic republic? Evidence on the impact of the Internet on citizenship and civic engagement in the U.S. *The International Journal of Social Education, 21*(1), 18–43.

VanFossen, P. J., & Shiveley, J. M. (2000). Using the Internet to create primary source teaching packets. *Social Studies, 91*(6), 244–252. doi:10.1080/00377990009602473

Whitworth, S. A., & Berson, M. J. (2003). Computer technology in the social studies: An examination of the effectiveness literature (1996-2001). *Contemporary Issues in Technology and Teacher Education, 2*(4), 472-509. Retrieved July 7, 2009, from http://www.citejournal.org/vol2/iss4/socialstudies/article1.cfm

Yan, J. (2008). Social technology as a new medium in the classroom. *New England Journal of Higher Education*, 27–30.

Yildirim, S. (2000). Effects of an educational computing course on preservice and inservice teachers: A discussion and analysis of attitudes and use. *Journal of Research on Computing in Education, 32*(4), 479–495.

Section 5
Framework and Application:
Learning Environment of Digital Age

Chapter 19
Increasing Teacher Candidates' Reflection with Technology

Chinwe H. Ikpeze
St. John Fisher College, USA

ABSTRACT

This chapter highlights the strategies that facilitated reflective thinking in teacher education through the integration of technology. Graduate students enrolled in a literacy course provided the data for the study. Major findings indicated that the reflective ability and quality of reflection among the teacher candidates increased because a structure that supported reflection was put in place. In addition, the teacher candidates engaged in a variety of multifaceted activities with new technologies in authentic contexts. The implications were discussed.

INTRODUCTION

Among the factors that contribute to successful teacher learning include collaboration, continued learning, as well as offering ample time and support for reflection, (Borko & Putnam, 1996). The need for continued learning and reflection by teachers cannot be overemphasized in the new media age, with the preponderance of new technologies. Technology promotes student learning by addressing a variety of learning styles, providing thought provoking challenges, and encouraging higher level thinking. It is therefore imperative that preservice and in-service teachers acquire the skills necessary to effectively integrate technology in their teaching in a way that would facilitate students' participation in the new global economy. According to the partnership for the 21st Century Skills (2006), teachers should be able to redesign and create curriculum and instruction to prepare their students with the skills of the 21st century literate citizens which include an expanded form of literacy as well as new information and communication technologies (ICTs). Teachers are also expected to develop the skills needed for a participatory culture, distributed expertise, collective intelligence, sharing, experimentation, innovation and evolution (Lankshear & Knobel, 2006).

DOI: 10.4018/978-1-61520-897-5.ch019

Copyright © 2010, IGI Global. Copying or distributing in print or electronic forms without written permission of IGI Global is prohibited.

Teachers for tomorrow's schools must be prepared to rethink, unlearn, relearn, revise and adapt the use of new technologies for instructional purposes (Niess, 2008). This includes being conversant with Web 2.0 tools (e.g., wikis, blogs, and social networking sites) which enable users to create, edit, manipulate, and collaborate online. Web 2.0 tools convey different expectations for participation, positioning users as authors or text producers (Hedberg & Brudvik, 2008; Jacobs, 2006). Currently, many teachers still see themselves as authority figures and might find it difficult to envisage a new role in which teachers and students are both designers of text. Research indicates that not enough teachers (novices or veterans), are developing sufficient knowledge required to effectively teach their subject matter with technology (Hughes & Scharber, 2008). One reason for that is the teachers' inability to become more metacognitively aware of their knowledge base with new technologies. Reflective thinking and writing would help teachers expose their old beliefs and practical theories of learning and teaching with technology in order to reconcile with new realities. In general, what is critically important for teachers is the knowledge of how, when and why to use technology effectively in teaching and how technology might change the way students actually learn to read and write (Schmidt & Gurbo, 2008). The emerging trend is to help teachers develop technological pedagogical content knowledge (TPCK) by integrating content, pedagogy and technology within the context of their content areas rather than in a separate, general technology skills course. Technological pedagogical content knowledge (TPCK) describes the interconnection and intersection of content, pedagogy (teaching and students' learning) and technology. TPCK involves a complex interplay of instructional decisions made by the teacher that includes content, pedagogy and technology. The question is "How do we as teacher educators support reflective thinking in our candidates especially as they learn to use various technologies for instruction? What role does reflective thinking play in teachers' development of the proficiency necessary to integrate their subject matter knowledge with technology and pedagogy (TPCK)?

I argue in this paper that teacher candidates need to engage with a wide range of technology-using opportunities in order to create genuine avenue for reflective thinking necessary to integrate technology into their content areas. To discuss the role of reflection in technology proficiency, I will first provide a historical overview of the theoretical and research basis for approaching reflective thinking in teacher education and the role of technology in promoting reflection, focusing on the types and roles of reflection in teacher education. Then I will highlight the result of an action research study in my teacher education class that provides evidence that (1) Reflection among teacher candidates increases within a course structure that supports reflection; (2) multiple technological projects and activities are essential for building reflective thinking; (3) Thought-provoking readings provide cognitive conflict that generates higher order reflective analysis; (4) collaborative teams working together on technology projects help build a community of learners, facilitate participatory culture and ultimately reflective ability of teachers; (5) an emphasis on experimentation rather than mere talking about technology help teacher candidates to better reflect on technology use; and (6) reflection increases within a problem-based and inquiry approach to technology integration.

REFLECTION AND TEACHER LEARNING

The importance of reflection in teacher learning and professional development is well recognized (Davis, 2006; Feisman & Nemser, 2001; Hatton & Smith, 1995; Schon, 1983). However, what is less certain and to a large extent debatable is how to support teacher reflection; the various roles that reflection plays in different teaching and learning situations; and the purposes it serves. Teacher reflection has a long standing history tracing back to John Dewey (1933). Dewey's sense of the term "reflection" involved a chain of thoughts or sequences of ideas leading to a consequence of action (i.e. reflection for action in the future). Dewey advocated that learning was contingent upon the integration of experiences with reflection and of theory and practice. Robin (2004) describes reflection as a cyclical process that requires teachers to select, describe, analyze, appraise, and transform their learning. Reflection promotes metacognition and involves teachers linking theory to practice, analyzing their own practice and learning from their experience (Feisman & Nemser, 2001). Although there have been diverse definitions and even occasional debates and implementation challenges, promoting teacher reflection remains a cornerstone of teacher education (Fendler, 2003). Schon (1983) differentiates between two types of reflection: reflection-in -action and reflection-on-action. Reflection-on-action involves looking back on and critiquing one's practice. Reflection-in-action involves dealing with on the spot professional problems as they arise and contextualization of multiple viewpoints within situations as they actually take place. Reflection-in-action guides teachers' in-the moment decision-making, and depends on their interaction with learners. Hatton and Smith (1995), building on Dewey and Schon's ideas created a developmental (not hierarchical) taxonomy of reflective practice beginning with the relatively simplistic or partial technical type (technical rationality), then working through different forms of reflection-on-action (descriptive, dialogic and critical), to the desired end-point of a professional able to undertake reflection-in-action. At this point, the teacher is able to contextualize multiple viewpoints and take on the spot decision.

Based on the developmental progression of reflective practice, Davies (2006) differentiates between what she calls productive and unproductive reflection. Unproductive reflection is mainly descriptive without much analysis or evaluation and involves listing ideas rather than connecting them logically. Teacher candidates who engage in such reflections do not provide evidence for their claims, generate alternatives to their decisions, or question their assumptions (LaBoskey, 1994). A productive reflection on the other hand provides reasons for decisions, evidence for claims, generate alternatives, question assumptions and identify the results of one's teaching decisions (Davis, 2006). Reflection either in-action or for-action is transformative and involve demanding rational and moral processes in making seasoned judgments about preferable ways to act (Hatton & Smith, 1995). In order to foster reflection, Hatton and Smith (1995) identify key questions that teacher educators must ask. These include: What patterns of reflection are identified and what factors seem important in fostering their development? In addition, what strategies appear to be effective in producing reflection and what are the salient characteristics of such approaches? How can more effective strategies be developed, and how can the conditions for encouraging reflective practice be improved? These questions suggest that teacher educators must reflect on their own practice even as they teach their teacher candidates to reflect. In order to foster effective reflection, what is needed is time and opportunity to work with authentic activities, so that the required essential metacognitive skills can be acquired (Hatton & Smith, 1995).

Efforts to promote teacher reflection often fall short for a variety of reasons. These include, but are not limited to, prospective teachers merely focusing on the logistical issues associated with teaching, ignoring the contextual factors in school-based environments, displaying shallow thought unaccompanied by action and failing to reflect in systematic and intentional ways (Dana & Silva, 2003). Because reflection is a key component of teacher learning, it also plays a significant role in helping teacher candidates' acquisition of technology skills needed for effective teaching in today's world. Teacher educators must capitalize on technology integration to help teacher candidates learn to effectively reflect on their use of technology. This is important because if teachers merely use technology without thinking deeply about it, if they merely allow their experiences to wash over without savoring and examining them for their significance, then growth will be greatly limited.

Technology and Teacher Reflection

A number of studies have examined the impact of technology on teacher reflection (Harford and MacRuairc, 2008; Kovalchick, 1998; Lin and Kinzer, 2003; Lin, 2008; Rich and Hannafin, 2009). Kovalchick (1998) argues that reflection can help teacher candidates articulate their awareness of the effectiveness of instructional methods supported by technology. Learning to use different technologies can be a thoughtful experience especially when it encourages teacher candidates to comment on their own learning as they use various technological tools, and as they work collaboratively in both learner and teacher roles by critiquing technology's educational functions. The integration of technology can also support teacher candidate's reflection by helping them highlight their emergent personal theories of technology use and their future plans (Lin, 2008). For example, the use of video and video annotation analysis have been identified as highly effective in teacher reflection because they aid scaffolding and structuring, thereby transforming the way teachers reflect on their learning (Harford and MacRuairc, 2008; Rich & Hannafin, 2009). Harford & MacRuairc (2008) advocate for a community of practice approach which involve student teachers engaging in peer videoing of class teaching in real time and subsequent analysis of their teaching in a tutorial session. This then facilitates working in a collaborative, collegial and supportive environment in which it is safe to speak the truth and ask hard questions. As noted by Harford and MacRuairc (2008), working in collaborative groups that study the use of technology can help teacher candidates demonstrate tangible evidence of the development of reflective skills. Lin and Kinzer (2003) argue that technology can be a valuable aid for making cultural values explicit if properly designed and implemented because it enables teachers to experience something new and non-routine and therefore allows them to see their own and students' values as well as problem-solving processes from new perspectives. Teachers, they argue need tools that facilitate access to specific and detailed knowledge about their own values and assumptions as well as others. Technology can provide teachers with such reflective tools. Therefore, a thoughtful reflection with educational technology would facilitate teachers' thinking, help make connections with prior learning and transform prior learning into active and authentic knowledge (Lin, 2008). An important step in developing TPCK therefore is to help teachers to critically reflect on their learning with technology and think deeply how their subject content can be effectively taught with new technologies (Mishra & Koehler, 2006).

Facilitating Reflective Thinking and Writing: Lessons from an Action Research

From May 2007 to July 2008, I conducted a teacher research (Cochran-Smith & Lytle, 1999) in which I served as researcher and course instructor. Transcripts for the study were obtained from a graduate-level introductory theory-based course in literacy. In four semesters, including summer, 65 preservice and in-service teachers consisting of four cohorts of teacher candidates who took this course were required to learn to use various technological tools. Course expectations included weekly reflections, group research projects and the completion of two major writing assignments which consisted of long essays. Because this course was primarily a literacy course, technology was not initially integrated into the course save for one or two articles on new literacies and technologies. However, changes were implemented to accommodate the integration of new technologies. This happened incrementally in that initial attempts were evaluated which necessitated subsequent changes and diversification of projects and activities. In the summer of 2007, the course was redesigned to include hands-on activities using various technological tools like the Interactive Whiteboard (IWB) or smart board as it is often called, blogs, podcasts, wikis, websites, iPod, virtual books, streaming videos, and other kinds of inquiry-based technology-enhanced projects. Teacher candidates (TCs), both pre-service and in-service teachers, were exposed to various technological tools during the course which required them to work either individually, in pairs, or in groups to research and teach lessons that demonstrate the use of particular technologies for instruction. Students participated in multiple technology projects which included teaching with the Interactive White Board (IWB), constructing/maintaining personal blogs and group wikis, and two open ended projects in which they chose from a variety of options or designed their own projects to suit their particular interests or classrooms. The teacher candidates (TCs) also prepared podcasts on their biographies which they uploaded to their wikis or blogs. Within each group wiki, each candidate maintained a personal folder and page which was used for e-portfolio. In-service teachers were encouraged to design projects that aligned with their classroom needs which they could immediately use with their students. For each technology project, the students were required to write reflections which included affordances or constraints of using that particular technological tool for instruction and suggestions for improvement. The teacher candidates were also required to write reflective papers on their group collaborations and experiences of working with partners. At the end of the semester, they wrote a culminating reflective paper that synthesized their entire course experiences with technology. In all, reflection was an integral part of the learning experiences provided for the teacher candidates in the course.

Primary data sources included reflections on each technology project and the end-of-semester technology reflections. Other sources of data which I used to make sense of the students' learning included focus group interviews, a reflective journal, where I recorded my thoughts, observations and insights from students' artifacts and a survey. The survey was used primarily to collect demographic information of the participants as well as some quantitative data that measured the perceptions of the teacher candidates on some selected activities. The survey included fill in the blank, yes/no, essay and Likert type questions. I approached the study through guiding questions such as: "How did various technology projects and activities enhance students' acquisition of technological pedagogical content knowledge?" Was reflective thinking enhanced? Was there evidence of critical or productive reflection? If so, what activities or scaffolds facilitated such reflections?

Data analysis was done through the creation of some coding schemes. Coding schemes were developed through an iterative process of individual coding, and re-checking against the data. Codes were also generated from the research literature. I developed three coding schemes for activity type, perceptions, and reflections. These codes were used to establish broad categories. For example, for the activity category, I sorted the students' technology projects into individual, partner and group projects. I also noted whether it was a mandatory or self-selected project. To analyze students' perceptions of their projects, I coded for positive and negative perceptions, and at the same time examined the interplay of perceptions on activity type. For each TC, I documented the type of reflection in each paper (descriptive or productive). At the end of each semester, I analyzed the data and used the findings to refine the activities for subsequent semesters. For example, findings from the first semester of the study indicated that students' reflections were unsystematic, shallow and merely descriptive. In addition, most TCs perceived their technology experiences as merely theoretical with little relevance in helping them develop technology proficiency. This, they attributed to inadequate hands-on experience. This finding helped me to refine the technology experiences provided students in subsequent semesters. It was clear from the students' reflection that the type of technology experiences they engaged with impacted their perception of the usefulness of technology and quantity and quality of their reflection.

Throughout the study, I continued annotation and recursive analysis of emerging data (LeCompte & Preissle, 1993), triangulating different data types and sources to identify salient themes or categories relevant to students' reflective writing. Themes identified in one semester were compared with those from other semesters. For example, using the systematic interpretive procedure (Fitzgerald, 995), I reread all categories and themes for clarification, confirmation or disconfirmation of emerging hypothesis. I looked for statements or ideas that were particularly revealing, expressive or outstanding. These were taken to the teacher candidates for verification and confirmation, including stimulated recall sessions with discussion transcripts. Based on the analysis and comparison of data for each semester, I collated themes that depicted the impact of technology integration on students' reflections. The themes that emerged in data analysis were those that were mostly consistent across semesters. The themes included those of structure, variety, theory, collaboration and experimentation. Through descriptive narrative accounts of classroom activities and interactions with various technological tools, I created patterned explanations of how the integration of technology can support opportunities for thoughtful reflections by teacher candidates. In the next session, I will highlight these key themes and findings that may contribute to our understanding of how technology can be used to increase teacher candidates' reflections.

The Impact of Structure on Reflection: Scaffolding and Modeling

Participants in this study were given guidelines for reflection. These guidelines were clearly communicated to the TCs so that they would easily conceptualize what they were required to consider and report in their reflective papers. For example, the guideline required candidates to describe the technological tool they used, how they learned to use the tool and how teacher modeling and interaction with peers helped them to navigate that particular technology. In addition, they must discuss the affordances and constraints of using that technology for instruction, the challenges they faced learning to use that particular technology and how they would envisage using the tool in their classrooms. Finally, candidates were also asked to examine if the technological tool can truly facilitate critical thinking or if teachers would likely use it in a way that supports "old wine in new wine bottle syndrome" (Stolle, 2008). However, candidates were not bound by these guidelines. They were instructed to not use the guidelines as a shopping list but as a guide to help direct their thinking. The guidelines provided the candidates with a structure to reflect on their learning in order to develop an insider mindset for technology integration. Lankshear and Knobel (2006) identified two divergent mindsets with regard to the ways technologies are conceived. The first assumes that the world remain essentially the same only that it is more technologized, while the second mindset recognizes that the contemporary world is different in many ways from the world we have known because of the uptake of digital electronic internetworked technologies (Lankshear & Knobel, 2006). The purpose of providing a structure was to help teacher candidates develop an insider mindset necessary to be proficient in technology use. Scaffolding teacher reflections ensured that the reflections were of high quality and enabled the candidates to be more meta-cognitively aware of their knowledge base. This finding corroborates Harford and MacRuairc's (2008) view that scaffolding teacher candidates' reflections would enable them think beyond their original ability. According to Schmidt and Gurbo (2008), the process of decision-making by the teacher is extremely complex and multifaceted as she must consider many classroom and instructional variables related to designing learning activities that incorporate different technological applications. Therefore, preparation and professional experiences for teachers should encourage observation, participation and reflection. Teachers need a structure that facilitate and scaffold reflection. Zeichner and Tabachnick (1991) underscored the relevance of analytic frameworks to scaffold and structure reflection when they noted that it would be senseless to encourage or to assess reflective practice in general without establishing clear priorities for the reflections that emerge from our pedagogies (p. 2). Creating a structure that supports reflection is possible because reflective processes are teachable (Scardamalia & Bereiter (1984). This can be done through instructor modeling, stimulating self-questioning, and showing examples of synthesis of conflicting ideas. Altogether, having a structure that supports reflection means that the instructor must clearly explain the kind of thinking needed for productive reflection, and how often reflections should be written.

Modeling technology use also spurred students' reflections. Many of the teacher candidates (TCs) indicated that they were initially intimidated by the requirements of the course but after observing the instructor demonstrations of different technologies, they were able to overcome the fear of learning to use these tools. Apart from my own modeling, classroom teachers were invited to demonstrate use of particular technologies. About 60% of the interns indicated that "listening to classroom teachers speak and share their personal experiences with technology was very helpful." In addition, the TCs indicated that reading "about exemplary teachers" from book chapters and articles helped them not only to experiment with new ideas but to reflect about the usefulness of technology in classroom context. Altogether, reading about or observing models of good practice provided the TCs with more avenues to reflect on their learning and how they envisaged technology integration.

Use of Multiple Projects and Activities

During the period of this study, teacher candidates were given multiple opportunities to reflect as they engaged in a variety of technological projects that involved working in collaborative groups, in pairs and individually. Candidates designed and taught lessons using the smart board, prepared podcasts, worked on wikis and blogs and carried out an inquiry project that involved designing and utilizing a suitable technological tool to teach a selected lesson in literacy. These projects gave them several opportunities to think deeply about their learning with various technologies. In assessing their learning, many candidates pointed to the influence of multiple tasks in helping them better understand the relationship between literacy and technology. One noted "my knowledge of technology integration has deepened because of the multiple projects that forced me to connect theory to practice." Another reflected; "I have realized that each of the projects I carried out added something new to my knowledge of using and analyzing different technologies." Students' reflections indicated that hands-on activities with various technologies helped the candidates to see several possibilities of using technology for instruction and the role of teachers in technology integration. One candidate observed that after working on four technology projects, she came to realize that it was crucial for teachers to help students "think critically about technology instead of just surfing the web and getting lost in cyberspace." In all, working with multiple technological projects not only increased the opportunity for reflections but also helped the TCs assess the affordances and constraints of different technologies and their usefulness for classroom instruction. In addition, the TCs were able to observe many ways of integrating technology and different purposes that technologies served. However, it is pertinent to point out that while all the TCs agreed that experience with various technologies helped them to learn and reflect about different technologies, a few, mostly in-service teachers, complained about course load and the multiple projects, because it was difficult for them to cope with the challenge of combining work and school.

Creating Cognitive Conflict with Thought-Provoking Readings

In order to promote reflections, students need to be confronted with readings that challenge their thinking, provide models of good practice and provoke their thinking about previously held beliefs. During the course of this study, the teacher candidates read about literacy learning theories such as the sociocultural, critical literacy and new technologies and literacy perspectives. These theories provided them with a background with which to talk about and discuss the relevance of technology integration and the need to connect theory to practice. The theories were relatively new to them, and created a cognitive conflict (Hughes & Scharber, 2008), which caused many of the candidates to question, accept or imagine several possibilities of applying these perspectives to issues around technology integration. Many candidates for example, described the sociocultural theory as an "eye opener" as far as understanding the need for technology integration is concerned. Because this theory advocates connecting in and out-of-school literacies, many of the TCs were able to make connection between this theory and technology integration. One candidate queried "What better way can teachers bring students' knowledge into the classroom than to bring in technology that they are being exposed to at home?" In addition to posing this question, this candidate critiqued some of the public schools' inability to equip teachers with the necessary skills to integrate technology, arguing that these schools have failed to understand the lives of children in the 21st century.

Critical literacy was another perspective that equipped the candidates with a tool for critical reflection. Critical perspective posits that students should be empowered to tackle sociopolitical issues pertaining to social inequities and analyze their social worlds to expose taken for granted issues as well as transform their worlds through social action like writing. This perspective gingered many of the candidates to critically analyze their course readings and question the perspectives taken by some of the authors of the books and articles that they read. After reading some book chapters and articles that promoted youth practices such as instant messaging (IM) and video games, many of the candidates rejected the argument of the authors. Eighty percent of the TCs believed that instant messaging (IM) was a hindrance to students' acquisition of academic literacies. One participant, whose views represented this group, argued that instant messaging had "affected students' spelling negatively" and made students' writing "more problematic." However, a contrary view was expressed by another participant, who represented 20% of the preservice teachers. She argued that IM is a social practice and part of children's functional literacy. In defending IM as a genuine social practice, she cited Rogoff's (2003) assertion that it was important to look at what people do with literacy in their everyday lives and instead of what they do not do when compared to a dominant group. In another reading, all teacher candidates (100%) rejected the view that video games promote learning and social interaction. For example, one intern argued that video games may be more detrimental than advantageous to children because children who play video games excessively will lack interpersonal skills and this may hinder their social development. Another intern equated video games with "addiction," adding that it was a "distraction" to children's learning. In many classrooms, argued another, "video games are no longer a proper choice to write about in writer's workshop." Some interns blamed the fast-paced, vivid colors and crazy sound effects of the Internet, television and video games for today's children's inability to adapt to the seemingly slow paced classroom learning. In all these examples, the candidates experienced a conflict between their prior beliefs and readings. Armed with a critical perspective, they questioned the assumptions of some authors while asserting their view points. These were aspects of productive reflection (Davies, 2006).

After reading about an exemplary teacher who used technology in a variety of ways, some candidates wondered if the teacher's practices were tenable in a school district with meager resources or if untenured teachers can afford to take the type of risk she took. Some also realized that they had a long way to go to achieve that type of proficiency. In their reflections, some candidates became more analytic by specifying the conditions that facilitated the teacher's successful technology use and how new teachers can cope or enhance such conditions. In all, both learning theories and thought-provoking readings facilitated reflections especially dialogic and critical reflections. Altogether, the more candidates read about issues that challenged their thinking, the more reflective they were. One candidate admitted "I think all of the readings challenged my view of literacy." Evidence from students' reflections showed that working with different technologies was instrumental to their growth in reflection. Another factor was collaboration.

Group Collaboration

Collaboration provided additional avenue for reflective thinking and writing. During the period of this study, the teacher candidates worked on some collaborative projects. First, each worked with a partner to learn to use the interactive white board and another self-selected inquiry project. In addition, they worked in groups to design and maintain group wikis as well as participate in a literacy artifact project. According to Niess (2008), the acquisition of TCPK is enhanced when teacher candidates form collaborative groups with similar interests and then identify a specific content area, design an inquiry around the topic and decide the technological tool suitable to teach the topic (Niess, 2008). Evidence from this study indicates that collaboration among teacher candidates offered them the opportunity to discuss their experiences with others, access their knowledge and exchange ideas with peers or more knowledgeable others. Ninety-three percent of the interns in this study indicated that collaborating with a peer or group members to carry out their technology projects facilitated their learning and their ability to better design and select appropriate technologies that suited their content. In the reflection guideline, they were told specifically to discuss the role their partner or group members played in the collaboration.

In their reflections, most of the TCs indicated that working with group members on various projects helped them to become better users of technology. Many observed that they initially felt intimidated by their more knowledgeable peers but later gained confidence and learned from them. The wiki for example allowed users to be both designers and mediators of text, which allowed for joint editing and revision of the wiki content. It was also easy to monitor individual participation on the wiki. Reflecting on their group wiki, one candidate wrote: "being a part of a team was gratifying and motivated me to do my best to be a contributing member." Another discussed the effect of collaboration on her writing skills using the wiki. "I made sure my grammar and spellings were properly written so that when my group members read my entry, it would be clear." Others simply extolled the value of working with others, like one candidate who noted: "working with a partner was extremely valuable; we played on each other's strengths and offset each other's weaknesses." Group projects, some noted, helped them better access their knowledge based when compared with others. There was no doubt from the teachers' reflections that collaborative projects helped them learn to work in a community and "bounce ideas off one another." This, in turn facilitated reflections. In all, collaboration is critical to reflecting on one's own practice (Halter, 2006), and has been identified as one of the dynamic thinking tools for developing declarative, procedural, schematic and strategic knowledge for TCPK (Niess, 2008). However, a few candidates, while acknowledging the benefit of collaboration, would rather work alone because of the perceived inconveniences of working with others. They cited the problem of finding time to meet with partners and the issue of non-cooperating partners or group members.

Authentic Hands-On Activities

Quality reflection depends on authentic experience and a combination of experience and reflection leads to professional growth (Posner, 2005). For students to get authentic experience, they need the opportunity for hands-on activities with multiple projects to strengthen their learning about new technologies. All participants (100%) indicated that having the opportunity to experiment with new technologies was the most powerful learning tool they had. As Lankshear & Knobel (1997) noted, "mastery, fruitful experimentation and testing the borders of contemporary usages" (P.178), inventing new social practices and technology-mediated literacies call for knowledge grasp of authentic social practices in which new technologies are embedded. One candidate quipped "I found that the projects that I actually researched and had hands-on experience served much more purpose for myself." Another observed "I am a very hands-on learner. When I am actually given the opportunity work with something, I tend to be more creative and learn much more from it." Another noted "I believe the best way to integrate technology successfully is to make more opportunities for hands-on interaction with certain technologies." It was clear that the hands-on experience helped the candidates to have much more purpose for their work. They made out more time to practice how to use these technologies which facilitated productive reflections.

Harris (2008) advocated for what he called "knowledge building activities" that would allow teacher candidates to build content related understanding through information-based processes. According to Harris (2008), divergent knowledge expression activities such as video production and analysis, digital storytelling, designing virtual books, creating websites, among others, promote reflective thinking because they involved the use of multimedia and are ubiquitous artifacts of modern culture. aHarris HH This view aligns with the findings of this study. Many candidates noted that "playing around" with different technologies such as setting up a wiki, designing smart board lessons, producing podcasts and creating inquiry-based activities were key knowledge building activities that helped them to effectively navigate new technologies and gain necessary confidence. They were also instrumental to a more productive reflection because they provided opportunity for the teacher candidates to design, discuss, select among, combine and apply different contents with appropriate pedagogies. These hands-on activities enabled the TCs to discuss the affordances and constraints of different technological tools. For example, the potential constraints of the Interactive White Board (IWB) were highlighted by some of the TCs. While they applauded the interactivity of the IWB, some pointed out that teachers might use it superficially without facilitating thoughtful learning. Another observed that while the Internet created many affordances "it has also robed teachers of creativity and innovation." Many teachers she noted, now depend on Internet lesson plans and other resources to teach rather than create custom-made lessons to suit the specific needs of their students. In all, opportunity for hands-on experience increased not only the quantity but quality of reflection by the teachers. However, many teacher candidates (TCs) indicated in their reflections that if they were not required to present their projects to their peers, they would not have been very serious about learning to use these technologies. Presenting and sharing their work with peers therefore motivated them to take their hands-on learning more serious and facilitated better reflection.

Inquiry and Problem-Based Approaches

Inquiry model of learning generally involves identifying a problem, generating questions, collecting the data, analyzing the data and deducing findings. During the period of this study, candidates had a choice to work on a number of inquiry projects. The questions were given in form of problem-solving projects in which candidates were given some scenarios. For example, one question asked candidates to assume they had many students who missed classes for one reason or the other. They were asked to find appropriate technological tool that would enable their students to listen to the lesson and answer some questions. To answer this question, they needed to think of possible technological tools and their affordances and constraints and then select the one they felt would be most appropriate. They also needed to evaluate their lesson effectiveness after they get a feedback from their peers. Because the entire project required deep thinking to plan, select and implement, most of the reflections were deep seated. Two students who prepared a podcast reflected on the challenge of choosing the right tool, deciding which lesson to podcast and how to simplify the lesson so that students listening to it at home can easily follow it. In her reflection, one TC wrote "podcasting a science lesson for students took a lot out of me in terms of deciding how to go about it." Another student wrote "it took me days to complete what I thought was a simple assignment. I realized that much thinking went into its planning and implementation." Some students chose other inquiry projects like webquest or mini unit plan. A pair that worked on a webquest project reflected on their learning:

I have heard and seen teachers who used webquest but I never used it nor designed one myself. During this project, we were asked to choose and prepare a tool that would enable our students to research on the Internet and we chose a webquest. However, it was not easy designing an original webquest. We brainstormed on a couple of ideas and topics and thought of how to write the introduction, the tasks, the process, resources e.t.c. The most challenging was finding websites that are kid friendly and would align with our 4th grade science unit. Then we had to create a rubric to evaluate students. Altogether, it was challenging because we created it from scratch. However, the experience has helped me to really understand how to design and use webquests

Like this TC pointed out, hands-on, inquiry-based learning spurred genuine reflections because the students had firsthand experience about the activity they engaged in. In all, the quality and quantity of students' reflections increased greatly as a result of their hands-on problem-based approach. Another important step that helped to increase students' reflection was the requirement that they write a reflection for each technology project they participated in. There was also a culminating reflection at the end of the semester where the candidates were required to reflect on all the projects and evaluate their learning, the challenges they faced and how they resolved their issues. Altogether, the inquiry model for technology integration was effective in helping teacher candidates reflect deeply and assess the affordances and constraints of each technological tool they used. Teacher inquiry around technology scaffolds prospective teachers as they systematically and intentionally explore their use of technology through a focused investigation. Dawson (2006) noted that technology-enhanced, project-based learning can support higher levels of cognitive processing and reflection, but only with substantial planning, support, and preparation on the part of the teacher. This observation is in line with findings from this study. Inquiry projects increased both the quality and quantity of students' reflection, because they designed and implemented the projects which gave them a repertoire of technological knowledge base to draw from. It also facilitated critical thinking as they analyzed the interplay among content, pedagogy and technology and as they evaluated the needs of the audience and configured their design to meet these needs.

DISCUSSIONS AND IMPLICATIONS

This study examined the role of technology in enhancing reflective thinking by teacher candidates (TCs). In addition, I examined the TCs' reflection to ascertain what type of reflection dominated their writing and which activities, pedagogical approach or scaffolding techniques promoted reflection. The literature on technology and teacher reflection indicates that reflection is critically important in helping teacher candidates develop technology proficiency especially their ability to think, plan, select, describe, analyze and implement lessons that take into account content, technology and pedagogy. According to Harford & MacRuairc (2008), if teacher candidates merely participate in technology learning and integration without thinking deeply about it and without examining their experiences for their significance, their growth in technology knowledge will be stymied. Findings from this study indicate that creating a structure that promotes reflection, use of multiple projects, thought-provoking readings, collaboration, hands-on activities and a problem-solving approach all enhanced the opportunity for teacher candidates to reflect as well as the quality of such reflection.

The TCs who participated in this study grew in their reflective ability partly because a structure that promoted reflection was put in place. Most of the candidates initially used the reflection guideline to articulate their thinking. Gradually, they not only internalized these guidelines but were also able to articulate and create theirs. In addition, instructor modeling and those from practicing teachers spurred the TCs to overcome fear and intimidation which many of them had at the inception of the study.

Because the TCs had varied contexts and experiences with various technologies, their reflective abilities increased because they had several experiences to draw from. This is not surprising because for some teacher candidates, their learning styles and the way they engage with technology vary according to: whether they worked on their own or in a group; whether they had a limited and extended knowledge base in the area; perceptions about their learning competence in the area and their beliefs. In addition, engaging with multiple projects facilitated cognitive flexibility (Spiro, Coulson, Feltovich, & Anderson (2004). Cognitive flexibility proposes that knowledge that will be used in many ways has to be "learned, represented and tried out (in application) in many ways" (Spiro et al., 1994), p.607), in order to capture the real-world complexities to which abstract conceptual knowledge must be applied. Central to the assumptions of cognitive flexibility theory are approaches to learning and instruction that places important roles for multiple knowledge representations, emphasizes knowledge assembly rather knowledge reproduction and promote active students' learning. Through different technology projects that the TCs participated in, they were better able to conceptualize different ways to use technology for classroom instruction which in turn increased the quality and quantity of their reflection.

In addition, it appeared that group learning helped the candidates to better work in their zone of proximal development and to reflect more deeply. It provided a social dynamics of working with others (Dawson, 2005; Mishra & Koehler, 2006). According to the partnership for the 21st Century Skills (2006), teachers should be able to redesign and create curriculum and instruction to prepare their students with the skills of the 21st century literate citizens such as collaboration, participatory culture, distributed expertise, collective intelligence, sharing, experimentation, innovation and evolution (Lankshear & Knobel, 2006). Working in groups to design and create units of study that integrated technology expanded the TCs repertoire of experience which became a vital tool for reflection. This finding is in line with Harford and MacRuairc (2008) observation that collaborative groups that are student-led, democratic, inclusive and sustainable foster a climate of reflective practice. By allowing the TCs to choose, design and implement units that involved use of new technologies with their peers, they were better able to conceptualize and reflect on how the new technologies impacted their learning.

Furthermore, a hands-on experience that involved problem-solving and inquiry oriented projects remained the most potent experience that spurred reflection. Without this concrete experience, it was doubtful if the TCs would have engaged in productive reflections. It appeared that planning, thinking about, designing, carrying out technology projects and teaching lessons with technology as opposed to merely learning about these technologies created genuine possibilities and challenges of using particular technologies for instruction (Niess, 2008; Schmidt & Gurbo, 2008). This, in turn spurred productive reflection in which candidates were able to reflect critically on their use of technology. This helped the teachers not only to monitor their progress in the development of TCPK but also to think, accept, reject, question, critique and imagine several possibilities of teaching and learning with various technologies. Evidence from this study indicates that there was a big difference between merely exposing students to different technologies or modeling their use versus making them teach with these technologies. During the first semester of this study, hands-on experience was highly limited and so were the TCs reflection. However, as soon as students engaged in more hands-on experiences, their reflective ability increased. Again, because they were required to present lessons with new technologies, most of the interns spent hours of their private time practicing how to use them thereby increasing their comfort level with these tools. This, in turn increased the quality and quantity of their reflections. They became more analytic, dialogic and critical about the usefulness of new technologies.

Certain implications for technology in teacher education can be deduced from the discussions above.

First, in order to help teachers to reflect, a structure that promotes reflection must be in place. The structure must allow the instructor to model reflective process and provide a clear guideline and expectations for students' reflection. Modeling should also extend to having practicing teachers demonstrate the use of technology. It is also important for teacher candidates to read well written articles about exemplary teachers who use technology. Productive reflection as opposed to merely descriptive reflection is not easy to achieve and needs practice and growth in reflective writing. By giving the teacher candidates a guideline as a general thinking tool, many educators can help the TCs improve the quality of their reflection. Candidates should also reflect on the interdependence of technology, pedagogy and content so that knowledge of each aspect is developed concurrently (Harris, 2008). By doing this, we help the candidates develop TPCK. In addition, selection of quality reading materials that would spur cognitive conflict and use of inquiry-based approach to technology analysis are some of the ways that educators can increase the reflective ability of teacher candidates.

Secondly, teacher candidates need sound theoretical knowledge, especially those from the sociocultural theory, new literacies and critical media literacy. These theories not only challenge their long-held beliefs and provide a necessary foundational knowledge but also spur them to greater reflection. When TCs encounters new information that does not align with their schemas, they are better able to think, question and analyze the new information, thereby increasing the quality of reflection. Ultimately, teacher educators should encourage hands-on, problem-based approach to learning in which different types of collaborative learning is encouraged.

Finally, teacher educators should create multifaceted opportunities and motivating contexts for teachers to experiment with new technologies so that current and prospective teachers are able to explore and synthesize their experiences as new technology users. This, in turn will facilitate cognitive flexibility. There should be a reflective requirement for each activity or project that students embarked on in the course of taking any course that integrates technology (Niess, 2008). Teacher candidates should be given the opportunity to work within authentic contexts in order to reflect on their learning and to determine the effects of their technology-using practices. In addition, they need robust hand-on, problem-based approach to learning with new technologies as well as the opportunity to observe models in authentic contexts.

REFERENCES

Albion, P. R. (2008). Web 2.0 in teacher education: Two imperatives for action [Electronic version]. *Computers in the Schools*, *25*, 181–198. doi:10.1080/07380560802368173

Attwell, G. (2007). *Web 2.0 and the changing ways we are using computers for learning: What are the implications for pedagogy and curriculum?* Retrieved February 20, 2009, from http://www.elearningeuropa.info/files/media/media13018.pdf

Cummins, J., Brown, K., & Sayers, D. (2007). *Literacy, technology, and diversity: Teaching for success in changing times*. Boston: Allyn and Bacon.

Dana, N. F., & Silva, D. Y. (2003). *The reflective educators' guide to classroom research: Learning to teach and teaching to learn through practitioner inquiry*. Thousand Oaks, CA: Corwin Press.

Davis, E. A. (2006). Characterizing productive reflection among preservice elementary teachers: Seeing what matters. *Teaching and Teacher Education*, *22*, 281–301. doi:10.1016/j.tate.2005.11.005

Dawson, K. (2006). Teacher inquiry: A vehicle to merge prospective teachers' experience and reflection during curriculum-based technology-enhanced field experiences. *Journal of Research on Technology in Education*, *38*(3), 265–292.

Feisman-Nemser, S. (2001). From preparation to practice: Designating a continuum to strengthen and sustain teaching. *The Teachers'. College Record*, *103*(6), 1013–1055. doi:10.1111/0161-4681.00141

Fendler, L. (2003). Teacher reflection in hall of mirrors: Historical influences and politic reverberations. *Educational Researcher*, *32*(3), 16–25. doi:10.3102/0013189X032003016

Harford, J., & MacRuaire, G. (2008). Engaging student teachers in meaningful reflective practice. *Teaching and Teacher Education*, *24*, 1884–1892. doi:10.1016/j.tate.2008.02.010

Hatton, N., & Smith, D. (1995). Reflection in teacher education: Toward definition and implementation. *Teaching and Teacher Education*, *11*(1), 33–49. doi:10.1016/0742-051X(94)00012-U

Hedberg, J. G., & Brudvik, O. C. (2008). Supporting dialogic literacy through mashing and modding of places and spaces. *Theory into Practice*, *47*(2), 138–149. doi:10.1080/00405840801992363

Hughes, J. E., & Scharber, C. M. (2008). Leveraging the development of English TPCK within the deictic nature of literacy. In AACTE committee on Innovation and Technology (Eds.), Handbook of Technological Pedagogical Content Knowledge (TPCK) for Educators (pp. 87-106). New York: Routeldge.

Kolalchick, A., & Milman, N. B. (1998). Instructional strategies for integrating Technology: Electronic journals and technology portfolios as facilitators for self-efficacy and reflection in preservice teachers. *Technology and Teacher Education Annual, 3-7.*

Lankshear, C., & Knobel, M. (2006). *New literacies: Changing knowledge in the classroom.* Maidenhead, UK: Open University Press.

LeCompte, M. D., & Preissle, J. (1993). *Ethnography and qualitative design in educational research*. New York: Academic Press.

Lin, Q. (2008). Preservice teachers' learning experiences of constructing e-portfolios online. *The Internet and Higher Education*, *2*, 194–200. doi:10.1016/j.iheduc.2008.07.002

Lin, X., & Kinzer, C. K. (2003). The importance of technology for making cultural values visible. *Theory into Practice*, *42*(3), 234–242. doi:10.1207/s15430421tip4203_10

Mishra, P., & Koehler, M. J. (2006). Technological Pedagogical content knowledge: A framework for teacher knowledge. *Teachers College Record*, *108*(6), 1017–1054. doi:10.1111/j.1467-9620.2006.00684.x

Niess, M. L. (2008). Guiding preservice teachers to develop TPCK. In AACTE committee on Innovation and Technology (Eds.), Handbook of Technological Pedagogical Content Knowledge (TPCK) for Educators (223-250). New York: Routledge.

Partnership for the 21st century. (2008). *Framework for the 21st century skills*. Retrieved September 30, 2007, from http://www.21stcenturyskills.org

Rich, P. J., & Hannafin, M. (2009). Video Annotation Tools: Technologies to scaffold, structure and transform teacher reflection. *Journal of Teacher Education*, *60*(1), 52–67. doi:10.1177/0022487108328486

Scardamalia, M., Bereiter, C., & Steinback, R. (1984). The teachability of reflective processes in written composition. *Cognitive Science*, *8*, 173–190.

Schon, D. A. (1987). *Educating the reflective practitioner: Toward a new design for teaching and learning in the profession*. San Francisco: Jossey Bass.

Spiro, R. J., Coulson, R. L., Feltovich, P. J., & Anderson, D. K. (2004). Cognitive Flexibility Theory: Advanced knowledge acquisition in ill-structured domains. In Ruddell, R. B., & Unrau, N. J. (Eds.), *Theoretical models and processes of reading* (5th ed., pp. 640–653). Newark, DE: International Reading Association.

Zeichner, K., & Tabachnick, B. R. (1991). Reflections on reflective thinking. In Tabachnick, B. R., & Zeichner, K. (Eds.), *Issues and practices in inquiry-oriented teacher education* (pp. 1–21). Bristol, PA: Falmer.

Chapter 20
The Professional Handbook:
Developing Professionalism and Reflective Skills while Connecting Theory and Practice through Technology

Sara Winstead Fry
Boise State University, USA

ABSTRACT

The Professional Handbook is a teacher education assignment that allows preservice teachers to use technology to connect theory and practice while also developing their reflective skills and professionalism. The assignment involves compiling information in an easy-to-use website that preservice teachers can access while engaged in their semester-long student teaching experience and once they are employed as inservice teachers. This chapter describes the Handbook's essential goals, discusses its use in an instructional methods course, and makes recommendations for modifying the Handbook's format for use in any teacher education course while preserving the framework provided by the assignment's essential goals. The chapter serves as a resource for teacher educators looking to use technology to enhance the quality of teacher preparation assignments.

INTRODUCTION

What kinds of assignments allow prospective teachers to *truly* learn sophisticated theoretical frameworks as well as research-based approaches for teaching so these approaches will not be overlooked in favor of invention or trial-and-error[1] when they enter the classroom? How can assignments be designed so they require positive interdependence among prospective teachers so they learn how to work as collegial professionals? What kinds of assignments allow prospective teachers to develop technology skills they can use with their students once they begin to work in public schools? How can reflection be meaningfully included in teacher education assignments? The search for answers to these questions led to the development and refinement of the Professional Handbook, a teacher education assignment that allows preservice teachers to use technology to develop reflective skills and professionalism while also connecting theory and practice. The assignment is pragmatic because it

DOI: 10.4018/978-1-61520-897-5.ch020

Copyright © 2010, IGI Global. Copying or distributing in print or electronic forms without written permission of IGI Global is prohibited.

involves compiling information into an easy-to-use website that preservice teachers can access while engaged in their semester-long student teaching experience and once they are employed as inservice teachers. The Handbook offers great potential but has yet to be formally validated, although preliminary action research evidence supports the efficacy of the assignment.

It is important to point out the distinction between the Professional Handbook and a teaching portfolio. Teaching portfolios are a holistic assessment that allows preservice teachers to demonstrate their professional competence, growth, and academic achievement through a thoughtfully prepared collection of materials (Hill, 2003). Hill also explained that portfolios are intended to be a more authentic source of information about preservice teachers' abilities to teach than their transcripts, scores on professional licensure exams, and check-list student teacher evaluations. In contrast, the Professional Handbook is a tool preservice teachers can use while student teaching and as inservice teachers. A Handbook might be a meaningful artifact to include in a teaching portfolio, but its primary purpose is utilitarian. It is not a holistic assessment of professional competence.

This chapter provides a background to issues related to the Professional Handbook; introduces readers to the context and components of the Professional Handbook, including the assignment's essential goals; and describes the results of preliminary action research about the assignment's effectiveness. The chapter also makes recommendations for modifying the Handbook's format for use in any teacher education course while preserving the framework provided by the essential goals; describes issues, problems, solutions, and recommendations; and discusses future research directions. The chapter serves as a resource for teacher educators looking to use technology to enhance the quality of teacher preparation assignments.

BACKGROUND

This chapter is grounded in two beliefs about teacher education assignments. First, assignments can have a pragmatic purpose yet also help preservice teachers learn sophisticated theoretical frameworks and research-based approaches for teaching. Second, one assignment can be designed to achieve multiple goals that support the preparation of beginning teachers. The Professional Handbook is such an assignment, and it has three overarching goals: 1) reduce the gap between theory-based teacher preparation experiences and inservice teachers' practice, 2) increase preservice teachers' technology skills, and 3) foster the development of preservice teachers' reflective skills and professionalism. These goals provide the overarching framework for the Handbook, and this section reviews related literature. The term "student teaching" is used throughout this chapter, and for the sake of clarity it is defined as a culminating, semester-long field experience in which a teacher candidate ultimately assumes responsibility for (nearly) all of the planning, curriculum, and instruction in a classroom under the supervision of a mentor teacher and a representative from the teacher preparation institution.

Goal 1: Reduce the Gap between Theory and Practice

The first goal is fundamental because of the gap between theory and practice that has been prominent in the literature for more than three decades (for examples, see Feiman-Nemser, 2001; Flores, 2007; Goodlad, 1990; Lortie, 1975). Lortie's seminal book *Schoolteacher* explored how teachers' professional isolation contributed to the gap between theory and practice, and many of the problems Lortie identified over thirty years ago remain. More recent studies reported how beginning inservice and preservice teachers often failed to implement teaching techniques they are taught in their preparation programs (Feiman-Nemser;

Gratch, 2000). For example, Gratch found preservice teachers prone to adopting their cooperating teachers' attitudes and approaches uncritically, with no consideration of their implications for students. This suggests that preservice teachers may fail to effectively implement reflective practice, a beneficial teaching behavior advocated by teacher preparation programs (literature related to reflective practice is discussed in the section for *Goal 3)*.

Hawley (as quoted in Lieb, 1992) explained the results of the gap between theory and practice:

Colleges of teacher education can train people to do anything. When teachers enter the schools, however, they do not do those things... Even in the most powerful programs, the slippage, the fadeout is pretty high. When teachers enter their classrooms, much of what they have learned dissipates (p. 13).

Related problems have been reported in more recent literature (Feiman-Nemser, 2001; Fry, 2007; McLeskey & Billingsley, 2008), suggesting that the slippage problem Hawley discussed nearly two decades ago remains. Such problems are not unique to the United States. Upon finding that contemporary teacher preparation reforms in Australia and England were undertaken with a sense of "historic amnesia," Vick (2006) documented teacher education models that were used from 1900-1950 to provide teacher educators with a historical context for their efforts to address contemporary issues. Al-Sharaf (2006) described how prospective teachers at Kuwait University encountered disconnect between theory and practice during student teaching because they were supervised by representatives from the government's Ministry of Education, and there was no coordination between the university and the Ministry. The literature indicates that the gap between theory and practice is a contemporary problem with historic precedence and international relevance.

Reducing the problem is possible; some studies report successful initiatives that used technology as a tool to bridge theory and practice. Recognizing that the gap begins in preparatory coursework, Barnett (2008) used a web-based professional development forum to allow preservice teachers to interact with inservice teachers who used the kinds of innovative inquiry-based instructional practices taught in a university's science methods courses. The forum facilitated preservice teachers' reflective practice by giving them the opportunity to "critically examine real classrooms through online videos of teaching practice, and engage in collaborative discussion with peers" (p. 3). Others have used technology such as email to help span the gap between theory and practice during student teaching and the first year of teaching (Brintnall, 2002; Roddy, 1999). Babinski, Jones, and DeWert (2001) found that discussion boards were a meaningful method of supporting first-year teachers. Fry and Bryant (2006-2007) found that the use of multiple forms of distance technology has the capacity to help preservice teachers make connections between their preparation program and student teaching experiences as well as increase their comfort with educational technology. The need to enhance preservice teachers' skills with technology is discussed further in the next section.

Goal 2: Increase Preservice Teachers' Technology Skills

Another literature-based impetus for the Handbook was the documented need to increase preservice teachers' instructional technology skills. Studies have indicated the inadequacy of the instructional technology preparation many preservice teachers receive. Problems stem from a lack of experience integrating technology into curriculum and instruction because many prospective teachers are only required to take one technology course, often in the first or second year of a teacher preparation program (Pope, Hare, & Howard, 2005). Some teacher preparation programs do not require any computer coursework (Austin, 2004; Whetstone & Carr-Chellman, 2001). Lei's (2009) investigation of confidence and competence using instructional technology in classroom settings among "digital natives" suggested that technology preparation will remain important even as the preservice teacher population grows more technology literate. Bansavich (2005) found that level of comfort, attitude towards, and proficiency with technology were positively correlated with preservice teachers' readiness to integrate technology into instruction. These findings underscore the importance of providing preservice teachers with experiences that increase their exposure to technology rather than leaving them to learn instructional technology skills on their own. Bansavich, Albee (2003), and Fleming, Motamedi, and May (2007) recommended integrating technology into teacher preparation courses and student teaching so skills are not learned in isolation.

Graham, Culatta, Pratt, and West (2004) also valued integration, but they recognized that complete integration of technology skills into teacher education coursework often poses logistical barriers. Their experience completely redesigning an instructional technology course at a large university underscored the importance of fundamental skills. They explained, "While we would have preferred to focus much more on integration, inadequate incoming technology literacy levels of many students made it essential to first teach basic technology skills" (p. 137). Likewise, Banister and Vannatta (2006) indicated that the technology skills many preservice teachers possess posed a barrier to integrating instructional technology into education coursework. Professors at their university often eliminated technology integration lessons because the time-consuming process of teaching technology skills left them with inadequate time for the pedagogy of technology integration. Banister and Vannatta indicated that a strong foundation in basic technology skills is needed before preservice teachers can be prepared to integrate technology in K-12 school settings.

Other studies have reported how using educational technology in meaningful contexts can increase preservice teachers' competence and confidence with technology (Fry & Bryant, 2006-2007; Lin, 2008). Lin used a yearlong case study to determine the impact that creating electronic online portfolios had on 38 preservice teachers. Creating the electronic portfolios was not a course or graduation requirement. The participants found the experience beneficial because it allowed them to review technology skills they already possessed as well as learn new ones. Results indicated that participants seemed to learn more because they were required to apply course-based learning to a new environment. Lin's participants also found that constructing the electronic portfolios fostered their reflective skills. The importance of reflective skills and professionalism among preservice teachers is discussed in the following section.

Goal 3: Foster the Development of Preservice Teachers' Reflective Skills and Professionalism

Professionalism is an essential quality among teachers, and it has multiple facets. Professionalism includes knowing how to seek help from and participate with colleagues in professional communities, which "can be especially powerful influences on learning [to teach]" (Hammerness, et al. 2005, p. 388). Bransford, Darling-Hammond, and LePage (2005) described dedication to student success as an essential component of professionalism among teachers. Demonstration of these and other professional qualities are often required for initial teacher certification in the United States, where individual states set certification requirements. For example, in Pennsylvania a teacher candidate has to demonstrate the "Ability to cultivate professional relationships with school colleagues" (Pennsylvania Department of Education, 2009, p. 4). The need to demonstrate professionalism continues in a teacher's inservice career, and research makes it clear that teachers value good colleagues. For example, in a study describing how early childhood educators in New Zealand defined professionalism, Dalli (2007) asked participants to describe professional qualities in a teacher. Seventy-five percent of the 594 participants included collaborative relationships in their descriptions, underscoring the importance of this aspect of teachers' professionalism.

Likewise, the ability to engage in reflective practice is another essential component of teachers' professional responsibilities. Like collegiality, it is a common requirement for initial teacher certification in the United States. Idaho's Standards for Initial Certification of Professional School Personnel (2005) require the candidate to be "a reflective practitioner who demonstrates a commitment to professional standards and is continuously engaged in purposeful mastery of the art and science of teaching" (p. V). Reflective practice has been defined as thoughtful consideration of classroom events that leads to plans for action; the plans can be implemented immediately or be long-term decisions about how to teach more effectively (Dicker & Monda-Amaya, 1995; Valli, 1997). Semantic variations in the meaning of reflective practice contribute to a fuller understanding of the concept. Specifically, Dewey (1933) defined reflective thought as: "*Action, persistent, and careful consideration of any belief or supposed form of knowledge in the light of the grounds that support it and the further conclusions to which it tends*" (p. 9, emphasis in original). Dewey believed reflective thinking leads to action as opposed to the contemplation that comes with mere thinking. Schön (1983) discussed the differences between reflection-in-action, which happens at the time of an event, and reflection-on-action, which happens after. Both are important skills for an educator, as one must be able to make quick decisions in the classroom as well as make thoughtful plans for long-term change.

Given the importance of professionalism and reflective practice in teachers, it is essential for teacher education programs to prepare novices to be reflective professionals. At the same time, teacher education programs also need to prepare new teachers who are able to bridge the gap between theory and practice and who also demonstrate proficiency with educational technology. Existing literature established the importance of these goals and documented efforts to promote their achievement. However, the use of well-designed teacher education assignments intended to address all of these goals simultaneously appears undeveloped in the literature. Therefore, the Professional Handbook was developed to address this gap and provide teacher candidates with an assignment that allowed them to engage in reflective practice in a professional manner while developing a technology-based tool they can use to help bridge the gap between theory and practice. The following section provides a more specific description of the Professional Handbook.

THE PROFESSIONAL HANDBOOK

A Professional Handbook consists of a website that organizes and preserves materials from teacher preparation coursework. The format described here does not require the instructor or prospective teachers to possess advanced or highly sophisticated technology skills. Indeed, the author's interest in giving students meaningful experiences with instructional technology often surpasses her own technological skill level. As a result, the author consulted with the instructional technology team where she worked to identify a format for the Handbook that the university could support. It was also important that Handbook development use technology that would not take a lot of time for preservice teachers to learn. Rather than recommending and providing an in-depth description of how use a specific technology platform, this section focuses on the kind of thinking about teaching and learning compiling a Professional Handbook facilitates. Issues, problems, solutions and recommendations related to the development and use of the Handbook are discussed in the subsequent sections. The solutions and recommendations section will be of particular interest to those teacher educators with limited instructional technology resources and support because it describes the use of a free and easy-to-use technology platform.

The author has used Professional Handbooks in two teacher preparation courses: social studies methods and child and adolescent development. The design can be modified for use in any teacher education course. In order to be effective, modifications should preserve the three essential goals of the handbook: 1) reduce the gap between theory-based teacher preparation experiences and inservice teachers' practice, 2) increase preservice teachers' technology skills, and 3) foster the development of preservice teachers' reflective skills and professionalism. The sub-sections that follow describe the context and components of the Handbook as it was used in the social studies methods course, present the results of preliminary action research about the Handbook, and offer guidelines for modifying the Handbook for use in other courses.

Context and Components

This section describes the how the Professional Handbook was initially used in a social studies methods course at a small liberal-arts university in the mid-Atlantic region of the United States. Because of the small size of the university, the author only taught the course during the spring semesters and candidate elementary teachers *and* secondary teachers seeking social studies certification enrolled in the course. Typically students took the course in their sophomore or junior year. The preservice teachers worked on the Professional Handbook throughout a 15-week semester and submitted the finished product as their summative assessment. Each preservice teacher prepared their Handbook as a multiple-page website that included: evaluations of and directions for instructional techniques; unit plans; evaluations of research articles; a collection of "brain breaks," short activities teachers use to help children focus; other resources such as helpful websites; and an analytical database of children's literature with social studies topics and themes. Prospective teachers also wrote a reflection about the Handbook that went beyond allowing them to make meaning of their growing skills as educators. The focus of the reflective writing helped preservice teachers develop vital skills that inservice teachers use daily: professionalism and collegiality.

Figure 1 provides an example of the home page for one student's Handbook. The homepage template used a table to organize the links to other pages, and perspective teachers had two empty squares they could fill with pictures, their university's logo, or in some other way. The author for the Handbook pictured in Figure 1 was a talented artist who used two examples of her own art to personalize the empty squares. Prospective teachers developed their handbooks using Adobe® Dreamweaver® [2] and a template the author developed. The handbooks were initially stored in a "www folder" provided to each student at the university where the Handbook was developed. Items in this folder were automatically posted on each individual preservice teacher's website, which was hosted on the university's server. Although it was easy for students to update or change Handbook content using this system, this approach was not without shortcomings. These are discussed in the *Issues and Problems* section and a new approach intended to address these problems is discussed in *Solutions and Recommendations.*

Figure 1 shows the final product of a semester's worth of work, but Handbook development begins on the first day of class when students learned that professionalism and collegiality are organizing themes for the social studies methods course. The syllabus states:

Inservice teachers share the majority of their writing publicly through documents that are prepared for students or shared with colleagues,

Figure 1. A professional handbook for teaching social studies: homepage

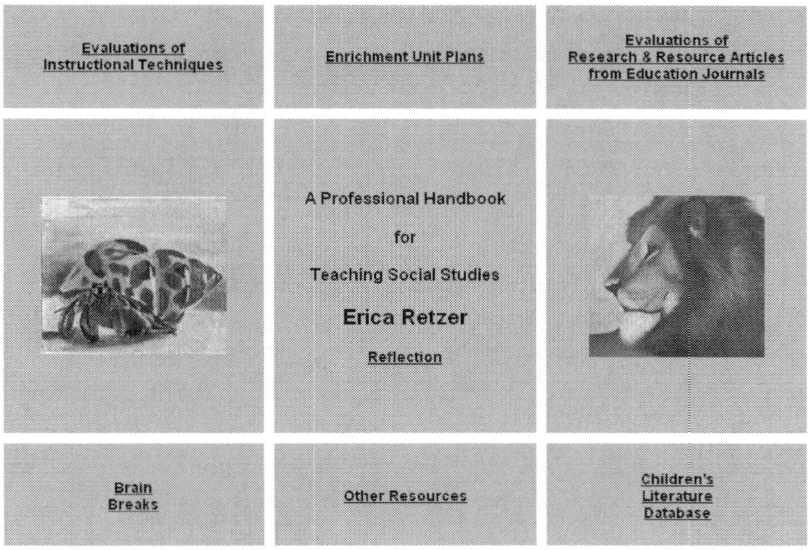

administrators, and parents. Given the nature of a teacher's professional writing, writing for this course will be shared publicly with your classmates. Your literature analysis, instructional technique write-ups, and unit plans should be prepared as public documents that you are proud to share with colleagues.

This public writing was compiled in each preservice teacher's Professional Handbook. Approximately half of each student's Handbook consisted of these common materials. Preparing professional-quality assignments to share with their classmates helped preservice teachers develop some of the professional skills required of inservice teachers. Part of the reflection component of the assignment asked the teacher candidates to explain the nature of the assignment, including how they created the Handbook in collaboration with their entire social studies methods class, and what that means about teaching in general and teaching social studies specifically. One student's words summarize the essence of the professional attitude and skills the assignment helped her to develop;

This handbook is especially reflective of the spirit of Social Studies teaching and learning. In Social Studies specifically, themes like community and democracy are central... we had to collaborate and work together to form working documents. We relied on one another for support and ideas in our work. We faced problems and challenges in a team atmosphere, and responded to suggestions for improvement through peer evaluation. These practices align well with Social Studies principles, while at the same time aligning with best practices in any teaching career. Professional educators rely on collaboration and teamwork to accomplish goals... It is in this spirit that this handbook was produced, helping to prepare us as pre-service teachers for a productive and collaborative career.

The reflections also described how the assignment was aligned with state standards for initial teacher certification and included the preservice teachers' personal thoughts about the meaning and usefulness of the assignment.

In addition to having a structured opportunity to reflect on the *process* of creating the Handbook, the preservice teachers reflected about the *content* of the Handbook throughout the semester. For example, part of the course involved learning about research-based instructional techniques. After learning how each instructional technique worked, the author led the preservice teachers in the class in a reflective discussion based on questions such as: When can teachers use this instructional technique in a K-12 the classroom? How can a teacher modify this technique for use with children in grades K-2, 3-5, 6-8, or 9-12? How can a teacher modify this technique for use with children who have a physical handicap, learning disability, or have limited English proficiency? What didn't you like about the technique that you would do differently in your own classroom? At the end of each discussion, preservice teachers were also given the opportunity to write about their personal response to the technique. This general model of learning an instructional technique and then debriefing it with a reflective discussion was repeated throughout the semester; a class typically learned 15-25 different instructional techniques.

Scaffolding this whole-class reflection prepared preservice teachers for an independent reflective component of the Handbook: each preservice teacher was required to include the directions for and evaluations of at least ten instructional techniques. For the evaluation, each preservice teacher had to briefly explain the technique in 1-2 sentences, and explain why she or he planned to use the technique in the future by clearly, explicitly, and accurately demonstrating the technique's connection to the nature and goals of social studies education. Preservice teachers need meaningful opportunities to engage in reflection early on in their preparation programs so fruitful reflective practice becomes a habit they are prepared to implement as student and inservice teachers. Assignments like the Handbook make teacher education courses laboratories for developing reflective skills by structuring pedagogical practices and assignments so they help preservice teachers learn to engage in meaningful reflective practice, which Dicker and Monda-Amaya (1995) and Valli (1997) described as the thoughtful consideration of classroom events that leads to plans for action.

Preliminary Research about the Efficacy of the Handbook

The Handbook offers great potential, but its overall impact has yet to be formally established through empirical studies using robust sample sizes. The lack of empirical studies is a result of the small size of the teacher education program where the author worked when she developed the assignment. Each year the program typically graduates between 15 and 30 elementary teacher candidates and five or fewer secondary social studies teacher candidates. Over a period of four years, approximately 35 preservice teachers developed professional handbooks; this was not a robust enough number of subjects with whom to conduct a valid quantitative study. Additionally, the many candidates prepared by the university went directly onto graduate school rather than into teaching positions. This trend limited the number of participants available for an investigation of how the Handbook is used by inservice teachers.

Even though the small program size made formal validation untenable, the author was able to use action research (Dana & Yendol-Silva, 2003) to obtain feedback about the Professional Handbook in order to improve the assignment. The Handbook was initially used in the social studies methods course during the spring 2005 semester and revised based on the author's reflections prior to the next time the course was offered in spring 2006. Most of the students in the revised course student taught in the 2006-2007 academic year. The author administered a Professional Handbook feedback questionnaire to that group of 14 elementary and 3 secondary social studies preservice teachers at the conclusion of their student teaching semester. The author also conducted in-depth interviews about Handbook use with two preservice teachers (one elementary and one secondary) who student taught during the fall 2007 semester.

Before describing the preservice teachers' reported use of their handbooks, it is necessary to explain the extent to which the elementary student teachers taught social studies. Throughout the United States the *No Child Left Behind* era has led many elementary schools and teachers to reduce the amount of instruction time available for social studies because of the pressures to improve scores on literacy and mathematics high-stakes assessments (Fry, 2009). Leming, Ellington, and Schug's (2006) survey of a nationally representative sample of elementary school teachers found that 70% "spent less than four hours per week teaching social studies" (p. 323). This discouraging statistic was actually *better* than the experiences of the 14 elementary teacher candidates who participated in the author's inquiry about the Professional Handbook. In the elementary schools where they student taught, five did not get to teach any social studies whatsoever. Another taught it "depending on the week, anywhere from 0-1 hour." Seven taught it between 1.5 and 2.5 hours a week. One student teacher got to teach the subject for five hours a week.

Despite these limited opportunities to teach social studies, the elementary student teachers who completed the questionnaire during the 2006-2007 academic year reported using their Handbooks for a variety of purposes. Although the elementary student teacher who got to teach social studies for five hours a week only reported consulting her Handbook two times, she used six of the instructional techniques and consulted two of the unit plans. A secondary social studies student teacher only reported visiting his handbook three times, but he used three instructional techniques, consulted four unit plans, and used between five and eight ideas from the unit plans. This suggests that the number of times a student teacher actually goes to the Handbook may not an indicator of how useful the candidate finds the resources it contains.

One item on the questionnaire asked, "What suggestions do you have for how the Professional Handbook could be improved to make it more useful for student teachers?" Instead of offering critical feedback, five student teachers offered praise for the Handbook and lamented not getting to teach social studies more. Nine left this question blank. Only two offered suggestions, which were: "perhaps more strategies" and "Make sure that the students' lessons are ones they could/will actually teach in student teaching, if possible." No student teachers provided critical feedback about the technology or indicated that they had difficulty using or accessing their Handbooks. The most interesting feedback came from two of the student teachers who spent a limited amount of time teaching social studies. The student teacher who only taught social studies for "approx. 1.5 hr. per week for about 5 weeks" used three instructional techniques, three books from the children's literature data base, and almost all of the ideas from one of the unit plans. The student teacher who got to teach social studies between 0-1 hours a week still reported consulting her Handbook four or more times during the semester. She used three teaching techniques from the Handbook. Most striking of all, she reported consulting the unit plans that were in her Handbook, not because she got to teach a social studies unit, but she "used them to help other [student teachers]." Since one of the goals of the Handbook was to foster professional skills, this reported use was encouraging. A similar use pattern was reported during the in-depth interview conducted with Eva, who student taught in an elementary classroom during the fall 2007 semester.

Eva described how her student teaching cohort acted as a professional community by sharing ideas for effective practice. She explained one specific day when:

[We] were throwing around ideas and someone brought up "Hey, I tried this, and it was from my Handbook." We actually ended up sharing everyone's links to different handbooks, so we could use those tools all around. Some of the student teachers didn't have handbooks [because they took the methods course with an adjunct professor], so they were appreciative, too.

This cohort demonstrated professionalism by sharing resources that could help their colleagues improve their instructional practice. Eva also explained how she consulted her Handbook when she wanted to use a specific technique that "we had talked about in a couple different classes [in the preparation program], but this was the only place where I actually had a how-to written up to tell me how to implement this." This was a typical pattern of use for Eva; she would remember the big idea behind an instructional technique and turn to her Handbook because she knew she could find the information easily. She explained:

I'm very glad that I took the time to organize [my Handbook] really well. So whenever I did have that little memory, "Hey I think we [learned] something about this two years ago," I knew exactly where to go to look for it, which I didn't do for my other classes. I think that is part of the reason I used this Handbook so much – because it was so accessible, and it was organized, and I knew exactly where to go to find things.

These reflections indicate how the Handbook helped Eva bridge theory and practice by making it easy to find the resources from her preparation experience.

Thus, although the Handbook has yet to be formally validated, the preliminary action research suggests that the assignment has the potential to help novice teachers bridge theory and practice and learn to act as a professional community. The *Future Research Directions* section near the conclusion of this chapter provides a discussion of research opportunities based on the refinement and expanded implementation of the Professional Handbook, while the next section describes how to modify the assignment for use in other courses.

Modifying the Professional Handbook for Use in Other Courses

The preceding sections described the context and content of and preliminary research about the Handbook for a social studies methods course. The Handbook has been used in a child and adolescent development course, and the requirements were adjusted according to the purposes and goals of that course. For example, the child and adolescent development course's curriculum did not include the examination of instructional techniques. Instead, prospective teachers considered typical and atypical influences on development. They created a synthesis of valuable information from required readings that they wanted to be able to reference again or share with others as inservice teachers.

Teacher educators reading this chapter are encouraged to modify the Handbook's design for use in other courses. Modifications to the assignment should be made within the framework of the essential goals of the assignment (see Table 1).

The Handbook is not a portfolio of best work, and Recommendation 1 means not every assignment prospective teachers complete should be placed in the Handbook. Three of the assignments in the social studies methods course do not go in the Handbook because, while they are meaningful, the assignments lack a utilitarian application to inservice practice. For example, the prospective teachers completed four hours of community service during the semester and wrote a reflection about how their service extended their understanding of the purposes and goals of social studies education. The reflections were thoughtful and well-written, but not pragmatic because re-reading the reflection in the context of student teaching or inservice practice would

Table 1. Recommendations for modifying the professional handbook within the framework of the assignment's essential goals

Essential Goal	Recommendation
1. Reduce the gap between theory-based teacher preparation experiences and inservice teachers' practice.	A Handbook needs to be a pragmatic collection of materials and resources teachers can use.
2. Increase preservice teachers' technology skills.	Build well-organized Handbooks using contemporary, up-to-date technology prospective teachers will be able to access as inservice teachers.
3. Foster the development of preservice teachers' reflective skills and professionalism.	Include reflection and a collaborative component in the design for Handbook development.

not help a teacher be more effective in planning and implementing curriculum and instruction.

Recommendation 2 is grounded in the understanding that teachers' access to technology in public schools does not keep pace with technology innovations. Using up-to-date technology that is available for free or at minimal cost helps preservice teachers develop technological skills they can use with their future students regardless of the financial resources of the school districts in which they work. It is also important to use technology to provide an organizational structure for Handbooks so the materials are easy to access. As Eva (the preservice teacher who was interviewed about how she used her Handbook during student teaching) explained, she used her handbook because it was easy to access and the materials were well-organized, while resources from her other preparatory classes were not. Regardless of the modifications that are made to the Handbook's design to make it useful in other courses, the end product needs to be organized and accessible. Technology plays an essential role in accomplishing that goal.

The second recommendation also has implications for the kind of technology used to develop a Handbook. The technological resources available to teacher educators and their students vary considerably. The overall model for the Professional Handbook should be modified to work using the technology that is supported by individual institutions and available to preservice teachers after they graduate. The author developed the model for the Handbook by consulting the instructional technology team at her university. During the spring 2009 semester, the author switched to a new technology platform that was supported by her university and available to users for free. This means the teacher candidates can continue to use the technology as inservice teachers, which is far more beneficial than relying on university-based technology that may not be replicable in K-12 public schools. The new technology platform is discussed further in the Solutions and Recommendations section.

The third recommendation is essential in order for the process of developing the Handbook to help prospective teachers become more reflective and professional practitioners. Sharing responsibility for authoring parts of the Handbook requires preservice teachers to collaborate, compromise, and trust one another to develop well-written, professional contributions to the assignment. This takes time and sometimes is difficult, but as an old proverb points out "Smooth seas don't make strong sailors." Overcoming challenges in appropriate ways helps the prospective teachers develop professional skills. The opportunity to reflect on the process, product, and utilitarian nature of the Handbook helps the preservice teachers make deeper meaning out of the assignment.

ISSUES AND PROBLEMS

The greatest issue that affects the use and development of a Professional Handbook is access to technology. This issue influences preservice teachers' development of the Handbook during their teacher education courses as well as their ability to use the Handbook while student teaching or as inservice teachers. Technology access also has an impact on teachers' abilities to make changes or additions to their Handbooks once they graduate from the university where they completed their teacher preparation program. As discussed in the *Context and Components* section, prospective teachers developed their handbooks using Adobe® Dreamweaver® and a pre-designed template. The handbooks were stored in a "www folder" provided to each student by their university, and items in this folder were automatically included on each preservice teacher's website that was hosted on the university's server. This approach presented two major problems for Handbook use and development.

The main problems were preservice teachers lost access to their student "www folder" and other technology resources one week after graduation. In order to stop this from meaning the complete loss of their Handbooks, preservice teachers were taught how to export a copy of their completed Handbook to a CD. They were also encouraged to store their Handbook on another server that they might be able to access in the future (e.g. at the public school where they eventually are employed). Preservice teachers were also told about other web-authoring tools in addition to Adobe® Dreamweaver® that they might have access to through their public schools, purchase, or the Internet. The preservice teachers were encouraged to look into these options so they could continue to add to their Handbooks. Creating a CD and being told about technology they "might" be able to access was a temporary fix while the author worked with an instructional technology support team to pursue other resources that would resolve this problem. Although no formal longitudinal data was gathered to determine whether students went on to update their Handbooks using another web-authoring tool and/or hosted it on another server, anecdotal evidence suggests this did not happen.

A lesser problem with using campus-based technology was preservice teachers needed to use a university-owned computer in order to work on their Handbooks. Even though the assignment was initially implemented at a residential 4-year university, this requirement posed an inconvenience because most of the students owned their own computers and would have preferred to work on them rather than in the university's labs. While this was only an inconvenience, it would be a greater problem at a primarily non-residential university where most students commute to campus. This problem confronted the author when she accepted a position at another university with the latter demographic; indeed, most of the author's students at her new university were non-traditional undergraduates with part- or full-time jobs and/or children. Making time to work in a campus computer lab was a significant challenge for these students. In response to this and the challenges described in the preceding paragraph, the author adopted a new technology format for the Handbook during the spring 2009 semester. It is discussed in the *Solutions and Recommendations* section.

SOLUTIONS AND RECOMMENDATIONS

In order to take advantage of a technological innovation that addressed the two problems discussed in the previous section, preservice teachers developed their Professional Handbooks using Google Sites during the spring 2009 semester. Google Sites became readily available to university students and faculty when the author's university switched to an e-mail system powered by Google Apps. Google Sites are stored on Google's server, so preservice teachers do not automatically lose access upon graduation. Google provides an "edit page" feature for each Google Site; thus, the site can be edited without a web-authoring program. The set up also facilitates collaboration on a website, which made it easier for preservice teachers to work together on the common parts of the Handbook. The change also allowed preservice teachers to make updates to their Handbooks from any computer with Internet access. For additional information about Google Sites and its features, see http://www.google.com/sites/overview.html.

Preservice teachers still lose access to their university email accounts within a year or two of graduation. Google Sites has a feature that addresses this potential problem, too: an owner of a Google Site can invite someone else to collaborate on or own a site. Website ownership is identified by email address. Therefore, preservice teachers need to set up a personal Google email account sometime before losing their university student account, and invite themselves to own the site at their new email address. As a result of this functionality, preservice teachers should be able to continue using and editing their Handbooks during their inservice teaching careers. Google email accounts and the resulting access to Google Sites are free. Therefore, this solution seemed to resolve many of the problems that affected earlier implementation of the Professional Handbook without attaching a hefty price tag that would inhibit some preservice teachers' continued use of their Handbook.

The switch to Google Sites necessitated some changes to the layout of the Professional Handbook to take advantage of the features this program provided. Google Sites provided its own template, so preservice teachers were no longer able to use the template presented in Figure 1. The author created the initial Handbook Google site and invited each member of the class to share its ownership. The preservice teachers worked together to create the Handbook's resources and add them to the appropriate pages of the website. The class was responsible for preparing and vetting all of the content; the author gave final approval for the finished products.

The platform change facilitated the addition of a new requirement for the Handbook: near the end of the semester, preservice teachers replicated the content from the class-compiled Handbook into an individual Handbook. This easy-to-complete process allowed the preservice teachers to have their own Google Site on which to post their reflection about the assignment. Thus they conclude the semester with a resource that no one else can modify. Preservice teachers can personalize their individual Handbook, adding to it as they learn about new resources that they wish to preserve and use in their inservice careers. Google Sites also has a feature that allows users to decide whether they want their site visible to everyone in the world or by invitation only. Creating an individual Handbook allowed students to determine their own level of security for the site.

It is important to note that technological advances will undoubtedly continue to provide additional alternatives for the format of the Professional Handbook. The author initially decided to use a website format because that was what the instructional technology department at her university was best able to support. Wikis or blogs are more common and sophisticated now than when the author first implemented the Handbook assignment in 2005. When the format change was made in 2009, wikis and blogs were considered but determined to be less appropriate than Google Sites for a Professional Handbook. Although wikis are a good way to compile large amounts of information from many people, ultimately the author requires prospective teachers to replicate the content of the class-compiled Handbook in an individual Handbook. This would be complicated with a wiki. Blogs do not allow for editing of another person's submission without leaving a long trail of editorial marks. This was an undesirable feature for the Handbook because there is no need to document changes and revisions. Overall, it is important for teacher educators to regularly consider innovative technologies that might better serve their students' needs and/or achieve the goals of their teacher preparation courses. It is useful to collaborate with instructional technology personnel whose professional focus involves being up to date on technological innovations. The switch to a new form of technology to host and prepare the Handbooks and the need to stay abreast of innovations that might further improve the Handbook are among the opportunities this teacher education assignment presents for future research.

FUTURE RESEARCH DIRECTIONS

There are extensive opportunities for future research through the refinement and expanded implementation of the Professional Handbook. Teacher educators who adopt the Handbook model can investigate how the assignment contributes to preservice teachers' achievement of course objectives. Another direction for future research is to validate the effectiveness of the assignment with a robust sample of preservice teachers *while* student teaching. Possible questions to be explored by such studies include: Do prospective teachers with Professional Handbooks make more or stronger connections between theory and practice than those who do not have Handbooks? What sorts of teaching situations lead prospective teachers to consult their Handbooks? How do prospective teachers apply information from their Handbooks to their student teaching? Similar questions can be asked in a longitudinal study of Handbook use among inservice teachers. The answers to these questions will help validate the efficacy of the Handbook and refine the design to make the assignment more useful in practice.

A related line of research involves examining if the enhanced confidence with technology that preservice teachers ideally develop as a result of completing a Handbook leads them to be more inclined to teach with technology as inservice teachers and/or have their K-12 students use technology more regularly. Since technology is in a constant state of innovation, the effectiveness of additional refinements to the Handbook model that take advantage of state-of-the-art technologies provides another area for future research. Future studies can also examine how to expand the Handbook design into an assignment that prospective teachers work on throughout their entire teacher preparation program instead of in specific courses. Once developed, studies could compare the efficacy of programmatic Handbooks and single-course Handbooks.

Finally, Burns (2005) raised an important question about technology use: "Why are schools using computers primarily to teach low-level skills when technology has the potential to deepen student learning?" (p. 48). Burns' questions indicates another possibility for future research about the Professional Handbook; studies should go beyond determining the Handbook's influence on preservice teacher learning and examine how and if teachers' access to a Handbook affects the learning of the K-12 children they teach in their inservice careers. Ultimately the true measure of teacher educators' effectiveness is in the academic achievement of the K-12 youth our former students go on to teach. Therefore, specific investigations that examine K-12 student proficiency in the kinds of skills and thinking their teachers were prepared to teach and have access to through their Professional Handbooks are appropriate. Because of the large number of factors that influence student learning, qualitative methods that provide rich details about student skills and levels of understanding may be more appropriate than quantitative studies that attempt to establish a causal relationship.

CONCLUSION

The Professional Handbook is a technology-based assignment that allows preservice teachers to develop their reflective skills as well as professional skills and attitudes. The pragmatic nature of the assignment provides prospective teachers with a tool that they can easily consult to select instructional approaches to help them teach in meaningful ways that connect their practice with educational theory. Preliminary action research suggests that the positive interdependence preservice teachers must demonstrate while developing the assignment helps them learn the invaluable professional skill of collegiality. The assignment also fosters reflective skills among preservice teachers, and reflective practice is an important component of meaningful teaching. Like other education initiatives involving technology, the Handbook is a work in progress that needs to be updated regularly to take advantage of affordable technology innovations that are accessible to public school teachers. Refinement and modifications to the assignment offer a variety of opportunities for future research studies. In summary, the Professional Handbook provides beginning teachers with an easy-to-access resource to help them effectively teach the children entrusted into their care.

Author's Note

Elliott Stoddard of Word Harvesters, Eric Orton of Boise State University, and Michael Weaver of Bucknell University provided invaluable technological assistance during the development and implementation of the Professional Handbook. Their professionalism, patience, and creativity are truly appreciated.

REFERENCES

Al-Sharaf, A. (2006). New perspectives on teacher education in Kuwait. *Journal of Education for Teaching*, *31*(1), 105–109. doi:10.1080/02607470500511108

Albee, J. J. (2003). A study of preserivce elementary teachers' technology skill preparedness and examples of how it can be increased. *Journal of Technology and Teacher Education*, *11*, 53–71.

Austin, D. S. (2004). New literacies: Are Colorado teacher education programs preparing pre-service teachers to use technology in their learning environments? *Dissertation Abstracts International*, *65*(07), 2570. (AAT 3138978).

Babinski, L. M., Jones, B. D., & DeWert, M. H. (2001). The roles of facilitators and peers in an online support community for first-year teachers. *Journal of Educational & Psychological Consultation*, *12*(2), 151–169. doi:10.1207/S1532768XJEPC1202_05

Banister, S., & Vannatta, R. (2006). Beginning with a baseline: Insuring productive technology integration in teacher education. *Journal of Technology and Teacher Education*, *14*(1), 209–235.

Bansavich, J. C. (2005). Factors influencing preservice teachers' readiness to integrate technology into their instruction. *Dissertation Abstracts International*, *66*(03), 966. (AAT 3169712).

Barnett, M. (2008). Using authentic cases through the use of a web-based professional development system to support preservice teachers in examining classroom practice. *The entity from which ERIC acquires the content, including journal, organization, and conference names, or by means of online submission from the author. Action in Teacher Education*, *29*(4), 3–14.

Boger, C., & Boger, D. (2000). Preservice teachers' explanations of their teaching behavior. *Journal of Instructional Psychology*, *27*(4), 217–223.

Bransford, J., Darling-Hammond, L., & LePage, P. (2005). Introduction. In Bransford, J., & Darling-Hammond, L. (Eds.), *Preparing teachers for a changing world* (pp. 1–39). San Francisco: Jossey Bass.

Brintnall, S. K. (2002). *E-mentoring: A case study of the viability and benefits of electronic mentoring with beginning teachers in rural schools*. Unpublished dissertation, University of Oklahoma, Norman. (AAT 3040838).

Burns, M. (2005). Tools for the mind. *Educational Leadership*, *63*(4), 48–53.

Dalli, C. (2008). Pedagogy, knowledge and collaboration: Towards a ground-up perspective on professionalism. *European Early Childhood Education Research Journal*, *16*(2), 171–185. doi:10.1080/13502930802141600

Dana, N. F., & Yendol-Silva, D. (2003). *The reflective educator's guide to classroom research: Learning to teach and teaching to learn through practitioner inquiry*. Thousand Oaks, CA: Corwin Press.

Dewey, J. (1933). *How We Think: A restatement of the relation of reflective thinking to the educative process*. New York: D. C. Heath and Company.

Dicker, L. A., & Monda-Amaya, L. E. (1995). Reflective teaching: A process for analyzing journals of preservice teachers. *Teacher Education and Special Education*, *18*(4), 240–252. doi:10.1177/088840649501800404

Feiman-Nemser, S. (2001). From preparation to practice: designing a continuum to strengthen and sustain teaching. *Teachers College Record*, *103*(6), 1013–1055. doi:10.1111/0161-4681.00141

Fleming, L., Motamedi, V., & May, L. (2007). Predicting preservice teacher competence in computer technology: Modeling and application in training environments. *Journal of Technology and Teacher Education*, *15*(2), 207–231.

Flores, M. T. (2007). Navigating contradictory communities of practice in learning to teach for social justice. *Anthropology & Education Quarterly*, *38*(4), 380–404. doi:10.1525/aeq.2007.38.4.380

Freiberg, H. J. (2002). Essential skills for new teachers. *Educational Leadership*, *59*(6), 56–60.

Fry, S. W. (2007). First-Year teachers and induction support: Ups, downs, and in-betweens. *Qualitative Report*, *12*(2), 216–237.

Fry, S. W. (2009). On borrowed time: How four elementary preservice teachers learned to teach social studies in the NCLB era. *Social Studies Research and Practice*, *4*(1), 31–41.

Fry, S. W., & Bryant, C. J. (2006-2007). Using distance technology to sustain teacher education for student teachers in isolated areas: The Technology Supported Induction Network. *Journal of Computing in Teacher Education*, *23*(2), 63–69.

Goodlad, J. I. (1990). *Teachers for our nation's schools*. San Francisco: Jossey-Bass Publishers.

Graham, C., Culatta, R., Pratt, M., & West, R. (2004). Redesigning the teacher education technology course to emphasize integration. *Computers in the Schools*, *21*, 127–148. doi:10.1300/J025v21n01_10

Gratch, A. (2000). Becoming teacher: student teaching as identity construction. *Teaching Education*, *11*(1), 119–126. doi:10.1080/10476210050020435

Hammerness, K., Darling-Hammond, L., Bransford, J., Berliner, D., Cochran-Smith, M., & McDonald, M. (2005). How teachers learn and develop. In Bransford, J., & Darling-Hammond, L. (Eds.), *Preparing teachers for a changing world* (pp. 358–389). San Francisco: Jossey Bass.

Hill, D. M. (2003). E-Folio and teacher candidate development. *Teacher Educator*, *38*(4), 256–266. doi:10.1080/08878730309555322

Idaho Standards for Initial Certification of Professional School Personnel. (2005). Retrieved March 2, 2009, from: http://www.sde.idaho.gov/site/teacher_certification/accredited.htm

Lei, J. (2009). Digital natives as preservice teachers: What technology preparation is needed? *Journal of Computing in Teacher Education, 25*(3), 87–97.

Leming, J. S., Ellington, L., & Schug, M. (2006). The state of social studies: A national random survey of elementary and middle school social studies teachers. *Social Education, 70*(5), 322–327.

Lieb, B. (1992). *Proceedings of the OERI study group on educating teachers for world class standards: The challenge for education teachers.* Washington, DC: US Department of Education.

Lin, Q. (2008). Preservice teachers' learning experiences of constructing e-portfolios online. *The Internet and Higher Education, 11*(3-4), 194–200. doi:10.1016/j.iheduc.2008.07.002

Lortie, D. C. (1975). *Schoolteacher: A sociological study*. Chicago, IL: University of Chicago Press.

McLeskey, J., & Billingsley, B. S. (2008). How does the quality and stability of the teaching force influence the research-to-practice gap?: A perspective on the teacher shortage in special education. *Remedial and Special Education, 29*(5), 293–305. doi:10.1177/0741932507312010

Pennsylvania Department of Education. (2009). *Form PDE-430 student teacher assessment.* Retrieved June 22, 2009, from http://www.pde.state.pa.us/teaching/cwp/view.asp?a=90&Q=32539&teachingNav=|93|87|&teachingNavPage=|

Pope, M., Hare, D., & Howard, E. (2005). Enhancing technology use in student teaching: A case study. *Journal of Technology and Teacher Education, 13*(4), 573–618.

Roddy, M. (1999). Using the Internet to unite student teaching and teacher education. *Journal of Technology and Teacher Education, 7*(3), 257–267.

Schön, D. (1983). *The reflective practitioner: How professionals think in action.* New York: Basic Books, Inc.

Valli, L. (1997). Listening to other voices: A description of teacher reflection in the United States. *Peabody Journal of Education, 72*(1), 67–88. doi:10.1207/s15327930pje7201_4

Veenman, S. (1984). Perceived problems of beginning teachers. *Review of Educational Research, 54*(2), 143–178.

Vick, M. (2006). It's a Difficult Matter: Historical perspectives on the enduring problem of the practicum in teacher preparation. *Asia-Pacific Journal of Teacher Education, 34*(2), 181–198. doi:10.1080/13598660600720579

Whetstone, L., & Carr-Chellman, A. A. (2001). Preparing preservice teachers to use technology: Survey results. *TechTrends, 45*(4), 11–17. doi:10.1007/BF02784820

ADDITIONAL READING

Ball, D., & Cohen, D. (1999). Developing practice, developing practitioners: Toward a practice based theory of professional education. In Sykes, G., & Darling-Hammond, L. (Eds.), *Teaching as the learning profession: Handbook of policy and practice* (pp. 3–32). San Francisco: Jossey-Bass.

Boger, C., & Boger, D. (2000). Preservice teachers' explanations of their teaching behavior. *Journal of Instructional Psychology, 27*(4), 217–223.

Chubbuck, S. M., Clift, R. T., Allard, J., & Quinlan, J. (2001). Playing it safe as a novice teacher: Implications for programs for new teachers. *Journal of Teacher Education, 52*(5), 369–376. doi:10.1177/0022487101052005003

Edens, K. M. (2000). Promoting communication, inquiry and reflection in an early practicum experience via an on-line discussion group. *Action in Teacher Education, 22*(2), 14–23.

Eisenman, G., & Thornton, H. (1999). Telementoring: Helping new teachers through the first year. *T.H.E. Journal, 26*(9), 79–82.

Heflich, D. A., & Putney, L. G. (2001). Intimacy and reflection: Online conversation in a practicum seminar. *Journal of Computing in Teacher Education, 17*(3), 10–17.

Ingersoll, R. M. (2001). Teacher turnover and teacher shortages: An organizational analysis. *American Educational Research Journal, 38*, 499–534. doi:10.3102/00028312038003499

Marzano, R. J. (2003). *What works in schools: translating research into action*. Alexandria, VA: Association for Supervision and Curriculum Development.

Risko, V. J., Vukelich, C., & Roskos, K. (2002). Preparing teachers for reflective practice: Intentions, contradictions and possibilities. *Language Arts, 80*(2), 134–144.

Roddy, M. (1996). Using the Internet to support preservice and novice teachers. In B. Robin, J. Price, J. Willis, J., & D. Willis (Eds.). Technology and Teacher Education Annual, 1996 (pp. 711-714). Charlottesville, VA: AACE.

Spalding, E., & Wilson, A. (2002). Demystifying reflection: A study of pedagogical strategies that encourage reflective journal writing. *Teachers College Record, 104*(7), 1393–1421. doi:10.1111/1467-9620.00208

Turley, S., Powers, K., & Nakai, K. (2006). Beginning teachers' confidence before and after induction. *Action in Teacher Education, 28*(1), 27–39.

Wepner, S. B., & Mobley, M. M. (1998). Reaping new harvests: Collaboration and communication through field experiences. *Action in Teacher Education, 20*(3), 50–61.

Yost, D. S. (2006). Reflection and self-efficacy: enhancing the retention of qualified teachers from a teacher education perspective. *Teacher Education Quarterly, 33*(4), 59–76.

ENDNOTES

[1] Veenman's (1984) seminal work on the problems faced by beginning teachers identified reliance on their "own ideas" and "trial and error" as common, and problematic, origins for teaching behavior. More recent literature indicated that these origins of teaching behavior remain problematic (Boger & Boger, 2002; Freiberg, 2002).

[2] Adobe® Dreamweaver® requires no knowledge of a web-programming language. It is a fairly user-friendly web-authoring program. The university where this Professional Handbook was initially developed had a site-license to the program, so it was available to preservice teachers on all campus computers.

Chapter 21
Game-Based Learning: A Strategy to Integrate Digital Games in Schools

Begoña Gros
Universitat Oberta de Catalunya, Spain

ABSTRACT

Children and young people today are introduced to the virtual world via video games, and the way that they interact with technology is changing ways of learning and the production of knowledge. The design of a learning environment based on the educational properties of games seems to be an ideal way of increasing learning. Digital games offer a very good example of the principles of successful learning environments; they are users-centered, and they promote challenge, co-operation, engagement and the development of problem-solving strategies. Games can help students learn to collaborate, solve problems, collect and analyse data, test hypotheses, and engage in debate. But there are differences between using digital games for play and using them in a formal context. For this reason, methodologies must be developed for their use in the classroom. In this chapter, the author proposes examples of methods that can be applied to the use of video games in formal education.

INTRODUCTION

In recent years, electronic games have assumed an important place in the lives of children and adolescents. As a result, researchers and educators pay particular attention to them. The presence of video games in the lives of children provokes concern. Games have been a constant source of criticism – and even alarm – among teachers and parents. The potentially harmful effects of videogames have been linked to problems associated with sedentary lifestyles among youth, childhood obesity, addiction, socialization problems, poor academic performance, and aggressive behavior (Vanderwater, 2004; Gailey, 1996). At the same time, there is a growing consensus that learning takes places when people use games (Gee, 2003; Prensky, 2005; Shaffer 2006).

DOI: 10.4018/978-1-61520-897-5.ch021

Support for the use of digital games as a medium for education is based on different approaches that

Copyright © 2010, IGI Global. Copying or distributing in print or electronic forms without written permission of IGI Global is prohibited.

we categorize as: (a) games as powerful context, (b) immersive learning, (c) development of soft skills, and (d) complex learning.

Games as a Powerful Context

The central argument of Gee (2003) regarding the potential contribution of video games to learning is the idea that semiotic domains are shared by groups of people, described as affinity groups, who share knowledge, skills, tools and resources to form complex systems of interrelated parts. Learners gain resources from fellow members which equip them to solve problems: "the learner needs to learn not only how to understand and produce meanings in a particular semiotic domain that are recognizable to those affiliated with the domain, but, in addition, how to think about the domain at a 'meta' level" (Gee, 2003: 23). Players have to understand the meaning of the internal design grammar and the ongoing social practice that determine the activity of play. This view makes players think about games as systems and designed spaces. "A video game is a set of experiences as player participates in from a particular perspective, namely the perspective of the character the player control" (Gee 2008: 23). In summary, digital games provide powerful contexts for learning because "they make it possible to create virtual worlds, and because acting in such worlds makes it possible to develop the situated understandings, effective social practices, powerful identities, shared values, and ways of thinking of important communities of practice" Shaffer &Clinton: 2005, 7).

Immersive Learning

According to Squire (2005), video games immerse learners in situations in which they use tools and resources in order to solve complex problems. As games become more complex, learners begin to use intelligent tutors, intelligent agents and scaffolding techniques.

An important point mentioned by Squire (2005) is that the main differences between e-learning and games are related to content. The most important element in e-learning is content, whereas in games it is experience. Games structure the entire experience around problem solving. For this reason, "learning through play, with games and with simulation is a part of more general process of learning in immersive worlds" (De Freitas&Oliver, 2006: 11).

Development of Soft Skills

School learning has traditionally focused on the transmission of knowledge from instructor to student. Schools do a reasonably good job preparing students in hard skills such as, mathematics, languages, and science. However, they have not done as well developing student competences in the soft skills such as, problem solving, communication, working in groups, and collaborative learning. Educators need to find ways of providing students meaningful experiences through which they can develop these skills in the context of their existing subject-matter. Videogames provide opportunities for students to develop soft skills and schools can take advantage of them to facilitate this work.

Complex Learning

The contexts that most video games provide are complex learning environments in which the player has to control many different variables, take decisions, establish strategies and constantly compare the effects of their actions on the system. Prensky (2005) establishes the levels of learning that summarize the complex learning environment provided by video games. The most basic level of learning that takes place during a video or computer game is learning how to control the interaction with the screen. In the case of games, this learning is always related to practice. One learns, gradually, after mastering the various stages of the game. The next level of learning is related to the rules of the game. The rules of the game teach what is permitted; players typically learn the rules by trial and error, by playing and discovering what they can or cannot do. The third level of learning is why one does something. Players learn the strategy of a game as they play it. The strategy applied may conform to many different approaches: cause and effect, order and chaos, second-order consequences, complex system behaviors, the value of persistence, and so on. Finally, learners acquire cultural metaphors about the world.

In this chapter, we consider digital games as a medium for education. The main emphasis is how to take advantage of characteristics in the gaming environment and to optimize the learning that the environment may engender. The paper explores how games may help students learn to collaborate, solve problems, collect and analyze data, test hypotheses, and engage in debate. These skills have to be built into game activities. For this reason, it is important to select games based on their pedagogical objectives.

CLASSIFICATION OF DIGITAL GAMES

There are many genres of digital games but there is no one standard classification. The industry, developers, and academics all use different taxonomies. We will categorize seven major genres (Gros,B, 2008):

1. **Action games (also called platform games).** These games are reaction-based. Most first-generation games correspond to this kind.
2. **Adventure games.** The player solves a series of tests in order to progress through a virtual world.
3. **Fighting games.** These involve fighting computer-controlled characters, or those controlled by other players.
4. **Role-playing games.** Here, players take on the characteristics of another person or creature.
5. **Simulations.** The player has to succeed in a simplified recreation of a place or situation.
6. **Sports games.** Based on sports.
7. **Strategy games.** Mainly games that recreate a historical situation.

This taxonomy helps to clarify the different types of games. However, it is not easy to apply to all products, because many games fall into more than one category. For instance, most of the sports games currently contain information needed to manage a team and combine simulation with characteristics of the strategy games. What is important is that most of the famous games (with their constantly updated versions) contain features of simulations and adventure. Elsewhere, strategy is also present in most historical simulations. In other words, there is a tendency to produce games that provide complex environments in which content, skills, and attitudes play an important role during the game.

Models and modeling are integral to games like *Civilization*, *Zoo Tycoon*, *Rise of Nations*, *The Sims*. In all these cases, the game stresses first and third person player experiences. In some games, the whole game is a model of the practice and culture of the particular topic. For instance, in *Tony Hawk's Pro Skater*, players can design their own skaters, clothes, boards, skate parks, and so on. They build a mode and interact with a set of more abstract models of environments that help to build a more realistic context.

Other games are educational rather than commercial. Most educational games are designed to transmit curricular content, and emphasize the material the student needs to learn rather than the context of experience. For this reason, educational games are not very popular among children; they are not immersive games. However, in recent years, there has been a resurgence of educational games due to the rise of the "serious games" movement. Michael and Chen (2006) consider that serious games are ones "in which education (in its various forms) is the primary goal, rather than entertainment'". These serious games may be differentiated from educational games by their focus on the post-secondary market and training.

Currently the production of games for handhelds and mobiles is increasing. This requires exploiting the platform and the context in which these games are used. According to Klopfer (2008: 38) the social component for mobile games allows the creation of flexible and ever-changing complex games, promotes the ability to adapt games to a number of different styles such as competition and collaboration, creates situations in which players learn specialized communication, and produces a social dynamic in which players need to construct arguments and strategies with and against other players.

Epistemic games are computer games (Shaffer&Gee, 2006) that can help players learn to think like professionals. This concept is based on the idea of "epistemic frames" — the way in which a profession or other community of practice thinks and works — and entails a situated and action-based form of learning based on the ways in which professionals develop these epistemic frames. Shaffer (2008) argues that this approach makes it possible to create epistemic games in which subjects learn to work as doctors, lawyers, architects, engineers, journalists, and other valued professionals; in this way they develop the skills, habits, and concepts of a post-industrial society. These games help them to develop ways of thinking and knowing that are valued in the world, giving them a way to imagine the future person they might someday become.

Squire (2008) provides a framework for examining different games (2008: 172) based on the type of narrative the game applies. The classification compares the differences in the time taken to complete the game, and the modes of creative expression.

In order to integrate a game in the classroom, the selection stage is very important. Teachers must be well acquainted with it in order to be able to plan the educational element. So they must be aware of the differences between games, the time needed to finish the game or part of it, and the style of interaction and problem-solving strategies that are required.

RESEARCH IN THE FIELD

Research in the fields of sociology, developmental psychology and neurobiology suggests that there are two profiles of people interacting in modern society. The differences between these two profiles weave together generational, social and cognitive factors. On the one hand are the *Digital Natives*, the *Network Generation*, people who have grown

Table 1. Framework for examining different games. Source: Squire (2008:172)

Game genre	Time to completion	Timescale	Open-endedness	Modes of creative expression	Educational examples
Targeted games (puzzle, minigames)	1-4 hours	Weeks	Low	Style of completion: level creation	Supercharged
Linear games	20-40 hours	Month	Low	Style of completion: machinema	Full spectrum, warrior, epistemic games
Open-ended, sandbox games	100 hours	2-24 months	High	Style of completion: multiple solution, paths	Civilization, Sim City, Sims
Persistent worlds	500 hours	6-48 months	High	Modding, social engineering, game play	Quest Atlantis

up with information and communications technology: computers, internet, mobile phones and video games. On the other are the *Digital Immigrants*, generally adults who were born and educated in non-digital environments (Prensky, 2001; 2007).

For digital natives, digital games on their different platforms are the main vehicle through which they enter digital culture, involving changes not only in the format of screens but also in their interaction. Video games, on the other hand, place the emphasis on action and interaction. The player is not passive but becomes the protagonist of the story and must act in consequence. The forms of interaction vary depending on the games, ranging from very simple interaction based on rapid reactions on the player's part (hand-eye games) to responses based on performing strategic and tactical activity (adventure games) or on realistic activities (simulators).

The informative and communicative features of on-line computers conform to the indicators of quality in education: dialogue, exchange of information and opinions, participation, intervention and collaborative authorship are essential principles in education for citizenship. However, the (first-generation) television model prevails in classrooms. Pupils cannot choose the channel; they all receive the same information. Traditionally, teachers have constructed a route for everybody to follow. The job of teachers today, however, is to build networks, to be able to design territories to be explored. Learning occurs precisely through exploration by pupils, just as players learn how to progress through the different screens and attain the goals set for them by the game.

In recent years digital games have received increased attention from researchers and educators. The use of computer games in education is not unexplored territory, but the studies so far are disjointed and the field lacks well-defined boundaries. The research has ranged over a number of disciplines with little in common, such as literature, psychology, media studies, anthropology, ethnography, sociology, history, business studies, military tactics, literary theory, educational, theory, instructional technology and computer games studies.

Although substantial progress has been made in the last five years. the research field of digital games is not yet well established. There is a lack of a common research language, and few basic and theoretical discussions.

Most of the studies have been concerned with what and how children learn in an informal context using video games. However, several recent studies of the use of computer games in schools have explored whether these games can have a role in supporting current educational objectives. In most cases (De Freitas&Oliver, 2006; Gros, 2005; Gros&Garrido, 2008) the most common obstacle facing the use of digital games in school is related to teachers. They identify aspects of the games as positive learning experiences, but mention a number of problems and limitations: the lack of time available for them to familiarize themselves with the game, the problem of selecting the game, and the difficulty in persuading other colleagues of the benefits.

The general perceptions about the usefulness of games to support learning are sure to improve over the next few years, as the generations learning with games in the classroom reach tertiary education and as tutors who are contemplating using games in their classroom practice receive tools and guidance for developing their own game-based learning activities with groups of learners different skills, levels and competencies.

Tutors surveyed in schools (Sandford et al., 2006) reported that fixed lesson duration was a constraint in both the planning and implementing of game-based learning. Teachers' lack of familiarity with the game was cited as another reason for failure (Sandford et al., 2006). Assisting teachers with game-based learning may therefore require more flexibility in terms of lesson duration, as well as measures to ensure adequate time for lesson preparation and good technical support. Teachers require guidelines and frameworks for supporting innovative practice. These authors report that while teachers need to be familiar with the game, the successful "achievement of educational objectives was more dependent upon a teacher's knowledge of the curriculum…than it was on their ability with the game" (Sandford et al., 2006: 3). In summary, the teacher played a central role in scaffolding and supporting students' learning.

INTEGRATING DIGITAL GAMES IN THE SCHOOL

It is important to distinguish between playing in an informal situation and playing in an educational context (see table 2). There is a differentiation between the direct interaction with the game, and the context in which we are using it. Teachers have to design the social setting inside which the game takes place and all the interaction produced around the game. All learning experiences have content, facts, principles, information and skills. In education, we need to create the context, that is, the social system that ensures that experiences will be integrated in game. This is the main role of the teachers and mentors. For this reason, reflection and interpretation are encouraged, not just through game-design features, but also through socially shared practices.

There are four aspects to bear in mind in the planning of the use of digital games in school: the context, the learner specification, the representation of the game, and the pedagogical approach.

The context of the game is central to the effectiveness of its use. Contextual factors include where a game is used, the technical support provided, and the game's general environment. For instance, the game might be used in the classroom, at home, or in both situations.

The learner or learner group is also central to the selection and use of the game. Aspects such as age, stage of study, demographics, use of ICT and games technologies and past learning experiences will all have an influence on the selection of the game.

The representation of the game itself, that is, the level of immersion and fidelity, familiarity of the learner group with the interface and the internal reality and narrative of the game will also have a bearing upon effective learning. Young learners are becoming accustomed to high levels of immersion and interactivity in leisure games, so different learner groups may require different levels.

The pedagogical model is particularly important for using games in learning contexts, rather than for leisure time activities. De Freitas- Olivier (2006) found that learning processes are supported by associative (instructivist and often task-centered), cognitive (constructivist) and situative (learning in communities of practice) modes of learning.

Learning to use a game is a learning experience in itself, which should be complemented with a set of activities which, according to the pedagogical approach adopted, may be more experiential or more problem-based. The role of debriefing is crucial because it allows participants to discuss and reflect on the experience with their peers and the teacher.

Here we present some examples based on two different approaches that can help to integrate the use of digital games in school: experiential learning and inquiry learning.

Experiential Learning

The first approach is based on experiential learning (Kolb 1984). Experiential learning takes place when students observe and reflect on a prior experience and reach some kind of abstraction by fitting these reflections in with their previous knowledge, which they then use for guidance in their subsequent actions. Thus, experiential learning describes the acquisition of knowledge in a learning cycle with four successive stages (Kolb 1984, figure 1):

Table 2. Differences between playing inside and outside school (source: Sandford-Williamson, 2005)

	Games outside the school	Games inside the school
Challenging & adaptable	Games tend to be at their most enjoyable when they are difficult but 'just do-able', rather than when they are too easy; they make demands that are at the edge of players' competence.	Games to be used in school should provide progressively complex challenges, which are clear and finite and can be repeated; players should be able to adapt the level of difficulty (from novice to expert) if necessary.
Absorbing & immersive	Playing a good game can immerse players in a state of 'flow', the condition in which they are completely absorbed in an activity that closely matches and stretches their abilities.	Players need to be absorbed in meaningful activities whose aims and goals they clearly understand and the accomplishment of which stretches their current competence.
Non-didactic & practice-based	Games do not have to be explained and players do not have to read manuals or practice activities before beginning to play; the rules are learned through practicing 'in the game'.	Using a game in the classroom should not necessarily need players to be 'trained' beforehand; players should be allowed to practice playing, often by failing and revising and re-trying tactics, but may need support from staff or peers.
Authentic & experiential	Tasks have immediate application; challenges must be overcome 'just in time' and are consistent with the experiences within the context of the game environment.	Tasks should be related closely to real-world practices and concrete experiences or be consistent with the fantasy, and not staged as practice for some later test or exam, or, worse still, as reward for completing a 'learning activity'.
Interacting with rules, alternatives & consequences	By interacting with the game system and its rules, players experience what it is like to exercise alternative forms of control and authority, and to experience the consequences of particular courses of action.	The game demands that players interact with the rule system, by taking responsibility for actions in alternative contexts, and by seeing their impact on the outcomes of the game as a whole.
Feedback & 'assessment'	Games provide immediate feedback on players' performance, offering scores, visual and audio cues, and notification when individual goals have been accomplished.	Players should be able to infer from the feedback supplied how their actions have caused particular effects, and whether these effects are the ones that were desired; scoring systems provide immediate and constant 'assessment' of progress and accomplishment, although cannot as yet provide any improvement or further progress.
Social & collaborative	Games are central to friendship cultures, where peers exchange their views and knowledge about games; these exchanges also occur over the internet amongst geographically and generationally dispersed groups.	Games to be used in classrooms should promote dialogue and the exchange of knowledge and opinions; they don't need to be multiplayer titles, but should have some cultural relevance to the participating players.
Material exchange	Verbal advice and material resources such as magazines and demo discs are a currency of exchange amongst game players; players are often not just playing a game, but gathering data and information and forming knowledge about it	Playing a game should be supported by the availability of additional resources such as walkthrough guides and hints and tips on the internet in order to promote wider understanding and knowledge about it.

continued on following page

Table 2. Continued.

	Games outside the school	Games inside the school
Expertise & apprenticeship	Some players are expert at particular games, while others are new to them; expert players can take on new players as apprentices, guiding them through titles by playing together, tutoring them online and sharing other materials with them.	It should not be assumed that all players in a classroom have the same expertise; some may be recruited to 'tutor' others how to play, including pointing them towards relevant resources or sources of information.
Identities	Players experience what it is like to inhabit particular alternative identities, such as military medics, warrior trolls, city planners, sportspeople or pregnant mothers; they experience and practice the actions peculiar to each.	Games in the classroom should allow players to take on new identities and to experience these identities' demands and challenges, and to consider their potential courses of action; players may begin to understand alternative perspectives in particular social and political contexts.
Literacies	Games situate players in particular literacy practices associated with the identities being played, immersing them in peculiar vocabularies and social customs; often these literacy practices are associated with real-world professional domains, or are consistent within the fantasy.	The literacy demands in games vary from the fantastical to the professional and are often as complex as the literacies of subject domains as diverse as science, literature and history; in-game literacy demands may extend and stretch players' linguistic repertoire in particular contexts.
New media literacy	Games prepare players to deal with complex electronic environments, to negotiate and handle data in multiple formats simultaneously, to interact with images, sounds and actions, and to interact with others through electronic channels.	Playing games in classrooms can prepare players for 21st century working and learning practices, by dealing with diverse media and complex data, multi-tasking, communicating and working with others, making decisions, analyzing pictures, audio and actions as well as written words, and to engage in ongoing development through 'on the job' practice.
Reflective practice	Players are often involved in reviewing and rethinking their performance in games, reconsidering the strategies they have employed to overcome challenges and thus reflecting on how well they are able to manipulate and exploit the system and rules of the game being played.	Space for reflection is rarely present in games; players in classrooms should be provided space to review their performance and what they have learned by playing.

1. “Concrete Experience”, (CE)
2. “Reflective Observation”, (RO)
3. “Abstract Conceptualization”, (AC) and
4. “Feedback or Active Experimentation” (AE),

The core of Kolb’s four-stage model is a simple description of the learning cycle which shows how experience (1) is translated by reflection (2) into concepts (3), which in turn are used as a guide to feedback or active experimentation and planning new experiences or creating alternative methods of action (4). In this way it helps learners to understand the process of acquisition of concepts, skills and attitudes from their own point of view.

Using this approach allows us to highlight a very important aspect: the experience of games is not the same in a formal context as outside the school setting. The inclusion of games in a learning context aims to use the advantages of the design of digital games to enhance learning. It is important to stress that pedagogical exploitation of video games involves bringing the game into the classroom under the guidance of teachers, who must work to make the experience of playing a reflective experience.

The video game used does not need to correspond to specific curriculum content, but may be used to work on digital skills and serve as a basis for a variety of activities. It is important to choose the right game in accordance with the aims proposed.

We illustrate the process with the example of the game *Age of Empires,* used with 13-14 year old students. This is an epic real-time strategy game spanning 10,000 years, in which players are the guiding spirit in the evolution of small Stone Age tribes. Starting with minimal resources, players are challenged to build their tribes into great civilizations. Players can choose from one of several ways to win the game, including: world domination by conquering enemy civilizations, exploration of the known world, and economic victory through the accumulation of wealth.

The first stage in using the game in the school (see figure 2) is to create a professional circle of reflection as a regular forum for professional dialogue, exchange, and decision-making. This includes roles for a specialist in educational technology, an expert player of the game and the teacher responsible for facilitating agreement and decision-making at each stage of the design of the sequence: purposes, activities, tasks, and resources.

The second strategy is to encourage teachers to learn to play the video game if they do not have previous knowledge of it. The aims

Figure 1. Experiential learning according to Kolb (1984)

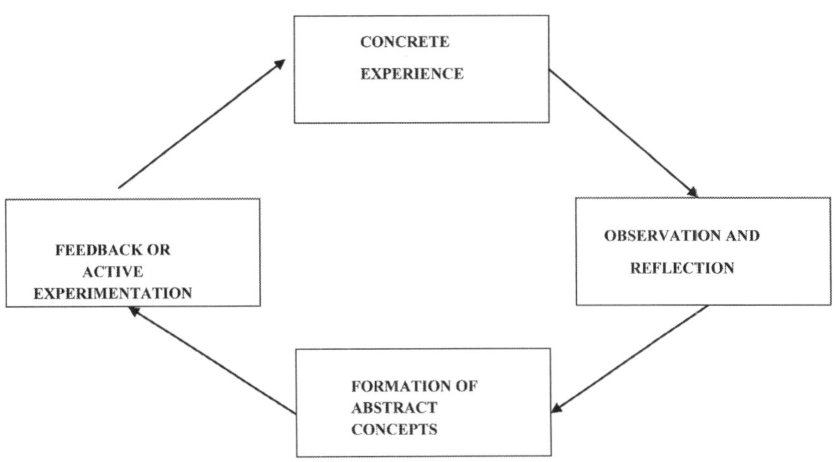

Figure 2. Diagram showing the strategies used to design the educational sequence

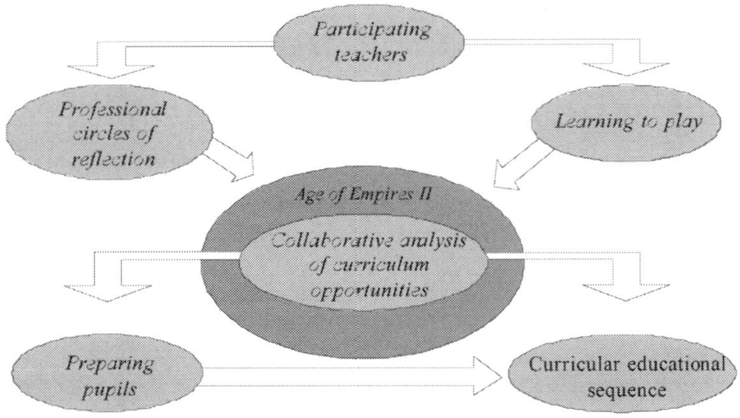

of this strategy are, on the one hand, to resituate the meaning and scope of the game-playing as a way of learning and, on the other, to help individual teachers to identify the opportunities offered by the video game *Age of Empires* II in order to link them up with learning within their curriculum areas.

The third strategy consists of collaborative agreement on the curriculum opportunity, which can be pursued through the use of the video game, taking into account the features of each subject area. The professional circle of reflection plays an important role in this process by mediating a shared framework of beliefs, opinions and ideas. In this example, three teachers were involved: social science, mathematics, and computer science teachers.

The product that emerges from these strategies is the preparation of a single plan for classes based on the interactive phase with a central core theme from the unit. For instance: "The western world: from the mediaeval period to the modern period" from the social science curriculum area on feudalism can be complemented by content belonging to the unit on ratios from the mathematics curriculum.

The video game was incorporated into learning activities using the William Wallace Learning Campaign as preparation for the work, especially stages 1, 2 and 5: "Marching and Fighting", "Feeding the Army" and the "Battle of Stirling", selected by the teachers as the most useful to link with the content of the course.

The contact and relations between the pairs of students are highly important because it is a space for teaching and learning from peers with regard to both the game and the way of organizing collaborative work. Typical of this interaction is the image of the pupil's finger pointing to the screen as a way of accompanying what they are saying, becoming a pointer and a "technique" for interactive practice between peers which reflects the processes of observation, dialogue, exchange and agreement on decision making with the video game. One aspect that should be noted and may be interpreted as a result of the interaction achieved is the consistently high level of attention and concentration displayed by the pupils working together in front of the screen, generating a degree of involvement that makes the classes work more easily. This impression is supported by many research studies (Salen, 2008)

The role played by the teachers is a key factor. They must:

- ensure that everybody works together for the first 15 minutes of each session (the transition from the start phase and the execution phase), preventing pairs of pupils from starting the game early.

- give clear instructions as a way of guiding pupils' activities; pupils must be attentive to what teachers say and to the information supplied at the various stages by the video game; and
- highlight the difference between playing and learning.

There is no doubt that teachers can exploit games as educational material to teach specific curriculum content on the basis of creating a learning environment that enables learners to confront a complex, multidimensional and interactive multimedia system. Bringing games into the classroom makes it possible to work with the entire class through cooperative groups and joint discussions, which provide space for analysis and critical reflection.

Involving and motivating learners is critical for educational purposes. In games, involvement is fundamental, as players will only invest time and effort in a game if it is relevant to them. So a video game can be a starting point for a gradual approach a subject, problem, or issue that is of interest to all or is among the aims teachers have to pursue. This approach must set out from the students' initial perceptions and open the way for constructing more elaborate problems, theories and practices for exploration or research.

Figure 3 shows a clear difference between the perspectives of the player and the student. It is especially important for teachers to analyze the concepts provided by the game that may challenge the scientific concepts of the area.

Inquiry Learning

This model for the sequence of learning is based on the concept of "progressive inquiry" developed by Hakkarainen (2003). The model describes the elements (see figure 4) of expert-like knowledge practices in the form of a cyclic inquiry process. In

Figure 3. Player perspective versus student perspective Source: Engenfeld (2005)

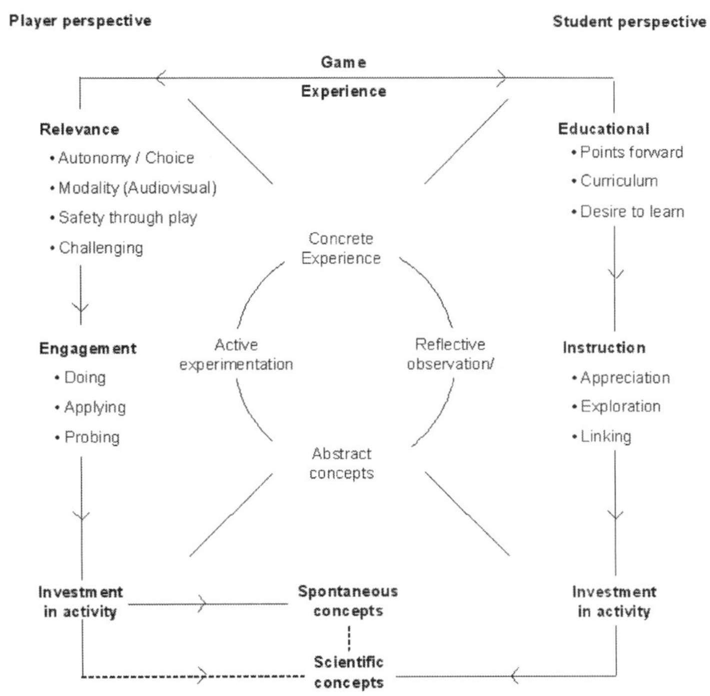

a progressive inquiry process, the teacher creates a context for inquiry by presenting a multidisciplinary approach to a theoretical or real-life phenomenon, after which the students start defining their own questions and intuitive working theories about it. Students' questions and explanations are shared and evaluated together, which directs the utilization of authoritative information sources, offering conceptual tools to describe, understand and take into account the critical elements in collaborative knowledge-advancing inquiry.

The use of a video game makes inquiry learning easier and serves to create a culture in which knowledge is treated as an object under development; the ideas presented are neither final nor immutable, but expressions of a constantly evolving discourse.

Critical reflection creates the need to assess the arguments behind the theories and explanations supplied. This is how the joint cognitive efforts of all those involved can be directed.

Assessment focuses on the research process rather than simply on the end result. It is therefore a question of assessing the group's efforts and giving learners a leading role in this process. It is important that this leading role and this way of working should help them to consolidate their previous learning and lead them to generate high-level syntheses using the results of the research process.

We have used Zoo Tycoon with children of 10-11 years old. The class members start to make questions about the construction of the Zoo: best area, types of vegetation, weather conditions, etc. Once the questions have been posed, the class organizes and selects two of them. The sequence begins by creating a context for everybody to work on: a context based around a specific theme, an issue to study, and a situation to resolve, among others. Once the question has been presented, the class group organizes itself on the basis of planning and establishing common goals and content. This process involves determining what needs to be known, planned and supervised on a collective basis throughout the research process.

The video game is a source of knowledge and experimentation that allows learners to experience simulations, test hypotheses, and so on. Moreover, the use of the game encourages learners to use other resources, including the Internet, books, and forum. By using a game in this way, students learn the cognitive value of social co-operation

Figure 4. Inquiry model Source: Hakkanairen (2003)

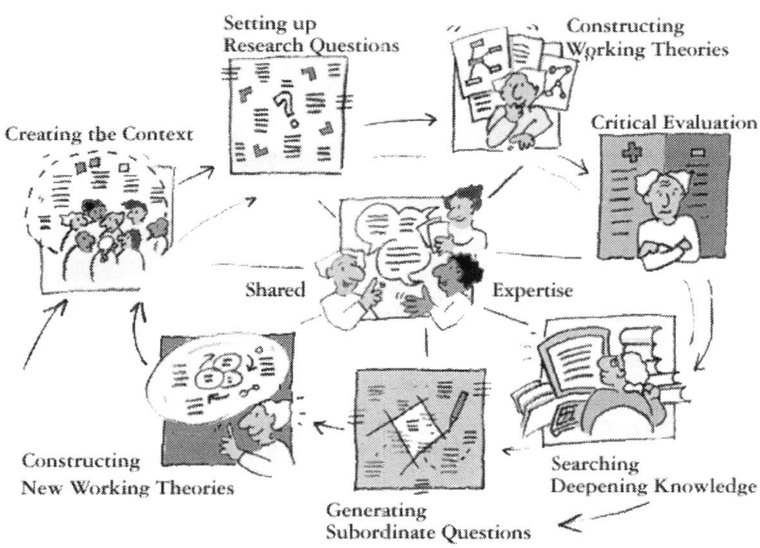

and build up their ability to use socially distributed cognitive resources.

The final result can be set down in the form of a dossier including all the work done and things learnt in the course of the exercise, a session diary including the results and assessments of all the exploratory work, a graphic or audiovisual presentation of the subject or a presentation of the exercise for the benefit of another group of learners. This end product or products, which form a part of the whole process, should be proposed by the group and must be appropriate to their level of competence with the tools they choose as a medium for it.

PROBLEMS AND CHALLENGES

An important problem for the integration of digital games is the time that is required to produce an activity. Generally, the games take hours to play and, on occasion, it is difficult to establish the sequences of play that would be significant for both the students and school curriculum. In this regard, the most efficient procedure is to leave the students to continue to playing outside the classroom, via access to the game in the school.

Teachers with little experience in the use of video games may express reticence. They may feel insecure and require significant support during the process. Our intervention in schools has always been more successful when we have been able to give staff support during experiments. Most teachers recognize that the games support the development of a wide range of strategies that can be very important for learning: the resolution of problems, the learning of sequences, deductive reasoning, and memorization. Furthermore, it turns out that it is quite easy to introduce pedagogical group strategies into collaborative and co-operative forms of work where learning is based on the resolution of exercises and so on. However, in spite of their generally favorable opinion, few teachers have decided to use video games in their classes. We hope that the general perceptions about the usefulness of games in support of learning will increase over the next few years, as the generations learning with games in the classroom reach tertiary education, and as the tutors who are thinking of using games in their practice are given tools and guidance to develop their own game-based learning activities for groups with differing skills, levels and competencies.

A critical aspect is the transfer of the learning experience. The research conducted so far has said little about this issue, which is perhaps one of the most important challenges we face.

Another crucial aspect is the conceptual learning that the games provide. In this regard, the figure of the teacher is fundamental in all games that use simulations based on scientific concepts. The designers of the games are not concerned with the accuracy of the contents and, on occasion, they may produce contradictions or misconceptions in the function of particular games.

Play is a fundamental activity in the life of the child and the adolescent. Digital games incorporate the essential elements of digital literacy. The digital culture exists outside the school and the school must incorporate it. The informal experiences that children already possess and the knowledge that they have already acquired can serve as the basis for its successful introduction.

The use of videogames involves not only mastering instrumental control of the tool but also control of the knowledge needed to live in the information society. As such, the concept of digital literacy that we use is broad-ranging: from purely instrumental aspects to cultural and social elements.

The adventure and simulation games provide complex learning environments which are appropriate for the acquisition of learning with "authentic" materials, and permit the construction of knowledge using the best suited models in contemporary society. The process involves the construction of games not to teach but to guide students to play and work with the educational aspects of play that require the intervention of the educator. This involvement of the educator means that the players are unlikely to become isolated.

Beyond the characteristics of the tool, we have to bear in mind the context of its use. The medium possesses attributes of its own that condition its use, but at the same time our activities condition the development of the medium. Therefore, only a profound knowledge of the tool, the programs and its forms of use can permit us to select the most suitable methods and media according to our needs and educational objectives. Therefore, it is very important to analyze the practices and the role of the game within its specific context. Whatever the analysis we carry out, we must take four fundamental aspects into account:

1. How the game is contextualized: does it form a part of a daily activity, is it based on something extraordinary, as a reward, as something without relation to a habitual practice, etc?
2. The type of exercises performed: the development of the sessions.
3. The type of interaction between the participants: the role of the teacher, competitive activity, collaborative activity, both, etc.
4. The qualities of the critical and reflexive elements of the game itself.

REFERENCES

De Freitas, S., & Griffiths, M. D. (2008). The convergence of gaming practices with other media forms: what potential for learning? A review of the literature. *Learning, Media and Technology*, *33*(1). doi:10.1080/17439880701868796

De Freitas, S., & Oliver, M. (2006). How can exploratory learning with games and simulations within the curriculum be most effectively evaluated. *Computers and Education. Special Issue on Gaming*, *46*, 249–264.

Engenfeld, S. (2005). *Beyond Eductaiment*. Doctoral dissertation. Copenhagen, Denmark: University of Copenhagen.

Gailey, C. W. (1996). Mediated messages: Gender, class, and cosmos in home video games. In E. Sigel (Series Ed.), P. M. Greenfield & R. R. Cocking (Vol. Eds.), Interacting with video (pp. 177-184). Norwood, NJ: Ablex Publishing.

Gee, A. (2003). *What video games have to teach us about learning and literacy*. New York: MacMillan.

Gee, A. (2008). Learning and Game. In Salen, K. (Ed.), *The ecology of games. Connecting youth, games and learning* (pp. 21–40). Cambridge, MA: MIT Press.

Griffiths, M. (1997). Friendship and social development in children and adolescents: The impact of electronic technology. *Educational and Child Psychology*, *14*, 25–37.

Gros, B. (2005). Digital Games in Education: The Design of Games-Based Learning Environments. *Journal of Research on Technology in Education*, *40*(1), 23–38.

Gros, B. (Ed.). (2008). Videojuegos y aprendizaje. Barcelona, España: Graó.

Gros, B., & Garrido, J. M. (2008). The Use of Video games to Mediate Curricular Learning. In *DIGITEL: Proceedings of the 2008 Second IEEE International Conference on Digital Game and Intelligent Toy Enhanced Learning* (pp. 170-176).

Hakkarainen, K. (2003). Emergence of Progressive-Inquiry Culture in Computer-Supported Collaborative Learning. *Science and Education*, *6*(2), 199–220.

Klopfer, E. (2008). *Augmented Learning Research and Design for Mobile Educational Games*. Cambridge, MA: MIT Press.

Kolb, D. A. (1984). *Experiential learning*. Englewood Cliffs, NJ: Prentice-Hall.

Michael, D., & Chen, S. (2006). *Serious games: games that educate, train and inform*. Boston, MA: Thomson Course Technology.

Prensky, M. (2001). *Digital game based learning*. New York: McGraw Hill Press.

Prensky, M. (2005, September). Engage Me or Enrage Me. What Today's Learners Demand. *EDUCAUSE Review*, *40*(5), 60–65.

Prensky, M. (2007). How to teach with technology: keeping both teachers and students comfortable in an era of exponential change. *Emerging Technologies for Learning*, *2*, 40–46.

Salen, K. (Ed.). (2008). *The ecology of games. Connecting youth, games and learning*. Cambridge, MA: MIT Press.

Sandford, R. (2006). *Teaching with Games: Using commercial off-the-shelf computer games in formal education*. Bristol: Futurelab.

Shaffer, D. W. (2006). Epistemic frames for epistemic games. *Computers & Education*, *46*, 223–234. doi:10.1016/j.compedu.2005.11.003

Shaffer, D. W., & Clinton, A. (2005). *Video Games and the Future of Learning*. University of Wisconsin-Madison. Working Paper No. 2005-4.

Shaffer, D. W., & Clinton, K. (2004). *Toolfor-thoughts: reexamining thinking in the digital age*. University of Wisconsin-Madison.

Shaffer, D. W., & Gee, A. (2006). *Before every child is left behind: How epistemic games can solve the coming crisis in education*. Working Paper No. *2005*-7, University of Wisconsin-Madison.

Squire, K. (2005). *Game-Based Learning: Present and Future State of the Field*. University of Wisconsin-Madison.

Squire, K. (2008). Open-Ended Video Games: A Model for Developing Learning for the Interactive Age. In Salen, K. (Ed.), *The ecology of games. Connecting youth, games and learning* (pp. 167–198). Cambridge, MA: MIT Press.

Vanderwater, E. A., et al. (2004). Digital Childhood: Electronic Media and Technology Use Among Infants, Toddlers and Preschoolers. *Pediatrics*. Retrieved October 20, 2008, from http://pediatrics.aappublications.org/cgi/content/full/119/5/e1006

Williamson, B., & Sandford, R. (2005). *Games and learning: A handbook from Futurelab*. Bristol: Futurelab.

Chapter 22
Teacher Candidates Learning through the Creation of Podcasts

Christian Penny
West Chester University of Pennsylvania, USA

ABSTRACT

As teacher educators it is imperative that we model the sound use of technology to enrich the teaching and learning process. Podcasting is enjoying phenomenal growth in mainstream society, alongside other new media that enable users to author and distribute content quickly and easily. The project reported on in this chapter focuses on teacher candidates creating their own podcasts for distribution on iTunes. The chapter explains the what of podcasting and how podcasting is being used in higher education, then details the podcast creation process and describes how engaging in the podcasting exercise promoted collaboration and knowledge building among the teacher candidate producers. Thus the focus is on teacher candidates learning through creating podcasts, in contrast to learning from podcasts.

INTRODUCTION

Podcasting is encountering phenomenal growth, alongside other new media that enable users to create and share content quickly and easily. According to Mindlin (2005), current estimates state that 30 to 57 million US citizens will be accessing and using podcasting technology by 2010. The increased popularity of iPods or similar mobile audio/video devices can help to explain this podcasting phenomenon. Analysts at The Diffusion Group, a consumer technology research firm, believe US demand for podcasts will grow from "less than fifteen percent" of portable digital music player owners today to "seventy-five percent by 2010." (PoducateMe, 2008).

In higher education, podcasting has been used to distribute information and to support learning at a number of institutions. However, the most popular use of podcasting in colleges and universities is the recording and dissemination of lectures. I believe the true potential of podcasting in teacher education lies in its knowledge creation value, and its use as a vehicle for disseminating learner-generated content.

DOI: 10.4018/978-1-61520-897-5.ch022

Copyright © 2010, IGI Global. Copying or distributing in print or electronic forms without written permission of IGI Global is prohibited.

This view is echoed by Lee, McLoughlin and Chan (2008) and Atkinson (2006), the latter of whom believes that podcasting has a limited impact as a mere method for distribution.

Creating podcasts at the K-12 level has many educational benefits. Teachers and students are able to create a product to share with a potentially world-wide audience. Their podcast can be listed in iTunes, right along with podcasts from The Discovery Channel, Disney and NPR. Knowing that there is a real-world audience gives teachers, and students, purpose and motivation to create a spectacular product. The process of putting together an audio recording is extremely valuable and is certainly a cross-curricular experience (Vincent, 2009).

With a focus on teacher candidates creating their own podcasts for distribution in the Apple iTunes Store, this chapter will explain what podcasting is and how podcasting is being used in teacher education. It will then explain in further detail the podcast creation process and describe how engaging in podcasting-related exercises has promoted collaboration and knowledge building among teacher candidate producers in one institution of higher learning. Thus, the focus will be on teacher candidates learning *through* creating podcasts, as opposed to learning *from* podcasts. Teacher candidates as producers of content, not just consumers.

BACKGROUND

Podcasts are audio or video digital-media files delivered over the Internet by syndicated download, through Real Simple Syndication (RSS), to personal computers and portable media players. The same digital media files may also be made available by direct download or streaming, but what makes a podcast unique is the way it can be syndicated, subscribed to, and downloaded automatically when new content is made available. Like the term "broadcast," podcast can refer either to the series of content itself or to the method by which it is syndicated; the latter is also known as podcasting. The host or author of a podcast is often called a podcaster.

Dave Winer, a software developer and an author of the RSS format, in addition to former MTV VJ Adam Curry are recognized as the originating force behind the podcasting phenomenon. Journalist Ben Hammersley coined the term *podcasting* in the February 12, 2004 issue of *The Guardian* (PoducateMe, 2008). The term podcast is a portmanteau of the words "iPod" and "broadcast", the Apple iPod being the brand of portable media player for which the first podcasts were developed. The term has been mildly controversial, since it privileges the Apple iPod and to some users, implies that one must own an iPod to listen to a podcast. But podcasting is not limited to the iPod, nor MP3s or even portable music players.

In some respects, podcasting is not even new: Both streaming and downloading audio are as old as the World Wide Web, and the RSS specification that enables podcasting has been around for several years. What's new about podcasting is the ease of publication, ease of subscription, and ease of use across multiple environments. The term *podcast* has quickly gained traction, and the New Oxford American Dictionary selected podcasting as the Word of the Year in 2005 (PoducateMe, 2008). The term has been redefined by some parties as a "Netcast" or "Personal On Demand broadCASTING". A complete history of podcasting would likely double the length of this chapter. Fortunately, there's already a good one available on *Wikipedia* at http://en.wikipedia.org/wiki/Podcast. For the visual learners, the Common Craft video that explains in "Plain English" what a podcast is (http://commmoncraft.com/podcasting) is highly recommended. I use this video, and others created by Common Craft, to introduce new technology tools and applications in my educational technology classes at West Chester University.

Podcasting-capable aggregators or 'podcatchers', such as Apple iTunes, are used to download podcasts. They are configured to do so by supplying them with the URL of the relevant RSS feed. The podcatcher monitors the feed for RSS 2.0 (RSS Advisory Board, 2005) "enclosure" elements. Once downloaded, podcasts can be transferred to a variety of portable devices, including but not limited to Apple's ipod, handheld computers, netbooks, as well as smart phones. Users without access to such devices can simply listen to the content on their desktop or laptop computers.

Podcasting in teacher education is still relatively new. While many of today's college students have a high rate of digital literacy, the use of digital media as a vehicle for students to express their understanding and demonstrate their skills is uncommon. While conducting a literature review, it was very difficult to find the use of podcasts in higher education for anything other than lecture redelivery. Since late 2002, Georgia College and State University (2005) have been offering 'iPod-enhanced' courses that deliver audio material ranging from lectures and audio books to language study material and music. In 2004, Duke University (2006) received media attention when it distributed iPods to its 1650 incoming freshman, preloaded with orientation material. Specific to teacher education, Drexel University began a pilot program in September 2005 that provided iPods to its School of Education freshman (Read, 2005).

Many universities, such as Stanford and Pennsylvania State University, have implemented podcasting at an institutional level through Apple iTunes U, a free hosted service that provides access to educational content, including lectures and interviews. Upon signing up, each university can add school colors, logos, and photographs to make iTunes U a familiar landing place for staff, students, and alumni. iTunes U uses the same technology as the iTunes Music Store (To learn more about iTunes, follow this link: http://www.apple.com/education/solutions/itunes_u).

In a recent study, that gained much media attention, researchers at the State University of New York in Fredonia looked at the effectiveness of podcasts in higher education. Within the study undergraduate general psychology students participated in one of two conditions. In the lecture condition, participants listened to a 25-min lecture given in person by a professor using PowerPoint slides. Copies of the slides were given to aid note-taking. In the podcast condition, participants received a podcast of the same lecture along with the PowerPoint handouts. Participants in both conditions were instructed to keep a running log of study time and activities used in preparing for an exam. One week from the initial session students returned to take an exam on lecture content. Results indicated that students in the podcast condition who took notes while listening to the podcast scored significantly higher than the lecture condition (McKinney et al, 2009).

As mentioned earlier, there have been only a few published examples of podcasting being used within higher education to empower students and encourage active learning. It has only been recently that studies chronicling learner-created content have emerged (e.g. Lazzari 2009, Lee et al. 2008, McLoughlin et al. 2006).

Leaver (2006) describes:

"For students, podcasting can be far more than a content-delivery mechanism; it can be part of their ongoing participation in knowledge communities in both tertiary settings and beyond. Student podcasting also levels the playing field in relation to ideas of content-creation and can be part of the processes of helping learners develop the tools of cultural interaction, not just consumption, which are increasingly an essential part of digital literacy. "

As a teacher educator, the idea of expanding students' digital literacy while reinforcing content sounded encouraging. Many of my students arrive in my class being proficient with the consumption of digital media, but few of them are proficient in the creation of digital media (podcasting, digital storytelling, web design, etc).

Campbell (2005) found that there are "good reasons for acquiring at least rudimentary skills in 'rich media' (or 'multimedia') authoring. More and more students come to school with these skills. This is a language they not only understand, but use often on a daily basis. Some of them have been blogging, shooting and editing video, creating Flash animations, manipulating photographs, and recording digital audio for many years. These are the tools of their native expressiveness, and with the right guidance and assignments, they can use these tools to create powerful analytical and synthetic work. Yet, even such digitally fluent students need to learn to manipulate their multimedia languages well, with conceptual and critical acumen, and we in higher education do them a disservice if we exclude their creative digital tools from their education."

So, the inclusion of creating and using podcasts on devices that students may currently own, use frequently, and enjoy may be an opportunity knocking on the teacher educator's door. Therefore, it is very important that our teacher candidates have a strong command of podcasting and other technological opportunities available for integration into their classrooms.

THE PODCAST PROJECT

According to Bastes and Khasawneh (2007), to increase a students' self-efficacy in using technologies, they must have successful and positive experiences. The aim of the project described in this chapter was to enable teacher candidates enrolled in an educational technology class to create radio-style audio 'shows,' and to publish them as podcasts in the Apple iTunes Store. Within the context of the educational technology course at West Chester University, the decision was made three years ago to turn what was a paper and pencil review of K-12 educational software into a podcasting project that would result in three outcomes: First, the teacher candidate producers would develop technology skills needed for 21st century schools. Second, the podcasting project would foster teamwork and collaboration. Lastly, podcasting would enable the teacher candidates to demonstrate and share their understanding of subject matter.

The design of the podcast project was based on the review of K-12 educational software titles. In groups of two or three, teacher candidates were given hands-on time with a popular software title designed for K-12 students, then asked to review it in a manner not dissimilar to *At the Movies* with Gene Siskel and Roger Ebert. After spending approximately an hour reviewing software and taking notes, the teacher candidates were directed to create a script for a 3-5 minute podcast review show. After careful revision, the audio-only review shows were recorded and edited on Mac laptops using Garageband audio editing software, then submitted for grading as an MP3 file before being published to iTunes. Later in this chapter the steps for creating podcasts will be discussed in more detail.

This podcasting project is consistent with the Digital Audio Learning Objects (DALO's). The concept of a DALOs (Middleton & McCarter, 2005) combines reusable learning object theory with theory pertaining to the pedagogically sound use of digital audio to enhance e-learning. The key features of a well-designed DALO are as follows:

- *Simple to produce*. They have a well-defined and limited scope, ensuring that they can be easily designed, produced and re-used with little technical knowledge.
- *Immediate*. As there is no need for high-end, studio-grade equipment and/or techniques, DALOs are inexpensive to produce and can be made available to students in a quick and timely fashion.

Figure 1. Teacher candidates evaluating educational software

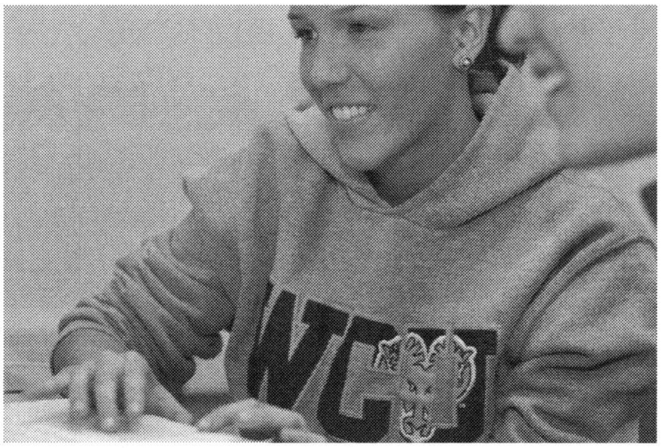

Figure 2. A teacher candidate editing a podcast script in Google Docs

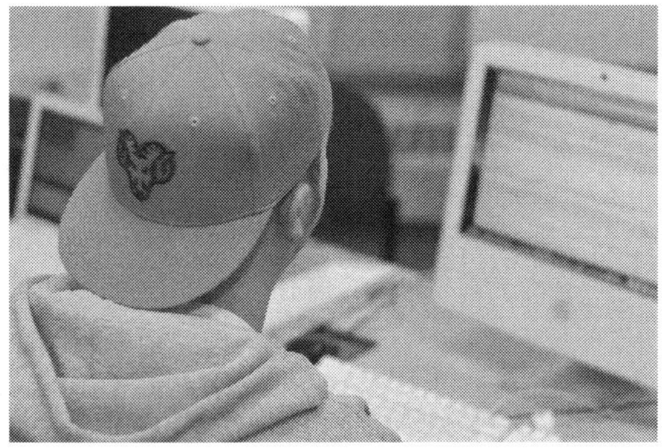

- *Educationally focused.* Designing to address a well-defined learning objective ensures that the DALO will serve its original purpose. However, as with other types of learning objects DALOs may be repurposed outside the original scenario for which they were designed.
- *Reusable.* Because a DALO does not *contain* a lecture, it can be interpreted according to the needs of different learning contexts, either within the same or in a different course.
- *Engaging.* This is of key importance because it is challenging to keep an audience's attention for extended periods of time by using audio alone. Audio is best used selectively, for example, to capture attention, summaries and 'add color' to the learning experience.

Through the application of these DALO design features the author anticipated that the podcasts produced by teacher candidates would improve their technology skills, foster teamwork and collaboration, and increase their understanding of K-12 software, including the need to carefully review titles before using them in the classroom.

For teacher candidates, podcasting will involve modest preparation, and a little editing, before they'll be ready for the world to hear their efforts. The good news is that once you get the hang of a few technical issues common to any kind of audio recording, you'll be on your way and ready to integrate podcasting into the teacher education classes you teach.

AUTHENTIC ASSESSMENT

Over the years I have reviewed multiple podcast rubrics. Most recently I came across a rubric created by Ann Bell from the University of Wisconsin-Stout. Upon identifying and selecting this rubric I obtained Ann's permission to modify and use it in my courses and in this book chapter (Bell, 2009). Table 1 includes the revised version of the rubric used in the project described in this chapter.

Pre-Production

Minimal training is needed to produce this type of assignment in teacher education courses. Podcasting is something students can do in all types of classes without committing too much instructional time for training, but before you begin students should be given an introduction to what podcasting is. The Common Craft video mentioned earlier works well as an introduction

Table 1. Podcast rubric. Adapted and used with permission from Ann Bell original at: http://www.uwstout.edu/soe/profdev/podcastrubric.html Updated by Chris Penny March 2009

CATEGORY	Exemplary - 6 points	Proficient - 4 points	Proficient - 2 points	Incomplete - 0 points
Introduction	Catchy and clever introduction. Provides relevant information and establishes a clear purpose engaging the listener immediately.	Describes the topic and engages the audience as the introduction proceeds.	Somewhat engaging (covers well-known topic), and provides a vague purpose.	Irrelevant or inappropriate topic that minimally engages listener. Does not include an introduction or the purpose is vague and unclear.
	Irrelevant or inappropriate topic that minimally engages listener. Does not include an introduction or the purpose is vague and unclear.	Tells most of the following: who is speaking, date of the podcast, and location of speaker.	Alludes to who is speaking, date of the podcast, and location of speaker.	Speaker is not identified. No production date or location of the speaker is provided.
Content	Creativity and original content enhance the purpose of the podcast in an innovative way. Accurate information and succinct concepts are presented.	Accurate information is provided succinctly.	Some information is inaccurate or long-winded.	Information is inaccurate.
	Vocabulary enhances content.	Vocabulary is appropriate.	Vocabulary is adequate.	Vocabulary is inappropriate for the audience.
	Includes a wide variety of appropriate, well-researched and informative sources and has well-edited quotes from "expert" sources. Quotes and sources of information are credited appropriately.	Includes appropriate and informative quotes from "expert" sources. Source quotes are credited appropriately.	Includes some variety of informative quotes from some "expert" sources, and one or more source quotes need some editing. One or more source quotes are not credited.	Includes no source quotes or includes source quotes with multiple citation errors.
	Keeps focus on the topic.	Stays on the topic.	Occasionally strays from the topic.	Does not stay on topic.
	Conclusion clearly summarizes key information.	Conclusion summarizes information.	Conclusion vaguely summarizes key information.	No conclusion is provided.
Delivery	Well rehearsed, smooth delivery in a conversational style.	Rehearsed, smooth delivery.	Appears unrehearsed with uneven delivery.	Delivery is hesitant, and choppy and sounds like the presenter is reading.
	Highly effective enunciation and presenter's speech is clear and intelligible, not distant and muddled. Expression, and rhythm keep the audience listening.	Enunciation, expression, pacing are effective throughout the podcast.	Enunciation, expression, rhythm are sometimes distracting during the podcast.	Enunciation of spoken word is distant and muddled and not clear. Expression and rhythm are distracting throughout the podcast.
	Correct grammar is used throughout the podcast.	Correct grammar is used during the podcast.	Occasionally incorrect grammar is used during the podcast.	Poor grammar is used throughout the podcast.
Music Enhancements	Music enhances the mood, quality, and understanding of the presentation.	Music provides supportive background to the podcast.	Music provides somewhat distracting background to the podcast.	Music is distracting to presentation.

continued on following page

Table 1. Continued

CATEGORY	Exemplary - 6 points	Proficient - 4 points	Proficient - 2 points	Incomplete - 0 points
Technical Production	Presentation is recorded in a quiet environment without background noise and distractions.	Presentation is recorded in a quiet environment with minimal background noise and distractions.	Presentation is recorded in a semi-quiet environment with some background noise and distractions.	Presentation is recorded in a noisy environment with constant background noise and distractions.
	Transitions are smooth and spaced correctly without noisy, dead space.	Transitions are smooth with a minimal amount of ambient noise.	Transitions are uneven with inconsistent spacing; ambient noise is present.	Transitions are abrupt and background noise needs to be filtered.
	Volume of voice, music, and effects enhance the presentation.	Volume is acceptable.	Volume is occasionally inconsistent.	Volume changes are highly distracting.
	Podcast length is 3-4 minutes, and keeps the audience interested and engaged.	Podcast length is 2-3 minutes and keeps audience listening.	Podcast length is somewhat long (4-5 minutes) or somewhat short (1-2 minutes) to keep audience engaged.	Podcast is either too long (over 5 minutes) or too short (under 1 minute) to keep the audience engaged.
Group Work	All team members contributed equally to the finished product and assist in editing process by offering critique and sharing in skill development.	Assisted group/partner in the editing process.	Finished individual task but did not assist group/partner during the editing process.	Contributed little to the group effort during the editing process.
	Performed all duties of assigned team role and contributed knowledge, opinions, and skills to share with the team. Always did the assigned work.	Performed nearly all duties of assigned team role and contributed knowledge, opinions, and skills to share with the team. Completed most of the assigned work.	Performed a few duties of assigned team role and contributed a small amount of knowledge, opinions, and skills to share with the team. Completed some of the assigned work.	Did not perform any duties of assigned team role and did not contribute knowledge, opinions or skills to share with the team. Relied on others to do the work.

to podcasting. It would also be useful for teacher candidates to listen to a few podcasts before they create their own. To help you get started a list of podcast directories is provided in table 2.

The podcast project we do in our educational technology class is based on the review and evaluation of educational software such as Math Blaster or Reader Rabbit. Although educational software is less troublesome that it used to be there is still a need for teachers to evaluate software (Roblyer, 2006). Many organizations and websites can help teachers select good software, but there is no substitute for hands-on personal reviews, so that is what we focus on for the content of our podcast project at West Chester University.

Before the candidates get their hands on the software we discuss software evaluation procedures. For this we use Roblyer's (2006) Essential Criteria Checklist for Evaluating Instructional Software. I find these criteria extremely helpful for my teacher candidates as they review K-12 software for the first time. The Essential Criteria Checklist covers four sets of qualities used to discriminate between acceptable and unacceptable software material. 1) Instructional design and pedagogical soundness. 2) Content. 3) User flexibility. 4) Technical soundness.

In groups of two or three, teacher candidates spend approximately one hour reviewing a title from the collection we have at West Chester University. The teacher candidates self-select their groups based upon their major and the software title they would like to evaluate. In my experience groupings of three work the best. One

Table 2. Podcast directories

Site Name	URL
iTunes	apple.com/itunes
Podcast Pickle	podcastpickle.com
Podcast Alley	podcastalley.com
Podcast Directory	podcastdirectory.com
Odeo	odeo.com

Figure 3. Teacher candidates reviewing K-12 software hands-on, and having a good time

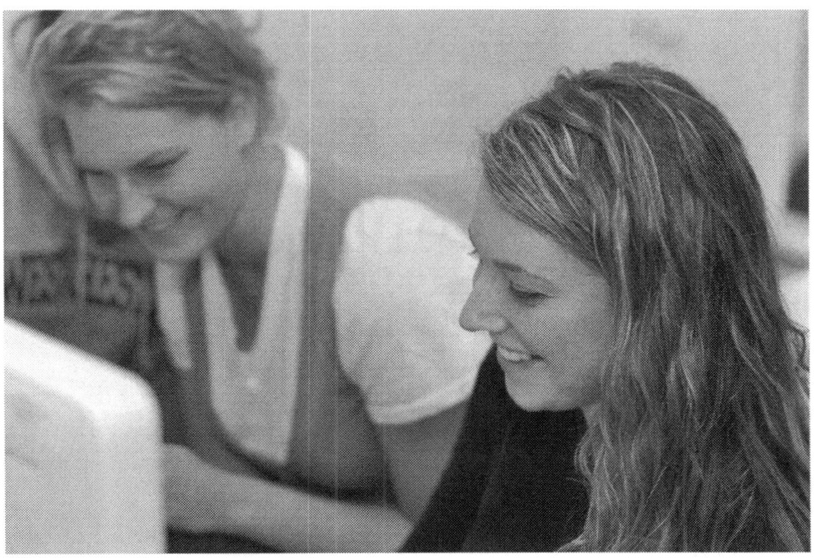

teacher candidate can run the software, the second group member can complete the Essential Criteria Checklist and take notes, and the third teacher candidate can be looking up information online as needed to complete the review. However, all of the group members should have an opportunity to "play" the game, and work hands-on with the software.

Chan *et al.* (2006) advises to "keep podcasts short, lively and entertaining", an idea supported by other authors (Hendron, 2008, Geoghegan & Klass, 2005). Thus our teacher candidates are challenged to create a script for a 3-5 minute software review podcast. I explain that we are aiming for high energy, up=tempo podcasts.

We use Google Docs as the word processing tool for the scripts. Google Docs is a free, Web-based word processor offered by Google. It allows users to create and edit documents online while collaborating in real-time with other users. Google Docs is the perfect tool for pre-production podcast script writing.

During the scriptwriting process the student producers are proactive and self-regulated in their work. They brainstorm, discuss and debate ideas for the podcast scripts during in-class meetings, with advice and guidance from me along the way. The scripts are then completed collaboratively out of class using Google Docs. Using an online word processor like Google Docs eliminates the need for groups to coordinate their schedules for face-to-face meetings. Input from all group members is required and part of the rubric presented earlier. This is easy to track because Google Docs includes a revision history tool. As a teacher educator you can see who has contributed what to the script and when they did so.

Production

Each group typically conducts informal rehearsals prior to each podcast recording, during which the script is tested and appropriate modifications made. Minor changes to wording and even swapping of roles often occurs as a result of this testing. The rehearsals are also especially helpful as a confidence building exercise for the teacher candidate presenters.

Like the script writing and editing process, the casting of roles for the presentation of each podcast episode is a democratic, team-based effort. I offer general guidance and assistance on request, but my involvment at this stage is minimal. All group members are required to have a speaking

Figure 4. Sample script created using Google Docs

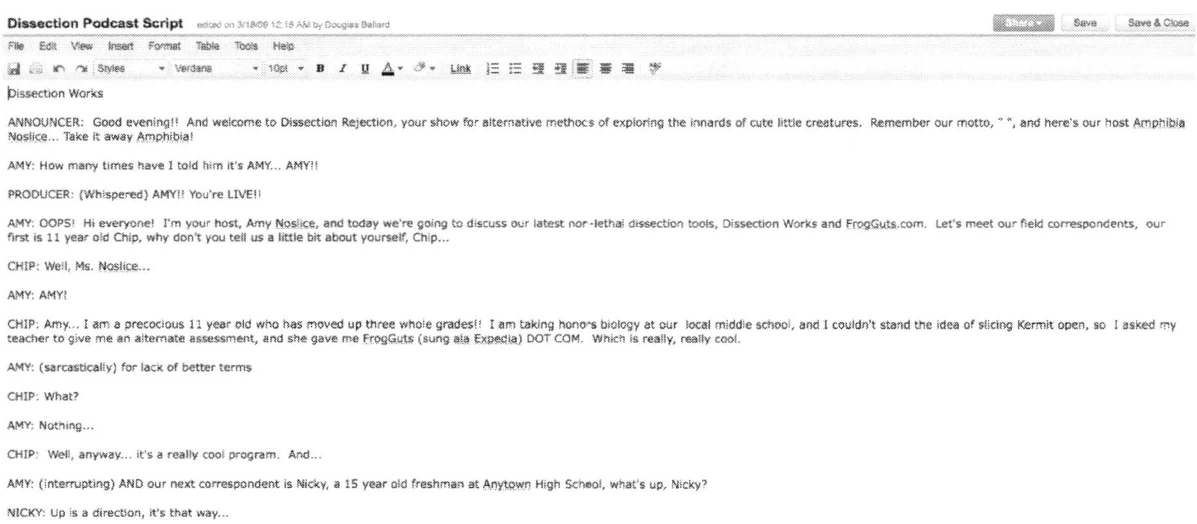
Dissection Podcast Script edited on 3/18/09 12:18 AM by Douglas Ballard

Dissection Works

ANNOUNCER: Good evening!! And welcome to Dissection Rejection, your show for alternative methocs of exploring the innards of cute little creatures. Remember our motto, " ", and here's our host Amphibia Noslice... Take it away Amphibia!

AMY: How many times have I told him it's AMY... AMY!!

PRODUCER: (Whispered) AMY!! You're LIVE!!

AMY: OOPS! Hi everyone! I'm your host, Amy Noslice, and today we're going to discuss our latest non-lethal dissection tools, Dissection Works and FrogGuts.com. Let's meet our field correspondents, our first is 11 year old Chip, why don't you tell us a little bit about yourself, Chip...

CHIP: Well, Ms. Noslice...

AMY: AMY!

CHIP: Amy... I am a precocious 11 year old who has moved up three whole grades!! I am taking honors biology at our local middle school, and I couldn't stand the idea of slicing Kermit open, so I asked my teacher to give me an alternate assessment, and she gave me FrogGuts (sung ala Expedia) DOT COM. Which is really, really cool.

AMY: (sarcastically) for lack of better terms

CHIP: What?

AMY: Nothing...

CHIP: Well, anyway... it's a really cool program. And...

AMY: (interrupting) AND our next correspondent is Nicky, a 15 year old freshman at Anytown High School, what's up, Nicky?

NICKY: Up is a direction, it's that way...

role in the production. During a recording session, scripts are often subject to impromptu variation and improvisation at the discretion of the presenters, who are encouraged to avoid simply reading the scripts.

Presentations of the completed scripts are recorded using Apple MacBook laptops with the built in mics and Garageband software. GarageBand is a Mac only software application that allows users to create podcasts or music. It is developed and marketed by Apple Inc., and is included as part of the iLife suite. For the Microsoft Windows operating system Acoustica's Mixcraft is a good alternative. Open-source tools such as Audacity are another option. Audacity is a free, easy-to-use alternative to Garageband and Mixcraft. It's an excellent choice for teacher candidate podcasters as it allows users to import, mix, edit and export audio. Audacity is available for download at http://audacity.sourceforge.net and is compatible with Windows, Macintosh, and Linux.

Detailed instructions on how to produce a podcast are beyond the scope of this chapter, but a Google search on "how to podcast" returned nearly 241,000 hits at the time of this writing, so there's no lack of free advice on how to get started.

Once the audio is recorded, editing tasks include deleting mistakes, splitting the audio to reduce the length of pauses or long periods of silence, and adding sound effects. Students are also expected to add bumpers/Jingles to the beginning and end of the recording during the editing process. The completed audio file is then exported into MP3 format to be submitted for grading

Post-Production

Publishing and distributing the teacher candidate created podcasts can be performed by the instructor to save time. MP3's can then subsequently be FTP'd to a University server. New blog entries and links can be created in Blogger, RSS feeds created using Feedburner, and Podcasts can then be listed in iTunes store. For me this is the most time consuming and frustrating part of the process.

At our institution we have a web server and professors are assigned web space on request. To get the podcasts online we use an File Transfer Protocol client called Fetch. If you are looking for a free Mac FTP client consider Cyberduck (http://www.cyberduck.ch/). Windows users can try Filezilla (http://sourceforge.net/projects/filezilla/). Once you've connected to the web server you drag and drop the podcasts. Double check that you've added the MP3's correctly by opening a browser window and typing the path

Figure 5. Using Garageband to record the podcast

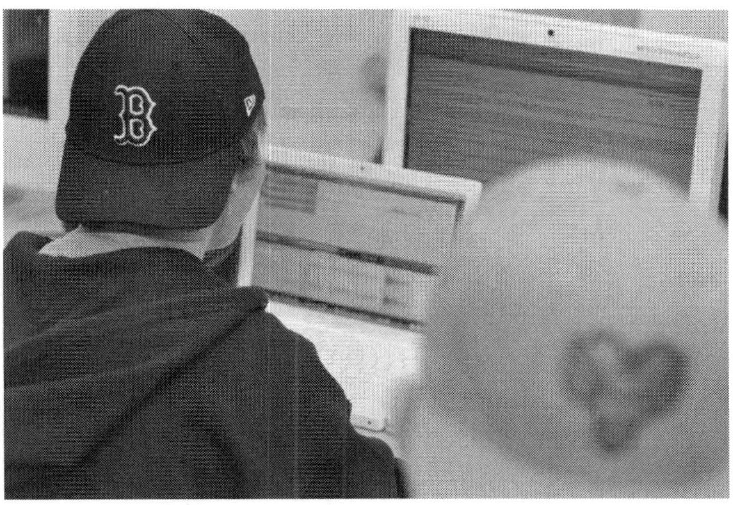

of one of the MP3 podcast episodes. The audio file should begin playing in the browser.

The next step is creating a web presence for your podcast. Many podcasters distribute their content via a blog. So if you're looking to spend the least amount of time publishing a podcast, look no further than the popular blogging software solutions such as blogger.com. Blogs are easy to set up, are often free, and ease the process of generating and updating the RSS feed by doing it automatically. Blogger (www.blogger.com) is a Google tool and holds the distinction of being one of the most widely used blogging systems. It's available only in a hosted model and is still the de-facto standard for most of the blogging world. Using Blogger we create a new blog post for each software review podcast, including a link to each MP3 that is hosted on our web server.

At this point you can stop here as your podcasts are officially published. But if you plan on submitting your podcast for inclusion in the iTunes Store podcast directory and would like to receive statistical information about who is listening to your podcasts it's worth taking the next step and using FeedBurner to create (burn) your feed for free. There are a few steps to burn a feed using Feedburner, but it is straightforward and you only need to run through the process once (PoducateMe, 2008).

With a free FeedBurner account, you can convert an existing RSS feed to a podcast-ready feed in three simple steps:

1. Sign up for a free FeedBurner account at www.feedburner.com.
2. Burn your existing feed. Enter the URL of your blog's feed into the easy-to-use interface and select the *I Am a Podcaster* option. Then click the Next button.
3. Confirm your feed title and address and then click the Activate Feed button. FeedBurner then converts any podcast media file links into an embedded <enclosure> element in a new feed, provided you link the podcast episode to the blog post. (Remember to provide a link to the MP3 in the post.)

FeedBurner is now watching your original blog feed. Simply post an entry into your blog, link your podcast's MP3 file to it, and FeedBurner will do the rest.

Submitting a podcast to the iTunes Store is the next step in the process. Having the teacher candidate created podcasts listed in the iTunes Store podcast directory provides potential listeners a quick and easy way to find and subscribe to the content. Step one is open iTunes, then look for the podcast submission button. Enter the feedburner feed URL into the form field, the after clicking continue you will be asked for additional information about the podcast. Once everything is submitted you'll receive a confirmation email from iTunes, then you sit and wait for your podcast to be officially accepted and listed. According to Apple the wait period is only a matter of hours. Once the podcast is accepted your teacher candidates will be thrilled that their work is actually published in the iTunes Store. Here is a link to some podcasts created in my Educational Technology classes that are published in the iTunes Store: http://tinyurl.com/qk6jpc

The post production steps appear more difficult than they really are. Once you have done this once or twice it is easy, but it can be time consuming. Other systems such as podOmatic (http://podomatic.com) provide an all-in-one solution where podcasters can post their content, describe it in a blog, and generate the RSS feed in just a few clicks.

OUTCOMES

The completed podcasts are submitted electronically and graded using the rubric included in Table 1. In my experience teacher candidates often loose points for delivery and technical production. Thus it is important to remind students to rehearse so the podcast is delivered in a more conversational style, as opposed to reading from a prepared script. With regards to production quality, finding a quiet place to record the audio podcast is critical. When we first started creating podcasts at West Chester University we used desktop computers. Having a class full of teacher candidates all recording podcasts in the same room, at the same time, was problematic. Now we use laptop computers and the groups are free to find a suitably quiet place anywhere in the education building. This has substantially improved the audio quality of the podcasts.

By applying DALO design features to the podcast project, it was anticipated that the learning objects produced by teacher candidates would improve their technology skills, foster teamwork and collaboration, and increase their understanding of K-12 software, including the need to carefully review titles before using them in the classroom.

In order to assess these outcomes, a survey was selected as the data collection method to elicit the views and experiences of the student-producers. A list of five questions was developed for the survey. What technology skills did you learn during this podcasting project? How did this podcasting project foster teamwork and collaboration? How did being involved in the scriptwriting, audio editing and presentation of your podcast support your understanding of educational software? What lessons have you learned from this assignment that might form the basis of advice/recommendations for educators pursuing similar podcasting projects? Do you have any further suggestions on how to make podcasting a really good experience for all those involved (producers, educators, listeners)?These questions were added to surveymonkey.com and responses were collected in class.

For the purpose of this project qualitative data analysis was employed to systematically review the survey responses, searching and rearranging them to increase understanding of them. Data analysis in qualitative research according to Bogdan & Biklen (1992) "...involves working with data, organizing them, searching for patterns, discovering what is important and what is to be learned, and deciding what and how to tell others." (p157)

Consistent with this definition I engaged in the prolonged and iterative process of data analysis. Patton (2002) writes that qualitative data analysis transforms the data into findings. Although no formula exists for this transformation, and methods for data analysis are unique for each researcher, it is imperative that you "do your very best with your full intellect to fully represent the data and communicate what the data reveal(p.433). Given the purpose of this study the steps of the constant comparison method provided by Glaser and Strauss (1967) and the operational refinements cited in Lincoln and Guba (1985) were followed. These operational steps were used to complement and enhance the data analysis before moving into the forth and final stage of the constant comparison method, reporting the results.

In this section of the chapter each question that was analyzed qualitatively will be presented followed by the emergent themes from the teacher candidate responses. A total of 93 teacher candidates responded to the survey.

Question 1. What technology skills did you learn during this podcasting project?

Our teacher candidates learned "what a podcast is, how you can subscribe to one through iTunes, why they're interesting/important, how to make one, how to post one, how to find ones that cater to your specific interests, etc." But they also "learned how to use garageband and google docs. I thought it was cool learning how to create audio files and post them as podcasts. it's like doing a presentation without having to stand in front of class" wrote one teacher candidate. Garageband and Google Docs was mentioned most frequently as the new technology skills. "I had never used the garageband software or recording device. It was a new multimedia application that challenged how I think about text and audience." Many of the teacher candidates used the word "easy" to describe the podcasting process. As one student put it "I was really surprised at how easy it was to make a podcast. I've been listening to them for a while, and always was impressed...little did I know!!"

Question 2. How did this podcasting project foster teamwork and collaboration?

Almost all of the responses to this question were positive."This project was a great assignment for fostering teamwork. I do not know how well it worked for other groups, but each of my group members did their part and the project turned out well." The fact that podcasting project had structure was an important consideration for our teacher candidates. "The Podcast project was a team effort from beginning to end. We each had to bring our own opinions of the software to the table. As a team we had to create a script then record our thoughts. It was one of the first group projects I had done where every group member had no choice but to contribute to the assignment." Another emergent theme was the usefulness and value of Google Docs as a collaborative tool. "Google docs was great because the three of us could work on it all the time." Another teacher candidate added "...we worked as a team in every aspect, drafting a Google doc, narrating the script, agreeing on our approach to the project.

Question 3. How did being involved in the script-writing, audio editing and presentation of your podcast support your understanding of educational software?

Responses to this question revolved around the theme you had to know it before you could record it. For example, "In order to express your opinion on the educational software, you had to investigate, research, and review the particular software. This process alone gave me a better understanding of the product." One teacher candidate added "I think it involved more thinking than a typical paper review...we really had to think about what we wanted to say in the podcast and then work together to make it happen." Said another, "It made the learning fun, it supported it because you had to analyze the material and make it into a script. It sparked a creative side in our group and is something that will probably stay with us for a while. Promotes high order thinking." Another illuminating and thoughtful response to the question was as follows. "The Podcast assignment provided us with a novel and contemporary method of expanding our knowledge about software. The overall point of the assignment was to delve deeper into the concepts of what makes software "good." By creating the podcast we were able to reinforce our learned notions about software criteria in a way that I had never done. Due to the uniqueness of this assignment the lessons we learned are ones that will stay with me."

Question 4. What lessons have you learned from this assignment that might form the basis of advice/recommendations for educators pursuing similar podcasting projects?

Podcasting is easy is a clear theme. Many of the responses included the word "easy" and/or "fun". For example one teacher candidate wrote, "Podcast[s] are really easy to create and could be used in a variety of ways in the classroom. It is definitely something new that students would find very enjoyable." Another commented "I thought this was a great tool that has many possibilities. For instance, instead of kids getting up in front of the class to give a book report, they can do a book report on a podcast with a partner, and this not only fosters group collaboration, but also gives students who are nervous speaking in front of groups to have a chance to do well and give a good book report." The decision to replace the previously paper and pencil software review assignment was probably a good one in light of the following response, "students would get a kick out of being able to create a pocast in place of a written project."

Question 5. Do you have any further suggestions on how to make podcasting a really good experience for all those involved (producers, educators, listeners)?

Having more time to complete the podcasting project was the common theme. Some of the advice included "practice practice practice", "have fun with it and don't be afraid!" and "listen to some professional [podcasts]." There were lots of positive comments, but the following quote best summed up the experience for many of the teacher candidates "I think podcasting could be an excellent exercise for students. They would be able to actually see the product of their research and work; it would become a living part of the internet. That could be extremely exciting for students to share their ideas with others. Most of the time, students do not have the opportunity to see each others' work. With a podcast, they would be able to appreciate and experience the projects of their fellow students."

CONCLUSION

As teacher educators it is imperative that we model the sound use of technology to enrich the teaching and learning process. Every semester the podcasting project gets a little easier, and the quality of the completed podcasts improves. That being said there is always room for improvement. Moving from the built in computer microphones to higher quality external units is something we are currently exploring. The inexpensive Snowflake USB mic by Blue Microphones looks promising. A concern that I have for this project is how well my teacher candidates understand podcasting, and to what extent will they be inclined to use podcasting when they start teaching. We have such a limited amount of time in the educational technology class that I teach, so the amount of time we devote to this project is an issue. The textbook we have used in the past only covers podcasting at a very cursory level. So next semester we will use Tony Vincent's excellent, and free, Podcasting for Teachers & Students booklet (http://www.learninginhand.com/podcasting/booklet.html). This free resource includes lots of useful tips, links and activities that will help our teacher candidates understand the potential of teacher created and students created media.

The true potential of podcasting in higher education and in K-12 education lies in its knowledge creation value, and its use as a vehicle for disseminating learner-generated content. It was anticipated that the podcasts produced by teacher candidates would improve their technology skills, foster teamwork and collaboration, and increase their understanding of K-12 software, including the need to carefully review titles before using them in the classroom.

Teacher candidates involved in this podcast project were exposed to methods of teaching and learning that utilized 21st century technology. Of the benefits afforded during the podcasting project, enthusiasm for, and engagement with, tools such as laptops, audio editing software and collaborative writing tools are perhaps the greatest. Post-experience comments indicated that not only are students receptive to learning and teaching with these cutting edge technologies, they welcome the possibility of incorporating these types of technologies into their future teaching practice.

In addition to attaining new technology skills, teacher candidate podcasters are uniquely positioned to develop advanced teamwork and collaboration skills. During the pre-production and production of their podcast episodes, teacher candidates developed interpersonal negotiation skills as they helped make strategic decisions about what to cover and how to organize ideas and best communicate them to their audience. Through their exchanges with each other, they gained valuable insights about managing their roles within a group. "Getting your way" gives way to meeting the needs of listeners. As Schmit (2007) writes, "collaborative podcasting teams learn to value the unique strengths of each member and to balance their own efforts with the priorities and inputs of their peers".

Our teacher candidates are learning about technology and course content in ways that mirror constructivism – frequently they have to build understanding for themselves, but in so doing, their understanding ends up being much stronger. At West Chester University the future for podcasting in teacher education looks bright.

Based on these findings, podcasting appears to be an effective and worthwhile learning activity in teacher education. Take some time to explore how this powerful new technology can support your personal and professional growth, supplement your curriculum, and provide your teacher candidates with a new expressive platform. Preparing our teacher candidates to use this emerging medium may have profound implications on their development as professionals.

REFERENCES

Atkinson, R. (2006). Podcasting: do they really need to know? *HERDSA News*, *28*(2), 20–22.

Bates, R., & Khasawneh, S. (2007). Self-efficacy and college students' perceptions and use of online learning systems. *Computers in Human Behavior*, *23*, 175–191. doi:10.1016/j.chb.2004.04.004

Bell, A. (2009). *A+ Rubric*. Retrieved February 16, 2009, from http://www.uwstout.edu/soe/profdev/podcastrubric.html

Bogdan, R., & Biklen, S. K. (1992). *Qualitative research for education: An introduction to theory and methods*. Boston: Allyn and Bacon.

Campbell, G. (2005). There's something in the air: podcasting in education. *EDUCAUSE Review*, *40*(6), 32–47.

Chan, A., & Lee, M. J. W. (2005). An MP3 a day keeps the worries away: Exploring the use of podcasting to address preconceptions and alleviate pre-class anxiety amongst undergraduate information technology students. In D. H. R. Spennemann & L. Burr (Eds.), *Good Practice in Practice: Proceedings of the Student Experience Conference* (pp. 58-70).

Duke University. (2006). *Duke digital initiative*. Retrieved December 2, 2008, from http://www.duke.edu/ddi/

Geoghegan, M. W., & Klass, D. (2005). *Podcast Solutions: The Complete Guide to Podcasting*. Berkeley, CA: Apress.

Georgia College & State University. (2005). *The iPod at GC&SU: a pocketful of learning*. Retrieved December 2, 2008, from http://ipod/gcsu.edu/

Glaser, B. G., & Strauss, A. L. (1967). *The discovery of grounded theory: strategies for qualitative research*. Chicago, IL: Aldine de Gruyter.

Hendron, J. (2008). *RSS for Educators: Blogs Newsfeeds, Podcasts and Wikis in the Classroom*. Eugene, OR: International Society for Technology in Education.

Lee, M. J. W., Chan, A., & McLoughlin, C. (2008). Talk the talk: Learner-generated podcasts as catalysts for knowledge creation. *British Journal of Educational Technology*, *39*(3), 501–521. doi:10.1111/j.1467-8535.2007.00746.x

Lincoln, Y. S., & Guba, E. G. (1985). *Naturalistic inquiry*. Beverly Hills, CA: Sage Publications.

McKinney, D., Dyck, J., & Luber, E. S. (2009, April). iTunes University and the classroom: Can podcasts replace Professors? *Computers & Education*, *52*(3), 617–623. doi:10.1016/j.compedu.2008.11.004

McLoughlin, C., Lee, M. J. W., & Chan, A. (2006). Using student generated podcasts to foster reflection and metacognition. *Australian Educational Computing, 21*(2), 34–40.

Middleton, A., & McCarter, R. (2005). Engaging solutions: a collaborative approach to digital audio learning object (DALO) production. Workshop presented at ALT-C 2005, Manchester, UK, September 6–8, 2005.

Patton, M. Q. (2002). *Qualitative evaluation and research methods* (3rd ed.). Thousand Oaks, CA: Sage Publications.

PoducateMe. (2008). *PoducateMe Podcasting Guide*. Retrieved March 16, 2009, from http://www.poducateme.com/

Read, B. (2005, March 2). Seriously, iPods Are Educational. *The Chronicle of Higher Education*. Retrieved December 2, 2008, from http://chronicle.com/weekly/v51/i28/28a03001.htm

Roblyer, M. D. (2006). *Integrating Educational Technology Into Teaching* (4th ed.). Upper Saddle River, NJ: Merrill Prentice-Hall.

RSS Advisory Board. (2005). *Really simple syndication: RSS 2.0.1 Specification (Rev. 6)*. Retrieved April 1, 2009, from http://www.rssboard.org/rss-2-0-1-rv-6

Schmit, D. (2007 January). Creating a Broadcast Empire...From the Corner of Your Classroom. *MultiMedia & Internet@Schools, 14*(1), 13-16.

Vincent, T. (2009). *Learning in Hand.* Retrieved June 18, 2009, from http://www.learninginhand.com/podcasting

Wagga Wagga. (2008). Digital Audio Learning Objects. In *Wikipedia, The Free Encyclopedia. Retrieved December 16, 2008, from.* Charles Sturt University.http://en.wikipedia.org/wiki/Digital_Audio_Learning_Objects

APPENDIX: ADDITIONAL READING

Podcasts--Created *By* Teachers, *For* Teachers

http://www.teachercreatedmaterials.com/podcasts/. Offers a variety of teacher-created podcasts designed for the purpose of helping busy teachers stay current on educational topics.

Helping Educators and Learners Harness the Power of Podcasting

http://www.intelligenic.com/blog/. A community of podcasters who are contributing innovative models and solutions for podcasting; includes podcasting project ideas, management tips, collaborative projects, contests and lots of resources to help you move into the podosphere for teaching, learning and building community.

Apple's Guide to Mobile Learning

http://www.apple.com/education/teachers-professors/mobile-learning.html. Website provided by Apple, geared towards educators

Exploiting the Educational Potential of Podcasting

http://recap.ltd.uk/articles/podguide.html. A brief guide to podcasting uses in education

Podcasting 101 for K-12 Librarians

http://www.infotoday.com/cilmag/apr06/Eash.shtml. Helping K-12 librarians turn podcasting into an opportunity to reach out to students and affect learning. Includes basic information about podcasting, how to access podcasts, reasons to use podcasts in school libraries, and how to create your own podcast.

Podcasting Tips and Ideas for Primary School Teachers

http://www.teachingideas.co.uk/index.shtml. Resource for primary school teachers illustrating how to develop podcasts catered to children.

Podcasting for Kids, by Kids

http://www.kid-cast.com/. A kid-safe forum for children to publish their own Podcasts for their peers to hear.

Teen Podcasters CEO Interview

http://videos.webpronews.com/2006/10/04/ceo-and-president-at-14-years-old/. Video interview with 14 year-old President and CEO of Teen Podcasters Network

Practical Solutions for Podcasting in Education

http://poducateme.com/guide/. A comprehensive how-to guide to Podcasting, including hot topics and statistics within Podcasting in education

Podcasting articles and Quotes

http://chatt.hdsb.ca/~magps/boylit/Podcasting%20in%20Education. A brief guide to Podcasting with a few podcasting topic ideas

Podcasting in Education Sources

http://www.stager.org/podcasting.html. Website that provides helpful resources to educators from tutorials to articles on Podcasting

K12 Handheld, Inc

http://www.k12handhelds.com/podcasting.php. K12 Handhelds, Inc offers solutions to mobile technology catered to the needs of individual school programs

Podcasting for Educators, Schools and Colleges

http://recap.ltd.uk/podcasting/. U.K. directory for podcasts, carefully chosen from 450 podcast channels for educational use

Adventures in Podcasting

http://www.shawnwheeler.name/workshops/adventuresnpodcastingpresentation/. Website of Director of Services and Training for a school district

Why Every School Should Be Podcasting

http://www.guardian.co.uk/education/2007/sep/18/link.link16. An article written about an educator who uses Podcasting to encourage creative learning-article includes links

Podcasting and Education Resources

http://www.shambles.net/pages/learning/infolit/edupodcast/. Useful links and articles for students and educators

How Do We Assess Student Podcasts?

http://www.mobile-learning.blog-city.com/how_do_we_assess_student_podcasts.htm. An article review regarding rubric for assessing podcasts

Chapter 23
Annotation Practices with Pen-Based Technologies

Kevin J. Reins
The University of South Dakota, USA

ABSTRACT

This chapter discusses pen-based technologies and their digital ink usage patterns. While traditional instructor inking practices provide opportunities for information to flow in a static unidirectional manner, pen-based computers can be combined with shared writing surfaces, real-time web interfacing, and software to increase the collaboration and interaction between students and the instructor's presentation through active learning. Suggestions of ways post-secondary faculty can utilize digital ink using sound pedagogical practices and a discussion of an experimental study testing the impact of one inking technique used to refine student thinking processes are included.

INTRODUCTION

One-to-one computing is the goal of a laptop initiative called *Classroom Connections* in the state of South Dakota. It is a part of the 2010 Education Initiative that provides incentive money for school districts to initiate one-to-one laptop programs for high school students. By fall 2007 there were 41 high schools with 9,600 students and over 1000 teachers participating in the program. Twenty-five percent of South Dakota high school students have tablet PCs 24/7 (24 hours per day, 7 days per week).

DOI: 10.4018/978-1-61520-897-5.ch023

South Dakota is not the only state with a plan to get a laptop or tablet PC into every student's hand. *Education Week* in an article by Rhea Borja estimated in 2006 that since Maine started their initiative, almost one-quarter of school districts nationwide and nine states have invested in one-to-one laptop programs. Additionally, the K-12 Computing Blueprint hosted by *Technology & Learning* (2007) stated the demand in all U.S. schools to create one-to-one access for all students is increasing exponentially.

There is a general belief in the potential of this next-generation technology to improve teaching and learning (Metiri Group, 2006). The goal of placing a laptop, notebook, tablet PC, or netbook in every

Copyright © 2010, IGI Global. Copying or distributing in print or electronic forms without written permission of IGI Global is prohibited.

student's hand is different for districts and states nationwide, most of which are centered on the development of 21st Century Skills (Center for Digital Education, 2004). But in broader terms, the goals of one-to-one computing can be summarized by what can be accomplished with one-to-one: creating learning environments that are more student-centered by using mobilized software that can accompany students and provide accessibility of technology for all students anytime/anywhere.

One-to-one computing infrastructures are changing constantly to maintain currency with the new technologies that are available. Many states and districts joining the one-to-one initiative or those previous participants now replacing technologies are contemplating moving away from the idea of simply placing a laptop into every student's hand and have begun to consider additional learning opportunities provided by tablet PCs (Milner, 2006) or less expensive alternatives, such as netbooks (Cramer, Beauregard, & Sharma, 2009). This chapter adds to the possibilities of technology-enhanced learning afforded to students through one pen-based technology, namely tablet PCs (see Orlando, 2008).

One advantage tablet PCs have over laptops and netbooks is their ability to digitally ink directly to the display by using a stylus. *Digital Inking* "is the ability to scrawl (i.e., to write or draw awkwardly, hastily, or carelessly) directly on the screen of a tablet PC or convertible laptop…much like writing on a sheet of paper with a pen" (Reins, 2007, p. 159). Inking capabilities built into software applications are considered to be *ink aware*, while other affordances are accomplished by providing an ink layer on top of the document or image. In either case, the ability to fully integrate the digital ink into the document or image is present by saving the file as a specified file type. Many of the applications used for instructional presentation purposes have some type of electronic slide or layer on which an instructor can write prior to, during, and/or post presentation as a way of accomplishing digital inking.

Now that tablet PCs and their ink applications have entered classrooms nationwide, instructors are presumably experimenting with understanding how to leverage the inking capabilities of this tool for (1) enhancement of instruction, (2) curricular changes, (3) affective changes in students and instructors, and/or (4) a noticeable, directed improvement in technology-mediated student learning. There have been many unique models and approaches toward tablet PC implementation, such as a 30-day electronic homework challenge (Dicken, 2008) in a high school mathematics classroom, an upside down teaching approach (Berque, Byers & Myers, 2008) used in a computer science course, or design research conducted since 2006 by the College of Engineering at Virginia Polytechnic Institute and State University in which each year the implementation team reviews and alters existing practices.

One can learn from each of these models as many can be adapted to situations where not all students have a tablet PC or ubiquitous access (i.e., everywhere, all the time). Teacher educators can make generalizations from different approaches, methods, and practices to their respective disciplines that need not be contextually tied to specific applications (e.g., *DyKnow, Classroom Presenter, Ubiquitous Presenter, WriteOn, and Microsoft OneNote*). Such perspectives speak to the versatility and adaptability of tablet PCs and their ink applications to various educational environments.

Post-secondary faculty should be concerned with modeling effective pedagogical practices using pen-based technologies based on sound educational theory. Preservice teachers, upon their graduation, should not only have a knowledge base of tablet PCs as tools, but also considerations of their appropriate field use as well as remaining current regarding these constantly changing technologies.

However, the integration of tablet PCs has not always been easy for many postsecondary faculties working with preservice teachers. Anecdotal conversations with the author have revealed a desire from faculty, practitioners, trainers, and administrators for tried-and-true *best practices*. Perhaps the strongest concern of those involved in a transition to teaching with a pen-based technology is the lack of sound professional development and scaffolding once given a tablet PC for course integration.

Overwhelmingly, these faculty report being given training for the tool itself (tablet PC and pen capabilities) or the workings of a piece of software, but not the professional development for introducing sound pedagogy with the tablet. As such, overloaded faculty are essentially required to "figure these things out" on their own or collaborate with others equally inexperienced to make adaptations or create new software. However, South Dakota provides ten days of technology training and implementation support. Other states may be providing similar professional development and support.

The driving forces behind this chapter and book are to introduce post-secondary teacher educators to effective and engaging pedagogical practices and software that support teaching and learning by using tablet PCs. By sharing the research, experiences, and trials of those using these new technologies, assistance will be provided for faculty just beginning to recontextualize their classroom in incorporating tablet PCs with additional doors opened for those seeking new and higher levels of engagement.

BACKGROUND

The intent of this background section is to present a classification of digital inking techniques and offer a few solid examples of each with their implications to the topic, rather than providing an exhaustive review of literature of digital ink practices. Exemplary practices draw attention to the author's new classification (i.e., augmentative versus collaborative-interactive) of ink usage patterns among faculty and organizes researchers' subsequent tried-and-true best practices. It also serves P-16 institutions in finding possible solutions and generating new ideas that work within their existing architecture and personnel.

Augmentative Inking

The most basic level of digital inking begins with an instructor compiling a series of electronic slides which are uploaded into software, allowing the instructor to write directly on them with digital ink via an active panel, slate, or tablet PC pen. The firmware and software communicates with a data projector that synchronously displays the slides and inking to an audience. Current choices for applications combining electronic slides and digital ink include *Tablet Mylar Slides* (TMS; University of Maryland); *Classroom Presenter* (University of Washington); *Microsoft Word, Journal, OneNote* or *PowerPoint*; *WriteOn*; *Smart Notebook* software; *Promethean* software; and a host of other small business and educational solutions. Available for educator use are commonly used Information and Communication Technology (ICT) solutions which assist mathematics, science, and engineering instructors in preparing formulas and equations for their electronic slides (e.g., *MathType, Multimedia MathJournal 2.1, LaTex*).

Using digital ink in this way affords instructors the ability to integrate it onto his/her notes or slides by writing, sketching, tracing, or annotating. This creates a more natural way for instructors to interact with his/her documents, respond to students' questions, and add extemporaneous thoughts to presentations. This type of inking is considered to *augment* prepared lecture notes, and the following studies depict unique augmentative practices meant to inspire new implementation ideas.

Engineering faculty at Virginia Polytechnic Institute and State University has embarked on longitudinal studies of the effectiveness of tablet PCs (See a video documenting the success of its implementation, click the Tablet PC Initiative link in the right top pane of the College of Engineering's

Web site at http://www.eng.vt.edu/main/index.php). All incoming freshmen in the College of Engineering are required to purchase tablet PCs with specific minimum hardware and software requirements. Each year faculty report their current practices to help create an ongoing analysis of best practices and their assessment system. In summaries and findings, faculty frequently reported the copious use of digital ink to annotate ready-made complex drawings, diagrams, and graphics along with creating incomplete drawings and figures and finishing them during presentations. For engineering faculty, these inking practices proved to engage the students more in question generation during instructors' lectures.

One practice by Tront and Scales (2007) described how instructors created drawings and diagrams prior to their lectures, then traced or recreated them during the lecture. The software allowed the lecturer to see the drawings and diagrams on the tablet PC in front of them, but not broadcast them for students to view on the projected image. This created the illusion that the instructor was creating each drawing from scratch, when in reality the instructor was meticulously tracing existing drawings with the pen stylus. An ink-based example of the recreation of a mathematical proof exists at http://www.cs.umd.edu/~egolub/TabletMylarSlides. Classroom Presenter also allows for hidden text and figures. This practice is made possible in many applications, including *Mylar Slides, Microsoft PowerPoint, Ubiquitous Presenter,* and *Classroom Presenter* through "instructor" or "hidden" ink. Instructors have more time to focus on finding better ways of captivating students with their lectures since they no longer needed to commit these drawings and diagrams to memory (Tront & Scales, 2007).

The implication of Tront and Scales's augmentative practice is that an instructor can draw more complex diagrams and create incomplete diagrams that *engage* students during their presentation. This practice may free up the instructor's thought processes during teaching for more intense focus on student thinking and the interpretation of student responses with respect to their thinking. The incomplete diagrams or inkings provide opportunities for questions and allow for student predictions before they are completed or fully disclosed. This brings students' existing knowledge to the forefront of the learning environment, and aids instructors in assisting students' assimilation and accommodation of new information.

Price and Simon (2007) explored the inking practices of three university-level physics classes by analyzing the saved lecture materials of three instructors at two different institutions. They found three ink usage patterns emerged from their study of the instructor's ink, "using ink to explicitly link multiple representations; making prepared figures dynamic by animating them with ink; and preparing slides with sparse text or figures, then adding extensive annotations during class" (Price & Simon, p. 108). All are examples of a unidirectional flow of information from instructor to students, which is typical of augmentative inking practices. The second and third in the list are consistent with Tront and Scales's practice, but the first ink usage pattern describe by Price and Simon is different.

In a tablet PC blog for teaching college mathematics teachingcollegemath.com, Maria H. Andersen depicted the first inking pattern described in Price and Simon's 2007 study, that is, using ink to explicitly link multiple representations (see Figure 1) for mathematics teaching.

The instantiation of this practice can be seen in Andersen's links between the graph and the locations along the graph where the slope of the derivative is positive or negative and between expressions and their expansions. The problem described was to find the derivative of[INSERT FIGURE 001]. Using a highlighter, Andersen and her students were able to use one color for the function and a different color for the derivative, and highlight the parts of f that had positive slopes in yellow. Likewise, they could highlight the parts of the function f and that had negative

Figure 1. Maria Andersen's example of explicitly linking representations with ink. (© 2008, Maria H. Andersen. Used with permission.)

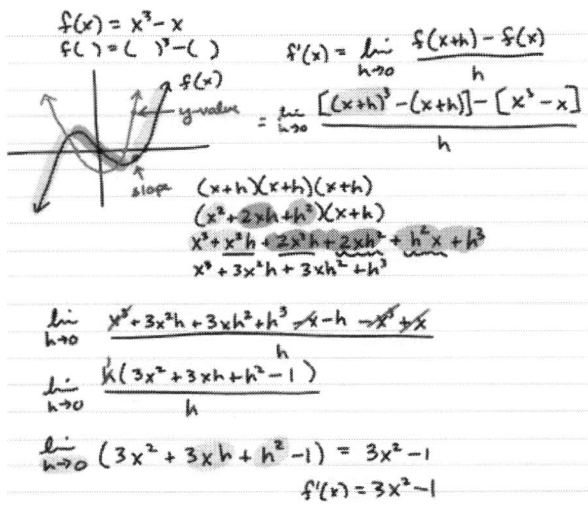

slopes in green. Andersen also used color to assist students in following the distribution of *(x+h)* to the expansion of *(x+h)(x+h)*. Andersen reported that the impact of doing this with digital ink is different visually for students; it focuses students' attention toward the mathematics rather than the lines added to the mathematical work. To see the colors in this figure, visit http://teachingcollegemath.com/?p=421.

The implication of Anderson's depiction of Price and Simon's usage pattern is that attention can be drawn to important mathematical connections and sense-making that one accomplishes during problem solving. Students do not always "see" the connections between mathematical ideas or how they build on one another and the connections to their existing knowledge. Instructors can leverage this augmentative digital inking practice as a sense-making tool.

Each of these examples uses digital ink as a way of augmenting prepared lecture notes and can be categorized as effective pedagogical practices in which the digital ink functions as *attentional ink*. Digital ink used in this way allows students to focus on what is of importance and what the instructor adds to the broadcasted content. With respect to ink usage patterns, this classification is consistent with older software applications that do not take advantage of *ConferenceXP* and/or faculty seeking simple ways to become comfortable with its use as a tool for teaching and learning.

Collaborative-Interactive Inking

A second class of digital ink usage designated by the author is *collaborative-interactive*. The main difference between the presentations of electronic slides and the collaborative-interactive ink usage pattern is the presence of a presentation system that allows for multi-channel, bidirectional inking on a shared electronic surface.

This type of a presentation system allows for higher levels of engagement among students and with their instructor. Small groups or individual students can ink their thoughts, musings, and solution strategies directly into the broadcasted presentation (i.e., the projected image). This allows the instructor and other students in the classroom to analyze written work, listen to explanations of written work, witness their peers' questions and thinking processes, and engage in formative assessment with immediate feedback. All of these allow for just-in-time teaching and scaffolds for student success.

This level of interaction with digital ink allows students to see and interact with presentations by inking their own work or ideas via a slate or tablet PC. The instructor can project student work or ideas and discuss positive and negative submissions without increasing student anxiety. Current choices for combining student inking to presentations include *SMART Notebook* in conjunction with *SynchonEyes* (SMART Technologies' classroom management software), and either tablet PCs or slates. Another is a Promethean whiteboard in conjunction with *SynchronEyes* or Activslates (individual slates made by Promethean) that teachers can activate or de-activate within its projection system, but only a few can be activated at a time; not every student can have one.

Also available as an inexpensive solution are Airprojectors in conjunction with standard 802.11b wireless cards, such as Komatsu's TriLink Airprojector with moderator and client software installed on tablet PCs, or computers accompanied by slates. Others included are software system solutions such as *OneNote*, *MessageGrid* (Clemson University), *Classroom Presenter* (University of Washington), *Ubiquitous Presenter* (University of San Diego) or *Classroom Learning Partner* (MIT) that are both built on top of and extend *Classroom Presenter*. All of these software solutions work with tablet PCs or computers accompanied by slates, some of which are freeware. Using digital ink in this collaborative-interactive manner has the potential to enhance the discourse in the classroom and provide more opportunities for interaction. This potential for interaction is accessibly described by Fischman (2007). Two points made by Fischman are that it prevents the class loud-mouth from deterring other students' participation and allows professorial talk from more of a "just starting" perspective of the concept. The following studies depict unique collaborative-interactive practices meant to inspire interaction and new implementation ideas.

Cantu used *OneNote 2007* and tablet PCs in conjunction with an online electronic textbook in her mathematics classroom (Cantu, Phillips, & Tholfsen, 2008), as the *OneNote* application by Microsoft contains many features allowing for collaboration and sharing. Using this application, small groups of students would be selected to participate in a notebook "live-sharing" activity. This feature of OneNote allows one notebook to be shared among a group of students, all of whom have the ability to add content which is updated and seen in the shared notebook of all its members on their individual tablets.

Permission can be granted by teachers for projecting rights of the classroom projector as students share their work. Cantu would many times connect one of the student tablet PCs, capturing the shared notebook to the wired projector, to free up her tablet PC for walk-around observations as the "expert" students presented. Cantu felt that both the expert student presenters and the others in the class were reportedly much more engaged in the lessons with this type of interactive sharing (Cantu, Phillips, & Tholfsen, 2008).

The implication of Cantu's (2008) study is students can now share one writing surface to serve as the basis of their collaboration. Students can come together in this environment and brainstorm and share ideas that can move the group as a whole toward their final resolution to the problem at hand. Their ability to see one another's inking on the shared writing surface may spur more alternative approaches and thinking and lead to the building of a solution from fragmented or incomplete ideas.

Berque, Byers, and Myers (2008) from DePauw University have taught many classes using pen-based technologies and *DyKnow* software. Their approach affords instructors more in-class time for active learning (AL). Students view on-line recorded audio or video files prior to class sessions in order to allow additional class time for in-class interactive activities. Berque and others (2008) have called this an "upside down" approach to teaching because the lecture portion of class is moved outside of class meeting time making way for active learning. Students used *DyKnow* software features to compile the mini-lectures, organize their class notes, and complete in-class activities. In small groups students would work on a shared electronic page in the *DyKnow* software on a collaborative design activity. Each group's work was then shared with the entire class for discussion and critique.

The implication of Berque and others (2008) is that in-class time can be more aptly used by moving some instructional experiences outside the classroom. Students might work on a performance task outside of regular class time and submit their work to the instructor so that the in-class time may be spent talking about the processes and solutions that were produced. This allows for greater exposure and coverage of more significant mathematical tasks that are open-ended and realistic.

Davis and others (2007) studied making note-taking public by using the web and software called *Ubiquitous Presenter*. Self-selected students take notes on the instructor's presentation for others in the class to view real-time as the noteblogger (person taking the notes) is actively taking notes on the presentation slides during class time. Their results show that the notebloggers predicted classmates might not have information that instructors assumed was known; as such they used more concrete entry points and presented background information. As a result, the blog watchers gained more confidence and had more success while problem solving in class.

This new real-time data has encouraged a unique engagement of students within the courses that it is being used. It has been found to have the most potential with more advanced students, but that the content of the notebloggers has potential to support a broad range of students. The researchers suggested that a teaching assistant (TA) might be introduced to the course as a "master blogger." The participants of the course are able to distinguish instructor from noteblogger ink by color, or by choosing to turn off the noteblogger ink. This more modern technology practice meshes well with the mantra of the current web culture of sharing everything (e.g., personal blogs, Twitter, YouTube, and DailyMotion).

The implication of Davis and others (2007) is that peer-tutoring and peer-coaching can now happen in real-time. More able students in the class can help one another understand the language and instructional techniques used by the instructor without interruption of the lesson. This allows for more collaboration between students during the learning process.

These examples are ways of creating more engagement through digital ink in prepared lecture notes and activities. They exemplify effective pedagogical practices in which the digital ink was used in a collaborative-interactive way. Thus producing an active learning environment in which students are more cognitively active.

USING DIGITAL INK FOR TEACHING AND LEARNING

Recently ubiquitous home usage has encouraged the use of computers for teaching and learning in the classroom. A report conducted by DeBell and Chapman (2006) from the National Center for Education Statistics found that computer use (91%) and Internet use (59%) were commonplace among PK-12 students, and that by high school 97% used computers and 80% used Internet mostly at home, with 72% of young Internet users exploiting it for schoolwork. Furthermore, a white paper from the Metiri Group (2006) depicted 13 to 18 year-olds spending on average six hours per day using digital media. Many of these students need to learn how to use technology for creative thinking, problem solving, and effective communicating and socializing, as well as its acceptable use through proper technology integration at school. Therefore, teacher educators and technology integrationists must make transitions in their courses from learning *about* computers to learning *with* computers.

Learning how to leverage digital inking in the mathematics classroom for teaching and learning is important. Using digital ink and tablet PCs has mostly been supported by the change in levels of engagement of students in the classroom, with engagement being described as having components of involvement, interactivity, perseverance, effort, and attitudes (Metiri Group, 2006). From an *Active Learning* (AL) perspective, engagement might also include a component of being cognitively active. Digital inking practices can also put mathematical authority on the shoulders of the student. Learning how to justify their work and solutions is an important mathematical process, as is overcoming reliance on teachers for having or knowing the correct answer. Using digital ink appropriately also typically results in more rigorous and authentic learning experiences. However, learning to use digital ink effectively does not come without trials and issues. The sections that follow help reader contemplate the use of digital ink and how one can better leverage it as a tool for teaching and learning in their classroom.

Issues, Controversies, and Problems

Each presentation system capable of leveraging digital ink technology and pedagogical practices mentioned in the Background section has its issues and disadvantages for K-16 education. For example, some presentation systems require faculty to create a series of slides that must be uploaded into a piece of software. For a discipline like mathematics, this can be seen as a prohibitive amount of frontloaded work required for a course. Having to create or convert a deck of slides and learn new software keeps many traditional mathematics teachers from using digital ink technology. One mathematics faculty member precisely describes the give and take of time constraints:

The face-to-face time increased substantially and along with it also the opportunity to judge and respond to student reactions during lectures. I definitely found that this model allows the lecturer to either cover more material in the same time period or to spend more time explaining and discussing the displayed material. This, however, must be seen against the backdrop of a substantial increase in the preparation time that was needed to prepare lectures for a first-time presentation. (Olivier, 2005, p. 178)

Today, however, there are many newer alternatives which address the constraints of an electronic slide-based system and the complexity of the processes which would allow transition from current practices to best practice implementation at a much quicker rate. For example, a mathematics instructor may choose to open only a whiteboard deck for a lecture in UP or TMS at the start of each class without having prepared any slides. This is similar to what one might do during a more traditional presentation of the content from a set of notes on a chalkboard or a set of transparencies. Glub (2004) realized that his transition from transparencies to TMS did not cause him to invest any additional time in classroom preparation.

The difference is that instructors may now take advantage of all of the collaborative-interactive aspects of using digital ink, especially in an environment where every student has a tablet PC or where there is an allocation of one tablet per small group. UP and DyKnow also allow for a digital archive of all of the lessons and a stroke-by-stroke playback option for students using a Web-based interface. This means that students can review the lecture from any computer, anytime, at a pace necessary to analyze each step or process. Using this presentation system, the instructor may be freed from the frontloading work of creating electronic slides to focus on only creating slides for specific performance tasks, or intense, in-class collaborative and interactive activities, as will be described later in this chapter. This moves the class toward a more active learning environment.

Some researchers believe that the amount of engagement from the students in using the tablet

PCs is mostly dependent upon the fit of the task to the aspects of a tablet PC that separate it from a laptop. For example, Bilen, Lee, Messner, Nyguyen, Simpson, Techatassanasoontorn, and Devon (2008) showed the level of task-technology fit influences the extent of the students' use of the tablet PC. They stated that instructors need to design classroom tasks that leverage unique features of tablet PCs, which will motivate students to explore the value and fruitfulness of using tablet PCs.

Further analysis of focus groups of students in this study (Bilen et al., 2008) resulted in a suggestion for instructors to consider whether or not their redesign of class materials takes advantage of unique tablet PC features. If instructors do not spend time thinking about this fit, it may be a detriment. Students have reported feeling like the tablet PCs were "forced" into the curriculum and that they could have learned the content just as well without the technology (Chidanandan et al., 2007). Instructors need to critically and precisely analyze the supporting structures of the technology and the task itself with respect to its fit for pen-based computing and explain its use to students.

During 2007 and 2008, DiStasi, Birmingham, and Welton investigated whether students' satisfaction with collaborative-interactive programs like *DyKnow* are impacted by individual differences in learning styles. In their treatment, students and faculty were using the software during the entire course, so in the second year most students and all faculty involved had prior exposure to the software. In their 2008 data evaluating the overall satisfaction of the software there were large groups of 20% or more students on both ends of the scale, decidedly positive and decidedly negative, which is against the notion that satisfaction should increase as the comfort of using the software increases. This large mass of overall satisfaction on both ends of the Likert scale ratings was attributed to students' learning styles, and evidence suggested that visual learners will value and be more satisfied with presentations using *DyKnow* and similar types of software. Qualitative data also supported the quantitative data on both ends of the spectrum.

Some students believed that the "actual process of writing down the notes facilitates their memory, and so they would prefer not to have so many notes delivered," while others felt the "provided notes freed them from the mundane need to copy, and hence they were given more time to think" (p. 44). This finding was not reflected in the analysis of the Active-Reflective learner type, but led researchers to an alternate hypothesis of the nature of the material and the inherent student motivation to learn the content may be related to higher satisfaction.

Price and Simon (2007) found a possibility that inking practices may be bound to certain disciplines. The commonality of ink usage patterns among physics instructors led them to believe that there may be "physics inking" patterns as well as inking patterns that are specific to other disciplines, although they were cautious about making overgeneralizations as only three instructors were studied. This finding supports the need for creating communities within disciplines for sharing inking techniques.

A final issue cannot be substantiated in great volume or detail by the review of literature for this chapter, but has been identified by the work of the author as researcher. When using a presentation system like UP where students are submitting large amounts of content via slides, it becomes difficult to sort through and manage the entire student submission list, especially if students are manually moving through the slides at their own pace.

Part of the reason for this difficulty stems from the size of the student submission slide in the instructor preview mode, and the time it takes for an instructor to peruse the filmstrip and find a slide that is worthy of or needing discussion. Two recommendations can be made to help alleviate this difficulty; first, label the prepared slide during its creation with an easily identifiable label in the corner of the slide that separates it from all other slides, and second, have students write their name or group name or number in the upper right hand corner of the slide. This is helpful, but the mundane work of finding correct and incorrect conceptions to discuss still needs the critical eye of the instructor.

One related study examined two sections of Algebra II students in a unique environment (Kamin, Capitanu, Twidale, & Peiper, 2008). The model classroom had a teacher's dashboard, which is an array of four monitors displaying each student's individual work on a portion of one of the monitors. This was accomplished via a networked set of slates. The teacher would regularly consult the NuPaper Dashboard, which was overwhelming at first, to passively monitor students' work on electronic worksheets and seek items needing attention. The software developers added an ability to sort the thumbnails of student work by student identification, current page, strokes created, strokes deleted, ink volume, writing time, erasing time, average pressure, average speed, and group number. This helped alleviate some of the challenge of scanning the dashboard to find something noteworthy that needed instructional attention. Ideas from this study led to recommendations provided to UP developers for the ability to sort the student submissions deck.

Solutions and Recommendations

Once the system that best suits one's unique environment is in place, the struggle begins. The next step becomes moving educators toward creating optimal environments for meaningful classroom interaction. One beneficial resource that assists in sharing knowledge in this area of focus has been ongoing for several years. The *Workshop on the Impact of Pen-based Technology on Education* (WIPTE) conferences brings together educators from all disciplines (www.wipte.org). All of the workshop participants displayed a serious commitment to sharing experiences and best practices of using tablet PCs and other pen-based technologies. Teacher educators also need to stimulate a community of shared ideas at their home institutions. It is difficult to remain current with the ever-changing state of technologies and their availability, but WIPTE is an excellent place to learn new practices, stimulate the creation of fresh ideas, and foster collegiality centered on this topic.

Currently there exists a dearth of research that examines best pedagogical practices of integrating digital ink technology into mathematics classrooms. Olivier's (2005) recommendation for further research pointed to the need for true experimental studies that determine possible best inking practices for teaching mathematics which give attention to the sequencing and systematic use of digital ink on tablet PCs. A study conducted by the author will now be described as a solution and recommendation for this topic and chapter.

A STUDY OF ONE COLLABORATIVE-INTERACTIVE TECHNIQUE

The study was conducted on one research-based activity. The problem under investigation was whether or not the use of digital ink affected the attitudes and learning that occurred during a mathematical investigation of area. It is described to provide flesh to the collaborative-interactive classification of digital inking practices. The study is also described so that the inking practice can be replicated and used for similarly structured activities. The inking practice can be generalized to mathematics teaching as well as other disciplines.

Introduction

One research-based practice from a list of nine types of high-quality inking techniques thought to improve instructor-learner dialogue from Reins (2007) was investigated. This study's main objective was to isolate and validate the effectiveness of a technique that can be classified as *collaborative-interactive*. The contextual example demonstrated an attempt to adapt pen-based technologies to enhance the teaching and learning of mathematics while affirming current mathematics reform efforts. It described a method of using digital ink and classroom discourse to *refine thinking processes*. This technique, first identified by the author (2007), demonstrated time and again to be a fruitful technique but needed further justification. Following Olivier's recommendation in 2005, this study was conducted to provide description of the sequencing and systematic use of the digital ink technique and measure its effectiveness.

Method

Fifty-three students in two sections of mathematics methods, one using UP and shared electronic writing surfaces, and the other a more traditional approach where students wrote with styli on an electronic worksheet and shared ideas via a classroom discussion, were studied. Students in both cohorts met twice a week for seventy-five minute classes in a model technology classroom for teacher preparation.

Several controls were employed or realized in the study. The teaching style was controlled by having the same instructor for both sections, so the activities' objectives, electronic worksheets, and information presented were also the same. The time of the day was also controlled as the sections met at the same scheduled time in the same classroom. There were 31 undergraduate senior elementary education majors in each of the two groups, with a total of nine students choosing to not complete all of the assessments and thus dropped from the study. The characteristics of the students in each of the sections were similar with respect to year in school and types of courses taken. The control group had a slightly higher but significantly different GPA, $F\ (1,52) = 6.124, p=.017$.

The classroom had one wireless Internet access point, an HD ceiling mounted EIKI projector connected to a 94-inch wall-mounted interactive whiteboard with a 16:9 aspect ratio (SMART Board 690), and a mobile computing cart filled with twelve Gateway M285E tablet PCs. Students in both semesters were accustomed to taking a tablet PC on their way into the classroom and working around them in small teams at tables that were powered. The students also worked within the same peer groups for in-class activities; the instructor never assigned groups. The course was a web-based one in which the instructor provided sessional notes for every class in an electronic html format which contained activities that allowed for digital inking.

The differences in treatment of the groups were only found in the techniques that were used to help facilitate students' refinements to their thinking processes. The design experiment was the same for each semester except for how the students shared their thinking. The control group shared and demonstrated their solution strategies via whole class discussions and a Sympodium. A Sympodium is a wired slate that is housed on a cabinet that contains a desktop station at the front of the classroom that allows for inking with a stylus on the broadcasted image coming from a ceiling mounted projector.

The experimental groups' work was facilitated in software called *Ubiquitous Presenter*. This allowed the experimental group to ink on electronic slides, which displayed the in-class task and submitted them with their inked solution strategies to the instructor that were collected in aggregate by a Web-based platform. The students could also synchronously review the student-generated submissions collected in the software in a browser (see Figure 2). The whole-class discussions were facilitated within the student deck of submissions.

The objective of the instructional lesson was to help students learn how to find the areas of basic 2D geometric shapes on a grid system. This was accomplished through first exploring the concept of area on a Geoboard. Instruction began by helping students understand that area is about cover-

Figure 2. Student submission slide in ubiquitous presenter. (©2008, Reins.)

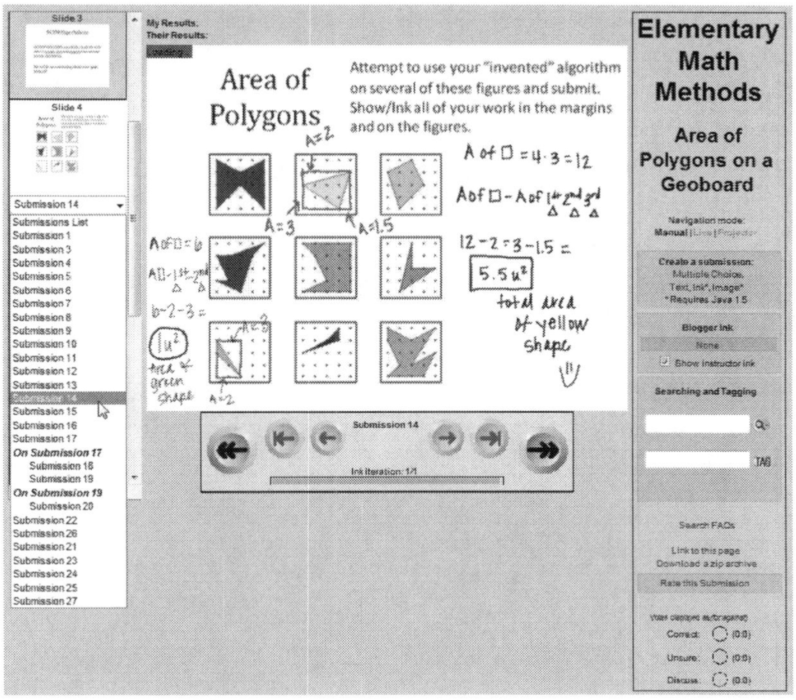

age and square units. Students created their own algorithms for finding the area of a rectangle on a Geoboard and used this knowledge to create an algorithm to find the area of right triangles on a Geoboard. This was discovered first since many preservice teachers and elementary students incorrectly apply a peg-counting algorithm for finding the area of a rectangle on a Geoboard versus looking at the number of segment lengths between two pegs represented on one of its sides. This results in an incorrect calculation of area since the number of segments along a side is one less than the number of pegs along the segment counting the end pegs. Once the non-existence of this misconception was realized, the students were introduced to the activity.

The Active Learning (AL) activity that was the focus of study required students to develop algorithms for finding the area of any polygon (simple closed curve; concave or convex) on a Geoboard. They were encouraged to use their knowledge gained from the in-class activities centered on developing algorithms for finding the area of a rectangle and a right triangle in the previous session.

Before the next class session, students were asked to create as many algorithms as they could that worked for all polygons including the nine cases on the *Area of Polygons* electronic worksheet (see Figure 3). They were to fully develop at least one algorithm that included a typed, written explanation that outlined a series of finite steps that would result in the correct area of any polygon when applied and meticulously followed. They were also asked to complete the *Area of Nine Polygons* electronic worksheet using their typed algorithm and search for other algorithms that always worked. Simultaneously they were to record in their mind algorithms that did not always work that they generated while tackling the homework exercise. The nine polygons that were presented as challenges to their algorithm development were presented in the electronic worksheet.

The in-class discussions that followed the homework assignments focused first on non-generalizable algorithms; i.e., ones that did not work for all polygons all of the time. Students were asked to give an example of when it worked and a counter example for when it did not while providing these solution strategies. Students were asked if they were capable of resolving the conflict or issues that the non-generalizable algorithms caused, and to instantiate their "invented" algorithms on several of the figures on the electronic worksheet and include as much ink as possible/necessary for others to make sense of what they were doing in their solution strategy.

The goal of the sharing process was to collaboratively refine as many different generalizable solution strategies as possible. Students at the end of the sharing and refinement processes were also asked to define their favorite algorithm, when it would be fruitful for one to use or apply this algorithm, and when they would apply a different one. This objective was initiated in response to National Council of Teachers of Mathematics' (NCTM, 2000) goal of students being able to create, test, and choose from among several algorithms.

Figure 3. Area of nine polygons electronic worksheet. (© 2008, Reins.)

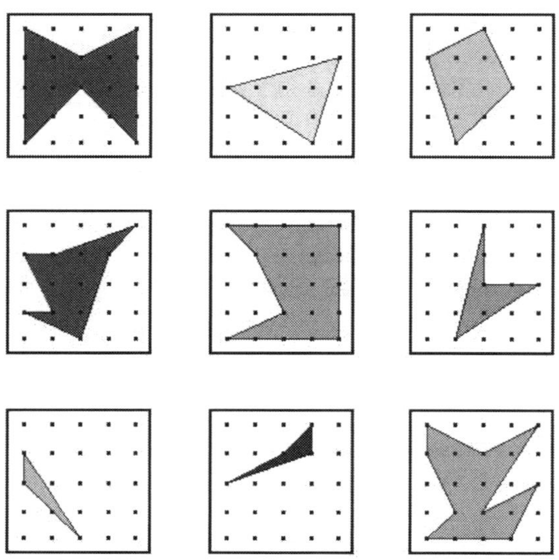

The control group was allowed to share and demonstrate their solution strategies by bringing their tablet PCs up to the Sympodium and changing out the projector's cable attached to the instructor's tablet PC to their tablet PC. They were able to describe their thinking processes and inking as they presented their solution strategies. The Sympodium was also leveraged to talk about refinements to a student-generated solution strategy.

The new ideas that added to an old way of thinking had to be re-inked on the *Area of Nine Polygons* electronic worksheet to assist talk about ways to resolve the conflict or issues with non-generalizable solution strategies. One example of which would be recognizing that the algorithm christened the "interior chunking" strategy seemed to not work on *all* polygons, especially some of those located on the electronic worksheet.

This is typically the belief of a majority of the teacher candidates because they tend to use square units and rectangles to fill the interior, which sometimes leaves small slivers of area that do not have vertices landing on pegs of the Geoboard whose areas are difficult to calculate. This usually manifests itself until someone suggests refining the interior chunking strategy by dividing up the interior of the polygon into triangles using only interior peg(s). This refinement of the interior chunking strategy was necessary by both the control and experimental groups, but was accomplished in different ways.

The experimental group was allowed a few minutes at the start of class to ink their solution strategies on a slide in UP that contained the *Area of Nine Polygons* electronic worksheet. The students were able to ink each of their ideas for a solution strategy on a separate slide and submit it to the instructor's presentation. These slides were compiled in the UP system and were used to discuss the different solutions produced and the refinements made by students to some of the strategies in real-time.

For the refinement example, a student-submitted slide was used which displayed an interior-triangles-chunking algorithm and broadcasted for the review and focus of the entire class. The small group that generated the solution strategy was then able to explain how they started with a more gross interior chunking strategy that included squares, rectangles, and triangles. It was refined by looking at a peer's submission slide containing the use of triangles as a solution for one of the more difficult shapes. The same result was achieved as the control groups', but the way in which it was achieved was different. The students in the experimental group used hints from looking at other submissions to help them revise their thinking in real-time.

The following types of data were collected and analyzed from both groups: an *Area of Nine Polygons* electronic worksheet, a typed algorithm for finding the area of a polygon on a Geoboard, a delayed post-test for recall of different solution strategies (a final exam question), and an online delayed-questionnaire of digital ink technologies. The students in the experimental group also completed an online delayed-questionnaire on the use of *Ubiquitous Presenter* for the activity. The students' GPAs were used as a covariate in the analysis of the final exam question. This chapter will focus on the questionnaire results which highlight ideas related to the classification of digital inking practices.

Several instruments were used to try to pick up demonstrated and affective differences between the techniques used with the control and experimental groups. The two instruments created to measure the affect of digital ink technologies and *Ubiquitous Presenter* software were modeled after related Lickert scale items from various instruments and designed to assess the impact of the digital inking practices on student attitudes toward the achievement of their learning objectives from the specific active learning activity. The two questionnaires were entitled *Digital Ink Technologies* and *Active Learning and Ubiquitous Presenter*.

Results

One question, number 9 of 10 on the *Digital Ink Technologies* questionnaire, contained Likert scale responses that were reversed in comparison to the other questions and statements on the questionnaire in order to establish reliability of the responses. The statement read, *I feel like the technology was forced; it was not a good fit for the activity.* 64.2% (34) of the students disagreed with the statement, 20.8% (11) somewhat disagreed, 5.7% (3) can't decide, 7.5% (4) somewhat agree, and 1.9% (1) agreed. This was the only question that displayed a reversed response rate from the respondents and thus corroborates that the students read each question and responded appropriately to each survey question.

Question three demonstrated that not all students in the study appreciated seeing their instructor's and peers' solution strategies for finding the area of a polygon on a Geoboard demonstrated in class on the SMART Board. The differences of means for the groups were not found to be significant with overall responses of 0% (0) disagree, 24.5% (13) somewhat disagree, 37.7% (20) can't decide, 24.5% (13) somewhat agree, and 13.2% (7) agree.

The only two questions that produced significant differences for the means of the control and experimental groups were questions six and seven on the *Digital Ink Technologies* questionnaire. The experimental group (M=3.79, SD=.50) significantly felt that the incorporation of the tablet PC into the activity helped them become a better communicator when compared to the control group (M=3.24, SD=1.01). A two-sample test of means assuming unequal variances shows that this difference was statistically significant at the 5% level (p=.020). The experimental group also thought that the tablet PC activity significantly enhanced, in comparison to the control, their learning of multiple algorithms and their understanding of multiple ways of finding area on a Geoboard (Experimental, M=4.07, SD=0.604; Control M=3.72,

SD=0.613, $t(1,52)=50.137, p=.041$). Summaries of the percentages and responses to the Likert scales for these two questions are displayed in Table 1.

It is also important for future studies to note the aspects of UP that the experimental group indicated as having a higher learning value. One question on the *Active Learning and Ubiquitous Presenter* questionnaire asked participants of the experimental group to rank order aspects of the UP environment. A little over half of the participants in this group rated the ability to view other students' work/submissions in-class in real-time during the activity as one of the most important aspects of UP, with the ability to view them outside of class coming in second. The rankings for the five aspects of UP are summarized in Table 2.

DISCUSSION

Interpreting the reversal of question nine on the *Digital Ink Technologies* questionnaire would mean that 85% of the students in either the control or the experimental group agreed or somewhat agreed that the use of technology was a good fit for the activity and that it did not seemed forced. Chidanandan and others (2007) were warned by their students that the tablet PCs felt forced into the curriculum. It is important to know, especially for replication purposes, that the sequencing and systematic use of the digital ink in this activity was well received by a majority of the students in both groups. This finding further substantiates the idea suggested by Bilen and others' (2008) about the importance of the task-technology fit. The incorporation of digital inking as a collaborative-interactive technique must take into account the fit of the task. If students do not see that the inking is benefitting them in the experience in any way, they are more apt to not fully engage themselves in the task.

Collaborative-interactive inking environments may be created with minimal frontloading work to a class. If the task-technology fit is appropriate for what is to be accomplished, the instructor can use a small amount of time to create a few slides to present the task to the students. For UP purposes, these two to four slides can be created in PPT and uploaded into the UP system. The flexibility of the UP system, and its ease of use from the student end, allows instructors to integrate this technology into their classrooms; UP does not have to be used on a daily basis. This software presentation system may be viewed as just another tool that

Table 1. Response rates to selected survey questions on the digital ink technologies questionnaire

		Percentage and Number of Students				
Item	**Group**	**not a result from its use (1)**	**a little (2)**	**can't decide (3)**	**a lot (4)**	**almost inevitable improvements (5)**
Q6. How much do you feel the incorporation of the tablet PC into the activity helped you become a better communicator?	Control	4% (1)	24% (6)	20% (5)	48% (12)	4% (1)
	Exp.	0% (0)	3.6% (1)	14.3%(4)	82.1% (23)	0% (0)
Item	Group	greatly impaired (1)	impaired (2)	can't decide (3)	enhanced (4)	greatly enhanced (5)
Q7. Did the tablet PC activity enhance your learning of multiple algorithms and your understanding of multiple ways of finding area on a Geoboard?	Control	0% (0)	4% (1)	24% (6)	68% (17)	4% (1)
	Exp.	0% (0)	0% (0)	14.3%(4)	64.3% (18)	21.4% (6)

Table 2. Response rates of the experimental group for the rank ordering of five aspects of the ubiquitous presenter (UP) environment with respect to their learning value

	Percentage and Number of Responses				
	1	**2**	**3**	**4**	**5**
• Ability to rate other students' submissions	0.0% (0)	4.8% (1)	9.5% (2)	38.1% (8)	**47.6% (10)**
• Ability to submit more than one response	13.0% (3)	**34.8% (8)**	13.0% (3)	30.4% (7)	8.7% (2)
• Ability to view other students' work/ submissions in-class in real-time during the activity	**54.5% (12)**	22.7% (5)	9.1% (2)	9.1% (2)	4.5% (1)
• Ability to view the in-class submissions and instructor ink outside of class	**33.3% (8)**	20.8% (5)	29.2% (7)	4.2% (1)	12.5% (3)
• Ability to follow (live) or not follow (manual) the instructor's slides	4.8% (1)	19.0% (4)	**38.1% (8)**	14.3% (3)	23.8% (5)

Note: Ranking were from most valuable (1) to least valuable (5).

can be used to enhance learning, and therefore, can be integrated when the tool-choice is appropriate. The question for technology integrationists to analyze then becomes, *How does the inking benefit the learner in the experience?*

The findings from Table 1, question 6, show that creating a collaborative-interactive inking environment in UP can make a difference in the belief that the experience helped students learn how to better communicate their ideas to peers and instructors. This question determined that the pedagogical technique for sharing student solution strategies in a UP environment was significantly better than a whole class discussion accomplished by swapping out the computer hooked up to the projector and/or using the Sympodium for *refining thinking processes*. UP does catalyze discussions simply because everyone participating can view in real-time others' thinking displayed on the submitted slides. Both instructors and students can view and select student submissions that they would like to discuss further. This UP environment can be set up for any well thought-out activity for which faculty would like some intense in-class interaction and discussion while still maintaining anonymity of responses. The UP environment also works well for interactive problem solving, and students appear more engaged in the learning objective as a result of the active learning happening within the activity.

With this understanding, a caveat to this technique of sharing ink-based solution strategies in UP might need to be considered based on the analysis of question three. It was found that not all students appreciated seeing their instructor's and peers' solution strategies demonstrated in class on the SMART Board. One possibility that might partially explain this result comes from DiStasi, Birmingham, and Welton's (2007, 2008) data showing visual learners are those that most appreciate this type of learning environment. It might also be partially explained by the possibility that the students' solution strategies that were analyzed and critiqued made their owners apprehensive of the display of their work. A milieu must be created by the instructor that helps students realize that the analysis of incorrect routes or solutions is beneficial for learning.

From a learning objective analysis, question seven shows that students also believed that the collaborative-interactive inking environment helped them learn multiple different ways to find the area of any polygon on a Geoboard. It showed the students in the UP group believed they were able to commit to memory more varied ways to solve the task at hand than those in the control group. This reinforces the power of sharing multiple approaches (i.e., various submission slides) whether in the mathematics classroom or if made available to the students via the Web interface outside of class time. It was important for students to review these submissions to help them make sense of their ideas.

Faculty in charge of leading the way with digital inking practices therefore should consider the fit of the task for digital inking and what the inking accomplishes for the learner. Regarding this study, it was shown that the inking practice was helpful in refining the thinking processes necessary for the mathematical task and for generating and recalling multiple alternative approaches, all of which are aligned directly to the goals of the research lesson.

FUTURE RESEARCH DIRECTIONS

Since this study has been conducted it has been refined by changing the timing of when the students perform the inking of their solution strategies and collaborative discussion. One suggestion if attempting replication of this inking technique is to have students submit their solution strategies at the end of one class or as homework with the discussion of their submitted work during the next class session. This allows the instructor more time to analyze the responses and plan how to use them more effectively. The students could also be encouraged to view the submissions through the Web interface outside of class in preparation for the next session's discussion.

Future research needs to continue to isolate possible best practices for using digital ink technologies and sound experimental studies need to be designed to test these newly developed pedagogical practices. Larger scale studies should replicate smaller studies like the one described in this chapter and include a series of significant tasks in the treatment. Promising data suggest visual learners are those who benefit most from shared writing experiences, so studies should be conducted to further investigate whose learning is impacted more in collaborative-interactive learning environments using digital ink.

Teacher educators must also make predictions as to what changes the future holds for digital ink and pen-based technologies. Such predictions are necessary from a teacher educator's perspective to help entrepreneurs see how their ideas can be better adapted for educational purposes. Software companies are quickly creating applications for new digital pens, such as *Microsoft's Magic Pen* or *IOGEAR's Mobile Digital Scribe.*

One example is how Adapx worked with digital pen and paper technology to produce its first product, *Capurx*, built for *OneNote*. Field notes can now be captured on regular paper printed with a certain dot pattern and stored in the pen and uploaded to a PC into *Microsoft Office OneNote 2007*. This could easily be adapted for capturing student work in a classroom.

Another possibility is having students perform their in-class work under some kind of document camera centered above a table which could isolate an individual's work through recognition and capture of notebooks for display. It may not be long before future mathematics students may simply purchase a special pen, pencil, or paper for math class that would enable their handwritten notes to be integrated into the presentation. Or, perhaps all of the necessary technology exists within the classroom environment that allows for sharing of student notes on regular paper in the classroom presentation. Regardless, suggestions for educational applications must be made by current users of the technology, removing the constraints that are not feasible within a classroom and adding additional features that serve educational purposes. Educators should seek to directly impact the directions taken and options provided by cutting edge companies.

CONCLUSION

Studies of positive effects of digital ink technologies in the teaching and learning of mathematics (Reba, 2007; Reba & Pargas, 2008; Mitchell, 2007) and mathematics pedagogy (Koshelva, Rusch, & Ioudina, 2007) have already been established at the collegiate level. The next step is to isolate the inking practices that have been and are making a significant difference in the integration of tablet PCs. More research on effective pedagogical practices needs to be conducted since tablet PCs and one-to-one computing are rapidly making their way into high school classrooms. Teacher leaders and technology integrationists can take best practices and the classification levels described in this chapter to their K-12 colleagues in any discipline and help them create more effective learning environments with digital ink. They can also help them analyze the task-technology fit and identify appropriate opportunities for its use.

Unless we desire to see this tool phased in and out of education due to poor professional development, studies must be designed to establish best practices for the use of digital ink technology in the mathematics classroom. Teacher educators and technology integrationists must become aware of these researched best practices, use them, and teach them to preservice candidates. As Stigler (2000) reported, "The key to long-term improvement [in teaching] is to figure out how to generate, accumulate, and share professional knowledge" (p. 23).

REFERENCES

Andersen, M. (2008). How tablets enhance the math. *Teaching College Math.* Retrieved June 30, 2009, from http://teachingcollegemath.com/?p=421

Berque, D., Byers, C., & Myers, A. (2008). Turning the classroom upside down using tablet PCs and DyKnow ink and audio tools. In Reed, R., Berque, D., & Prey, J. C. (Eds.), *The Impact of Tablet PCs and Pen-based Technology on Education: Evidence and Outcomes* (pp. 3–9). West Lafayette, IN: Purdue University Press.

Bilen, S. G., Lee, D., Messner, J. I., Nguyen, H. T., Simpson, T. W., Techatassanasoontorn, A. A., & Devon, R. F. (2008). Tablet PC use and impact on learning in technology and engineering classrooms: A preliminary study. In Reed, R., Berque, D., & Prey, J. C. (Eds.), *The Impact of Tablet PCs and Pen-based Technology on Education: Evidence and Outcomes* (pp. 11–19). West Lafayette, IN: Purdue University Press.

Cantu, P., Phillips, J., & Tholfsen, M. (2008). Three is not a crowd: The pedagogical power of tablet PCs, digital organizers, and digital textbooks in middle school mathematics. In Reed, R., Berque, D., & Prey, J. C. (Eds.), *The Impact of Tablet PCs and Pen-based Technology on Education: Evidence and Outcomes* (pp. 21–29). West Lafayette, IN: Purdue University Press.

Center for Digital Education. (2004). One-to-one laptop initiatives: Providing tools for 21st century learners. Folsom, CA: eRepublic, Inc.

Chidanandan, A., DeVasher, R., Ferro, P., Fisher, D., Mitra-Kirtley, S., & Merkle, L. D. (2007). Evaluating the symbiosis of DyKnow software and pen-based computing in the Rose-Hulman classroom. In Reed, R., Berque, D., & Prey, J. C. (Eds.), *The Impact of Tablet PCs and Pen-based Technology on Education: Evidence and Outcomes* (pp. 21–31). West Lafayette, IN: Purdue University Press.

Cramer, M., Beauregard, R., & Sharma, M. (2009). An investigation of purpose built netbooks for primary school education. In *Proceedings of the 8th International Conference on Interaction Design and Children* (pp. 36-43). Como, Italy: Association for Computing Machinery.

Davis, K. M., Kelly, M., Malani, R., Griswold, W. G., & Simon, B. (2007). Preliminary evaluation of NoteBlogger: Public note taking in the classroom. In Prey, J. C., Reed, R. H., & Berque, D. A. (Eds.), *The Impact of Tablet PCs and Pen-based Technology on Education: Beyond the Tipping Point* (pp. 33–42). West Lafayette, IN: Purdue University Press.

DeBell, M., & Chapman, C. (2006). *Computer and Internet use by students in 2003. (Issue Brief No. 065)*. Washington, DC: National Center for Education Statistics.

Dicken, C. (2008). The 30-day challenge: Digital homework in a high school mathematics classroom. In Reed, R., Berque, D., & Prey, J. C. (Eds.), *The Impact of Tablet PCs and Pen-based Technology on Education: Evidence and Outcomes* (pp. 31–37). West Lafayette, IN: Purdue University Press.

DiStasi, V. F., Birmingham, W. P., & Welton, G. L. (2008). Evaluating learning software in the classroom: A continuing study. In Reed, R., Berque, D., & Prey, J. C. (Eds.), *The Impact of Tablet PCs and Pen-based Technology on Education: Evidence and Outcomes* (pp. 39–45). West Lafayette, IN: Purdue University Press.

Fischman, J. (2007). Talking back to teacher. *The Chronicle of Higher Education, 53*(48), A.27.

Glub, E. (2004, March). *Handwritten slides on a tablet PC in a discrete mathematics course*. Paper presented at the 35th SIGCSE technical symposium on Computer Science Education, Norfolk, VA.

Kamin, S. N., Capitanu, B., Twidale, M., & Peiper, C. (2008). A "teacher's dashboard" for a high school algebra class. In Reed, R., Berque, D., & Prey, J. C. (Eds.), *The Impact of Tablet PCs and Pen-based Technology on Education: Evidence and Outcomes* (pp. 63–71). West Lafayette, IN: Purdue University Press.

Kosheleva, O., Medina-Rusch, A., & Ioudina, V. (2007). Pre-service teacher training in mathematics using tablet PC technology. *Informatics in Education, 6*(2), 321–334.

Metiri Group. (2006). *1:1 Learning: A review and analysis by the Metiri group*. Retrieved June 30, 2009, from http://www.k12blueprint.com/k12/blueprint/story_11_learning_a_review.php

Milner, J. (2006). Tablet PCs: The write approach. *T.H.E. Journal, 33*(9), 20–26.

Mitchell, R. S. (2007, May). PC Tablet Project. *Reprint of the Proceedings of the 1st International Workshop on Pen-Based Learning Technologies, Enabling Advanced Graphical, Multimodal and Mobile Learning Interactions (PLT 2007),* Aula Magna, Universita' degli Studi di Catania, Catania, Italy.

National Research Council. (2000). *Principles and standards for school mathematics*. Reston, VA: National Council of Teachers of Mathematics.

Olivier, W. (2005). Teaching mathematics: Tablet PC technology add a new dimension. In *Proceedings of the Mathematics Education into the 21st Century Project Eighth International Conference, Reform, Revolution and Paradigm Shifts in Mathematics Education* (pp. 176-181). Johor Bahru, Malaysia: Univeriti Teknologi Malaysia.

Orlando, D. (2008). *Advantages of tablets over laptops.* Retrieved June 30, 2009, from http://schoolcomputing.wikia.com/wiki/Advantages_of_Tablets_Over_Laptops

Price, E., & Simon, B. (2007). Instructor inking in physics classes with Ubiquitous Presenter. In Prey, J. C., Reed, R. H., & Berque, D. A. (Eds.), *The Impact of Tablet PCs and Pen-based Technology on Education: Beyond the Tipping Point* (pp. 107–117). West Lafayette, IN: Purdue University Press.

Reba, M. (2007). Tablet PCs and web-based interaction in the mathematics classroom. *The Mathematics Education into the 21st Century Project, Programme of the Ninth International Conference Mathematics Education in a Global Community* (pp. 549-554). Charlotte, NC: The University of North Carolina.

Reba, M., & Pargas, R. (2008, May). Using tablet PCs as interactive web-based instruction tools in freshman calculus [Monograph]. In *Second International Workshop on the Impact of Pen-Based Technology on Education, PLT 2008* (pp. 1-6).

Reba, M., & Weaver, B. (2007, May). Tablet PC-enabled active learning in mathematics: A first study. In *The Impact of Tablet PCs and Pen-based Technology on Education, 2007* (pp. 1–6). Beyond the Tipping Point.

Reins, K. J. (2007). Digital tablet PCs as new technologies of writing and learning: A survey of perceptions of digital ink technology. *Contemporary Issues in Technology & Teacher Education, 7*(3), 158–177.

Stigler, J. (1999, September). *Briefing for the National Commission on Mathematics and Science Teaching for the 21st Century*. Washington, DC.

Technology & Learning. (2007). *K-12 Computing Blueprint: Leadership.* Retrieved June 30, 2009, from http://www.k12blueprint.com/k12/blueprint/leadership.php?menu=leadership

Tront, J. G., & Scales, G. R. (2007). Keynote address implementing a large-scale tablet PC deployment. In Prey, J. C., Reed, R. H., & Berque, D. A. (Eds.), *The Impact of Tablet PCs and Pen-based Technology on Education: Beyond the Tipping Point* (pp. 1–10). West Lafayette, IN: Purdue University Press.

SOFTWARE REFERENCES

Classroom Learning Partner (CLP) Web site. http://projects.csail.mit.edu/clp/software/ (accessed June, 2009).

Classroom Presenter (CP) Web site. http://classroompresenter.cs.washington.edu (accessed June, 2009).

DyKnow Web site. http://www.dyknow.com (accessed June, 2009).

Tablet Mylar Slides (TMS) Web site. http://www.cs.umd.edu/~egolub/TabletMylarSlides (accessed June, 2009).

Ubiquitous Presenter (UP) Web site. http://up.ucsd.edu (accessed June, 2009).

WriteOn Web site. http://filebox.ece.vt.edu/~jgtront/tabletpc/writeon.html (accessed June, 2009).

Compilation of References

Abell, S., Bryan, L., & Anderson, M. (1998). Investigating preservice elementary science teacher reflective thinking using integrated media case-based instruction in elementary science teacher preparation. *Science Education*, *6*(4), 491–510. doi:10.1002/(SICI)1098-237X(199807)82:4<491::AID-SCE5>3.0.CO;2-6

Abraham, L. M. (2002). What do high school science students gain from field-based research apprenticeship programs? *Clearing House (Menasha, Wis.)*, *75*(5), 229–232. doi:10.1080/00098650209603945

Adler, J., Ball, D., Krainer, K., Fou-Lai, L., & Novotna, J. (2005). Reflections on an emerging field: Researching mathematics teacher education. *Educational Studies in Mathematics*, *60*, 359–381. doi:10.1007/s10649-005-5072-6

Akengin, H. (2008). Opinions of prospective social studies teachers on the use of information technologies in teaching geographic subjects. *Journal of Instructional Psychology*, *35*(2), 127–139.

Albee, J. J. (2003). A study of preserivce elementary teachers' technology skill preparedness and examples of how it can be increased. *Journal of Technology and Teacher Education*, *11*, 53–71.

Albion, P. R. (2008). Web 2.0 in teacher education: Two imperatives for action [Electronic version]. *Computers in the Schools*, *25*, 181–198. doi:10.1080/07380560802368173

Alias, N. A., & Alias, N. A. (2009). Improving the affective learning outcomes of trainees in teacher education: An immersive approach. In Nygaard, C., & Holtham, C. (Eds.), *Improving Students Learning Outcomes in Higher Education*. Copenhagen: Copenhagen Business School Press.

Ally, M. (2004). Foundations of educational theory for online learning. In Anderson, T., & Elloumi, F. (Eds.), *Theory and practice of online learning* (pp. 3–31). Athabasca, Alberta, Canada: Athabasca University.

Al-Sharaf, A. (2006). New perspectives on teacher education in Kuwait. *Journal of Education for Teaching*, *31*(1), 105–109. doi:10.1080/02607470500511108

Altun, T. (2007). Information and communications technology (ICT) in initial teacher education: What can Turkey learn from range of international perspectives? *Journal of Turkish Science Education*, *4*(2), 45–60.

Alvarez, J. (1995). *In the time of the butterflies*. New York: Plume.

American Association of Colleges for Teacher Education. (2008). *Handbook of technological pedagogical content knowledge (TPCK) for educators*. New York: Routledge for the American Association of Colleges for Teacher Education.

Andersen, M. (2008). How tablets enhance the math. *Teaching College Math*. Retrieved June 30, 2009, from http://teachingcollegemath.com/?p=421

Anderson, D. (2007). The role of cooperating teachers' power in student teaching. *Education*, *128*(2), 307–323.

Anderson, J. (2005). *School bullying, a review of the research*. Crime prevention and criminal Justice policy, [CRIM 420], Amber MacDonald, Spring 2005

Copyright © 2010, IGI Global, distributing in print or electronic forms without written permission of IGI Global is prohibited.

Anderson, J. B., Swick, K., & Yff, J. (2001). *Service learning in teacher education: Enhancing the growth of new teachers, their students, and communities.* Washington, DC: American Association of College for Teacher Education.

Andriessen, J. (2002). Arguing to learn. In Sawyer, R. K. (Ed.), *Cambridge handbook of learning science* (pp. 443–444). Cambridge, UK: Cambridge University Press.

Andriessen, J., Baker, M., & Suthers, D. (2003). Argumentation, computer support, and the educational context of confronting cognitions. In Andriessen, J., Baker, M., & Suthers, D. (Eds.), *Arguing to learn. Confronting cognitions in computer supported collaborative learning environments* (pp. 3–25). Dordrecht, The Netherlands: Kluwer.

Angeli, C. (2005). Transforming a teacher education method course through technology: Effects on preservice teachers' technology competency. *Computers & Education, 45*, 383–398. doi:10.1016/j.compedu.2004.06.002

Angeli, C., & Valanides, N. (2009). Epistemological and mythological issues for the conceptualization, development, and assessment of ICT-TPCK: Advances in technological pedagogical content knowledge (TPCK). *Computers & Education, 52*, 154–168. doi:10.1016/j.compedu.2008.07.006

Angeli, C., Valanides, N., & Bonk, C. J. (2003). Communication in a web-based conferencing system: The quality of computer-mediated interactions. *British Journal of Educational Technology, 34*(1), 31–43. doi:10.1111/1467-8535.00302

Angelova, M. (2001, December 22). Impact of service learning on the cognitive and affective development of pre-service teachers. *The Free Library*. Retrieved April 7, 2009, from http://www.thefreelibrary.com/Academic+Exchange+Quarterly/2001/December/22-p568

Anthony, R., & Coghill-Behrends, W. (2009). Teachers of the future: Report on a national survey. In C. Crawford et al. (Eds.), *Proceedings of Society for Information Technology and Teacher Education International Conference 2009* (pp. 1696-1697). Chesapeake, VA: AACE.

Antonijevic, R. (2007). *Usage of computers and calculators and students' achievement: Results from TIMSS 2003.* Paper presented at the International Conference on Informatics, Educational Technology and New Media in Education. ERIC Document Reproduction Services ED497737.

Antstey, M., & Bull, G. (2006). *Teaching and learning multiliteracies: Changing times, changing literacies.* Kensington Gardens, Australia: International Reading Association and Australian Literacy Educator's Association.

Archambault, L., & Oh-Young, C. (2009). Putting the T in PCK: exploring the nature of the TPCK framework among K-12 online educators. In C. Crawford et al. (Eds.), *Proceedings of Society for Information Technology and Teacher Education International Conference 2009* (pp. 4008-4014). Chesapeake, VA: AACE.

Artigue, M. (2010). The future of teaching and learning mathematics with digital technologies. In Hoyles, C., & Lagrange, J. (Eds.), *Mathematics education and technology-rethinking the terrain. The 17th ICMI Study* (pp. 463–476). New York: Springer.

Assaf, L. (2005). Staying connected: Student teachers' perceptions of computer-mediated discussions. *Teacher Educator, 40*(4), 221–237. doi:10.1080/08878730509555363

Association for the Advancement of Computing in Education (AACE). 2003). *A study of preservice elementary teachers' technology skill preparedness and examples of how it can be increased.*

Association of Mathematics Teacher Educator (2009). *Mathematics TPACK Framework.*

Association of Mathematics Teacher Educators. (2006). *Preparing teachers to use technology to enhance the learning of mathematics: A position statement of the Association of Mathematics Teacher Educators.* Retrieved June 14, 2008, from http://www.amte.net

Atkinson, R. (2006). Podcasting: do they really need to know? *HERDSA News, 28*(2), 20–22.

Attwell, G. (2007). *Web 2.0 and the changing ways we are using computers for learning: What are the implications for pedagogy and curriculum?* Retrieved February 20, 2009, from http://www.elearningeuropa.info/files/media/media13018.pdf

Austin, D. S. (2004). New literacies: Are Colorado teacher education programs preparing pre-service teachers to use technology in their learning environments? *Dissertation Abstracts International, 65*(07), 2570. (AAT 3138978).

Australian Association of Mathematics Teachers. (2002). *Standards for Excellence in Teaching Mathematics in Australian Schools.* Retrieved on February 19, 2009 from http://www.aamt.edu.au/Standards

Ba, H., Admon, N., & Anderson, L. (2002). *A quantitative investigation of teachers and the JASON Multimedia Science Curriculum: Reported use and impact: Year Two Evaluation Report.* New York: Center of Children and Technology, Education Development Center.

Ba, H., Martin, W., & Diaz, O. (2001). *The JASON Project's Multimedia Science Curriculum Impact on Student Learning: Final Evaluation Report Year One.* New York: Center of Children and Technology, Education Development Center.

Babinski, L. M., Jones, B. D., & DeWert, M. H. (2001). The roles of facilitators and peers in an online support community for first-year teachers. *Journal of Educational & Psychological Consultation, 12*(2), 151–169. doi:10.1207/S1532768XJEPC1202_05

Baggott LaVelle, L., McFarlane, A., & Brawn, R. (2003). Knowledge transformation through ICT in science education: A case study in teacher-driven curriculum development - case study 1. *British Journal of Educational Technology, 32*(2), 183–189. doi:10.1111/1467-8535.00319

Bailey, F. (1996). The role of collaborative dialogue in teacher education. In Freeman, D., & Richards, J. C. (Eds.), *Teacher Learning in Language Teaching* (pp. 260–280). Cambridge, UK: Cambridge University Press.

Baker, D. (1998). Equity issues in science education. In Fraser, B., & Tobin, K. (Eds.), *International handbook of science education* (pp. 869–895). Dordrecht, Netherlands: Kluwer Academic.

Baldwin, S. C., Buchanan, A., & Rudisill, M. (2007). What teacher candidates learned about diversity, social justice, and themselves from service learning experiences. *Journal of Teacher Education, 58*(4), 315–327.. doi:10.1177/0022487107305259

Banister, S., & Vannatta, R. (2006). Beginning with a baseline: Insuring productive technology integration in teacher education. *Journal of Technology and Teacher Education, 14*(1), 209–235.

Bannasch, S. (1999). The electronic curator: Using a hand-held computer at the Exploratorium. *Concord Consortium Newsletter.* Retrieved August 10, 2003 from http://www.concord.org/library/1999fall/electronic-curator.html

Bansavich, J. C. (2005). Factors influencing preservice teachers' readiness to integrate technology into their instruction. *Dissertation Abstracts International, 66*(03), 966. (AAT 3169712).

Barab, S., Barnett, M., & Squire, K. (2002). Developing an empirical account of a community of practice: Characterizing the essential tensions. *Journal of the Learning Sciences, 11*(4), 489–542. doi:10.1207/S15327809JLS1104_3

Barab, S., MaKinster, J., & Scheckler, R. (2003). Designing system dualities: Characterizing a web-supported professional development community. *The Information Society, 19*(1), 237–256. doi:10.1080/01972240309466

Barnett, M. (2006). Using a web-based professional development system to support preservice teachers in Examining Authentic Classroom Practice. *Journal of Technology and Teacher Education, 14*(4), 701–729.

Barnett, M. (2008). Using authentic cases through the use of a web-based professional development system to support preservice teachers in examining classroom practice. *The entity from which ERIC acquires the content, including journal, organization, and conference names, or by means of online submission from the author. Action in Teacher Education, 29*(4), 3–14.

Baron, G. L., & Bruillard, E. (2007). ICT, educational technology and educational instruments. Will what has worked work again elsewhere in the future? *Education and Information Technologies*, *12*, 71–81. doi:10.1007/s10639-007-9033-9

Barton, R. (2004). Why use computers in practical science? In Barton, R. (Ed.), *Teaching secondary science with ICT* (pp. 27–39). Maidenhead, UK: Open University Press.

Bates, A. (2008). Learning to design WebQuests: An exploration in preservice social studies education. *Journal of Social Studies Research*, *32*(1), 10–21.

Bates, A. W. (2000). *Managing Technological Change*. San Francisco: Jossey-Bass.

Bates, R., & Khasawneh, S. (2007). Self-efficacy and college students' perceptions and use of online learning systems. *Computers in Human Behavior*, *23*, 175–191. doi:10.1016/j.chb.2004.04.004

Battey, D., Kafai, Y., & Franke, M. (2005). Evaluation of mathematical inquiry in commercial rational number software. In Vrasidas, C., & Glass, G. (Eds.), *Preparing teachers to teach with technology* (pp. 241–256). Greenwich, CT: Information Age Publishing.

Bauman, V. (2008, January 29). N.Y. legislation targets Internet predators. *MSNBC*. Retrieved March 29, 2009, from http://www.msnbc.msn.com/id/22903731/

Bazler, J. A., Spokane, A. R., Ballard, R., & Fugate, M. S. (1993). The Jason Project Experience and Attitudes Toward Science as an Enterprise and Career. *Journal of Career Development*, *20*(2), 101–112.

Becker, H. J. (2000). Who's wired and who's not: Children's access to and use of computer technology. *The Future of Children: Children and Computer Technology*, *10*, 44–75. doi:10.2307/1602689

BECTA. (2005). The BECTA review: Evidence on the progress of ICT in education. *ICT in Schools Research and Evaluation Series*. Retrieved September, 2005, from http://www.becta.org.uk/page_documents/research/becta_review_feb05.pdf

Bednar, A., & Charles, M. (1999). A constructivist approach for introducing pre-service teachers to educational technology: Online and classroom education. In J. Price et al. (Eds.), *Proceedings of Society for Information Technology and Teacher Education International Conference 1999* (pp. 1796-1801). Chesapeake, VA: AACE

Beijaard, D., Meijer, P. C., & Verloop, N. (2004). Reconsidering research on teachers' professional identity. *Teaching and Teacher Education*, *20*, 107–128. doi:10.1016/j.tate.2003.07.001

Bell, A. (2009). *A+ Rubric*. Retrieved February 16, 2009, from http://www.uwstout.edu/soe/profdev/podcastrubric.html

Benedict, R. (1934). *Patterns of culture*. Boston: Houghton Mifflin Company.

Benson, A., Lewler, C., & Whitworth, A. (2008). Rules, roles, and tools: Activity theory and the comparative study of e-learning. *British Journal of Educational Technology*, *39*(3), 456–467. doi:10.1111/j.1467-8535.2008.00838.x

Bereiter, C. (2005). Design research: The way forward. *Education Canada*, *46*(1), 16–19.

Berge, Z. L. (1995). The role of the online instructor/facilitator in facilitating computer conferencing: Recommendations from the field. *Educational Technology*, *35*(1), 22–30.

Berger, H., Eylon, B., & Bagno, E. (2008). Professional Development of Physics Teachers in an Evidence-Based Blended Learning Program. *Journal of Science Education and Technology*, *17*(4), 399–409. doi:10.1007/s10956-008-9109-3

Berque, D., Byers, C., & Myers, A. (2008). Turning the classroom upside down using tablet PCs and DyKnow ink and audio tools. In Reed, R., Berque, D., & Prey, J. C. (Eds.), *The Impact of Tablet PCs and Pen-based Technology on Education: Evidence and Outcomes* (pp. 3–9). West Lafayette, IN: Purdue University Press.

Berson, M. J. (2004). Digital images: Capturing America's past with the technology of today. *Social Education*, *68*(3), 214–219.

Betrus, A. K., & Molenda, M. (2002). Historical evolution of instructional technology in teacher education programs. *TechTrends*, *46*(5), 18–21. doi:10.1007/BF02818303

Bewick, V., Cheek, L., & Ball, J. (2004). Statistics review 8: Qualitative data–tests of association. *Critical Care (London, England)*, *8*(1), 46–53. doi:10.1186/cc2428

Bielaczyc, K., & Collins, A. (1999). Learning communities in classrooms: A reconceptualization of educational practice. In Reigeluth, C. M. (Ed.), *Instructional-design theories and models: A new paradigm of instructional theory* (2nd ed., pp. 269–292). Mahwah, NJ: Lawrence Erlbaum Associates.

Biesenbach-Lucas, S. (2003). Asynchronous discussion groups in teacher training classes: Perceptions of native and non-native students. *Journal of Asynchronous Learning Networks*, *7*(3), 24–33.

Biesenbach-Lucas, S. (2004). Asynchronous web discussions in teacher training courses: Promoting collaborative learning - or not? *AACE Journal*, *12*(2), 155–170.

Biggs, J. (2003). *Teaching for Quality Learning at University – what the Student Does.* Buckingham, UK: The Society for Research into Higher Education and Open University Press.

Bigum, C., & Rowan, L. (2008). Landscaping on shifting ground: Teacher education in a digitally transforming world. *Asia-Pacific Journal of Teacher Education*, *36*(3), 245–255. doi:10.1080/13598660802232787

Bilen, S. G., Lee, D., Messner, J. I., Nguyen, H. T., Simpson, T. W., Techatassanasoontorn, A. A., & Devon, R. F. (2008). Tablet PC use and impact on learning in technology and engineering classrooms: A preliminary study. In Reed, R., Berque, D., & Prey, J. C. (Eds.), *The Impact of Tablet PCs and Pen-based Technology on Education: Evidence and Outcomes* (pp. 11–19). West Lafayette, IN: Purdue University Press.

Blackwell, P., Applegate, J., Earley, P., & Tarule, J. (2000). *Education reform and teacher education: the missing discourse of gender.* Washington, DC: American Association of Colleges for Teacher Education.

Bland, M. (1988). *An introduction to medical statistics.* Oxford, UK: Oxford University press.

Blatchford, P., Kutnick, P., Baires, E., & Galton, M. (2003). Toward a social pedagogy of classroom group work. *International Journal of Educational Research*, *39*(1–2), 153–172. doi:10.1016/S0883-0355(03)00078-8

Bleed, R. (2006, January). The IT leader as alchemist: Finding the true gold. *EDUCAUSE Review*, 33–42.

Boal, A. (1992). *Games for actors and non-actors* (Jackson, A., Trans.). London: Routledge.

Bogdan, R., & Biklen, S. K. (1992). *Qualitative research for education: An introduction to theory and methods.* Boston: Allyn and Bacon.

Boger, C., & Boger, D. (2000). Preservice teachers' explanations of their teaching behavior. *Journal of Instructional Psychology*, *27*(4), 217–223.

Bolick, C. M., Berson, M. J., Friedman, A. M., & Porfeli, E. J. (2007). Diffusion of technology innovation in the preservice social studies experience: Results of a national survey. *Theory and Research in Social Education*, *35*(2), 174–195.

Bolin, A., Khramtsova, I., & Saarnio, D. (2005). Using student journals to stimulate authentic learning: Balancing Bloom's cognitive and affective domains. *Teaching of Psychology*, *32*(3), 154–159. doi:10.1207/s15328023top3203_3

Bomar, L. (2006). iPods as Reading Tools. *Principal*, *85*(5), 52–53.

Bonk, C. J., & Graham, C. R. (Eds.). (2006). *Handbook of blended learning: Global perspectives, local designs.* San Francisco, CA: Pfeiffer Publishing.

Borgen, W., & Hiebert, B. (2006). Career guidance and counseling for youth: What adolescents and young adults are telling us? *International Journal for the Advancement of Counseling*, *28*(4), 389–400. doi:10.1007/s10447-006-9022-5

Borko, H. (2004). Professional Development and Teacher Learning: Mapping the Terrain. *Educational Researcher*, *33*(8), 3–15. doi:10.3102/0013189X033008003

Borko, H., & Putnam, R. T. (1995). Expanding a Teacher's Knowledge Base. In Guskey, T. R., & Huberman, M. (Eds.), *Professional development in education* (pp. 35–65). New York: Teachers College Press.

Borko, H., & Putnam, R. T. (1996). Learning to teach. In Berliner, D. C., & Calfee, R. C. (Eds.), *Handbook of educational psychology* (pp. 673–708). New York: Macmillan.

Borsheim, C., Merritt, K., & Reed, D. (2008). Beyond technology for technology's sake: advancing multiliteracies in the twenty-first century. *Clearing House (Menasha, Wis.)*, *82*(2), 55–59. doi:10.3200/TCHS.82.2.87-90

Bower, M., Woo, K., Roberts, M., & Watters, P. (2006). *Wiki Pedagogy – A Tale of Two Wikis*. Paper presented at the 7th conference on Information Technology based Higher Education and Training, Sydney, Australia.

Boyd, D., & Ellison, N. (2007). Social Network Sites: Definition, History, and Scholarship. *Journal of Computer-Mediated Communication, 13*(1). Retrieved February 22, 2009, from http://jcmc.indiana.edu/vol13/issue1/boyd.ellison.html

Brandon, P. R., Taum, A. K. H., Ayala, C. C., Young, D. B., Gray, M. E., Speitel, T. T., et al. (2007). *Phase I study of fast implementation, outcomes, and scaling up: Final report*. Retrieved June 2007, from http://www.hawaii.edu/crdg/programs/pre/scup.html

Bransford, J. D., & Schwartz, D. L. (1999). Rethinking transfer: A simple proposal with multiple implications. In Iran-Nejad, A., & Pearson, P. D. (Eds.), *Review of research in education* (pp. 61–100). Washington, DC: American Educational Research Association.

Bransford, J., Brown, A., & Cocking, R. (2000). *How People Learn: Brain, Mind, and Experience & school*. Washington, DC: National Academy Press.

Bransford, J., Darling-Hammond, L., & LePage, P. (2005). Introduction. In Bransford, J., & Darling-Hammond, L. (Eds.), *Preparing teachers for a changing world* (pp. 1–39). San Francisco: Jossey Bass.

Braun, J., & Risinger, F. (1999). *Surfing social studies*. Washington, DC: National Council for the Social Studies.

Brent, D. (2005). Teaching performance in the electronic classroom. *First Monday*, *10*(4).

Brickhouse, N. (1990). Teachers' beliefs about the nature of science and their relationship to classroom practice. *Journal of Teacher Education*, *41*, 52–62. doi:10.1177/002248719004100307

Brigden, D. (2004). Becoming a reflective practitioner. *The Newsletter of Itsn-0*. Retrieved March 29, 2009, from http://www.medev.ac.uk/newsletter/01.6.html

Brinkerhoff, J. (2006). Effects of a long-duration, professional development academy on technology skills, computer self-efficacy, and technology integration beliefs and practices. *Journal of Research on Technology in Education*, *39*(1), 22–43.

Brintnall, S. K. (2002). *E-mentoring: A case study of the viability and benefits of electronic mentoring with beginning teachers in rural schools*. Unpublished dissertation, University of Oklahoma, Norman. (AAT 3040838).

Britten, J., & Clausen, J. (2009). Using what they bring with them. In C. Crawford et al. (Eds.), *Proceedings of Society for Information Technology and Teacher Education International Conference 2009* (pp. 1744-1747). Chesapeake, VA: AACE.

Britten, J., Estridge, M., Volmer, K., & Clausen, J. (2009). The digital natives are speaking. In C. Crawford et al. (Eds.), *Proceedings of Society for Information Technology and Teacher Education International Conference 2009* (pp. 1741-1743). Chesapeake, VA: AACE.

Brookfield, S. (1995). Adult learning: An overview. In Tuinjman, A. (Ed.), *International Encyclopedia of Education* (pp. 265–269). Oxford, UK: Pergamon Press.

Brown, S., Boyer, M., Mayall, H., Johnson, P., Ming, L., & Butler, M. (2003). The GlobalEd Project: Gender differences in a problem-based learning environment of international negotiations. *Instructional Science*, *31*(4–5), 255–276. doi:10.1023/A:1024677708501

Brunner, C. (2003 April). Approaching technology. *Women's Educational Equity Act Resource Center Digest*, 1-16. Retrieved November 7, 2007, from http://www.edc.org/WomensEquity

Brush, T., & Appelman, R. (2003). Transforming the Pre-service Teacher Education Technology Curriculum at Indiana University: An Integrative Approach. In C. Crawford et al. (Eds.), *Proceedings of Society for Information Technology and Teacher Education International Conference 2003* (pp. 1613-1619). Chesapeake, VA: AACE

Brush, T., & Saye, J. W. (2009). Strategies for preparing preservice social studies teachers to integrate technology effectively: Models and practices. *Contemporary Issues in Technology and Teacher Education, 9*(1). Retrieved July 7, 2009, from http://www.citejournal.org/vol9/iss1/socialstudies/article1.cfm

Brush, T., Glazewski, K., Rutowski, K., Berg, K., Stromfors, C., & Hernandez Van-Nest, M. (2003). Integrating technology in a field based teacher training program: The PT3@ASU Project. *ETR&D, 51*(1), 57–72. doi:10.1007/BF02504518

Bulbeck, C. (1997). *Reorienting western feminisms*. Cambridge, UK: Cambridge University Press. doi:10.1017/CBO9780511552151

Bulger, S. (2006). A web-enhanced approach to undergraduate internship supervision. *Physical Educator, 63*(3), 114–125.

Bullen, A. (2008). The 'long tale': Using Web 2.0 concepts to enhance digital collections. *Computers in Libraries*, 31–35.

Burns, M. (2005). Tools for the mind. *Educational Leadership, 63*(4), 48–53.

Butterfield, L. (2005). Cybersafety: an intrinsic part of the online experience. In Lai, K.-W. (Ed.), *E-learning communities: teaching and learning with the Web* (pp. 179–197). Dunedin, New Zealand: University of Otago Press.

Campbell, A. P. (2004). Using LiveJournal for Authentic Communication in EFL Classes. *The Internet TESL Journal, 10*(9). Retrieved February 22, 2009, from http://iteslj.org/Techniques/Campbell-LiveJournal/

Campbell, G. (2005). There's something in the air: podcasting in education. *EDUCAUSE Review, 40*(6), 32–47.

Canadian Teacher's Federation. (2003). *Kids take on media: Summary of finding*. Retrieved January 15, 2007, from www.ctf-ee.ca/en/projects/MERP/summaryfindingd.pdf

Cantu, P., Phillips, J., & Tholfsen, M. (2008). Three is not a crowd: The pedagogical power of tablet PCs, digital organizers, and digital textbooks in middle school mathematics. In Reed, R., Berque, D., & Prey, J. C. (Eds.), *The Impact of Tablet PCs and Pen-based Technology on Education: Evidence and Outcomes* (pp. 21–29). West Lafayette, IN: Purdue University Press.

Capobianco, B. M. (2007). A self-study of the role of technology in promoting reflection and inquiry-based science teaching. *Journal of Science Teacher Education, 18*(2), 271–296. doi:10.1007/s10972-007-9041-z

Capobianco, B. M., & Lehman, J. D. (2006). Integrating technology to foster inquiry in an elementary science methods course: An action research study of one teacher educator's initiatives in a PT3 project. *Journal of Computers in Mathematics and Science Teaching, 25*(2), 123–146.

Capobianco, B. M., Horowitz, R., Canuel-Browne, D., & Trimarchi, R. (2004). Action research for teachers: Understanding the steps for developing and implementing productive action plans. *Science Teacher (Normal, Ill.), 71*(3), 48–53.

Carlson, M. P., & Bloom, I. (2005). The cyclic nature of problem solving: An emergent multidimensional problem-solving framework. *Educational Studies in Mathematics, 58*, 45–75. doi:10.1007/s10649-005-0808-x

Carr, W., & Kemmis, S. (1986). *Becoming critical: Education, knowledge, and action research*. London: Falmer Press.

Carroll, T. (2005). Forward. In Rhine, S., & Bailey, M. (Eds.), *Integrated technologies, innovative learning: Lessons from the PT3 program*. Eugene, OR: International Society for Technology in Education.

Carter, K. (1990). Teachers' knowledge and learning to teach. In Houston, W. R., Huberman, M., & Sikula, J. (Eds.), *Handbook of research on teacher education* (pp. 291–310). New York: MacMillan.

Cashion, J., & Palmieri, P. (2002). *The secret is the teacher. The learner's view of online learning. Australian National Training Authority*. Adelaide, South Australia: NCVER.

Center for Digital Education. (2004). One-to-one laptop initiatives: Providing tools for 21st century learners. Folsom, CA: eRepublic, Inc.

Chamblee, G. E., Slough, S. W., & Wunsch, G. (2008). Measuring high school mathematics teachers' concerns about graphing calculators and change: A yearlong study. *Journal of Computers in Mathematics and Science Teaching, 27*(2), 183–194.

Chan, A., & Lee, M. J. W. (2005). An MP3 a day keeps the worries away: Exploring the use of podcasting to address preconceptions and alleviate pre-class anxiety amongst undergraduate information technology students. In D. H. R. Spennemann & L. Burr (Eds.), *Good Practice in Practice: Proceedings of the Student Experience Conference* (pp. 58-70).

Chang, V., & Fisher, D. L. (2001). A new learning instrument to evaluate online learning in higher education. In Kulski, M., & Herrmann, A. (Eds.), *New horizons in university teaching and learning* (pp. 23–34). Perth, Western Australia.

Charles, C. M. (1974). *Teacher's petite Piaget*. Belmont, CA: David S. Lake Publishers.

Chen, C. (2008). Why do teachers not practice what they believe regarding technology integration? *The Journal of Educational Research, 102*(1), 65–75. doi:10.3200/JOER.102.1.65-75

Cheney, A., Matzen, N., Sanders, R., Bronack, S., Riedl, R., & Tashner, J. (2008). Social constructivism in a 3D immersive world. In K. McFerrin et al. (Eds.), *Proceedings of Society for Information Technology and Teacher Education International Conference 2008* (pp. 2922-2929). Chesapeake, VA: AACE.

Cheung, W. S., & Hew, K. F. (2004). Evaluating the extent of ill-structured problem-solving process among pre-service teachers in an asynchronous online discussions and reflection log learning environment. *Journal of Educational Computing Research, 30*(3), 197–227. doi:10.2190/9JTN-10T3-WTXH-P6HN

Chidanandan, A., DeVasher, R., Ferro, P., Fisher, D., Mitra-Kirtley, S., & Merkle, L. D. (2007). Evaluating the symbiosis of DyKnow software and pen-based computing in the Rose-Hulman classroom. In Reed, R., Berque, D., & Prey, J. C. (Eds.), *The Impact of Tablet PCs and Pen-based Technology on Education: Evidence and Outcomes* (pp. 21–31). West Lafayette, IN: Purdue University Press.

Chiu, C.-M., Hsu, M.-H., Sun, S.-Y., Lin, T.-C., & Sun, P.-C. (2005). Usability, quality, value and e-learning continuance decisions. *Computers & Education, 45*(4), 399–416. doi:10.1016/j.compedu.2004.06.001

Christopher, M. M., Thomas, J. A., & Talent-Runnels, M. K. (2004). Raising the bar: Encouraging high level thinking in online discussion forums. *Roeper Review, 26*(3), 166–171. doi:10.1080/02783190409554262

Clausen, J. M. (2007). Beginning teachers' technology use: First-year teacher development and the institutional context's affect on new teachers' instructional technology use with students. *Journal of Research on Technology in Education, 39*(3), 245–261.

Clausen, J., & Mallaby, M. (2008). Immersive learning and effective technology integration: Educational foundations redefined. In K. McFerrin et al. (Eds.), *Proceedings of Society for Information Technology and Teacher Education International Conference 2008* (pp. 1987-1991). Chesapeake, VA: AACE

Clayton, J. (2007). *Development and validation of an instrument for assessing online learning environments in tertiary education: The Online Learning Environment Survey (OLLES).* PhD thesis, Curtin University of Technology.

Cleaves, A., & Toplis, R. (2008). Pre-service science teachers and ICT: Communities of practice? *Research in Science & Technological Education, 26*(2), 203–213. doi:10.1080/02635140802037344

Clegg, S. (2001). Theorising the machine: Gender, education, and computing. *Gender and Education, 13*(3), 307–324. doi:10.1080/09540250120063580

Clements, D. H. (2000). From exercises and tasks to problems and projects: Unique contributions of computers to innovative mathematics education. *The Journal of Mathematical Behavior, 19,* 9–47. doi:10.1016/S0732-3123(00)00036-5

Cleveland-Innes, M., & Mohamed Ally (2007). Learning to feel: Education, affective outcomes and the use of online teaching and learning. *EURODL 2007, 2.* Retrieved December 12, 2008 from http://www.eurodl.org/materials/contrib/2007/Cleveland_Ally.htm

Cochran-Smith, M. (2000). *The outcomes question in teacher education.* AERA Vice Presidential Address for Division K (Teaching and Teacher Education), AERA Annual Meeting, April 2000. Retrieved 15 November, 2008 from http://www2.bc.edu/~cochrans/default.html

Cochran-Smith, M., & Lytle, S. L. (1993). *Inside/Outside: Teacher research and knowledge.* New York: Teachers College Press.

Cochran-Smith, M., & Lytle, S. L. (1999). Relationships of knowledge and practice: Teacher learning in communities. In A. Iran- Nejad & P. D. Pearson (Eds.), Review of research in education (Vol. 24, pp. 249-306). Washington, DC: American Educational Research Association.

Coffland, D. A., & Strickland, A. (2004). Factors related to teacher use of technology in secondary geometry instruction. *Journal of Computers in Mathematics and Science Teaching, 23*(4), 347–365.

Cohen, A. (2001). Two reactions to the mathematical education of teachers. *Notices of the AMS*, 985-991.

Cohen, D. J., & Rosenzweig, R. (2006). *Digital history: A guide to gathering, preserving, and presenting the past on the Web.* Philadelphia, PA: University of Pennsylvania Press.

Cole, H., & Stanton, D. (2003). Designing mobile technologies to support co-present collaboration. *Personal and Ubiquitous Computing, 7,* 365–371. doi:10.1007/s00779-003-0249-4

Coley, R., Cradler, J., & Engel, P. K. (1997). Computers and classrooms: The status of technology in U.S. schools. *Educational Testing Service.* Retrieved February 2, 2006, from http://www.ets.org/Media/Research/pdf/PICCOMPCLSS.pdf

Collins, R. (2004). *Interaction Ritual Chains.* Princeton, NJ: Princeton University Press.

Cooper, J. M., & Bull, G. L. (1997). Technology and teacher education: Past practice and recommended direction. *Action in Teacher Education, 19*(2), 97–106.

Coppola, E. (2005). *Powering up: Support for constructivist teaching with technology.* Paper presented in Philadelphia, PA at the National Educational Computing Conference. Retrieved from http://www.iste.org/Content/NavigationMenu/Research/ NECC_Research_Paper_Archives/NECC_2005/Coppola-Eileen-NECC05.pdf

Cornford, I. R. (2002). Reflective teaching: Empirical research findings and some implications for teacher education. *Journal of Vocational Education and Training, 54,* 219–235. doi:10.1080/13636820200200196

Cortes, W. (2008). Comic Life. Oral history presentation, New York.

Cortes-Figueroa, J. E., & Moore, D. A. (1999). Using CBL technology and a graphing calculator to teach the kinetics of consecutive first-order reactions. *Journal of Chemical Education, 76*(5), 635–638. doi:10.1021/ed076p635

Costa, A., & Loveall, R. (2002). The legacy of Hilda Taba. *Journal of Curriculum and Supervision, 18,* 56–62.

Cowan, J. (2008). The Strategies for planning technology–enhanced learning experiences. *Clearing House (Menasha, Wis.)*, *82*(2), 55–59. doi:10.3200/TCHS.82.2.55-59

Cox, M. J., & Marshall, G. (2007). Effects of ICT: Do we know what we should know? *Education and Information Technologies*, *12*, 59–70. doi:10.1007/s10639-007-9032-x

Cox, M., Webb, M., Abbott, C., Blakeley, B., Beauchamp, T., & Rhodes, V. (2003). ICT and pedagogy: A review of the research literature. *ICT in Schools Research and Evaluation Series.* Retrieved September 2005, from http://www.becta.org.uk/page_documents/research/ict_pedagogy_summary.pdf

Cramer, M., Beauregard, R., & Sharma, M. (2009). An investigation of purpose built netbooks for primary school education. In *Proceedings of the 8th International Conference on Interaction Design and Children* (pp. 36-43). Como, Italy: Association for Computing Machinery.

Criswell, C. (2008). What Web 2.0 means for teachers. *Teaching Music*, *16*(3), 1–2.

Crocco, M. S. (2001). Leveraging constructivist learning in the social studies classroom: A response to Mason, Berson, Diem, Hicks, Lee, and Dralle. *Contemporary Issues in Technology and Teacher Education, 1*(3), 386-394. Retrieved April 7, 2009, from http://www.citejournal.org/vol1/iss3/currentissues/socialstudies/article2.ht

Crocco, M. S. (2005). Teaching *Shabanu*: The challenges of using world literature in the social studies classroom. *Journal of Curriculum Studies*, *37*(5), 561–582. doi:10.1080/0022027042000310692

Crocco, M. S., & Cramer, J. (2005). Women, WebQuests, and controversial issues in the social studies. *Social Education*, *69*(3), 143–148.

Crocco, M. S., Cramer, J., & Meier, E. (2008). (Never) Mind the gap! Gender equity in social studies research on technology in the twenty-first century. *Multicultural Education & Technology Journal*, *2*(1), 19–36. doi:10.1108/17504970810867133

Crocco, M., & Cramer, J. (2004). A virtual hall of mirrors? Confronting the digital divide in urban social studies teacher education. *Journal of Computing in Teacher Education*, *20*(4), 133–137.

Crocco, M., & Cramer, J. (2005). Technology use, women, and global studies in social studies teacher education. *Contemporary Issues in Technology & Teacher Education*, *5*(1), 38–49.

Cuban, L. (1986). *Teachers and machines.* New York: Teachers College Press.

Cuban, L. (1993). Computers meet classroom: Classroom wins. *Teachers College Record*, *95*, 185–210.

Cuban, L. (2001). *Oversold and underused computers in the classroom.* Cambridge, MA: Harvard University Press.

Cummins, J., Brown, K., & Sayers, D. (2007). *Literacy, technology, and diversity: Teaching for success in changing times.* Boston: Allyn and Bacon.

Curtis, M. (2005). The rise of the handheld computer in schools. *Media and Methods*, *41*(6), 14.

Dalli, C. (2008). The name assigned to the document by the author. This field may also contain sub-titles, series names, and report numbers.Pedagogy, knowledge and collaboration: Towards a ground-up perspective on professionalism. *The entity from which ERIC acquires the content, including journal, organization, and conference names, or by means of online submission from the author. European Early Childhood Education Research Journal*, *16*(2), 171–185. doi:10.1080/13502930802141600

Dana, N. F., & Silva, D. Y. (2003). *The reflective educators' guide to classroom research: Learning to teach and teaching to learn through practitioner inquiry.* Thousand Oaks, CA: Corwin Press.

Dana, N. F., & Yendol-Silva, D. (2003). *The reflective educator's guide to classroom research: Learning to teach and teaching to learn through practitioner inquiry.* Thousand Oaks, CA: Corwin Press.

Danesh, A., Inkpen, K., Lau, E., Shu, K., & Booth, K. (2001). Geney: Designing a collaborative activity for the Palm handheld computer. In *Proceedings of CHI, Conference on Human Factors in Computing Systems*, Seattle, WA.

DaPonte, J. P., Oliveira, H., & Varandas, J. M. (2002). Development of pre-service mathematics teachers' professional knowledge and identity in working with information and communication technology. *Journal of Mathematics Teacher Education*, *5*, 93–115. doi:10.1023/A:1015892804607

Darling-Hammond, L., Holtzman, D. J., Gatlin, S. J., & Heilig, J. V. (2005). Does teacher preparation matter? Evidence about teacher certification, Teach for America, and teacher effectiveness. *Education Policy Analysis Archives*, *13*(42), 1–48.

Davidson, C. (2007, March 23). We can't ignore the influence of digital technologies. *Chronicle of Higher Education, 53*(29). eTalkinghead.com. (2003-2008). *Etalkinghead's political blog directory*. Retrieved April 1, 2009, from http://directory.etalkinghead.com/

Davis, B., & Simmt, E. (2006). Mathematics-for-teaching: An ongoing investigation of the mathematics that teachers (need) to know. *Educational Studies in Mathematics*, *61*(3), 293–319. doi:10.1007/s10649-006-2372-4

Davis, E. A. (2006). Characterizing productive reflection among preservice elementary teachers: Seeing what matters. *Teaching and Teacher Education*, *22*, 281–301. doi:10.1016/j.tate.2005.11.005

Davis, E., & Krajcik, J. (2005). Designing educative curriculum materials to promote teacher learning. *Educational Researcher*, *34*(3), 3–14. doi:10.3102/0013189X034003003

Davis, J. E. (1997). *Categories of technology use in education*. Retrieved December 18, 2008, from http://www.quasar.ualberta.ca/edpy485/edtech/category.htm#category

Davis, K. M., Kelly, M., Malani, R., Griswold, W. G., & Simon, B. (2007). Preliminary evaluation of NoteBlogger: Public note taking in the classroom. In Prey, J. C., Reed, R. H., & Berque, D. A. (Eds.), *The Impact of Tablet PCs and Pen-based Technology on Education: Beyond the Tipping Point* (pp. 33–42). West Lafayette, IN: Purdue University Press.

Dawson, K. (2006). Teacher inquiry: A vehicle to merge prospective teachers' experience and reflection during curriculum-based technology-enhanced field experiences. *Journal of Research on Technology in Education*, *38*(3), 265–292.

De Freitas, S., & Griffiths, M. D. (2008). The convergence of gaming practices with other media forms: what potential for learning? A review of the literature. *Learning, Media and Technology*, *33*(1). doi:10.1080/17439880701868796

De Freitas, S., & Oliver, M. (2006). How can exploratory learning with games and simulations within the curriculum be most effectively evaluated. *Computers and Education. Special Issue on Gaming*, *46*, 249–264.

DeBell, M., & Chapman, C. (2006). *Computer and Internet use by students in 2003. (Issue Brief No. 065)*. Washington, DC: National Center for Education Statistics.

Dede, C., Ketelhut, D., Whitehouse, P., Breit, L., & McCloskey, E. (2006). *Research Agenda for Online Teacher Professional Development*. Cambridge, MA: Harvard Graduate School of Education.

Demetriou, O. (2004). Prioritizing ethnicities: the uncertainty of Pomak-ness in the urban Greek Rhodopi. *Ethnic and Racial Studies*, *27*(1), 95–119. doi:10.1080/0141987032000147959

Denzin, N. K., & Lincoln, Y. S. (2000). Introduction: The discipline and practice of qualitative research. In Denzin, N. K., & Lincoln, Y. S. (Eds.), *Handbook of qualitative research* (2nd ed.). Thousand Oaks, CA: Sage Publications.

Design-Based-Research-Collective. (2003). Design-based research: An emerging paradigm for educational inquiry. *Educational Researcher*, *32*(1), 5–8. doi:10.3102/0013189X032001005

Devins, D., Darlow, A., Burdens, T., & Petrie, A. (2003). *Connecting communities to the Internet: Evaluation of the Wired Up Communities programme (2000-2002)*. London: Department for Education and Skills. [DFES]

Devlin-Scherer, R., & Daly, J. (2001). Living in the present tense: Student teaching telecommunications connect theory and practice. *Journal of Technology and Teacher Education*, *9*(4), 617–634.

Dewey, J. (1933). *How We Think: A restatement of the relation of reflective thinking to the educative process*. New York: D. C. Heath and Company.

Dexter, S. L., Anderson, R. E., & Becker, H. J. (1999). Teachers' views of computers as catalysts for changes in their teaching practice. *Journal of Research on Computing in Education*, *31*, 221–238.

Dicken, C. (2008). The 30-day challenge: Digital homework in a high school mathematics classroom. In Reed, R., Berque, D., & Prey, J. C. (Eds.), *The Impact of Tablet PCs and Pen-based Technology on Education: Evidence and Outcomes* (pp. 31–37). West Lafayette, IN: Purdue University Press.

Dicker, L. A., & Monda-Amaya, L. E. (1995). Reflective teaching: A process for analyzing journals of preservice teachers. *Teacher Education and Special Education*, *18*(4), 240–252. doi:10.1177/088840649501800404

Diem, R. A., & Katims, D. S. (2002). The introductioni of computers in an at-risk learning environment: A seven-year retrospectice view. *Computers in the Schools*, *19*, 19–32. doi:10.1300/J025v19n01_03

Dietz-Uhler, B., & Bishop-Clark, C. (2002). The psychology of computer-mediated communication: Four classroom activities. *Psychology Learning & Teaching*, *2*(1), 25–31.

Digiovanni, L., Schwartz, S., & Greer, C. (2009). I think, iPod(cast), I learn: using digital media and podcasting in teacher education. In C. Crawford et al. (Eds.), *Proceedings of Society for Information Technology and Teacher Education International Conference 2009* (pp. 1812-1819). Chesapeake, VA: AACE.

Dillenbourg, P. (2008). Integrating technologies into educational ecosystems. *Distance Education*, *29*(2), 127–140. doi:10.1080/01587910802154939

Dillenbourg, P., & Hong, F. (2008). The mechanics of CSCL macro-scripts. *International Journal of Computer-Supported Collaborative Learning*, *3*(1), 5–23. doi:10.1007/s11412-007-9033-1

Dillenbourg, P., & Jermann, P. (2007). Designing integrative scripts. In Fischer, F., Kollar, I., Mandl, H., & Haage, J. M. (Eds.), *Scripting computer-supported collaborative learning. Cognitive, computational, and educational perspectives* (pp. 275–301). New York: Springer. doi:10.1007/978-0-387-36949-5_16

Dillenbourg, P., & Tchounikine, P. (2007). Flexibility in macro-scripts for computer-supported collaborative learning. *Journal of Computer Assisted Learning*, *23*(1), 1–11. doi:10.1111/j.1365-2729.2007.00191.x

Dillenbourg, P., Järvelä, S., & Fisher, F. (2009). The evolution of research on computer-supported collaborative learning: From design to orchestration. In Balacheff, N., Ludvigsen, S., de Jong, T., Lazonder, T. A., & Barnes, S. (Eds.), *Technology enhanced learning: Principles and products* (pp. 3–19). Amsterdam: Springer.

DiStasi, V. F., Birmingham, W. P., & Welton, G. L. (2008). Evaluating learning software in the classroom: A continuing study. In Reed, R., Berque, D., & Prey, J. C. (Eds.), *The Impact of Tablet PCs and Pen-based Technology on Education: Evidence and Outcomes* (pp. 39–45). West Lafayette, IN: Purdue University Press.

Doering, A. (2006). Adventure learning: Transformative hybrid online education. *Distance Education*, *27*(2), 197–215. doi:10.1080/01587910600789571

Doering, A. (2007). Adventure learning: Situated learning in an authentic context. *Innovate 3*(6).

Doering, A., & Veletsianos, G. (2008). Hybrid online education in the K-12 classroom: Identifying integration models using adventure learning. *Journal of Research on Technology in Education*, *41*(1), 101–119.

Doerr, H. M., & Zangor, R. (2000). Creating meaning for and with the graphing calculator. *Educational Studies in Mathematics*, *41*(2), 143–163. doi:10.1023/A:1003905929557

Doolittle, P., & Hicks, D. (2003). Constructivism as a theoretical foundation for use of technology in social studies. *Theory and Research in Social Education*, *3*(1), 72–105.

Dreon, O., & McDonald, A. S. P. (2006). *Using an online community of practice to foster inquiry as pedagogy amongst student teachers.* Paper presented at the Proceedings of the 7th International Conference on Learning Sciences: International Society of the Learning Sciences, Bloomington, Indiana.

Drier, H. S. (2001, March). *Beliefs, experiences, and reflections that affect the development of techno-Mathematical knowledge.* Paper presented at the SITE, Orlando, FL.

Dudeney, G., & Hockly, N. (2007). *How to teach English with technology.* Harlow, UK: Pearson/Longman.

Duke University. (2006). *Duke digital initiative.* Retrieved December 2, 2008, from http://www.duke.edu/ddi/

Dun, A., Feldman, A., & Rearick, M. (2000, April). *Teaching and learning with computers in schools: The development of instructional technology pedagogical content knowledge.* Paper presented at the American Educational Research Association (AERA), New Orleans, LA.

Dunkel, C., & Kerpelman, J. (Eds.). (2006). *Possible selves: Theory, research and applications.* New York: Nova Science Publishers, Inc.

Durkheim, E., & Emirbrayer, M. (2003). *Sociologist of modernity.* San Francisco: Wiley-Blackwell.

Duschl, R. A., Schweingruber, H. A., & Shouse, A. W. (Eds.). (2007). *Taking Science to School: Learning and Teaching Science in Grades K-8.* Washington, DC: The National Academies Press.

Dusick, D. M. (1998). What social cognitive factors influence faculty members' use of computers for teaching? A literature review. *Journal of Research on Computing in Education*, *31*, 123–137.

Dutta, S., & Mia, I. (2009). *The global information technology report 2008-2009.* Retrieved April 1, 2009, from http://www.insead.edu/v1/gitr/wef/main/fullreport/index.html

Dwyer, C., Hiltz, S. R., & Passerini, K. (2007). Trust and privacy concern within social networking sites: A comparison of Facebook and MySpace. In *Proceedings of the Thirteenth Americas Conference on Information Systems*, Keystone, Colorado. Retrieved on February 2, 2009, from http://csis.pace.edu/~dwyer/research/DwyerAMCIS2007.pdf

Edens, K. M., & Gallini, J. K. (2000). Developing a discourse community of preservice teachers in a technology-mediated context. *Teacher Educator*, *34*(4), 64–82. doi:10.1080/08878730009555238

Education and Manpower Bureau. (2004). *Reforming the academic structure for secondary education and higher education- actions for investing in the future.* Retrieved March 5, 2009, from http://www.edb.gov.hk/FileManager/EN/content_4034/main.pdf

Ellison, N., & Wu, Y. (2008). Blogging in the Classroom: A Preliminary Exploration of Student Attitude and Impact on Comprehension. *Journal of Educational Media and Hypermedia*, *17*(1), 99–122.

Engenfeld, S. (2005). *Beyond Eductaiment.* Doctoral dissertation. Copenhagen, Denmark: University of Copenhagen.

Engstrom, M. E., & Jewett, D. (2005). Collaborative learning the wiki way. *TechTrends*, *49*(6), 12–15. doi:10.1007/BF02763725

Enyedy, N., Goldberg, & Welsh, K. (2006). Complex dilemmas of identity and practice. *Science Education*, *90*(1), 68–93. doi:10.1002/sce.20096

Ertmer, P. A. (1999). Addressing first- and second-order barriers to change: Strategies for technology integration. *Educational Technology Research and Development, 47*(4), 47–61. doi:10.1007/BF02299597

Ertmer, P. A. (2005). Teacher pedagogical beliefs: The final frontier in our quest for technology integration? *Educational Technology Research and Development, 53*(4), 25–39. doi:10.1007/BF02504683

Ertmer, P. A., Addison, P., Lane, M., Ross, E., & Woods, D. (1999). Examining teacher's beliefs about the role of technology in the elementary classroom. *Journal of Research on Computing in Education, 32*(1), 54–72.

European Commission. (2007). *Improving the Quality of Teacher Education. Communication from the Commission to the Council and the European Parliament.* Brussels, Belgium: European Commission. Retrieved February 18, 2009, from http://ec.europa.eu/education/com392_en.pdf

Evans, R. W., & Saxe, D. W. (Eds.). (1996). *Handbook for teaching controversial issues: NCSS bulletin 93.* Washington, DC: NCSS.

Ewell, P. T. (1985). *Assessing educational outcomes. New Directions for Institutional Research, 47.* San Francisco, CA: Jossey-Bass.

Farrell, T. (2008). *Reflective practice in the professional development of teachers of adult English language learners.* Washington, DC: Center for Applied Linguistics. Retrieved February 3, 2009, from http://www.cal.org/caelanetwrok/pd_resources/reflectivepractice.html

Fauske, J., & Wade, S. E. (2003). Research to practice online: Conditions that foster democracy, community, and critical thinking in computer-mediated discussions. *Journal of Research on Technology in Education, 36*(2), 137–154.

Feiman-Nemser, S. (2001). From preparation to practice: designing a continuum to strengthen and sustain teaching. *Teachers College Record, 103*(6), 1013–1055. doi:10.1111/0161-4681.00141

Felton, M., & Kuhn, D. (2001). The Development of Argumentative Discourse Skill. *Discourse Processes, 32*(2–3), 135–153. doi:10.1207/S15326950DP3202&3_03

Fendler, L. (2003). Teacher reflection in hall of mirrors: Historical influences and politic reverberations. *Educational Researcher, 32*(3), 16–25. doi:10.3102/0013189X032003016

Fenstermacher, G. D. (1994). The knower and the known: The nature of knowledge in research on Teaching. In Darling-Hammond (Ed.), Review of research in education (Vol. 20, pp. 3-56). Washington, DC: American Educational Research Association.

Ferdig, R. E., & Roehler, L. (2004). Student uptake in electronic discussions: Examining online discourse in literacy preservice classrooms. *Journal of Research on Technology in Education, 36*(2), 119–136.

Ferdig, R. E., & Roehler, L. R. (2003). Student uptake in electronic discussions: Examining online discourse in literacy preservice classrooms. *Journal of Research on Technology in Education, 36*(2), 119–136.

Fiege, K., Peacock, K., & Geelan, D. (2004). Professional Development: A Rural School District's Experience with Videoconferencing. In C. Crawford et al. (Eds.), *Proceedings of Society for Information Technology and Teacher Education International Conference 2004* (pp. 2150-2157). Chesapeake, VA: AACE.

Fischer, F., Kollar, I., Haake, J. M., & Mandl, H. (2007). Perspectives on collaboration scripts. In Fischer, F., Kollar, I., Mandl, H., & Haage, J. M. (Eds.), *Scripting computer-supported collaborative learning. Cognitive, computational and educational perspectives* (pp. 1–10). New York: Springer. doi:10.1007/978-0-387-36949-5_1

Fischman, J. (2007). Talking back to teacher. *The Chronicle of Higher Education, 53*(48), A.27.

Fleming, L., Motamedi, V., & May, L. (2007). Predicting preservice teacher competence in computer technology: Modeling and application in training environments. *Journal of Technology and Teacher Education, 15*(2), 207–231.

Flick, L., & Bell, R. (2000). Preparing tomorrow's science teachers to use technology: Guidelines for science educators. *Contemporary Issues in Technology & Teacher Education, 1*(1), 39–60.

Flores, A., Knaupp, J. E., Middleton, J. A., & Staley, F. A. (2002). Integration of technology, science, and mathematics in the middle grades: A teacher preparation program. *Contemporary Issues in Technology & Teacher Education, 2*(1). Retrieved from http://www.citejournal.org/vol2/iss1/mathematics/article1.cfm.

Flores, M. T. (2007). Navigating contradictory communities of practice in learning to teach for social justice. *Anthropology & Education Quarterly, 38*(4), 380–404. doi:10.1525/aeq.2007.38.4.380

Flores-Marti, I. (2008). Reflection as a critical component in the preparation of teacher candidates. *Strategies, 21*(6), 15–18.

Foreign Language Resource Center. Retrieved March 2, 2009, from http://nflrc.hawaii.edu/NetWorks/NW44

Forgasz, H. (2006). Factors that encourage or inhibit computer use for secondary mathematics teaching. *Journal of Computers in Mathematics and Science Teaching, 25*(1), 77–93.

Foucault, M. (1994). *The Order of Things: An Archaeology of the Human Sciences*. New York: Vintage Books.

Freiberg, H. J. (2002). Essential skills for new teachers. *Educational Leadership, 59*(6), 56–60.

Freidhoff, J. (2008). Reflecting on the affordance and constraints of technologies and their impact on pedagogical goals. *Journal of Computing in Teacher Education, 24*(4), 117–122.

French, D. (2006). iPods: informative or invasive? *Journal of College Science Teaching, 36*(1), 58–59.

Friedman, A. M. (2006). State standards and digital primary sources: A divergence. *Contemporary Issues in Technology and Teacher Education, 6*(3). Retrieved July 6, 2009, from http://www.citejournal.org/vol6/iss3/socialstudies/article1.cfm

Friedman, A. M. (2008). Social studies teachers' use of the Internet to foster democratic citizenship. In VanFossen, P. J., & Berson, M. J. (Eds.), *The electronic republic? The impact of technology on education for citizenship* (pp. 173–195). West Lafayette, IN: Purdue University Press.

Friedman, A. M., & Heafner, T. L. (2006, March). *Student creation of social studies-specific websites to enhance historical understandings*. Roundtable presented at the annual meeting of the Society for Information Technology and Teacher Education (SITE), Orlando, FL.

Friedman, A. M., & Heafner, T. L. (2007). You think for me, so I don't have to. *Contemporary Issues in Technology and Teacher Education, 7*(3). Retrieved July 7, 2009, from http://www.citejournal.org/vol7/iss3/socialstudies/article1.cfm

Friedman, A. M., & Heafner, T. L. (2008). Finding and contextualizing resources: A digital literacy tool's impact in ninth grade world history. *Clearing House (Menasha, Wis.), 82*(2), 82–86. doi:10.3200/TCHS.82.2.82-86

Friedman, A. M., & Hicks, D. (2006). The state of the field: Technology, social studies, and teacher education. *Contemporary Issues in Technology and Teacher Education* [Online serial], *6*(2). Retrieved July 7, 2009, from http://www.citejournal.org/vol6/iss2/socialstudies/article1.cfm

Fry, S. W. (2007). First-Year teachers and induction support: Ups, downs, and in-betweens. *Qualitative Report, 12*(2), 216–237.

Fry, S. W. (2009). On borrowed time: How four elementary preservice teachers learned to teach social studies in the NCLB era. *Social Studies Research and Practice, 4*(1), 31–41.

Fry, S. W., & Bryant, C. J. (2006-2007). Using distance technology to sustain teacher education for student teachers in isolated areas: The Technology Supported Induction Network. *Journal of Computing in Teacher Education, 23*(2), 63–69.

Fuchs, C. (2005). CMC-based model learning in language teacher education: A German-American telecollaboration. In I. Thompson & D. Hiple (Eds.), Selected papers from the 2004 NFLRC symposium: Distance Education, Distributed Learning and Language Instruction (pp. 141-156). Honolulu. HI: University of Hawai'i, National

Fuller, F. F., & Manning, B. A. (1973). Self-Confrontation Reviewed: A Conceptualization for Video Playback in Teacher Education. *Review of Educational Research*, *43*(4), 469–528.

Fulton, K., Glenn, A. D., & Valdez, G. (2003). *Three preservice programs preparing tomorrow's teachers to use technology: a study in partnerships.* Retrieved April 2, 2009, from http://www.learningpt.org/pdfs/tech/preservice.pdf

Fulton, K., Glenn, A. D., & Valdez, G. (2004). Teacher education and technology planning guide. Naperville, IL: Learning Point Associates. (ERIC document Reproduction Service No. ED489530).

Gado, I., Ferguson, M., & Van't Hooft, M. (2006). Using handheld-computers and probeware in a Science Methods course: Preservice teachers' attitudes and self-efficacy. *Journal of Technology and Teacher Education*, *14*(3), 501–529.

Gagne, R. (1985). *The Conditions of Learning and the Theory of Instruction* (4th ed.). New York: Holt, Rinehart, and Winston.

Gagné, R. M., Wager, W. W., Golas, K. C., & Keller, J. M. (2005). *Principles of instructional design*. Belmont, CA: Wadsworth/ Thomson Learning.

Gailey, C. W. (1996). Mediated messages: Gender, class, and cosmos in home video games. In E. Sigel (Series Ed.), P. M. Greenfield & R. R. Cocking (Vol. Eds.), Interacting with video (pp. 177-184). Norwood, NJ: Ablex Publishing.

Gall, M. D., Borg, W. R., & Gall, J. P. (1996). *Educational research. An introduction* (6th ed.). New York: Longman.

Garofalo, J., Drier, H., Harper, S., Timmerman, M. A., & Shockey, T. (2000). Promoting appropriate uses of technology in mathematics teacher preparation. *Contemporary Issues in Technology and Technology Education*, *1*, 66–88.

Garrison, D. R. (1997). Self-directed learning: Toward a comprehensive model. *Adult Education Quarterly*, *48*(1), 18–33. doi:10.1177/074171369704800103

Garrison, D. R., & Kanuka, H. (2004). Blended learning: Uncovering its transformative potential in higher education. *The Internet and Higher Education*, *7*(2), 95–105. doi:10.1016/j.iheduc.2004.02.001

Garrison, D. R., & Vaughan, N. D. (2008). *Blended learning in higher education - Framework, principles and guidelines.* CA: Jossey-Bass - A Wiley Imprint.

Garrison, D., Anderson, T., & Archer, W. (2000). Critical inquiry in a text-based environment: Computer conferencing in higher education. *The Internet and Higher Education*, *2*(2-3), 87–105. doi:10.1016/S1096-7516(00)00016-6

Garrison, R., & Kanuka, H. (2004). Blended Learning: Uncovering its transformative potential in higher education. *The Internet and Higher Education*, *7*(2), 95–105. doi:10.1016/j.iheduc.2004.02.001

Garthwait, A., & Wellwer, H. G. (2005). A year in the life: Two seventh grade teachers implementing one-to-one computing. *Journal of Research on Technology in Education*, *37*(4), 361–377.

Gee, A. (2003). *What video games have to teach us about learning and literacy.* New York: MacMillan.

Gee, A. (2008). Learning and Game. In Salen, K. (Ed.), *The ecology of games. Connecting youth, games and learning* (pp. 21–40). Cambridge, MA: MIT Press.

Gee, J. P. (2003). *What video games have to teach us about learning and literacy.* New York: Palgrave Macmillan.

Gentry, C. G. (1995). Educational technology: A question of meaning. In Anglin, G. J. (Ed.), *Instructional technology: Past, present, and future* (pp. 1–10). Englewood, CO: Libraries Unlimited, Inc.

Geoghegan, M. W., & Klass, D. (2005). *Podcast Solutions: The Complete Guide to Podcasting.* Berkeley, CA: Apress.

Georgia College & State University. (2005). *The iPod at GC&SU: a pocketful of learning.* Retrieved December 2, 2008, from http://ipod/gcsu.edu/

Georgiadis, F., & Zisimos, A. (2005). Migrants', refugees' and minorities' children in European Education: the Greek experience. In *Proceedings from the Conference Diversity in Education in an International Context*, 20-23 April. (Verona, International Association of Intercultural Education (IAIE)).

Gilbert, P. K., & Dabbagh, N. (2005). How to structure online discussions for meaningful discourse: a case study. *British Journal of Educational Technology, 36*(1), 5–18. doi:10.1111/j.1467-8535.2005.00434.x

Glaser, B. G., & Strauss, A. L. (1967). *The discovery of grounded theory: strategies for qualitative research.* Chicago, IL: Aldine de Gruyter.

Glub, E. (2004, March). *Handwritten slides on a tablet PC in a discrete mathematics course.* Paper presented at the 35th SIGCSE technical symposium on Computer Science Education, Norfolk, VA.

Gningue, S. M. (2003). The effectiveness of long term vs. short term training in selected computing technologies on middle and high school mathematics teachers' attitudes and beliefs. *Journal of Computers in Mathematics and Science Teaching, 22*(3), 207–224.

Goffman, E. (1963). *Stigma: notes on the management of spoiled identity.* New York: Prentice Hall.

Goldenberg, L., Ba, H., Heinze, J., & Hess, A. (2003). *JASON Multimedia Science Curriculum Impact on student learning: Final Evaluation Report.* New York: Center of Children and Technology, Education Development Center.

Goodlad, J. I. (1984). *A place called school: Prospects for the future.* New York: McGraw Hill.

Goodlad, J. I. (1990). *Teachers for our nation's schools.* San Francisco: Jossey-Bass Publishers.

Goodnough, K. (2004). *Learning in communities of practice: The science across the curriculum project.* Retrieved June, 2006, from http://www.mun.ca/educ/faculty/mwatch/fall05/goodnough.htm

Goodson, I. V., & Mangan, J. M. (1995). School cultures and the introduction of classroom computers. *British Educational Research Journal, 21*(5), 613–628. doi:10.1080/0141192950210505

Goos, M. (2005). A sociocultural analysis of the development of pre-service and beginning teachers' pedagogical identities as users of technology. *Journal of Mathematics Teacher Education, 8*, 35–59. doi:10.1007/s10857-005-0457-0

Goos, M., Galbraith, P., Renshaw, P., & Geiger, V. (2000). Reshaping teacher and student roles in technology-enriched classrooms. *Mathematics Education Research Journal, 12*, 303–320.

Goos, M., Galbraith, P., Renshaw, P., & Geiger, V. (2003). Perspectives on technology mediated learning in secondary school mathematics classrooms. *The Journal of Mathematical Behavior, 22*(1), 73–89. doi:10.1016/S0732-3123(03)00005-1

Gorski, P., Heidlebach, R., Howe, B., Jackson, M., & Tell, S. (2000). Forging communities for educational change with e-mail discussion groups. *Multicultural Perspectives, 2*(4), 37–42. doi:10.1207/S15327892MCP0204_8

Govaris, Ch., Kaplanoglou, M., Skourtou, E., & Vratsalis, K. (2003). The Construction of the Substantialist Obstacle in Education through promoting the 'Substance' of Culture. *International Journal of Learning, 10*, 1219–1230.

Graham, C. R. (2006). Blended learning systems: definition, current trends, and future directions. In Bonk, C. J., & Graham, C. R. (Eds.), *Handbook of blended learning: Global perspectives, local designs* (pp. 3–21). San Francisco, CA: Pfeiffer Publishing.

Graham, C. R., Allen, S., & Ure, D. (2005). Benefits and challenges of blended learning environments. In Khosrow-Pour, M. (Ed.), *Encyclopedia of information science and technology* (pp. 253–259). Hershey, PA: Idea Group.

Graham, C., Culatta, R., Pratt, M., & West, R. (2004). Redesigning the teacher education technology course to emphasize integration. *Computers in the Schools, 21*, 127–148. doi:10.1300/J025v21n01_10

Gratch, A. (2000). Becoming teacher: student teaching as identity construction. *Teaching Education, 11*(1), 119–126. doi:10.1080/10476210050020435

Gredler, M. E. (2005). *Learning and instruction - theory into practice.* Upper Saddle River, NJ: Pearson Education, Inc.

Griffiths, M. (1997). Friendship and social development in children and adolescents: The impact of electronic technology. *Educational and Child Psychology, 14*, 25–37.

Grion, V., & Varisco, B. (2007). On line collaboration for building a teacher professional identity. *PsychNology, 5*(3), 271–284.

Groff, J., & Haas, J. (2008). Web 2.0: Today's technologies, tomorrow's learning. *Leading and Learning with Technology*, 12-15.

Gros, B. (2005). Digital Games in Education: The Design of Games-Based Learning Environments. *Journal of Research on Technology in Education, 40*(1), 23–38.

Gros, B. (Ed.). (2008). Videojuegos y aprendizaje. Barcelona, España: Graó.

Gros, B., & Garrido, J. M. (2008). The Use of Video games to Mediate Curricular Learning. In *DIGITEL: Proceedings of the 2008 Second IEEE International Conference on Digital Game and Intelligent Toy Enhanced Learning* (pp. 170-176).

Grossman, P. L. (1988). *A study in contrast: Sources of pedagogical content knowledge for secondary English.* Unpublished Doctoral Dissertation, Stanford University, Palo Alto, CA.

Guerrero, S., Walker, N., & Dugale, S. (2004). Technology in support of middle grade mathematics: What have we learned? *Journal of Computers in Mathematics and Science Teaching, 23*(1), 5–20.

Gueudet, G. (2007). Investigating the secondary-tertiary transition. *Educational Studies in Mathematics, 67*, 237–254. doi:10.1007/s10649-007-9100-6

Hakkarainen, K. (2003). Emergence of Progressive-Inquiry Culture in Computer-Supported Collaborative Learning. *Science and Education, 6*(2), 199–220.

Häkkinen, P., & Mäkitalo-Siegl, K. (2007). Educational perspectives on scripting CSCL. In Fischer, F., Kollar, I., Mandl, H., & Haage, J. M. (Eds.), *Scripting computer-supported collaborative learning. Cognitive, computational and educational perspectives* (pp. 263–271). New York: Springer. doi:10.1007/978-0-387-36949-5_15

Hale, A. (2008). Service learning with Latino communities: Effects on preservice teachers. *Journal of Hispanic Higher Education, 7*(1), 54–69. doi:10.1177/1538192707310511

Hämäläinen, J. (2003). The concept of social pedagogy in the field of social work. *Journal of Social Work, 3*(1), 69–81. doi:10.1177/1468017303003001005

Hämäläinen, R. (2008). *Pedagogical scripts to facilitate computer-supported collaborative learning.* Jyväskylä, Finland: University of Jyväskylä, Finnish Institute for Educational Research.

Hammerness, K., Darling-Hammond, L., Bransford, J., Berliner, D., Cochran-Smith, M., & McDonald, M. (2005). How teachers learn and develop. In Bransford, J., & Darling-Hammond, L. (Eds.), *Preparing teachers for a changing world* (pp. 358–389). San Francisco: Jossey Bass.

Hanson, K. (1997). *Gender, discourse, and technology.* Center for Equity and Diversity Working Paper No. 5. Retrieved June 9, 2009, from http://www.eric.ed.gov/ERICWebPortal/custom/portlets/recordDetails/detailmini.jsp?_nfpb=true&_&ERICExtSearch_SearchValue_0=ED418913&ERICExtSearch_SearchType_0=no&accno=ED418913

Hara, N., Bonk, C. J., & Angeli, C. (2000). Content analysis of online discussion in an applied educational psychology course. *Instructional Science, 28*(2), 115–152. doi:10.1023/A:1003764722829

Harford, J., & MacRuaire, G. (2008). Engaging student teachers in meaningful reflective practice. *Teaching and Teacher Education*, *24*, 1884–1892. doi:10.1016/j.tate.2008.02.010

Hargittai, E., & Shafer, S. (2006). Differences in actual and perceived online skills: The role of gender. *Social Science Quarterly*, *87*(2), 432–448. doi:10.1111/j.1540-6237.2006.00389.x

Harschbarger, R. J. (1995). Training pre-service and in service teachers in the use of technology. In *Electronic Proceedings of the Eighth Annual International Conference on Technology in Collegiate Mathematics*, Houston, Texas, November 16-19, 1995. Retrieved January 10, 2009 from http://archives.math.utk.edu/ICTCM/i/08/C085.html

Hart, S. M., & King, J. R. (2007). Service learning and literacy tutoring: Academic impact on preservice teachers. *Teaching and Teacher Education*, *23*(4), 323–338. doi:10.1016/j.tate.2006.12.004

Hasan, H. (2001). An overview of techniques for applying activity theory to information systems. In H. Hasan, E. Gould, & P. Larkin (Eds.), Information systems and activity theory: Vol. 2, Theory and practice (pp. 2-33). New South Wales, Australia: Wollongong University Press.

Hassard, J., & Dias, M. (2000, May). *Experiences in a constructivist community of practice: An inquiry into TEEMS: A science teacher education program.* Paper presented at the Annual Meeting of the National Association for Research in Science Teaching, New Orleans, LA.

Hastings, N., & Tracey, M. (2005). Does media affect learning? Where are we now? *TechTrends*, *49*(2), 28–30. doi:10.1007/BF02773968

Hatton, N., & Smith, D. (1995). Reflection in teacher education: Toward definition and implementation. *Teaching and Teacher Education*, *11*(1), 33–49. doi:10.1016/0742-051X(94)00012-U

Hawkes, M., & Rosmiszowski, A. (2001). Examining the reflective outcomes of asynchronous computer-mediated communication on inservice teacher development. *Journal of Technology and Teacher Education*, *9*(2), 285–308.

Hazzan, O. (2000). Attitudes of prospective high school mathematics teachers towards integrating information technologies into their future teaching. In. *Proceedings of the Society for Information Technology and Teacher Education*, *11*, 1582–1587.

Hazzan, O. (2003). Prospective high school mathematics teachers' attitudes toward integrating computers in their future teaching. *Journal of Research on Technology in Education*, *35*, 213–225.

Heafner, T. L., & Friedman, A. M. (2008). Wikis and constructivism in social studies: Fostering a deeper understanding. *Computers in the Schools*, *25*(3-4), 288–302. doi:10.1080/07380560802371003

Hedberg, J. G., & Brudvik, O. C. (2008). Supporting dialogic literacy through mashing and modding of places and spaces. *Theory into Practice*, *47*(2), 138–149. doi:10.1080/00405840801992363

Hedges, L. V., Konstantopoulos, S., & Thompson, A. (2003). *NAEP validity studies: Computer use and its relation to academic achievement in mathematics, reading, and writing* (Working paper no. 2003-15). Retrieved March 12, 2009 from http://nces.ed.gov/pubsearch/pubsinfo.asp?pubid=200315

Heflich, D. A., Dixon, J. K., & Davis, K. S. (2001). Taking it to the field: The authentic Integration of mathematics and technology in inquiry-based science instruction. *Journal of Computers in Mathematics and Science Teaching*, *20*(1), 99–112.

Hellmig, L. (2008). Blended Learning for Teachers' Professional Development. Paper presented in the conference E-Learning Baltics, Rostock, Germany.

Helms, J. (1998). Science and me: Subject matter and identity in secondary science teachers. *Journal of Research in Science Teaching*, *35*(7), 811–834. doi:10.1002/(SICI)1098-2736(199809)35:7<811::AID-TEA9>3.0.CO;2-O

Henderson, M. (2007). Sustaining online teacher professional development through community design. *Campus-Wide Information Systems*, *3*(24), 162–173. doi:10.1108/10650740710762202

Hendron, J. (2008). *RSS for Educators: Blogs Newsfeeds, Podcasts and Wikis in the Classroom*. Eugene, OR: International Society for Technology in Education.

Hennessy, S., Ruthven, K., & Brindley, S. (2005). Teacher perspectives on integrating ICT into subject teaching: Commitment, constraints, caution, and change. *Journal of Curriculum Studies*, *37*(2), 155–192. doi:10.1080/0022027032000276961

Hesse, H. (2007). Being told to do something or just being aware of something? An alternative approach to scripting in CSCL. In Fischer, F., Kollar, I., Mandl, H., & Haage, J. M. (Eds.), *Scripting computer-supported collaborative learning. Cognitive, computational and educational perspectives* (pp. 91–98). New York: Springer. doi:10.1007/978-0-387-36949-5_6

Hew, K., & Brush, T. (2007). Integrating technology into K-12 teaching and learning: Current knowledge gaps and recommendations for future research. *Educational Technology Research and Development*, *55*(3), 223–252. doi:10.1007/s11423-006-9022-5

Hicks, D., & Ewing, E. T. (2003). Bringing the world into the classroom with online global newspapers. *Social Education*, *67*(3), 134–139.

Hied, M. K., & Blume, G. W. (2008). Research on technology and the teaching and learning of mathematics: *Vol. 1. Research syntheses*. Charlotte, NC: Information Age Publishing, Inc.

Hill, D. M. (2003). E-Folio and teacher candidate development. *Teacher Educator*, *38*(4), 256–266. doi:10.1080/08878730309555322

Hill, H. C., Blunk, M. L., Charalambous, C. Y., Lewis, J. M., Phelps, G. C., Sleep, L., & Ball, D. L. (2008). Mathematical knowledge for teaching and the mathematical quality of instruction: An exploratory study. *Cognition and Instruction*, *26*(4), 430–511. doi:10.1080/07370000802177235

Hin, L. T. W., & Subramaniam, R. (Eds.). (2009). *Handbook of research on new media literacy at the K-12 level: Issues and challenges*. Hershey, PA: IGI Global.

Hirsch, J. (2005). Applying Students' Own Devices in the Classroom. [from Education Full Text database.]. *School Administrator*, *62*(10), 8. Retrieved February 27, 2007.

Hirsch, L., Saeedi, M., Cornillon, J., & Litosseliti, L. (2004). A structured dialogue tool for argumentative learning. *Journal of Computer Assisted Learning*, *20*(1), 72–80. doi:10.1111/j.1365-2729.2004.00068.x

Hojsholt-Poulsen, L. (2007). *Current Trends in Teachers' Professional Development - 21 Cst Teachers Need Digital Competences and Digital Learning Resources*. The Sixth Open Classroom Conference, Real Learning in Virtual Worlds, Stockholm, Sweden.

Holly, M. (1989). Reflective writing and the spirit of inquiry. *Cambridge Journal of Education*, *19*(1), 71–80. doi:10.1080/0305764890190109

Holmes, A., Polhemus, L., & Jennings, S. (2005). CATIE: A blended approach to situated professional development. *Journal of Educational Computing Research*, *32*(4), 381–394. doi:10.2190/F97W-QUJ4-G7YG-FPXC

Hong, W. (2008). Exploring educational use of blogs in U.S. education. *U.S.-China Education Review*, *5*(10), 47, 34-38.

Hord, S. M., Rutherford, W. L., Huling-Austin, L., & Hall, G. E. (1987). *Taking charge of change*. Alexandria, VA: ASCD Publications.

Hough, B. W., Smithey, M. W., & Evertson, C. M. (2004). Using computer-mediated communication to create virtual communities of practice for intern Teachers. *Journal of Technology and Teacher Education*, *12*(3), 361–386.

Houndoymani, A., & Pateraki, L. (2001). Bullying and Bullies in Greek Elementary schools: Pupils attitudes and teachers - parents' awareness. *Educational Review*, *53*(1), 19–26. doi:10.1080/00131910120033619

Hoyles, C., & Lagrange, J. (2010) (Eds.). Mathematics education and technology-rethinking the terrain. The 17th ICMI Study. New York: Springer.

Hsiang, M. Y. (1999). *Technology assisted reflection: A study of pre-service teacher education in middle school Language Arts and Social Studies and secondary school English and Social Studies*. Unpublished Dissertation, North Carolina State University.

Huang, R., & Zhou, Y. (2006). Designing blended learning focused on knowledge category and learning activities. In Bonk, C. J., & Graham, C. R. (Eds.), *Handbook of blended learning: Global perspectives, local designs* (pp. 296–310). San Francisco, CA: Pfeiffer Publishing.

Hughes, J. E. (2000). *Teaching English with technology: Exploring teacher learning and practice*. Unpublished Doctoral Dissertation, Michigan State University, East Lansing, MI.

Hughes, J. E. (2005). The role of teacher knowledge and learning experiences in forming technology-Integrated pedagogy. *Journal of Technology and Teacher Education, 13*(2), 277–302.

Hughes, J. E., & Scharber, C. (2008). Leveraging the development of English TPCK within the deictic Nature of literacy. In Technology, T. A. C. I. a. (Ed.), *Handbook of Technological Pedagogical Content Knowledge (TPCK) for Educators* (*Vol. 1*, pp. 87–106). New York: Lawrence Erlbaum.

Hughes, J., & Purnell, E. (2008). Blogging for beginners? Using blogs and eportfolios in teacher education. In *Proceedings of the 6th International Conference on Networked Learning* (pp. 144-152).

Huitt, W. (2001, April). Krathwol et al.'s taxonomy of the affective domain. In *Educational Psychology Interactive*. Valdosta, GA: Valdosta State University. Retrieved October 4, 2008, from http://chiron.valdosta.edu/whuitt/col/affsys/affdom.html

Hull, D. M., & Saxon, T. F. (2009). Negotiation of meaning and co-construction of knowledge: An analysis of experimental analysis of asynchronous online instruction. *Computers & Education, 52*, 624–639. doi:10.1016/j.compedu.2008.11.005

Hussein, J. (2007). Experience gained through engaging student teachers in a developmental reflective process. *Teacher Development, 11*(2), 189–201. doi:10.1080/13664530701414852

Idaho Standards for Initial Certification of Professional School Personnel. (2005). Retrieved March 2, 2009, from: http://www.sde.idaho.gov/site/teacher_certification/accredited.htm

Inkpen, K. (2001). Designing handheld technologies for kids. In *Proceedings of CHI, Conference on Human Factors in Computing Systems*, Seattle, WA.

Inkpen, K. M., Ho-Ching, W., Kuederle, O., Scott, S., & Shoemaker, G. (1999). *'This is fun! We're all best friends and we're all playing': Supporting children's synchronous collaboration*. Paper presented at the Computer Support for Collaborative Learning Conference '99, Stanford, U.S.

International Society for Technology in Education. (1999). *National education technology standards*. Retrieved February 2, 2006, from http://www.iste.org/Template.cfm? Section=NETS&CONTENTID=4963&TEMPLATE=/ContentManagement/ContentDisplay.cfm

International Society for Technology in Education. (2008). *National Educational Technology Standards for Teachers*. (http://www.iste.org/AM/Template.cfm?Section=NETS)

International Society for Technology in Education. (2008). *National Education Technology Standards for Teachers*. Online document. Retrieved July 16, 2008, from http://www.iste.org/Content/NavigationMenu/NETS/ForTeachers/2008Standards/NETS_for_Teachers_2008.htm

Isiksal, M., & Askar, P. (2005). The effect of spreadsheet and dynamic geometry software on the achievement and self-efficacy of 7th-grade students. *Educational Research, 47*(3), 333–350. doi:10.1080/00131880500287815

ISTE. (2008). *International Society for Technology Education teacher standards*. Retrieved April 10, 2009, from http://www.iste.org/Content/NavigationMenu/NETS/ForTeachers/2008Standards/NETS_ or_Teachers_2008.htm

Jaworski, B. (2006). Theory and practice in mathematics teaching development: Critical inquiry as a mode of learning in teaching. *Journal of Mathematics Teacher Education*, *9*(2), 187–211. doi:10.1007/s10857-005-1223-z

Jegede, O., Fraser, B. J., & Fisher, D. L. (1998). *The distance and open learning environment scale: Its development, validation and use.* Paper presented at the 69th Annual Meeting of the National Association for Research in Science Teaching, San Diego, USA.

Jenkins, H., Clinton, K., Purushotma, R., Robison, A. J., & Weigel, M. (2006). Confronting the challenges of participatory culture: media education for the 21st century. *The MacArthur Report: Building the Field of Digital Media and Learning.* Retrieved February 7, 2008, from http://digitallearning.macfound.org/site/c.enJLKQNlFiG/b.2029291/k.97E5/ Occasional_Papers.htm

Jenkins, S. (2008) *The impact of in-class service-learning on cognitive and affective learning outcomes.* Paper presented at the 2008 Annual Meeting of the American Political Science Association in Boston, MA. Kikin-Gil, R. (2006). Affective is effective: How information appliances can mediate relationships within communities and increase one's social effectiveness. *Personal and Ubiquitous Computing, 10*(2006), 77-83.

Jenning, H. (2005). Increasing value without increasing effort? The use of WebCT in accompanying face-to-face lectures under the constraint of low budget. *Journal of Distance Education*, *20*(2), 78–84.

Jetton, T. L. (2004). Using computer-mediated discussion to facilitate preservice teachers' understanding of literacy assessment and instruction. *Journal of Research on Technology in Education*, *36*(2), 171–191.

Jimoyiannis, A., & Komis, V. (2007). Examining teachers' beliefs about ICT in education: Implications of a teacher preparation programme. *Teacher Development*, *11*(2), 149–173. doi:10.1080/13664530701414779

Johnson, K. E., & Golombek, P. R. (2002). Inquiry into experience: Teachers' personal and professional growth. In Johnson, K. E., & Golombek, P. R. (Eds.), *Teachers' Narrative Inquiry as Professional Development* (pp. 1–14). Cambridge, UK: Cambridge University Press.

Johnston, C. J. (2009). *Pre-service elementary teachers planning for mathematics instruction: The role and evaluation of technology tools and their influence on lesson design.* Unpublished doctoral dissertation, George Mason University.

Jonassen, D. (1996). *Computers in the Classroom: Mind tools for Critical Thinking.* Englewood Cliffs, NJ: Prentice-Hall, Inc.

Jonassen, D. (2000). Instructional design model for well-structured and ill-structured problem solving learning outcomes. *Educational Technology Research and Development*, *45*(1), 65–95. doi:10.1007/BF02299613

Jonassen, D. H. (1997). Instructional design models for well-structured and ill-structured problem-solving learning outcomes. *Educational Technology Research and Development*, *45*(1), 1043–1629. doi:10.1007/BF02299613

Jonassen, D. H. (1999). Designing constructivist learning environments. In Reigeluth, C. M. (Ed.), *Instructional Theories and Models: A New Paradigm of Instructional Theory* (2nd ed., pp. 215–239). Mahwah, NJ: Lawrence Erlbaum Associates.

Jonassen, D. H. (2002). Integration of problem solving into instructional design. In Reiser, R. A., & Dempsey, J. V. (Eds.), *Instructional Design and Technology* (pp. 107–122). Upper Saddle River, NJ: Merrill Prentice Hall.

Jonassen, D. H., Carr, C., & Yueh, H. (1998). Computers as mindtools for engaging learners in critical thinking. *TechTrends*, *43*(2), 24–32. doi:10.1007/BF02818172

Jones, P. D. (2008). Using ePortfolios. *Modern English Teacher*, *17*(4), 53–59.

Jung, I. (2005). ICT-Pedagogy Integration in Teacher Training: Application Cases Worldwide. *Educational Technology &Society*, *8*(2), 94–101.

Kafai, Y., Franke, M., & Battey, D. (2002). Educational software reviews under investigation. *Education Communication and Information*, *2*, 163–180. doi:10.1080/1463631021000025349

Kamin, S. N., Capitanu, B., Twidale, M., & Peiper, C. (2008). A "teacher's dashboard" for a high school algebra class. In Reed, R., Berque, D., & Prey, J. C. (Eds.), *The Impact of Tablet PCs and Pen-based Technology on Education: Evidence and Outcomes* (pp. 63–71). West Lafayette, IN: Purdue University Press.

Kante, C. (2002). E-training: The new frontier of the teacher professional development. *TechKnowLogia*, *4*(4), 12–14.

Kaplan, R. M., & Sacusso, D. P. (1993). *Psychological testing: Principles, applications, and issues.* Belmont, CA: Wadsworth.

Kastberg, S., & Leatham, K. (2005). Research on graphing calculators at the secondary level: Implications for mathematics teacher education. *Contemporary Issues in Technology & Teacher Education*, *5*, 25–37.

Kay, R. H. (2006). Evaluating Strategies Used to Incorporate Technology into Preservice Education: A Review of the Literature. *Journal of Research on Technology in Education*, *38*(4), 383–408.

Kersaint, G. (2007). Toward technology integration in mathematics education: A technology-integration course planning assignment. *Contemporary Issues in Technology & Teacher Education*, *7*, 256–278.

Kersaint, G., Horton, B., Stohl, H., & Garofalo, J. (2003). Technology beliefs and practices of mathematics education faculty. *Journal of Technology and Teacher Education*, *11*(4), 567–595.

Kian-Sam, H., & Lee, J. C. (2008). Postgraduate students' knowledge construction during asynchronous computer conferences in a blended learning environment: A Malaysian experience. *Australasian Journal of Educational Technology*, *24*(1), 91–107.

Kim, K., Sachin, J., Westhoff, G., & Rezabek, L. (2008). A quantitative exploration of preservice teachers' intent to use computer-based technology. *Journal of Instructional Psychology*, *35*(3), 275–287.

King, K. (2007). *New technology to revolutionize teaching and learning.* Charlotte, NC: Information Age Publishing.

Klecker, B., Lennex L., & Lackner, K. (2004). *Evaluating the integration of technology in a teacher preparation program.* (ERIC Document Reproduction Service No. ED 481667).

Klein, S. (Ed.). (2007). *Handbook of gender equity* (2nd ed.). New York: Lawrence Erlbaum.

Klopfer, E. (2008). *Augmented Learning Research and Design for Mobile Educational Games.* Cambridge, MA: MIT Press.

Knox, K. L., Moynihan, J. A., & Markowitz, D. G. (2003). Evaluation of short-term impact of a high school summer science program on students' perceived knowledge and skills. *Journal of Science Education and Technology*, *12*(4), 471–478. doi:10.1023/B:JOST.0000006306.97336.c5

Koehler, M. J., & Mishra, P. (2005). What happens when teachers design educational technology? The development of technological pedagogical content knowledge. *Journal of Educational Computing Research*, *32*(2), 131–152. doi:10.2190/0EW7-01WB-BKHL-QDYV

Koehler, M. J., & Mishra, P. (2008). Introducing TPCK. In AACTE Committee on Innovation and Technology (Ed.), Handbook of technological pedagogical content knowledge (TPCK) for educators (pp. 3-29). New York: Routledge.

Koehler, M., & Mishra, P. (2006). Introducing tpck. In AACTE committee on innovation and technology (Eds.), Handbook of technological pedagogical content knowledge (tpck) for educators (pp. 3-31). London: Routledge Press.

Kolaitis, M., Mahoney, M. A., & Pomann, H. (2006). Training ourselves to train our students for CALL. In Hubbard, P., & Levy, M. (Eds.), *Teacher Education in CALL* (pp. 317–314). Philadelphia, PA: John Benjamins Publishing Company.

Kolalchick, A., & Milman, N. B. (1998). Instructional strategies for integrating Technology: Electronic journals and technology portfolios as facilitators for self-efficacy and reflection in preservice teachers. *Technology and Teacher Education Annual, 3-7.*

Kolb, D. A. (1984). *Experiential learning.* Englewood Cliffs, NJ: Prentice-Hall.

Kollar, I., Fischer, F., & Slotta, J. (2007). Internal and external scripts in computer-supported collaborative inquiry learning. *Learning and Instruction, 17*(6), 708–721. doi:10.1016/j.learninstruc.2007.09.021

Kolstø, S. D. (2006). Patterns in students' argumentation controlled with a risk-focused socio-scientific issue. *International Journal of Science Education, 28*(14), 1689–1716. doi:10.1080/09500690600560878

Korthagen, F. A. J. (2001). *Linking practice and theory: the pedagogy of realistic teacher education.* Paper presented at the Annual Meeting of the American Educational Research Association, Seattle, April 2001.

Kosheleva, O., Medina-Rusch, A., & Ioudina, V. (2007). Pre-service teacher training in mathematics using tablet PC technology. *Informatics in Education, 6*(2), 321–334.

Krajcik, J. S., & Blumenfeld, P. C. (1994). A collaborative model for helping middle grade science teachers learn project-based instruction. *The Elementary School Journal, 94*(5), 483. doi:10.1086/461779

Krathwohl, D. R. (1997). *Methods of educational and social science research: An integrated approach.* New York: Addison-Wesley.

Kress, T., & Silva, K. (2009). Using digital video for professional development and leadership: understanding and initiating teacher learning communities, In C. Crawford et al. (Eds.), *Proceedings of Society for Information Technology and Teacher Education International Conference 2009* (pp. 2841-2847). Chesapeake, VA: AACE.

Krueger, K., Hansen, L., & Smaldino, S. (2000). Preservice teacher technology competencies: A model for preparing teachers of tomorrow to use technology. *TechTrends, 44*(3), 47–50. doi:10.1007/BF02778227

Kuhn, D. (1991). *The skills of argument.* Cambridge, UK: Cambridge University Press.

Kuhn, D. (1999). A developmental model of critical thinking. *Educational Research, 28*(2), 16–25.

Kumar, D. D., & Altshuld, J. W. (2002). Complimentary approaches to evaluating technology in science teacher education. In Kumar, D. D., & Altshuld, J. W. (Eds.), *Evaluation of Science and Technology Education at the dawn of the new millennium* (pp. 165–185). New York: Kluwer Academics. doi:10.1007/0-306-47560-X_7

Kumar, S. (2007). Professor Use, Facilitation, and Evaluation of Asynchronous Online Discussions in On-campus Courses. In C. Montgomerie & J. Seale (Eds.), *Proceedings of World Conference on Educational Multimedia, Hypermedia and Telecommunications 2007* (pp. 2855-2863). Chesapeake, VA: AACE.

Kurz, T. L., Middleton, J. A., & Yanik, H. B. (2005). A taxonomy of software for mathematics education. *Contemporary Issues in Technology & Teacher Education, 5,* 123–137.

Kurz, T., & Middleton, J. A. (2006). Using a functional approach to change preservice teachers' understanding of mathematics software. *Journal of Research on Technology in Education, 39,* 45–65.

Kurz, T., Middleton, J., & Yanik, H. B. (2004). Preservice teachers' conceptions of mathematics-based software. In. *Proceedings of the International Group for the Psychology of Mathematics Education, 28,* 313–320.

Kurz, T., Middleton, J., & Yanik, H. B. (2004). Preservice teachers' conceptions of mathematics-based software. In. *Proceedings of the International Group for the Psychology of Mathematics Education, 28,* 313–320.

Kuutti, K. (1996). Activity theory as a potential framework for human-computer interaction research. In

Lacey, M. (December 7, 2008). A lifestyle distinct: The muxe of Mexico. *The New York Times, Week in Review,* 4.

Lam, W. (2004). Encouraging on-line participation. *Journal of Information Systems Education, 15*(4), 345–349.

Lampert, M., & Ball, D. (1999). Aligning teacher education with contemporary K-12 reform visions. In Darling-Hammond, L., & Sykes, G. (Eds.), *Teaching as the learning professions: Handbook of policy and practice* (pp. 33–53). San Francisco, CA: Jossey Bass.

Lankshear, C., & Knobel, M. (2006). *New literacies: Changing knowledge in the classroom*. Maidenhead, UK: Open University Press.

Laurinen, L., & Marttunen, M. (2007). Written arguments and collaborative speech acts in practicing the argumentative power of language though chat debates. *Computers and Composition*, *24*(3), 230–246. doi:10.1016/j.compcom.2007.05.002

Lave, J., & Wenger, E. (1991). *Situated learning: Legitimate peripheral participation*. Cambridge, UK: Cambridge University Press.

Lavooy, M. J., & Newlin, M. H. (2003). Computer Mediated Communication: Online Instruction and Interactivity. *Journal of Interactive Learning Research*, *14*(2), 157–165.

Lawrenz, F., Gravely, A., & Ooms, A. (2006). Perceived helpfulness and amount of use of technology in science and mathematics classes at different grade levels. *School Science and Mathematics*, *106*, 133–137. doi:10.1111/j.1949-8594.2006.tb18170.x

Leckie, M., St. John, K., Peart, L., Klaus, A., Slough, S., & Niemitz, M. (2006). The School of Rock Expedition: Education and Science Connect at Sea Aboard the U.S. Scientific Drilling Vessel: A model for integrating cutting-edge ocean-going science with educational initiatives. *EOS*, *87*(24), 240–241.

LeCompte, M. D., & Preissle, J. (1993). *Ethnography and qualitative design in educational research*. New York: Academic Press.

Lederman, N. (2007). Nature of science: Past, present, and future. In Abell, S. K., & Lederman, N. G. (Eds.), *Handbook of research on science education* (pp. 831–879). Mahwah, NJ: Lawrence Erlbaum Associates.

Lee, J. K. (2008). Toward democracy: Social studies and TPCK. In the AACTE Committee on Innovation and Technology (Ed.), Handbook of technological pedagogical content knowledge (TPCK) for educators (pp. 129-144). New York: Routledge.

Lee, M. J. W., Chan, A., & McLoughlin, C. (2008). Talk the talk: Learner-generated podcasts as catalysts for knowledge creation. *British Journal of Educational Technology*, *39*(3), 501–521. doi:10.1111/j.1467-8535.2007.00746.x

Lee-Baldwin, J. (2005). Asynchronous discussion forums: A closer look at the structure, focus and group dynamics that facilitate reflective thinking. *Contemporary Issues in Technology & Teacher Education*, *5*(1), 93–115.

Lehman, J. D., Richardson, J., Malewski, E., & Phillion, J. (2005). Technology connections in teacher education: Lessons from faculty development, electronic portfolios, and virtual field experiences involving distant locations. In Rhine, S., & Bailey, M. (Eds.), *Integrated technologies, innovative learning: Insights from the PT3 program* (pp. 129–141). Eugene, OR: International Society for Technology in Education.

Lei, J. (2009). Digital natives as preservice teachers: What technology preparation is needed? *Journal of Computing in Teacher Education*, *25*(3), 87–97.

Leming, J. S., Ellington, L., & Schug, M. (2006). The state of social studies: A national random survey of elementary and middle school social studies teachers. *Social Education*, *70*(5), 322–327.

Lenhart, A. (2003). The ever-shifting Internet population: A new look at Internet access and the digital divide. *Pew Internet & American Life Project*. Retrieved November 7, 2007, from http://www.pewinternet.org/report_display.asp?r=88

Lenhart, A., & Madden, M. (2005). Teen content creators and consumers. *Pew Internet & American Life Project*. Retrieved November 7, 2007, from http://www.pewinternet.org/PPF/r/166/report_display.asp

Lenhart, A., & Madden, M. (2007). Social networking websites and teens: An overview. *Pew Internet & American Life Project*. Retrieved November 7, 2007, from http://www.pewinternet.org/PPF/r/198/report_display.asp

Lennex, L. (2006). Is this on the test? Technology integration perception in teacher education classes. In C. Crawford et al. (Eds.), *Proceedings of Society for Information Technology and Teacher Education International Conference 2006* (pp. 1695-1700). Chesapeake, VA: AACE.

Lennex, L. (2007). The faculty Web page: contrivance or continuation? *TechTrends*, *51*(5), 32–37. doi:10.1007/s11528-007-0067-z

Lennex, L. (2008). Digital natives and the use of video iPods: a Lewis and Clark expedition. In C. Crawford et al. (Eds.), *Proceedings of Society for Information Technology and Teacher Education International Conference 2008* (pp. 4913-4915). Chesapeake, VA: AACE.

Lennex, L., & Flynn, H. (2009). Wisely using cyberspace: needs analysis of P-12 teacher Web pages. In C. Crawford et al. (Eds.), *Proceedings of Society for Information Technology and Teacher Education International Conference 2009* (pp. 3473-3480). Chesapeake, VA: AACE.

Lennex, L., & Nettleton, K. (2009). *Ipods & the iLRN theory: A new vision for classroom Connections*. Unpublished raw data.

Lerner, G. (1985). *The creation of patriarchy*. New York: Oxford University Press.

Lerner, G. (1992). *The creation of feminist consciousness*. New York: Oxford University Press.

Lesh, R., & Zawojewski, J. S. (2007). Problem solving and modeling. In F. K. Lester, Jr. (Ed.). The Second Handbook of Research on Mathematics Teaching and Learning (pp. 763-804). National Council of Teachers of Mathematics. Charlotte, NC: Information Age Publishing.

Leuhmann, A. (2007). Identity development as a lens to science teacher preparation. *Science Education*, *91*(5), 822–839. doi:10.1002/sce.20209

Lever-Duffy, J., McDonald, J. B., & Mizell, A. P. (2005). *Teaching and learning with technology* (2nd ed.). Boston, MA: Pearson Education, Inc.

Levin, B. B. (1995). Using the case method in teacher education: The role of discussion and experience in teachers' thinking about cases. *Teaching and Teacher Education*, *11*(1), 63–79. doi:10.1016/0742-051X(94)00013-V

Levin, D., & Arafeh, S. (2002). *The digital disconnect: The widening gap between Internet-savvy students and their schools*. Washington, DC: Pew Internet & American Life Project. Retrieved March 14, 2007, from http://www.pewinternet.org/pdfs/PIP_Schools_Internet_Report.pdf

Li, Q. (2005). Infusing technology into a mathematics methods course: Any impact? *Educational Research*, *47*, 217–233. doi:10.1080/00131880500104341

Lieb, B. (1992). *Proceedings of the OERI study group on educating teachers for world class standards: The challenge for education teachers*. Washington, DC: US Department of Education.

Lightbody, P., & Durndell, A. (1996). The masculine image of careers in science and technology: Fact or fantasy? *The British Journal of Educational Psychology*, *66*, 231–246.

Lin, C.-Y. (2008). Beliefs about using technology in the mathematics classroom. Interviews with preservice elementry teachers. *Eurasia Journal of Mathematics, Science, and Technology Education*, *4*(2), 135–142.

Lin, J. M. (2008). ICT education: To integrate or not to integrate? *British Journal of Educational Technology*, *39*(6), 1121–1123. doi:10.1111/j.1467-8535.2008.00825.x

Lin, Q. (2008). Preservice teachers' learning experiences of constructing e-portfolios online. *The Internet and Higher Education*, *11*(3-4), 194–200. doi:10.1016/j.iheduc.2008.07.002

Lin, X., & Kinzer, C. K. (2003). The importance of technology for making cultural values visible. *Theory into Practice*, *42*(3), 234–242. doi:10.1207/s15430421tip4203_10

Lincoln, Y. S., & Guba, E. G. (1985). *Naturalistic Inquiry*. Beverly Hills, CA: Sage Publications.

Lipper, D., & Sagehorn, E. (2007). How to hire tech-savvy teachers. Interactive educator, (Winter), 28-32.

Lipsman, A. (2007). *Social Networking Goes Global*. Retrieved March 22, 2009, from http://www.comscore.com/press/release.asp?press=1555

Little, J. W. (1993). Professional community in comprehensive high schools: The two worlds of academic and vocational teachers. In Little, J. W., & McLaughlin, M. W. (Eds.), *Teachers' work: Individuals, colleagues, and contexts*. New York: Teachers College Press.

Lockyer, L., & Patterson, J. (2007). Technology use, technology views: Anticipating ICT use for beginning physical and health education teachers. *Issues in Informing Science and Information Technology*, *4*, 261–267.

Löfström, E., & Nevgi, A. (2008). University teaching staffs' pedagogical awareness displayed in ICT-facilitated teaching. *Interactive Learning Environments*, *16*(2), 101–116. doi:10.1080/10494820701282447

Lohr, L. L. (2000). Designing the instructional interface. *Computers in Human Behavior*, *16*, 161–182. doi:10.1016/S0747-5632(99)00057-6

Lord, G., & Lomicka, L. (2007). Foreign language teacher preparation and asynchronous CMC: Promoting reflective teaching. *Journal of Technology and Teacher Education*, *15*(4), 513–532.

Lord, G., & Lomicka, L. (2008). Blended learning in teacher education: An investigation of classroom community across media. *Contemporary Issues in Technology & Teacher Education*, *8*(2), 158–174.

Lortie, D. C. (1975). *Schoolteacher: A sociological study*. Chicago, IL: University of Chicago Press.

Lowther, D., & Morrison, G. (1998). The NTeQ model: a framework for technology integration. [from Education Full Text database.]. *TechTrends*, *43*, 33–38. Retrieved April 9, 2009. doi:10.1007/BF02818173

Lowther, D., Ross, S., & Morrison, G. (2003). When Each One Has One: The Influences on Teaching Strategies and Student Achievement of Using Laptops in the Classroom. [from Education Full Text database.]. *Educational Technology Research and Development*, *51*(3), 23–44. Retrieved April 9, 2009. doi:10.1007/BF02504551

Luke, N., Moore, J. L., & Sawyer, S. B. (1998). *Authentic approaches to encourage technology-using teachers*. Paper presented at the Society for Information Technology & Teacher Education International Conference, Washington, DC. ERIC Document #ED421083.

Lund, K., Molinari, G., Séjourné, A., & Baker, M. (2007). How do argumentation diagrams compare when student pairs use them as a means to debate or as a tool for representing debate? *International Journal of Computer-Supported Collaborative Learning*, *2*(2–3), 273–295. doi:10.1007/s11412-007-9019-z

Lyons, N. (1998). Reflection in teaching: Can it be developmental? A portfolio perspective. *Teacher Education Quarterly*, *25*(1), 115–127.

Lyublinskaya, I. (2003a). *Connecting Mathematics with Science: Experiments for Precalculus*. Emeryville, CA: Key Curriculum Press.

Lyublinskaya, I. (2003b). *Connecting Mathematics and Science: Experiments for Calculus*. Emeryville, CA: Key Curriculum Press.

Lyublinskaya, I. (2009). *Technology Activities for Elementary Mathematics and Science* (2nd ed.). Long Island, NY: Whittier Publications.

Lyublinskaya, I., & Zhou, G. (2008). Integrating Graphing Calculators and Probeware into Science Methods Courses: Impact on Preservice Elementary Teachers' Confidence and Perspectives on Technology for Learning and Teaching. *Journal of Computers in Mathematics and Science Teaching*, *27*(2), 163–182.

MacArthur, C. A. (2006). The effects of new technologies on writing and writing processes. In MacArthur, C. A., Graham, S., & Fitzgerald, J. (Eds.), *Handbook of writing research* (pp. 248–262). New York: Guilford.

MacDonald, R. J. (2008). Professional development for information communication technology integration: Identifying and supporting a community of practice through design-based research. *Journal of Research on Technology in Education*, *40*(3), 429–445.

MacDonald, R. J., & Larter, A. (2007, October). A professional learning community in senior high science: Data logging and learner-centeredness. In. *Proceedings of World Conference on E-Learning in Corporate, Government, Healthcare, and Higher Education, 2007*, 1044–1049.

Mackey, J. (2008). *Blending real work experiences and virtual professional development.* Paper presented at ASCILITE 2008 conference, Institute of Teaching and Learning, Deakin University, Melbourne, Australia

MacKinnon, G. R., Aylward, M. L., & Bellafontaine, J. (2006). Electronic discussion: A case study of the range of applications in a laptop university. *Computers in the Schools, 23*(1/2), 59–71. doi:10.1300/J025v23n01_06

Magenheim, J. (2003). Social, affective and normative aspects of learning in ICT-enriched learning environments: collaborative exploration of societal aspects of ICT. In. *Proceedings of the Conferences in Research and Practice in Information Technology Series, 23*, 85–88.

Maher, M., & Jacob, E. (2006). Peer computer conferencing to support teachers' reflection during action research. *Journal of Technology and Teacher Education, 14*(1), 127–150.

Malinowski, B. (1944). *A scientific theory of culture and other essays.* Chapel Hill, NC: University of North Carolina Press.

Mandryk, R. L., Inkpen, K. M., Bilezkjian, M., Klemmer, S. R., & Landay, J. A. (2001). Supporting children's collaboration across handheld computers. In *Proceedings of CHI, Conference on Human Factors in Computing Systems*, Seattle, WA.

Manfra, M. M., Friedman, A. M., Hammond, T. C., & Lee, J. K. (2009, March). *Peering behind the curtain: Digital history, historiography, and secondary social studies methods.* Presentation at the annual meeting of the Society for Information Technology and Teacher Education (SITE), Charleston, SC.

Marcum-Dietrich, N. I., & Ford, D. J. (2002). The place for the computer is in the laboratory: An Investigation of the effect of computer probeware on student learning. *Journal of Computers in Mathematics and Science Teaching, 21*, 361–379.

Margerum-Leys, J., & Marx, R. W. (2002). Teacher knowledge of educational technology: a case study of student/mentor teacher pairs. *Journal of Educational Computing Research, 26*(4), 427–462. doi:10.2190/JXBR-2G0G-1E4T-7T4M

Markauskaite, L. (2007). Exploring the structure of trainee teachers' ICT literacy: The main components of, and relationships between, general cognitive and technical capabilities. *Educational Technology Research and Development, 55*, 547–572. doi:10.1007/s11423-007-9043-8

Market Data Retrieval. (2005). The K-12 [Shelton, CT: Author.]. *Technology Review*, 2004–2005.

Markowitz, D. G. (2004). Evaluation of the long-term impact of a university high school summer science program on students' interest and perceived abilities in science. *Journal of Science Education and Technology, 13*(3), 395–407. doi:10.1023/B:JOST.0000045467.67907.7b

Markus, H., & Nurius, P. (1986, September). Possible selves. *The American Psychologist, 41*(9), 954–969. doi:10.1037/0003-066X.41.9.954

Martin, B. L., & Reigeluth, C. M. (1999). Affective education and the affective domain: Implications for instructional-design theories and models. In Reigeluth, C. M. (Ed.), *Instructional-design theories and models: A new paradigm of instructional theory* (*Vol. 2*, pp. 485–509). London: Lawrence Erlbaum Associates.

Martindale, T., & Wiley, D. A. (2005). Using weblogs in scholarship and teaching. *Techtrends Linking Research and Practice to Improve Learning, 49*(2), 55–61.

Martorella, P. H. (1997). Technology and social studies: Which way to the sleeping giant? *Theory and Research in Social Education, 25*(4), 511–514.

Marttunen, M., & Laurinen, L. (2001). Learning of argumentation skills in networked and face-to-face environments. *Instructional Science, 29*(2), 127–153. doi:10.1023/A:1003931514884

Marttunen, M., Laurinen, L., Litosseliti, L., & Lund, K. (2005). Argumentation skills as prerequisites for collaborative learning among Finnish, French and English secondary school students. *Educational Research and Evaluation, 11*(4), 365–384. doi:10.1080/13803610500110588

Martyn, M. (2003). The hybrid online model: Good practice. *EDUCAUSE Quarterly, 6*(1), 18–23.

Mason, C., Berson, M., & Diem, R. Hicks, Lee, J., & Dralle, T. (2000). Guidelines for using technology to prepare social studies teachers. *Contemporary Issues in Technology and Teacher Education, 1*(3), 386-394. Retrieved April 7, 2009, from http://www.citejournal.org/vol1/iss1/currentissues/socialstudies/article1.htm

Mason, C., Berson, M., Diem, R., Hicks, D., Lee, J., & Dralle, T. (2000). Guidelines for using technology to prepare social studies teachers. *Contemporary Issues in Technology and Teacher Education, 1*(1). Retrieved July 7, 2009, from http://www.citejournal.org/vol1/iss1/currentissues/socialstudies/article1.htm

Matzen, N. J., & Edmunds, J. A. (2007). Technology as a catalyst for change: the role of professional development. *Journal of Research on Technology in Education, 39*(4), 417–430.

Mayer, D. (2002). An electronic lifeline:Information and communication technologies in a teacher education internship. *Asia-Pacific Journal of Teacher Education, 30*(2), 181–195. doi:10.1080/13598660220135685

Mayer, R. E. (2001). *Multimedia learning.* New York: Cambridge University Press.

Mc Gee, P., & Diaz, V. (2007). Wikis, and podcasts and blogs! Oh, my! What is a faculty member supposed to do? *Educause, 42*(5), 28–41.

McAlister, M., Dunn, J., & Quin, L. (2005). Student teachers' attitudes to and use of computers to teach mathematics in primary mathematics classrooms. *Technology, Pedagogy and Education, 14*(1), 77–105. doi:10.1080/14759390500200194

McCarthy, S., & Youens, B. (2005). Strategies used by science student teachers for subject knowledge development: A focus on peer support. *Research in Science & Technological Education, 23*(2), 149–162. doi:10.1080/02635140500266377

McCloud, S. (1993). *Understanding comics.* Northampton, MA: Kitchen Sink Press.

McCloud, S. (2000). *Re-inventing comics.* Northampton, MA: Kitchen Sink Press.

McConnell, D. (2006). *E-learning groups and communities.* Berkshire, UK: Open University Press.

McFarlane, A., & Sakellariou, S. (2002). The role of ICT in science education. *Cambridge Journal of Education, 32*(2), 219–232. doi:10.1080/03057640220147568

McKernan, J. (1988). The countenance of curriculum action research: Traditional, collaborative, and emancipatory-critical conceptions. *Journal of Curriculum and Supervision, 3*(3), 173–200.

McKinney, D., Dyck, J., & Luber, E. S. (2009, April). iTunes University and the classroom: Can podcasts replace Professors? *Computers & Education, 52*(3), 617–623. doi:10.1016/j.compedu.2008.11.004

McLeskey, J., & Billingsley, B. S. (2008). How does the quality and stability of the teaching force influence the research-to-practice gap?: A perspective on the teacher shortage in special education. *Remedial and Special Education, 29*(5), 293–305. doi:10.1177/0741932507312010

McLoughlin, C., Lee, M. J. W., & Chan, A. (2006). Using student generated podcasts to foster reflection and metacognition. *Australian Educational Computing, 21*(2), 34–40.

McNeir, G. (1993). Outcome Based Education: Tool for restructuring. *Oregon School Study Council (OSSC). Bulletin, 36*(8).

Means, B., Penuel, W. R., & Padilla, C. (2001). *The connected school: Technology and learning in high school.* San Francisco: Jossey-Bass.

Means, M. L., & Voss, J. F. (1996). Who reasons well? Two studies of informal reasoning among children of different grade, ability, and knowledge level. *Cognition and Instruction, 14*(2), 139–178. doi:10.1207/s1532690xci1402_1

Medcalf-Davenport, N. (1999). Historical and current attitudes toward uses of educational technology. In Price, J. D., Willis, J., Willis, D. A., Jost, M., & Boger-Mehall, S. (Eds.), *The information technology and teacher education annual* (pp. 1424–1428). Charlottesville, VA: Association for the Advancement of Computers in Education.

Meel, D. E. (1997). Calculator-available assessment: The why, what, and how. *Educational Assessment, 4*(3), 149–174. doi:10.1207/s15326977ea0403_1

Meier, D. (2002). Standardization versus standards. *Phi Delta Kappan, 84*(3), 190–198.

Meiers, M., & Ingvarson, L. (2004). *Investigating the links between teacher professional development and student learning outcomes. Australian Government Quality Teacher Programme over 2001–2003. Australia council of educational research.* Commonwealth of Australia.

Merriam, S. B. (2001). Andragogy and self-directed learning. *New Directions for Adult and Continuing Education, 89,* 3–14. doi:10.1002/ace.3

Metiri Group. (2006). *1:1 Learning: A review and analysis by the Metiri group.* Retrieved June 30, 2009, from http://www.k12blueprint.com/k12/blueprint/story_11_learning_a_review.php

Meyer, K. A. (2002). *Quality in distance education: Focus on on-line learning.* Hoboken, NJ: Jossey-Bass.

Meyer, K. A. (2003). Face-to-face versus threaded discussions: the role of time and higher-order thinking. *JALN, 3*(7), 55–65.

Mezirow, J. (1990). *Fostering critical reflection in adulthood: A guide to transformative and emancipatory learning.* San Francisco: Jossey-Bass.

Mezirow, J. (1991). *Transformative dimension of adult learning.* San Francisco: Jossey-Bass.

Mezirow, J. (2003). Transformative Learning as Discourse. *Journal of Transformative Education, 1*(1), 58–63. doi:10.1177/1541344603252172

Michael, D., & Chen, S. (2006). *Serious games: games that educate, train and inform.* Boston, MA: Thomson Course Technology.

Middleton, A., & McCarter, R. (2005). Engaging solutions: a collaborative approach to digital audio learning object (DALO) production. Workshop presented at ALT-C 2005, Manchester, UK, September 6–8, 2005.

Milken Family Foundation. (2001). *Information technology underused in teacher education.* Retrieved February 2, 2006, from http://www.mff.org/edtech/article.taf?_function=detail&Content_uid1=131

Miller, C. V., & Doering, A. (2008). Curriculum at forty below: a phenomenological inquiry of an educator/explorer's experience with adventure learning in the Arctic. *Distance Education, 29*(3), 253–267. doi:10.1080/01587910802395789

Milner, J. (2006). Tablet PCs: The write approach. *T.H.E. Journal, 33*(9), 20–26.

Minnebo, J., & Eggermont, S. (2007). Watching the young use illicit drugs: Direct experience, exposure to television and the stereotyping of adolescents' use substance use. *Young, 15*(2), 129–144. doi:10.1177/110330880701500202

Mio, A. (2006). Effect of experience in immersive vr on application image. In C. Crawford et al. (Eds.), *Proceedings of Society for Information Technology and Teacher Education International Conference 2006* (pp. 1385-1392). Chesapeake, VA: AACE

Mishra, P., & Koehler, M. J. (2006). Technological pedagogical content knowledge: A framework for teacher knowledge. *Teachers College Record, 108*(6), 1017–1054. doi:10.1111/j.1467-9620.2006.00684.x

Mitchell, R. S. (2007, May). PC Tablet Project. *Reprint of the Proceedings of the 1st International Workshop on Pen-Based Learning Technologies, Enabling Advanced Graphical, Multimodal and Mobile Learning Interactions (PLT 2007),* Aula Magna, Universita' degli Studi di Catania, Catania, Italy.

Mizuko, I., Horst, H., & Bittanti, M. boyd, D., Herr-Stephenson, B., Lange, P. G., Pascoe, C. J., & Robinson, L. (2008). Living and Learning with New Media: Summary of Findings from the Digital Youth Project. *The MacArthur Report: Building the Field of Digital Media and Learning.* Retrieved March 28, 2009, from http://

digitallearning.macfound.org/site/c.enJLKQNlFiG/b.2029291/k.97E5/ Occasional_Papers.htm

Moja, T. (2004). Policy responses to global transformation by African higher education systems. In Zeleza, P. T., & Olukoshi, A. (Eds.), *African universities in the twenty-first century* (*Vol. 1*, pp. 21–41). Dakar, Senegal: CODESRIA.

Monaghan, J. (2004). Teachers' activities in technology-based mathematics lesson. *International Journal of Computers for Mathematical Learning*, *9*, 327–357. doi:10.1007/s10758-004-3467-6

Montgomerie, T. C., & Irvine, V. (2001). Computer skill requirements for new and existing teachers: Implications for policy and practice. *Journal of Teaching and Learning*, *1*(1), 43–55.

Morken, E. M., Divitini, M., & Haugalokkent, O. K. (2007). Enriching spaces in practice-based education to support collaboration while mobile: The case of teacher education. *Journal of Computer Assisted Learning*, *23*(4), 300–311. doi:10.1111/j.1365-2729.2007.00235.x

Moursand, D., & Bielefeldt, T. (1999). *Will new teachers be prepared to teach in a digital age?* Research study by the International Society for Technology in Education, commissioned by the Milken Exchange on Educational Technology. Milken Exchange on Educational Technology. Retrieved March 16, 2009, from http://www.mff.org/pubs/ME154.pdf

Moursund, D., & Bielefeldt, T. (1999). Will new teachers be prepared to teach in a digital age? A national survey on information technology in teacher education. Santa Monica, CA: Miliken Exchange on Education Technology (ERIC Document Reproduction Service No. ED 428 072).

Mouzakis, C. (2008). Teachers' perceptions of the effectiveness of a blended learning approach for ICT teacher training. *Journal of Technology and Teacher Education*, *16*(4), 459–481.

Moyer, P. S., Bolyard, J. J., & Spikell, M. A. (2002). What are virtual manipulatives? *Teaching Children Mathematics*, *8*, 372–377.

Munby, H., Russell, T., & Martin, A. K. (2001). Teachers' knowledge and how it develops. In Richardson, V. (Ed.), *Handbook of research on teaching* (*Vol. 4*, pp. 877–904). Washington, DC: American Educational Research Association.

Murphie, A., & Potts, J. (2003). *Culture & Technology*. New York: Palgrave Macmillan.

Murray, O., & Zembal-Saul, C. (2008). Educate at Penn State: Preparing beginning teachers with powerful digital tools. *Journal of Computing in Higher Education*, *20*, 48–58. doi:10.1007/s12528-008-9000-5

Nardi, B. (Ed.), *Context and consciousness: Activity theory and human-computer interaction* (pp. 17–44). Cambridge, MA: MIT Press.

Nardi, B. A. (1996). Activity theory and human-computer interaction. In Nardi, B. A. (Ed.), *Context and Consciousness* (pp. 7–16). Cambridge, MA: The MIT Press.

Nardi, B. A., & O'Day, V. L. (1999). *Information ecologies: Using technology with heart*. Cambridge, MA: The MIT Press.

National Center for Education Statistics. (2001). *The nation's report card: Mathematics 2000 (NCES Publication 2001-517)*. Washington, DC: US Department of Education.

National Center for Education Statistics. (2003, October). *Internet access in U.S. public schools and classrooms: 1994–2002* (Report No. NCES 2004-011). Washington, DC: U.S. Department of Education.

National Center for History in the Schools. (2005). *Overview of standards in historical thinking*. Retrieved January 23, 2009, from http://nchs.ucla.edu/standards/thinking5-12.html

National Council for the Accreditation of Teacher Education. (1997). *Technology and teacher education: New standards*. Washington, DC: Author.

National Council for the Social Studies. (2006). *Technology Position Statement and Guidelines*. Retrieved on February 19, 2009, from http://www.socialstudies.org/positions/technology

National Council of Teachers of English. (2008). *The NCTE Definition of 21st Century Literacies*. Retrieved on February 19, 2009, from http://www.ncte.org/positions/statements/21stcentdefinition

National Council of Teachers of Mathematics. (2000). *Principles and standards for school mathematics*. Reston, VA: Author.

National Council of Teachers of Mathematics. (2009). *Illuminations*. Retrieved from http://illuminations.nctm.org/

National Institute for Health and Welfare. (2008). *School Health Promotion Study*. Retrieved February 1, 2009, from http://info.stakes.fi/kouluterveys/tulokset/koko2008pk.pdf.

National Professional Development Center on Inclusion. (2008). *What do we mean by professional development in the early childhood field?* Chapel Hill, NC: The University of North Carolina, FPG Child Development Institute. Retrieved January 10, 2009, from http://community.fpg.unc.edu/resources/articles/NPDCI-ProfessionalDevelopment-03-04-08.pdf

National Research Council [NRC]. (1996). *National science education standards*. Retrieved January 10, 2006, from http://www.nap.edu/readingroom/books/nses/

National Research Council. (1996). *National Science Education Standards*. Washington, DC: National Academy Press.

National Research Council. (2000). *Principles and standards for school mathematics*. Reston, VA: National Council of Teachers of Mathematics.

National Science Teacher Association. (1999, January). *Use of Computers in Science Education*. Retrieved on February 19, 2009, from http://www.nsta.org/about/positions/computers.aspx

NCSESA & NRC. (1996). *National Science Education Standards*. Washington, DC: National Academy Press.

NCTM. (2000). *Principles and standards for school mathematics*. Reston, VA: Author.

NCTM. (2009). *Focus on high school mathematics: Reasoning and sense making*. Reston, VA: The Council.

Neiss, M. L. (2008a). Knowledge needed for teaching with technologies – Call it TPACK. *AMTE Connection, 17*(2), 9–10.

Neiss, M. L. (2008b). Teaching with technology: Standards for mathematics teachers. *AMTE Connection, 18*(1), 9–10.

Nguyen, T., & Katz, J. (2007). Learning Contract for Online Course Design. In C. Crawford et al. (Eds.), *Proceedings of Society for Information Technology and Teacher Education International Conference 2007* (pp. 2377-2380). Chesapeake, VA: AACE.

Nicholson, S. A., & Bond, N. (2003). Collaborative reflection and community building: An analysis of preservice teachers' use of an electronic discussion board. *Journal of Technology and Teacher Education, 11*(2), 259–279.

Niemitz, M., Slough, S., Peart, L., Klaus, A., Leckie, M., & St. John, K. (2008). Interactive Virtual Expeditions as a Learning Tool: The School of Rock Expedition. *Journal of Educational Multimedia and Hypermedia, 17*(4), 561–580.

Niess, M. (2001). A Model for Integrating Technology in Preservice Science and Mathematics Content-Specific Teacher Preparation. *School Science and Mathematics, 101*(2), 102–109. doi:10.1111/j.1949-8594.2001.tb18011.x

Niess, M. L. (2005). Preparing teachers to teach science and mathematics with technology: Developing a technology pedagogical content knowledge. *Teaching and Teacher Education, 21*(5), 509–523. doi:10.1016/j.tate.2005.03.006

Niess, M. L. (2008). Guiding preservice teachers to develop TPCK. In AACTE committee on Innovation and Technology (Eds.), Handbook of Technological Pedagogical Content Knowledge (TPCK) for Educators (223-250). New York: Routledge.

Niess, M. L., Ronau, R. N., Driskell, S. O., Kosheleva, O., Pugalee, D., & Weinhold, M. W. (2008). Technological pedagogical content knowledge (TPCK), Preparation of mathematics teachers for 21st century teaching and learning. In Arbaugh, F., & Taylor, P. M. (Eds.), *Inquiry into mathematics teacher education. Association of Mathematics Teacher Educators (AMTE)* (*Vol. 5*). Monograph Series.

Niess, M. L., Ronau, R. N., Shafer, K. G., Driskell, S. O., Harper, S. R., & Johnston, C. (2009). Mathematics teacher TPACK standards and development model. *Contemporary Issues in Technology & Teacher Education*, *9*(1). Retrieved from http://www.citejournal.org/vol9/iss1/mathematics/article1.cfm.

Niess, M. L., Ronau, R. N., Shafer, K. G., Driskell, S. O., Harper, S. R., & Johnston, C. (2009). Mathematics teacher TPACK standards and development model. *Contemporary Issues in Technology & Teacher Education*, *9*(1). Retrieved from http://www.citejournal.org/vol9/iss1/mathematics/article1.cfm.

Niess, M. L., Suharwoto, G., Lee, K., & Sadri, P. (2006, April). *Guiding inservice mathematics teachers in developing TPCK*. Paper presented at the annual meeting of the American Education Research Association, San Francisco, CA.

Niesz, T. (2007). Why teacher networks (can) work. *Phi Delta Kappan*, *88*(8), 605–610.

Norris, C., Sullivan, T., Poirot, J., & Soloway, E. (2003). No access, no use, no impact: Snapshot surveys of educational technology in K-12. *Journal of Research on Technology in Education*, *36*, 15–27.

Northfield, J., & Loughran, J. (1997). *The nature of knowledge development in self-study practice*. A paper presented at the annual meeting of the American Educational Research Association, Chicago, IL, March 24-28, 1997.

Norton, S., McRobbie, C. J., & Cooper, T. J. (2000). Exploring secondary mathematics teachers' reasons for not using computer in their teaching: Five case studies. *Journal of Research on Technology in Education*, *33*(1), 87–109.

Oblinger, D. (2005). Learners, learning and technology. *EDUCAUSE*, *40*(5), 66–75.

OECD. (2005). *Teachers matter: Attracting, Developing and Retaining Effective Teachers. Education and Training Policy*. Paris: OECD Publications.

OECD. (2006). *Science competencies for tomorrow's world. Analysis. Volume 1. Programme for International Student Assessment (PISA)*. Organization for Economic Co-operation and Development. Retrieved November 28, 2008, from http://www.oecd.org/dataoecd/30/17/39703267.pdf

OECD. (2009). *Equally prepared for life? How 15 year old boys and girls perform in schools*. Retrieved June 20, 2009, from http://www.oecd.org/

Office for Standards in Education. (2002). *ICT in schools: Effects of government initiatives – Secondary Mathematics*. London: Author.

Office of Technology Assessment. (1995, April). *Teachers and technology: Making the connection* (Report No. OTA-EHR-616). Washington, DC: U.S. Congress, Office of Technology Assessment.

Olitksy, S. (2007). Promoting student engagement in science: Interaction rituals and the pursuit of a community of practice. *Journal of Research in Science Teaching*, *44*(1), 33–56. doi:10.1002/tea.20128

Oliver, D. W., & Shaver, J. P. (1966). *Teaching public issues in the high school*. Boston: Houghton Mifflin Company.

Oliver, M., & Trigwell, K. (2005). Can 'Blended Learning' be redeemed? *E-learning*, *2*(1), 17–26.

Oliver, R., & Herrington, J. (2001). *Teaching and learning online. Mt. Lawley*. Perth, Australia: Centre for Research in Information Technology and Communication, Edith Cowan University.

Olivier, W. (2005). Teaching mathematics: Tablet PC technology add a new dimension. In *Proceedings of the Mathematics Education into the 21st Century Project Eighth International Conference, Reform, Revolution and Paradigm Shifts in Mathematics Education* (pp. 176-181). Johor Bahru, Malaysia: Univeriti Teknologi Malaysia.

Olkun, S., Altun, A., & Smith, G. (2005). Computers and 2D geometric learning of Turkish fourth and fifth graders. *British Journal of Educational Technology, 36*(2), 317–326. doi:10.1111/j.1467-8535.2005.00460.x

One Laptop per Child (OLPC). (n.d.). Retrieved April 2, 2009, from http://www.laptop.org/en/?gclid=CPi7w_y72pkCFQ9JagodgnhNXw

Organisation for Economic Cooperation and Development. (2000). *Schooling for tomorrow: Learning to bridge the digital divide.* Paris: Author.

Orlando, D. (2008). *Advantages of tablets over laptops.* Retrieved June 30, 2009, from http://schoolcomputing.wikia.com/wiki/Advantages_of_Tablets_Over_Laptops

Osborne, J., Erduran, S., & Simon, S. (2004). Enhancing the quality of argumentation in school science. *Journal of Research in Science Teaching, 41*(10), 994–1020. doi:10.1002/tea.20035

Osguthorpe, R. T., & Graham, C. R. (2003). Blended learning environments: definitions and directions. *The entity from which ERIC acquires the content, including journal, organization, and conference names, or by means of online submission from the author. Quarterly Review of Distance Education, 4*(3), 227–233.

Otliksy, S. (2007). Facilitating identity formation, group membership, and learning in science classrooms: What can be learned from out-of-field teaching in an urban school? *Science Education, 91*(2), 201–221. doi:10.1002/sce.20182

Overbaugh, R. C. (2002). Undergraduate education majors' discourse on an electronic mailing list. *Journal of Research on Technology in Education, 35*(1), 117–139.

Owston, R., Wideman, H., Murphy, J., & Lupshenyuk, D. (2008). Blended Teacher Professional Development: A Synthesis of Three Program Evaluations. *The Internet and Higher Education, 11*(3/4), 201–210. doi:10.1016/j.iheduc.2008.07.003

Pahl, R. H. (2003). *Assessment traps in K-12 social studies. Social Studies, 94*(5), 212–215. doi:10.1080/00377990309600209

Palloff, R., & Pratt, K. (1999). *Building learning communities in cyberspace.* San Francisco: Jossey-Bass.

Panel on Educational Technology. (1997, March). *Report to the President on the use of technology to strengthen K-12 education in the United States.* Washington, DC: President's Committee of Advisors on Science and Technology.

Parsad, B., & Jones, J. (2005). *Internet access in U.S. public schools and classrooms: 1994-2003. (NCES 2005-015). U.S. Department of Education.* Washington, DC: National Center for Education Statistics.

Partnership for 21st Century Skills. (2007). *Building 21st century skills.* Retrieved on February 17, 2009, from http://www.21stcenturyskills.org/route21/index.php?option=com_content&view=article&id=5&Itemid=2

Partnership for 21st Century Skills. (2009). *Framework for 21st century learning.* Retrieved on February 17, 2009, from http://www.21stcenturyskills.org/documents/framework_flyer_updated_jan_09_final-1.pdf

Partnership for the 21st century. (2008). *Framework for the 21st century skills.* Retrieved September 30, 2007, from http://www.21stcenturyskills.org

Passey, D., Rogers, C., Machell, J., McHugh, G., & Allaway, D. (2003). *The motivational effect of ICT on pupils.* Retrieved September 2005, from http://www.dfes.gov.uk/research/data/uploadfiles/rr523new.pdf

Patton, M. Q. (2002). *Qualitative evaluation and research methods* (3rd ed.). Thousand Oaks, CA: Sage Publications.

Paulus, T., & Scherff, L. (2008). Can anyone offer any words of encouragement? Online dialogue as a support mechanism for preservice teachers. *Journal of Technology and Teacher Education, 16*(1), 113–136.

Pcmag.com. (2009). *Definition of podcast.* Retrieved on April 1, 2009 from http://www.pcmag.com/encyclopedia_term/0,2542,t=podcast&i=49433,00.asp#

Peacock, L. (2000). Thinking skills to creatively enhance information competence. *Academic Exchange Quarterly, 4*(3).

Peavy, V. (2003). *Sociodynamic counseling. A constructivist perspective.* Victoria, Canada: Trafford.

Pedersen, J. E., & Yerrick, R. K. (2000). Technology in science teacher education: Survey of current uses and desired knowledge among science educators. *Journal of Science Teacher Education, 11*(2), 131–153. doi:10.1023/A:1009468808876

Pedretti, E. (2003). Teaching science, technology, society and environment (STSE) education: Preservice teachers' philosophical and pedagogical landscapes. In Zeidler, D. (Ed.), *The role of moral reasoning and socioscientific discourse in science education* (pp. 219–239). Dortecht, The Netherlands: Kluwer.

Pedretti, E., Bencze, L., Hewitt, J., Romkey, L., & Jivraj, A. (2006). Promoting issues-based STSE perspectives in science teacher education: Problems of identity and ideology. *Science and Education, 17*, 941–960. doi:10.1007/s11191-006-9060-8

Pena, C. M., & Almaguer, I. (2007). Asking the right questions: Online mentoring of student teachers. *International Journal of Instructional Media, 34*(1), 105–113.

Pennsylvania Department of Education. (2009). *Form PDE-430 student teacher assessment.* Retrieved June 22, 2009, from http://www.pde.state.pa.us/teaching/cwp/view.asp?a=90&Q=32539&teachingNav=|93|87|&teachingNavPage=|

Phelps, R., & Graham, A. (2008). Developing technology together, together: A whole-school metacognitive approach to ICT teacher professional development. *Journal of Computing in Teacher Education, 24*(4), 125–134.

Phillipson, M., & Hamilton, D. (2004). *The romantic audience project: A wiki experiment.* Retrieved November 22, 2007, from http://www.rc.umd.edu/pedagogies/commons/innovations/rap/toc.htm

Pierson, M. E. (2001). Technology integration practices as function of pedagogical expertise. *Journal of Research on Computing in Education, 33*(4), 413–429.

PoducateMe. (2008). *PoducateMe Podcasting Guide.* Retrieved March 16, 2009, from http://www.poducateme.com/

Poff, J. (2008 December). Don't void our voices. *Edutopia*, 10.

Polya, G. (1945). *How to solve it.* Princeton, NJ: Princeton University Press.

Poole, D. M. (2000). Student participation in a discussion-oriented online course: A case study. *Journal of Research on Computing in Education, 33*(2), 112–130.

Pope, M., Hare, D., & Howard, E. (2005). Enhancing technology use in student teaching: A case study. *Journal of Technology and Teacher Education, 13*(4), 573–618.

Pratt, N. (2008). Multipoint e-conferencing with initial teacher training students in England: Pitfalls and potential. *Teaching and Teacher Education, 24*, 1476–1486. doi:10.1016/j.tate.2008.02.018

Prensky, M. (2001). *Digital game based learning.* New York: McGraw Hill Press.

Prensky, M. (2001). Digital natives, digital immigrants. *On the Horizon, 9*(5), 1-6. Retrieved April 8, 2009, from http://www.marcprensky,com/writing/Prensky-DigitalNatives, DigitalImmigrants-Part1.pdf doi:10.1108/10748120110424816

Prensky, M. (2005, September). Engage Me or Enrage Me. What Today's Learners Demand. *EDUCAUSE Review, 40*(5), 60–65.

Prensky, M. (2007). How to teach with technology: keeping both teachers and students comfortable in an era of exponential change. *Emerging Technologies for Learning, 2*, 40–46.

Price, E., & Simon, B. (2007). Instructor inking in physics classes with Ubiquitous Presenter. In Prey, J. C., Reed, R. H., & Berque, D. A. (Eds.), *The Impact of Tablet PCs and Pen-based Technology on Education: Beyond the Tipping Point* (pp. 107–117). West Lafayette, IN: Purdue University Press.

Putnam, R. T., & Botko, H. (2000). What do new views of knowledge and thinking have to say about research on teacher learning? *Educational Researcher, 29*(1), 4–15.

Rainie, L., & Hitlin, P. (2005). The Internet at school. *Pew Internet & American Life Project.* Retrieved November 7, 2007, from http://www.pewinternet.org/PPF/r/163/report_display.asp

Raman, M., Ryan, T., & Olfman, L. (2005). Designing knowledge management systems for teaching and learning with wild technology. *Journal of Information Systems Education, 16*(3), 311–320.

Ramsey, C. (2003). Using virtual learning environments to facilitate new learning relationships. *The International Journal of Management Education, 3*(2), 31–41. doi:10.3794/ijme.32.62

Rao, Z. (2008). Reflecting on Native-English-speaking teachers in China. *Essential Teacher, 5*(1), 23–25.

Read, B. (2005). Duke U. Assess iPod Experiment and Finds It Worked--in Some Courses. [from Education Full Text database.]. *The Chronicle of Higher Education, 51*(43), A28. Retrieved February 27, 2007.

Read, B. (2005, March 2). Seriously, iPods Are Educational. *The Chronicle of Higher Education.* Retrieved December 2, 2008, from http://chronicle.com/weekly/v51/i28/28a03001.htm

Reba, M. (2007). Tablet PCs and web-based interaction in the mathematics classroom. *The Mathematics Education into the 21st Century Project, Programme of the Ninth International Conference Mathematics Education in a Global Community* (pp. 549-554). Charlotte, NC: The University of North Carolina.

Reba, M., & Pargas, R. (2008, May). Using tablet PCs as interactive web-based instruction tools in freshman calculus [Monograph]. In *Second International Workshop on the Impact of Pen-Based Technology on Education, PLT 2008* (pp. 1-6).

Reba, M., & Weaver, B. (2007, May). Tablet PC-enabled active learning in mathematics: A first study. In *The Impact of Tablet PCs and Pen-based Technology on Education, 2007* (pp. 1–6). Beyond the Tipping Point.

Reimer, K., & Moyer, P. S. (2005). Third-graders learn about fractions using virtual manipulatives: A case study. *Journal of Computers in Mathematics and Science Teaching, 24*, 5–25.

Reins, K. J. (2007). Digital tablet PCs as new technologies of writing and learning: A survey of perceptions of digital ink technology. *Contemporary Issues in Technology & Teacher Education, 7*(3), 158–177.

Reiser, R. A. (2007). Trends and issues in instructional design. In R. A. Reiser, & J. V. Dempsey, A history of instructional design and technology (2nd ed., pp. 27-45). Upper Saddle River, NJ: Pearson.

Reynolds, A., & Lennex, L. (in press). Can you read this? 508 compliance among Kentucky schools?

Reznichenko, N. (2007). *Learning mathematics with graphing calculator: A study of students' experiences.* Paper presented at the Annual Meeting of the Eastern Educational Research Association. ERIC Document Reproduction Services ED497715.

Rich, P. J., & Hannafin, M. (2009). Video Annotation Tools: Technologies to scaffold, structure and transform teacher reflection. *Journal of Teacher Education, 60*(1), 52–67. doi:10.1177/0022487108328486

Richardson, W. (2006). *Blogs, wikis, podcasts, and other powerful web tools for the classroom.* Thousand Oaks, CA: Corwin Press.

Roblyer, M. D. (2006). *Integrating Educational Technology Into Teaching* (4th ed.). Upper Saddle River, NJ: Merrill Prentice-Hall.

Roddy, M. (1999). Using the Internet to unite student teaching and teacher education. *Journal of Technology and Teacher Education, 7*(3), 257–267.

Rogers, E. V. (1995). *Diffusion of innovation* (4th ed.). New York: The Free Press.

Rogoff, B. (2003). *The cultural nature of human development.* Oxford, UK: Oxford University.

Romano, M., & Schwartz, J. (2005). Exploring technology a s a tool for eliciting and encouraging beginning teacher reflection. *Contemporary Issues in Technology and Teacher, 5*(2), 149–168.

Ronau, B. (2009). Technology committee update. *AMTE Connections*, *18*(2), 12–13.

Roschelle, J., & Pea, R. (2002). A walk on the WILD side: How wireless handhelds may change computer-supported collaborative learning. *International Journal of Cognitive Technology*, *1*(1), 145–272. doi:10.1075/ijct.1.1.09ros

Roth, W.-M., & Lee, Y.-J. (2006). Computers and cognitive development at work. *Educational Media International*, *43*(4), 331–346. doi:10.1080/09523980600926325

Rovai, A. P., & Jordan, H. M. (2004). Blended learning and sense of community: A comparative analysis with traditional and fully online graduate courses. *International Review of Research in Open and Distance Learning*, *5*(2), 1–13.

RSS Advisory Board. (2005). *Really simple syndication: RSS 2.0.1 Specification (Rev. 6).* Retrieved April 1, 2009, from http://www.rssboard.org/rss-2-0-1-rv-6

Russell, A., & Wineburg, M. (2007). Towards a national framework for evidence of effectiveness of teacher education programs. *Perspectives.* Policy Papers published by the American Association of State Colleges and Universities.

Russell, M., Bebell, D., O'Dwyer, L. M., & O'Connor, K. M. (2003). Examining Teacher Technology Use: Implications for Preservice and In-Service Teacher Preparation. *Journal of Teacher Education*, *54*(4), 297–310. doi:10.1177/0022487103255985

Russell, T., McPherson, S., & Martin, A. K. (2001). Coherence and collaboration in teacher education reform. *Canadian Journal of Education*, *26*(3), 14.

Sacristan, A. I., Calder, N., Rojano, T., Santos-Trigo, M., Friedlander, A., & Meissner, H. (2010). The influence and shaping of digital technologies on the learning –and learning trajectories- of mathematical concepts. In Hoyles, C., & Lagrange, J. (Eds.), *Mathematics education and technology-rethinking the terrain. The 17th ICMI Study* (pp. 179–226). New York: Springer.

Salen, K. (Ed.). (2008). *The ecology of games. Connecting youth, games and learning.* Cambridge, MA: MIT Press.

Salili, F. (2001). Teacher-Student Interaction: Attributional Implications and Effectiveness of Teachers' Evaluative Feedback. In Watkins, D., & Biggs, J. (Eds.), *Teaching the Chinese Learner: Psychological and Pedagogical Perspectives. Comparative Education Research Centre.* Hong Kong: The Chinese University of Hong Kong.

Salmon, G. (2000). *E-moderating: The key to teaching and learning online.* London: Kogan Press.

Samarawickrema, G. (2009). Blended learning and the new pressures on the academy: Individual, political and policy driven motivators for adoption. In Stacey, E., & Gerbric, P. (Eds.), *Effective Blended Learning Practices: Evidence-Based Perspectives in ICT- Facilitated Education.* Hershey, PA: IGI Publishing.

Sanders, J. (2002). Something is missing from teacher education: attention to two genders. *Phi Delta Kappan, 84*(3), 241-44. Retrieved November 2002, from http://www.pdkintl.org/kappan/k0211san.htm

Sanders, J. (2005). *Gender and technology in education: A research review.* Retrieved November 7, 2007, from http://www.josanders.com/pdf/gendertech0705.pdf

Sandford, R. (2006). *Teaching with Games: Using commercial off-the-shelf computer games in formal education.* Bristol: Futurelab.

Sandholz, J., Ringstaff, C., & Dwyer, D. (1997). *Teaching with technology: Creating student-centered classrooms.* New York: Teachers College Press.

Sandoval, W. A., & Bell, P. (2004). Design-based research methods for studying learning in context: Introduction. *Educational Psychologist*, *39*(4), 199–201. doi:10.1207/s15326985ep3904_1

Sanford, K., & Madill, L. (2006). Resistance through video games: It's a boy thing. *Canadian Journal of Education*, *29*(1), 287–306.

Santos-Trigo, M. (2007). Mathematical problem solving: An evolving research and practice domain. *ZDM - The International Journal on Mathematics Education*, 523-536.

Santos-Trigo, M. (2008). On the use of technology to represent and explore mathematical objects or problems dynamically. *Mathematics and Computer Education Journal*, *42*(2), 123–139.

Santos-Trigo, M., & Camacho, M. (2009). Towards the construction of a Framework to deal with routine problems to foster mathematical inquiry. *PRIMUS: Problems, Resources, and Issues in Mathematics Undergraduate Studies Journal*, *19*(3), 260–279.

Saraceni, M. (2003). *The language of comics*. London: Routledge.

Scardamalia, M. (2003). The knowledge society network (KSN): Toward an expert society for democratizing knowledge. *Journal of Distance Education*, *17*(3), 63–66.

Scardamalia, M., Bereiter, C., & Steinback, R. (1984). The teachability of reflective processes in written composition. *Cognitive Science*, *8*, 173–190.

Schaff, M. (2003). Student perceptions of technology and how it impacts their learning: A technology integration experience. In *Proceedings of World Conference on Educational Multimedia, Hypermedia and Telecommunications* (pp. 1764-1768). Chesapeake, VA: AACE.

Scharf, E., & Cramer, J. (2002). Desktop poetry project. *Learning and Leading with Technology*, *29*(6), 28–31, 50–51.

Schellens, T., & Valcke, M. (2006). Fostering knowledge construction in university students through asynchronous discussion groups. *Computers & Education*, *46*(4), 349–370. doi:10.1016/j.compedu.2004.07.010

Schlagal, B., Trathen, W., & Blanton, W. (1996). Structuring telecommunication to create instructional conversations about student teaching. *Journal of Teacher Education*, *47*(3), 175–183. doi:10.1177/0022487196047003003

Schlager, M. S., & Fusco, J. (2003). Teacher professional development, technology, and communities of practice: Are we putting the cart before the horse? *The Information Society*, *19*(3), 203. doi:10.1080/01972240309464

Schmidt, M. E. (1999). Middle grades teacher's beliefs about calculator use: Pre-project and two-years later. *Focus on Learning Problems in Mathematics*, *21*, 18–34.

Schmit, D. (2007 January). Creating a Broadcast Empire...From the Corner of Your Classroom. *MultiMedia & Internet@Schools*, *14*(1), 13-16.

Schoenfeld, A. H. (1985). *Mathematical Problem Solving*. New York: Academic Press.

Schoenfeld, A. H. (1992). Learning to think mathematically: Problem solving, metacognition, and sense making in mathematics. In Grows, D. A. (Ed.), *Handbook of Research on Mathematics Teaching and Learning* (pp. 334–370). NY: Macmillan.

Schön, D. (1983). *The reflective practitioner: How professionals think in action*. New York: Basic Books, Inc.

Schon, D. A. (1987). *Educating the reflective practitioner: Toward a new design for teaching and learning in the profession*. San Francisco: Jossey Bass.

Schwarz, C. V., Meyer, J., & Sharma, A. (2007). Technology, pedagogy, and epistemology: Opportunities and challenges of using computer modeling and simulation tools in elementary science methods. *Journal of Science Teacher Education*, *18*, 243–269. doi:10.1007/s10972-007-9039-6

Seager, J. (1997). *State of women of the world atlas* (2nd ed.). New York: Penguin.

Seels, B. B., & Richey, R. C. (1994). *Instructional technology: The definition and domains of the field*. Bloomington, IN: Association for Educational Communications and Technology.

Serim, F., & Schrock, K. (2007). *The Horizon Report*. Stanford, CA: The New Media Consortium.

Shaffer, D. W. (2006). Epistemic frames for epistemic games. *Computers & Education*, *46*, 223–234. doi:10.1016/j.compedu.2005.11.003

Shaffer, D. W., & Clinton, A. (2005). *Video Games and the Future of Learning*. University of Wisconsin-Madison. Working Paper No. 2005-4.

Shaffer, D. W., & Clinton, K. (2004). *Toolforthoughts: reexamining thinking in the digital age.* University of Wisconsin-Madison.

Shaffer, D. W., & Gee, A. (2006). *Before every child is left behind: How epistemic games can solve the coming crisis in education.* Working Paper No. *2005*-7, University of Wisconsin-Madison.

Sharples, M. (2000). The design of personal mobile technologies for lifelong learning. *Computers & Education, 34*, 177–193. doi:10.1016/S0360-1315(99)00044-5

Shodor. (2008). Retrieved from http://www.shodor.org/home/

Shulman, L. (1986). Those who understand: Knowledge growth in teaching. *Educational Researcher, 15*(2), 4–14.

Shulman, L. (1987). Knowledge and teaching: Foundations of the new reform. *Harvard Educational Review, 57*(1), 1–22.

Shulman, L. S. (1986). Those who understand: Knowledge growth in teaching. *Educational Researcher, 15*(2), 4–14.

Shumba, O. (1999). Relationship between secondary science teachers' orientation to traditional culture and beliefs concerning science instructional ideology. *Journal of Research in Science Teaching, 36*(3), 333–355. doi:10.1002/(SICI)1098-2736(199903)36:3<333::AID-TEA7>3.0.CO;2-Z

Silverman, J., & Thompson, P. W. (2008). Toward a framework for the development of mathematical knowledge for teaching. *Journal of Mathematics Teacher Education, 11*, 499–511. doi:10.1007/s10857-008-9089-5

Simkins, T., Coldwell, M., Close, P., & Morgan, A. (2009). Outcomes of In-School Leadership Development Work: A Study of Three NCSL Programmes. *Educational Management Administration & Leadership, 37*(1), 29–50. doi:10.1177/1741143208098163

Simon, M. (2006). Key developmental understandings in mathematics: A direction for investigating and establishing learning goals. *Mathematical Thinking and Learning, 8*(4), 359–371. doi:10.1207/s15327833mtl0804_1

Simonneaux, L. (2001). Role-play or debate to promote students' argumentation or justification on an issue in animal transgenesis. *International Journal of Science Education, 23*(9), 903–927. doi:10.1080/09500690010016076

Simonson, M., & Maushak, N. (2001). Instructional technology and attitude change. In Jonassen, D. (Ed.), *Handbook of research for educational communications and technology* (pp. 984–1016). Mahwah, NJ: Lawrence Erlbaum Associates.

Sinclair, M. (2004). Working with accurate representations: The case of pre-constructed dynamic geometry sketches. *Journal of Computers in Mathematics and Science Teaching, 23*(2), 191–208.

Sinclair, M., & Owston, R. (2006). Teacher Professional Development in Mathematics and Science: A Blended Learning Approach. *Canadian Journal of University Continuing Education, 32*(2), 43–66.

Singer, N. R., & Zeni, J. (2004). Building bridges: Creating an online conversation community for preservice teachers. *English Education, 37*(1), 30–49.

Singh, H. (2003). Building effective blended learning programs. *Educational Technology, 43*(6), 51–54.

Slavit, D. (2002). Expanding classroom discussion with an online medium. *Journal of Technology and Teacher Education, 10*(3), 407–423.

Smeaton, P. S., & Waters, F. H. (2000). Keeping connected: An asynchronous communication system to support student teachers. *T.H.E. Journal, 28*(2), 106–115.

Smerdon, B., Cronen, S., Lanahan, L., Anderson, J., Iannotti, N., & Angeles, J. (2000). *Teachers' tools for the 21st Century: A report on teacher's use of technology* (NCES Publication 2000-102). Retrieved February 26, 2009 from www.nces.ed.gov/pubsearch/pubsinfor.asp?pubid=2000102

Snider, S. L. (2002). Exploring technology integration in a field-based teacher education program: implementation efforts and findings. *Journal of Research on Technology in Education, 34*, 230–249.

Snoek, M., Uzerli, U., & Schratz, M. (2008, February). *Developing teacher education policies through peer learning.* Paper presented at the TEPE conference, Ljubljana, Slovenia.

Soloway, E., Norris, E., Blumenfeld, P., Fishman, B., Krajcik, J., & Marx, R. (2001). Log on education: Handheld devices are ready-at-hand. *Communications of the ACM, 44*(6), 15–20. doi:10.1145/376134.376140

Song, L., & Hill, J. (2007). A conceptual model for understanding self-directed learning in online environments. *Journal of Interactive Online Learning, 6*(1), 27–42.

Sowder, J. T. (2007). The mathematical education and development of teachers. In F. K. Lester, Jr. (Ed.), Second Handbook of Research on Mathematics Teaching and Learning (pp. 157-223). The National Council of Teachers of Mathematics. Charlotte, NC: Information Age Publishing.

Spillane, J. P. (2000). Cognition and policy implementation: District policy makers and the reform of mathematics education. *Cognition and Instruction, 18*(2), 141–179. doi:10.1207/S1532690XCI1802_01

Spiro, R. J., Coulson, R. L., Feltovich, P. J., & Anderson, D. K. (2004). Cognitive Flexibility Theory: Advanced knowledge acquisition in ill-structured domains. In Ruddell, R. B., & Unrau, N. J. (Eds.), *Theoretical models and processes of reading* (5th ed., pp. 640–653). Newark, DE: International Reading Association.

Spooner, M., Flowers, C., Lambert, R., & Algozzine, R. (2008). Is more really better? Examining perceived benefits of an extended student teaching experience. *Clearing House (Menasha, Wis.), 81*(6), 263–270. doi:10.3200/TCHS.81.6.263-270

Squire, K. (2005). *Game-Based Learning: Present and Future State of the Field.* University of Wisconsin-Madison.

Squire, K. (2008). Open-Ended Video Games: A Model for Developing Learning for the Interactive Age. In Salen, K. (Ed.), *The ecology of games. Connecting youth, games and learning* (pp. 167–198). Cambridge, MA: MIT Press.

St. John, K., Leckie, M., Slough, S., Peart, L., Niemitz, M., & Klaus, A. (in press). *Field Geoscience Education – The Pilot School or Rock Program at Sea for Teachers.* Geological Society of America Special Paper.

Stacey, E., & Gerbic, P. (2009). Introduction to Blended Learning Practices. In Stacey, E., & Gerbic, P. (Eds.), *Effective Blended Learning Practices: Evidence-Based Perspectives in ICT-Facilitated Education* (pp. 1–19). Hershey, PA: IGI Publishing.

Stager, G. (2000). Portable probeware: Science education's next frontier. *Curriculum Administrator, 36*(3), 32–36.

Staudt, C., & Hsi, S. (1999). *Synergy projects and pocket computers.* Concord Consortium Newsletter.

Stegman, S. (2007). An exploration of reflective dialogue between student teachers in music and their cooperating teachers. *Journal of Research in Music Education, 55*(1), 65–82. doi:10.1177/002242940705500106

Stephens, M. (2005). The iPod Experiments. [from Education Full Text database.]. *Library Journal Net Connect, 22*, 24–25. Retrieved February 27, 2007.

Stigler, J. (1999, September). *Briefing for the National Commission on Mathematics and Science Teaching for the 21st Century.* Washington, DC.

Stokes, D., Jenkins, C., Huhnke, L., Grey, G., & Manning, C. (2000). Math and Science Curriculum Revision: A Collaborative Approach to Improving Preservice Teachers' Use of Technology Knowledge and Instructional Skills. In *Proceedings of World Conference on Educational Multimedia, Hypermedia and Telecommunications 2000* (pp. 1832). Norfolk, VA: AACE.

Strauss, A., & Corbin, J. (1990). *Basics of qualitative research: Grounded theory procedures and techniques.* Newbury Park, CA: Sage Publications.

Strauss, A., & Corbin, J. (1998). *Basics of qualitative research: Techniques and procedures for developing grounded theory* (2nd ed.). Thousand Oaks, CA: Sage.

Strudel, N., & Wetzel, K. (1999). Lessons from exemplary colleges of education: Factors affecting technology integration in preservice programs. *Educational Technology Research and Development*, *47*(4), 63–81. doi:10.1007/BF02299598

Suh, J., & Moyer, P. S. (2007). Developing students' representational fluency using virtual and physical algebra balances. *Journal of Computers in Mathematics and Science Teaching*, *26*, 155–173.

Sun Associates. (2001). *Evaluating technology integration*. Retrieved January 11, 2009, from http://www.sun-associates.com/resources/categories.html#anchor237232

Syh-Jong, J. (2008). Innovations in science teacher education: Effects of integration technology and team-teaching strategies. *Computers & Education*, *41*, 646–659.

Taba, H. (1962). *Curriculum Development: Theory and Practice*. New York: Harcourt Brace and World.

Teaching and Learning Research Programme – TLRP. (2008). *Education 2.0? Designing the web for teaching and learning*. Retrieved March 20, 2009, from http://www.tlrp.org/tel/files/2008/11/tel_comm_final.pdf

Tearle, P. (2003). ICT implementation: What makes the difference. *British Journal of Educational Technology*, *34*(5), 567–583. doi:10.1046/j.0007-1013.2003.00351.x

Tech Trends.

Technology & Learning. (2007). *K-12 Computing Blueprint: Leadership*. Retrieved June 30, 2009, from http://www.k12blueprint.com/k12/blueprint/leadership.php?menu=leadership

Templin, M. A., Doran, R. L., & Engemann, J. F. (1999). A locally based science mentorship program for high achieving students: Unearthing issues that influence affective outcomes. *School Science and Mathematics*, *99*(4), 205–211. doi:10.1111/j.1949-8594.1999.tb17475.x

Thomas, J. A., & Cooper, S. B. (2000). Teaching technology: A new opportunity for pioneers in teacher education. *Journal of Computing in Teacher Education*, *17*(1), 13–19.

Thomas, L., Larson, A., Clift, R. T., & Levin, J. (1996). Integrating technology in teacher education programs: Lessons from the teaching tele-apprenticeships project. *Action in Teacher Education*, *17*(4), 1–8.

Tillma, H. (2000). Belief change towards self-directed learning in student teachers: Immersion in practice or reflection on action. *Teaching and Teacher Education*, *16*, 575–591. doi:10.1016/S0742-051X(00)00016-0

Tinker, R., & Krajcik, J. (Eds.). (2001). *Portable Technologies: Science Learning in Context*. New York: Kluwer Academic/Plenum Publishers.

Tomei, L. A. (2003). *The taxonomy for the technology domain*. Retrieved June 24, 2009, from http://academics.rmu.edu/~tomei/taxonomy/

Törner, G., Schoenfeld, A. H., & Reiss, K. M. (2007). Problem solving around the World: Summing up the state of the art. *ZDM Mathematics Education*, *39*(5-6), 353. doi:10.1007/s11858-007-0053-0

Toulmin, S. (1958). *The uses of argument*. Cambridge, UK: Cambridge University Press.

Tront, J. G., & Scales, G. R. (2007). Keynote address implementing a large-scale tablet PC deployment. In Prey, J. C., Reed, R. H., & Berque, D. A. (Eds.), *The Impact of Tablet PCs and Pen-based Technology on Education: Beyond the Tipping Point* (pp. 1–10). West Lafayette, IN: Purdue University Press.

Tynjälä, P. (2001). Writing, learning and the development of expertise in higher education. In G. Rijlaarsdarn, P. Tynjälä, L. Mason, & K. Lonka (Volume Eds.), Studies in writing. Writing as a learning tool: integrating theory and practice (Vol. 7, pp. 37–56). Dordrecht, Netherlands: Kluwer.

U.S. Department of Education. (2000). *E-Learning: Putting a world-class education at the fingertips of all children*. Washington, DC: U.S. Department of Education.

U.S. Department of Education. (2004). *National Educational Technology Plan*. Washington, DC: Author.

United Nations Educational, Scientific and Cultural Organization. (2008a). *ICT competency standards for teachers, policy framework*. London: UNESCO.

United Nations Educational, Scientific and Cultural Organization. (2008b). *ICT competency standards for teachers implementation guidelines*. London: UNESCO.

Vahey, P., & Crawford, V. (2002). *Palm Education Pioneers Program: Final evaluation report.* Menlo Park, CA: SRI International.

Valcke, M., Rots, I., Verbeke, M., & van Braak, J. (2007). ICT teacher training: Evaluation of the curriculum and training approach in Flanders. *Teaching and Teacher Education, 23*, 795–808. doi:10.1016/j.tate.2007.02.004

Valdez, G., McNabb, M., Foertsch, M., Anderson, M., Hawkes, M., & Raack, L. (1999). *Computer-based technology and learning: Evolving uses and expectations.* Oak Brook, IL: North Central Regional Educational Laboratory.

Valli, L. (1997). Listening to other voices: A description of teacher reflection in the United States. *Peabody Journal of Education, 72*(1), 67–88. doi:10.1207/s15327930pje7201_4

van Bruggen, J. M., Kirschner, P. A., & Jochems, W. (2002). External representation of argumentation in CSCL and the management of cognitive load. *Learning and Instruction, 12*(1), 121–138. doi:10.1016/S0959-4752(01)00019-6

van't Hooft, M., Diaz, S., & Swan, K. (2004). Examining the potential of handheld computers: Findings from the Ohio PEP project. *Journal of Educational Computing Research, 30*(4), 295–312. doi:10.2190/M1W6-A94D-3NKM-KBUU

Vanderwater, E. A., et al. (2004). Digital Childhood: Electronic Media and Technology Use Among Infants, Toddlers and Preschoolers. *Pediatrics.* Retrieved October 20, 2008, from http://pediatrics.aappublications.org/cgi/content/full/119/5/e1006

VanFossen, P. (1999). An analysis of the use of the Internet and World Wide Web by secondary social studies teachers in Indiana. *The International Journal of Social Education, 14*(2), 87–109.

VanFossen, P. J. (2006). The electronic republic? Evidence on the impact of the Internet on citizenship and civic engagement in the U.S. *The International Journal of Social Education, 21*(1), 18–43.

VanFossen, P. J., & Shiveley, J. M. (2000). Using the Internet to create primary source teaching packets. *Social Studies, 91*(6), 244–252. doi:10.1080/00377990009602473

Vaughan, N., & Garrison, D. R. (2005). Creating cognitive presence in a blended faculty development community. *The Internet and Higher Education, 8*(1), 1–12. doi:10.1016/j.iheduc.2004.11.001

Veenman, S. (1984). Perceived problems of beginning teachers. *Review of Educational Research, 54*(2), 143–178.

Veerman, A., & Treasure-Jones, T. (1999). Software for problem solving through collaborative argumentation. In Andriessen, J., & Coirier, P. (Eds.), *Foundations of argumentative text processing* (pp. 203–229). Amsterdam: Amsterdam University Press.

Veerman, A., Andriessen, J., & Kanselaar, G. (2002). Collaborative argumentation in academic education. *Instructional Science, 30*(3), 155–186. doi:10.1023/A:1015100631027

Velden, M. (2008). *Usability of web 2.0 functionalities for information dissemination organizations.* Unpublished Master Thesis. Erasmus University Rotterdam.

Vess, D. (2006). History to go: why I teach with iPods. *The History Teacher, 39*(4), 479–492.

Vess, D. L. (2005). Asynchronous discussion and communication patterns in online and hybrid history courses. *Communication Education, 54*(4), 355–364. doi:10.1080/03634520500442210

Vick, M. (2006). It's a Difficult Matter: Historical perspectives on the enduring problem of the practicum in teacher preparation. *Asia-Pacific Journal of Teacher Education, 34*(2), 181–198. doi:10.1080/13598660600720579

Vincent, T. (2009). *Learning in Hand.* Retrieved June 18, 2009, from http://www.learninginhand.com/podcasting

Volkmann, M. J., & Anderson, M. A. (1998). Creating professional identity: Dilemmas and metaphors of a first-year chemistry teacher. *Science Education, 82*(3), 293–310. doi:10.1002/(SICI)1098-237X(199806)82:3<293::AID-SCE1>3.0.CO;2-7

Volman, M., & von Eck, E. (2001). Gender equity and information technology in education: The second decade. *Review of Educational Research*, *71*(4), 614–634. doi:10.3102/00346543071004613

von Aufschnaiter, C., Erduran, S., Osborne, J., & Simon, S. (2008). Arguing to learn and learning to argue: case studies of how students' argumentation relates to their scientific knowledge. *Journal of Research in Science Teaching*, *45*(1), 101–131. doi:10.1002/tea.20213

Vrasidas, C., & Glass, G. (2007). Teacher professional development and ICT: Strategies and models. *Yearbook of the National Society for the Study of Education*, *106*(2), 87–102.

Vygotsky, L. S. (1978). *Mind in society: The development of higher psychological processes* (Cole, M., John-Steiner, V., Scribner, S., & Souberman, E., Eds.). Cambridge, MA: Harvard University Press.

Wachira, P., Keengwe, J., & Onchwari, G. (2008). Mathematics preservice teachers' beliefs and conceptions of appropriate technology use. *AACE Journal*, *16*(3), 293–306.

Wagga Wagga. (2008). Digital Audio Learning Objects. In *Wikipedia, The Free Encyclopedia. Retrieved December 16, 2008, from*. Charles Sturt University.http://en.wikipedia.org/wiki/Digital_Audio_Learning_Objects

Walker, S. L. (2002). *Development and Validation of an Instrument for Assessing Distance Education Learning Environments in Higher Education: The Distance Education Learning Environments Survey*. Unpublished doctoral dissertation, University of Curtin, Curtin.

Wallace, J., & Louden, W. (1992). Science teaching and teachers' knowledge: Prospects for reform of elementary classrooms. *Science Education*, *76*(5), 507–521. doi:10.1002/sce.3730760505

Warschauer, M. (2004). Technology and Writing. In Davison, C., & Cummins, J. (Eds.), *Handbook of English Language Teaching*. Dordrecht, Netherlands: Kluwer.

Warschauer, M., & Meskill, C. (2000). Technology and second language teaching and learning. In Rosenthal, J. W. (Ed.), *Handbook of undergraduate second language education: English as a second language, bilingual, and foreign language instruction for a multilingual world* (pp. 303–318). Mahwah, NJ: Erlbaum.

Watson, A., & Mason, J. (2006). Seeing an exercise as a single mathematical object: Using variation to structure sense-making. *Mathematical Thinking and Learning*, *8*(2), 91–111. doi:10.1207/s15327833mtl0802_1

Webb, E., Jones, A., Barker, P., & van Schaik, P. (2005). Perspectives of Faculty on the Use of e-Learning Dialogues. In P. Kommers & G. Richards (Eds.), *Proceedings of World Conference on Educational Multimedia, Hypermedia and Telecommunications 2005* (pp. 2354-2361). Chesapeake, VA: AACE

Weinberger, A., Stegmann, K., Fischer, F., & Mandl, H. (2007). Scripting argumentative knowledge construction in computer-supported learning environments. In Fischer, F., Kollar, I., Mandl, H., & Haage, J. M. (Eds.), *Scripting computer-supported collaborative learning. Cognitive, computational and educational perspectives* (pp. 191–211). New York: Springer. doi:10.1007/978-0-387-36949-5_12

Wellington, J. J. (1995). The role of new technology in teacher-education - A case-study of hypertext in a PGCE Course. *Journal of Education for Teaching*, *21*(1), 37–50. doi:10.1080/02607479550038734

Wenger, E. (1999). *Communities of practice: Learning, meaning, and identity*. New York: Cambridge University Press.

Wenger, E., McDermott, R., & Snyder, W. M. (2002). *Seven principles for cultivating communities of practice*. Retrieved June, 2006, from http://hbswk.hbs.edu/item.jhtml?id=2855&t=organizations

Wenglinsky, H. (1998). *Does it compute? The relationship between educational technology and student achievement in mathematics*. Princeton, NJ: Educational Testing Service (ETS). Retrieved February 20, 2006, from ftp://ftp.ets.org/pub/res/technolog.pdf

Wentworth, N., & Earle, R. (2003). Trends in computer uses as reported in *Computers in Schools*. *Computers in the Schools*, *20*(1/2), 77–90. doi:10.1300/J025v20n01_06

Whetstone, L., & Carr-Chellman, A. A. (2001). Preparing preservice teachers to use technology: Survey results. *TechTrends*, *45*(4), 11–17. doi:10.1007/BF02784820

Whitley, B. (1997). Gender differences in computer-related attitudes and behavior: A meta-analysis. *Computers in Human Behavior*, *13*(1), 1–22. doi:10.1016/S0747-5632(96)00026-X

Whitworth, S. A., & Berson, M. J. (2003). Computer technology in the social studies: An examination of the effectiveness literature (1996-2001). *Contemporary Issues in Technology and Teacher Education*, *2*(4), 472-509. Retrieved July 7, 2009, from http://www.citejournal.org/vol2/iss4/socialstudies/article1.cfm

Wideman, H., Owston, R., & Sinitskaya, N. (2007). Transforming teacher practice through blended professional development: Lessons learned from three initiatives. In C. Crawford et al. (Eds.), *Proceedings of Society for Information Technology and Teacher Education International Conference 2007* (pp. 2148-2154). Chesapeake, VA: AACE.

Wiesenberg, F., & Stacey, E. (2009). Blended Learning and Teaching Philosophies. Implications for Practice. In Stacey, E., & Gerbic, P. (Eds.), *Effective Blended Learning Practices: Evidence-Based Perspectives in ICT-Facilitated Education* (pp. 204–221). Hershey, PA: IGI Publishing.

Wiggins, G., & McTighe, J. (2005). *Understanding by Design*. Alexandria, VA: Association for Supervision and Curriculum Development.

Wilkerson, T. L. (2003). A triad model for preparing preservice teachers for the integration of technology in teaching and learning. *Action in Teacher Education*, *24*(4), 27–32.

Williams, P. (2006). MySpace, Facebook attract online predators. *MSNBC*. Retrieved February 3, 2009 from http://msnbc.msn.com/id/11165576

Williamson, B., & Sandford, R. (2005). *Games and learning: A handbook from Futurelab*. Bristol: Futurelab.

Willis, J., Thompson, A., & Sadera, W. (1999). Research on technology and teacher education: Current status and future directions. *ETR&D*, *47*(4), 29–45. doi:10.1007/BF02299596

Winters, R. (2004). Differentiated tech use: under what conditions, for what purposes? In C. Crawford et al. (Eds.), *Proceedings of Society for Information Technology and Teacher Education International Conference 2004* (pp. 2750-2754). Chesapeake, VA: AACE

Wirght, N., Dewstow, R., Topping, M., & Tappenden, S. (2006). New Zealand examples of Blended Learning. In Bonk, C. J., & Graham, C. R. (Eds.), *The Handbook of Blended Learning: Global Perspectives, Local Designs* (pp. 169–181). San Francisco: Pfeiffer.

Wong, E. M. L., & Li, S. C. (2008). Framing ICT implementation in a context of educational change: a multilevel analysis. *School Effectiveness and School Improvement*, *19*(1), 99–120. doi:10.1080/09243450801896809

Wormnaes, S. (2008). Cross-cultural collaboration in Special Education: An arena for facilitating reflection? *International Journal of Disability Development and Education*, *55*(3), 205–225. doi:10.1080/10349120802268305

Wu, D., & Hiltz, S. R. (2004). Predicting learning from asynchronous online discussions. *Journal of Asynchronous Learning Networks*, *8*(2), 139–152.

Wubbles, T. (2007). Do we know a community of practice when we see one? *Technology, Pedagogy and Education*, *16*(2), 225–233. doi:10.1080/14759390701406851

Center for Civic Education. (1994). *National standards for civics and government*. Retrieved January 23, 2009, from http://www.civiced.org/index.php?page=stds_toc_intro

International Society for Technology in Education (ISTE). (2008a). *National educational technology standards (NET•S) and performance indicators for students*. Retrieved on February 20, 2009, from http://www.iste.org/

International Society for Technology in Education (ISTE). (2008b). *National educational technology standards*

(NET•T) and performance indicators for teachers. Retrieved on February 20, 2009, from http://www.iste.org/

National Council for the Social Studies. (1994). *Expectations for excellence: Curriculum standards for social studies.* Washington, DC: National Council for Social Studies.

National Council for the Social Studies. (2006). *Technology position statement and guidelines.* Retrieved on February 11, 2009, from http://www.socialstudies.org/positions/technology

National Library of Virtual Manipulatives. (2007). Utah State University. Retrieved from http://nlvm.usu.edu/

National Research Council (NRC). (1996). *National science education standards.* Washington, DC: National Academic Press.

National Research Council (NRC). (2001). Adding it up: Helping children to learn mathematics. (J. Kilpatrick, J. Swafford, & B. Findell, Eds.). Mathematical Learning Study Committee, Center for Education, Division of Behavioral and Social Sciences and Education. Washington, DC: National Academic Press.

Yamagata-Lynch, L. (2007). Confronting analytical dilemmas for understanding complex human interactions in design based research from a cultural-historical activity theory (CHAT) framework. *Journal of the Learning Sciences, 16*(4), 451–484.

Yan, J. (2008). Social technology as a new medium in the classroom. *New England Journal of Higher Education,* 27–30.

Yildirim, S. (2000). Effects of an educational computing course on preservice and inservice teachers: A discussion and analysis of attitudes and use. *Journal of Research on Computing in Education, 32*(4), 479–495.

Young, J. R. (2002). Hybrid teaching seeks to end the divide between traditional and online instruction. *The Chronicle of Higher Education, 48*(28), A33.

Zapanta, J. T. (2004). *Can we count past two?* Zittleman, K., & Sadker, D. (2002). Gender bias in teacher education texts. *Journal of Teacher Education, 53*(1), 168–180.

Zbiek, R., Heid, M. K., Blume, G. W., & Dick, T. P. (2007). Research on technology in mathematics education: A perspective of constructs. In Lester, F. K. (Ed.), *Second handbook of research on mathematics teaching and learning* (pp. 1169–1206). Reston, VA: National Council of Teachers of Mathematics.

Zeegers, M. (2008). Beyond cognition: Affective learning and undergraduate education student engagement in learning. In ECER 2008, Göteborg, Sweden 10-12 September, 2008.

Zeichner, K., & Tabachnick, B. R. (1991). Reflections on reflective thinking. In Tabachnick, B. R., & Zeichner, K. (Eds.), *Issues and practices in inquiry-oriented teacher education* (pp. 1–21). Bristol, PA: Falmer.

Zgaga, P. (2008). Mobility and the European Dimension in Teacher Education. In Hudson, B., & Zgaga, P. (Eds.), *Teacher Education Policy in Europe: a Voice of Higher Education Institutions.* Umeå, Sweden: University of Umeå, Faculty of Teacher Education.

Zhao, Y. (2003). *What Teachers should Know about Technology: Perspectives and Practices.* Greenwich, CT: Information Age Publishing.

Ziob, L., & Mosher, B. (2006). Putting customers first at Microsoft. In Bonk, C. J., & Graham, C. R. (Eds.), *The Handbook of Blended Learning: Global Perspectives, Local Designs* (pp. 92–104). San Francisco: Pfeiffer.

Zucker, A. A., Tinker, R., Staudt, C., Mansfield, A., & Metcalf, S. (2008). Learning science in grades 3-8 using probeware and computers: Findings from the TEEMSS II project. *Journal of Science Education and Technology, 17*(1), 42–48. doi:10.1007/s10956-007-9086-y

Zurita, G., & Nussbaum, M. (2007). A conceptual framework based on activity theory for mobile CSCL. *British Journal of Educational Technology, 38*(2), 211–235. doi:10.1111/j.1467-8535.2006.00580.x

About the Contributors

Junko Yamamoto teaches Instructional Technology, World Language Teaching Methodology, and English Language Learners Teaching Methodology at Secondary Education/ Foundations of Education Department, Slippery Rock University. She also supervises student teachers. She earned her doctorate degree in Instructional Technology from Duquesne University. She is a reviewer for the American Council on the Teaching of Foreign Languages / National Council for Accreditation of Teacher Education institutional accreditation for teacher education programs. She also reviews papers for multiple international conferences.

Joseph C. Kush, Ph.D. is an Associate Professor and Director of the Doctoral Program in Instructional Technology at Duquesne University in Pittsburgh, PA. His research interests include over 40 publications and 70 presentations on topics related to test bias and test fairness for children from minority backgrounds, with a current focus on technological tools that will assist in reducing test bias. He is also strongly committed to issues of social justice. He received his Ph.D. from Arizona State University.

Ron Lombard earned his BS degree in secondary education with a major in the social studies from California University of PA 1969, MA degree in History California University 1972, M. Ed in secondary administration California University 1979, Ed. D in educational leadership Nova University 1987, post graduate work West Virginia University for superintendence certification 1988 -89. He has thirty years of educational experience in the public schools as a secondary classroom teacher, building principal, district assistant superintendent, and administrative certification at the elementary and secondary levels. He worked as a participant in New American Schools national group with CoNect Schools – dealing with integration of technology into the classroom environment, researched and created curricular materials for online work for Bell & Howell – in creation of online American history text / presented by Big Chalk. He has presented a number of papers at international education/technology Conferences and created materials and conducted research dealing with aspects of assessment and the classroom teacher for administrators and teachers. Dr. Lombard has been an Assistant Professor of Education for Chatham University since 2000. His has served as an instructor at both graduate and undergraduate levels and served as a student adviser for both levels. During his tenure at Chatham he has been involved in the development of online courses for the Education Department and Continuing Education.

C. Jay Hertzog, retired Dean of Education at Slippery Rock University of Pennsylvania, has spent 19 years as a public school teacher and administrator and 22 years in teacher/administrator preparation at higher education institutions in Georgia and Pennsylvania. During his 10 years as dean he also served as

Copyright © 2010, IGI Global, distributing in print or electronic forms without written permission of IGI Global is prohibited.

the chair of the Pennsylvania Deans of Education Forum representing all 95 teacher preparation institutions in the Commonwealth. In 2009 he was elected as President-Elect of the Pennsylvania Association of Colleges and Teacher Education (PAC-TE). Through his involvement with teacher education he has worked closely with the Pennsylvania State Board of Education, Pennsylvania's Secretaries of Education, the Pennsylvania House of Representatives Education Committee and several key legislators in crafting legislation regarding teacher certification. In 2006 he received the "Excellence in Education Award" for Distinguished Contributions in the Field of Education from the Pennsylvania State University College of Education Alumni Society and in 2007 received the "Teacher Educator of the Year Award" from PAC-TE. In 2006, he received an appointment from the Pennsylvania Department of Labor and Industry, Bureau of Mediation as a mediator/arbitrator for the Commonwealth in school-related cases. Hertzog and his research partner, Dr. P. Lená Morgan, are nationally recognized as leaders on the effects of student transition from middle school to high school. Together, they have presented at national and regional conferences, published numerous articles and have consulted with schools across the country on this topic. He also has co-authored two textbooks on Educational Leadership.

* * *

Nor Aziah Alias is an Associate Professor and currently the Deputy Dean at the Faculty of Education, Universiti Teknologi MARA, Malaysia. She holds a bachelor and Master's degree in Physics from Indiana University, Bloomington and a doctoral degree in Instructional Design and Technology from the International Islamic University Malaysia (IIUM). She also has a Graduate Certificate in Open and Distance Learning (USQ, Australia). Her current research interest is mainly in educational design research and the use of ICT for development. She has also published in areas of online and distance learning, teacher education and technology supported learning environment. She can be contacted at this e-mail: noraz112@salam.uitm.edu.my

Nor Aiza Alias is the Vice Principal and Senior English Teacher at Kepong Secondary School, Malaysia. She is also a socio-psychologist whose research focus is in school engagement and the affective outcomes of teacher training. She can be contacted at this e-mail: noraiza.alias@gmail.com

Constantinos Bourletidis is project manager for the Special Account for Research Grants of the National and Kapodistrian University of Athens. He is a doctoral candidate in distance learning at the Aegean University. He earned his MA in Money Banking and Finance, London UK and also M.A. in Adults Education from Greek Open University. He has been teaching business, marketing, and advertising courses for almost a decade and he has co-authored articles on distance education. He is currently researching factors influencing the effectiveness of business school courses.

Brenda M. Capobianco is an Associate Professor of Science Education in the Departments of Curriculum and Instruction and Engineering Education (courtesy) and Affiliated Faculty in Women's Studies at Purdue University. She is one of the coordinators of Purdue's elementary science teacher education program. Before entering academia, she was an award-winning middle science teacher for over ten years in Connecticut and an adjunct instructor of university science elementary and secondary methods courses. Brenda writes and teaches in the field of science and engineering education with interests in teacher action research and issues of gender and culture in science education. Her research and publications focus on teachers' development of practice through collaborative action research; teachers' attempts at integrating inclusive pedagogies using action research; and the construct of identity among young women in science and engineering. She currently serves as an associate editor of the Journal of Science Teacher Education.

Judith Cramer is the Educational Technology Specialist at Teachers College, Columbia University (TC), where she helps faculty members integrate new media into their research and pedagogy. Cramer spent five years developing projects across the curriculum for middle and high school students at Trinity School and The United Nations International School in New York City, where she also taught journalism and advised the award winning school paper. In 2006, with a seed grant from TC, Cramer developed We Media, a new MA level course focused on citizen journalism as a curriculur model. She led the Media Literacy team on TC's award winning "Teaching the Levees" project (www.teachingthelevees.org). Cramer's research interests include technology and gender, citizen media and democratic education, and, most recently, digital comics and graphic novels in the curriculum.

Margaret Smith Crocco is Professor and Coordinator of the Program in Social Studies at Teachers College, Columbia University and Chair of the Department of Arts and Humanities. She taught high school social studies for eight years as well as American Studies, Women's Studies, and American history at the college level. At Teachers College, where she has worked since 1993, she teaches doctoral and master's courses. Her research interests include gender, technology, and urban education as they relate to social studies. She has recently been involved in several award winning curriculum development projects including "Teaching The Levees," based on Spike Lee's When the Levees Broke about Hurricane Katrina in 2007. The project's Web site can be seen at http://www.teachingthelevees.org

Adam M. Friedman is an Assistant Professor and Director of Social Studies Education at Wake Forest University. He teaches undergraduate and graduate secondary social studies methods, undergraduate elementary social studies methods, a course in descriptive research in social studies, and conducts student teaching supervision. His research interests include the effect and impact of technology use in social studies teacher education and on student learning in secondary social studies. Dr. Friedman has published his research in various social studies and technology journals and book chapters, and was formerly the co-chair of the technology committee of the National Council for the Social Studies.

Sara Winstead Fry is an assistant professor of education in the department of Curriculum, Instruction, and Foundational Studies at Boise State University in Boise, Idaho. She earned her Ph.D. in curriculum and instruction at the University of Wyoming. Her research interests include beginning teacher induction, social studies education, and enhancing preservice teacher and K-12 student learning through educational technology. Sara teaches courses in social studies methods and qualitative research, and also serves as a liaison to local elementary schools that host student teachers. Prior to her university career, Sara taught middle school social studies and language arts in Colorado and Trinidad & Tobago.

Begoña Gros hold a Ph.D. in Education from the University of Barcelona (Spain). She has taught courses about the use of technology to enhanced learning as a Professor at the University of Barcelona. Currently, she is the Vice-Rector of Innovation and the Director of the eLearn Center at the Universitat Oberta de Catalunya (Spain). She has spent more than twenty years doing research about the use of

ICT in education with especial focus in the use of video games, collaborative learning and e-learning in higher education. She has published ten books and many articles about these topics and she has participated in a number of research and innovation projects at national level (R+D Programme of the Ministry for Education and Science) and at international level (Fifth Framework Programme, E-learning Programme, etc). She sits on a number of scientific committees of national and international journals (Human Computer Behaviour, International Journal of Web Based Communities, Educational Research and Development, etc.).

Tina L. Heafner is an Associate Professor in the Department of Middle, Secondary, and K-12 Education in the College of Education at the University of North Carolina at Charlotte. Dr. Heafner is the program coordinator for the social studies graduate and undergraduate programs in addition to the Minor in Secondary Education. She teaches undergraduate courses in social studies methods, instructional technology, content area literacy, graduate courses in advanced social studies content, and doctoral courses exploring the history of urbanization and its impacts on schooling. Her research interests include pedagogical and policy issues in social studies education, effective strategies for integrating technology in social studies teaching and learning, and strategic reading in social studies. Dr. Heafner has served on the Board of Directors for National Council for the Social Studies and for the North Carolina Council for the Social Studies.

Chinwe H. Ikpeze is an Assistant Professor of Literacy at St John Fisher College in Rochester, New York. She teaches undergraduate and graduate courses in literacy assessment and instruction, literacy methods, literacy acquisition and capstone project (research in education). Her research interests include use of new literacies and technologies across spaces, online and distance learning, teacher learning and self-study research. She has published articles in The Reading Teacher, Journal of Literacy Research, Journal of Technology and Teacher Education, Journal of literacy and Technology, the Language and Literacy Spectrum, among others.

Karen Johnson teaches elementary education majors at West Chester University in West Chester, Pennsylvania. Her main focus at West Chester has been supervising student teachers and teaching social studies methods courses. Her research interests center around technology and teacher education. Prior to teaching at the college level in PA and NY, Dr. Johnson taught elementary school for ten years in NJ and NY. She obtained her B.S. in elementary education from The College of New Jersey, her M. Ed. from Rutgers University, and her Ph.D. from the University at Albany. Her doctorate was in Curriculum and Instruction with a focus on Instructional Design and Technology.

Christopher J. Johnston is Assistant Professor of Mathematics Education at George Mason University, Fairfax, VA. He earned his Ph.D. in Mathematics Education Leadership at George Mason University in 2009. Christopher earned a Bachelor of Arts in Elementary Education with a specialization in Mathematics at Concordia University, River Forest, IL and a Master of Arts in Computer Science and Mathematics Education at Concordia University. For eight years, Christopher taught middle school math at two different private schools in Chicago, IL and Falls Church, VA. In addition to his teaching and research, Christopher has served as the lead consultant for Illuminations, a project of the National Council of Teachers of Mathematics. He is an active member of the Technology Committee of the

Association of Mathematics Teacher Educators, and he regularly attends and presents at conferences. Christopher has also served as the Managing Editor of the Journal of Technology and Teacher Education.

Gladis Kersaint, an Associate Professor of Mathematics Education K-12 at the University of South Florida, has taught in various levels including public school, community college and university and has provided provide professional development for teachers at all levels, K-12, both locally and nationally. Her interests include factors that the influence mathematic teacher education, teacher practices, access and opportunities for at-risk children, and technology for learning and teaching mathematics. She has authored over 30 manuscripts that include books, book chapters, and journal articles related to her areas of interests. She is active in several mathematics professional organizations, including the National Council of Teachers of Mathematics and the Association of Mathematics Teacher Educators.

Ann D. Klaus is the Associate Director for the European Union Center, International Programs Office at Texas A&M University. Previously, she worked for the Integrated Ocean Drilling Program (IODP) and Ocean Drilling Program (ODP) for 16 years where she held the positions of IODP Deputy Director of Data Services (2003-2009), ODP Publication Services Manager (1995-2003), ODP Chief Editor (2003-1995), and ODP Assistant Public Information Coordinator (1993). Ann has an MA in Marine Biology. Before working for the drilling program, Ann's career focused on marine science education. She held exciting jobs at an aquarium in Tokyo, Japan; served as Education Director at Bishop Museum, Hawaii; started the outreach education program for the Monterey Bay Aquarium, California; and worked as a naturalist on marine mammal observing cruises in the western Pacific.

Swapna Kumar is currently a Clinical Assistant Professor in the Educational Technology Program at the School of Teaching and Learning, University of Florida, USA. She has 15 years of experience in teaching, technology integration, professional development, and training evaluation. Prior to her current appointment, Dr. Kumar was an Instructor and Coordinator of Online Education at the School of Education, Boston University, MA, where her responsibilities included faculty development in the use of new technologies. Her teaching and research interests include the use of Web 2.0 technologies to supplement classroom teaching and learning, professional development for teachers and faculty, blended learning, online course design and facilitation, collaborative learning, and learning communities.

Leena Laurinen (PhD, professor in Education, special field: Research on learning and development) has been working at the Department of Educational Sciences in the University of Jyväskylä since year 1989. She started her research activity in 1976 in the University of Helsinki concerning psycholinguistic research on sentence elaboration (i.e. verbal inferences) and text understanding. On the basis of her results she developed teaching methods for schools concerning reading strategies in mother tongue (Finnish) and foreign language learning. Thereafter she has concentrated on collaborative learning and writing as well as argumentative interaction both in secondary school classrooms and in university lecture rooms.

R. Mark Leckie has been Professor of Geology, University of Massachusetts since 1985. He co-led the scientific instruction of the JOI/IODP School of Rock expedition in 2005. Since 2006, he has taught numerous workshops about teaching with authentic scientific ocean drilling data for both teachers and students, including the Urbino (Italy) Summer School for Paleoclimatology. Leckie is a marine micropaleontologist and specializes in paleoceanography, particularly reconstructing ocean-climate history of the past 120 million years, and has published >40 peer-reviewed papers. He has participated in 7 DSDP/ODP scientific expeditions. Leckie has served on the Education Subcommittee of US Advisory Committee, as well as other service panels of the Ocean Drilling Program. He has served as an associate editor of the Geology, Paleoceanography, and the Journal of Foraminiferal Research. Leckie is co-author of a classroom activity book: Investigating the Oceans, an Interactive Guide to the Science of Oceanography (Leckie and Yuretich, 2003).

James D. Lehman is Professor of Educational Technology and Head of the Department of Curriculum and Instruction at Purdue University. He teaches and does research on educational technology integration in the classroom, interactive multimedia design, and distance learning. He is a co-author of the book Educational Technology for Teaching and Learning, published by Pearson Education, and he has written numerous articles about the uses of technology in education. He has previously served as an associate editor of the Journal of Research in Science Teaching and the Journal of Computers and Mathematics in Science Teaching. He was the Project Director of P3T3: Purdue Program for Preparing Tomorrow's Teachers to use Technology, a PT3 implementation project funded by the U. S. Department of Education designed to enhance the preparation of future teachers to use technology.

Lesia Lennex received her doctorate in curriculum and instruction from the University of Tennessee, Knoxville. She is currently an Associate Professor of Education in the department of Middle and Secondary Education at Morehead State University, Morehead Kentucky. Dr. Lennex holds degrees in biology, anthropology, and education. She researches, presents, and publishes in technology issues and integration for P-16 schools, NCATE accreditation Web sites, biology curriculum, and ethnobotany. Dr. Lennex is a former high school science teacher in biology, chemistry, physics, and ecology. She is the Chair of Information Technology Education SIG for the Society for Information Technology and Teacher Education (SITE) 2008-2011.

Irina Lyublinskaya received Ph.D. in Theoretical and Mathematical Physics in 1991 from the Leningrad State University and has published substantially in that field. She has over 20 years of teaching experience in secondary and higher education. In recent years she has directed her professional endeavors to the curriculum development and research in the area of integrating technology into mathematics and science education and to the professional development of mathematics and science teachers, conducting grant-funded workshops to help teachers learn to use educational technology. She has received grants for these projects from such agencies as the Geraldine R. Dodge Foundation, the Bell Telephone Company, the Federal Eisenhower Professional Development program, The Clay Mathematics Institute, New York State Department of Education, US Department of Education, and National Science Foundation. Lyublinskaya is a recipient of Radioshack/Tandy Prize for Teaching Excellence Mathematics, Science, and Computer Science, NSTA Distinguished Science Teaching Award and citation, Education's Unsung Heroes Award for innovation in the classroom, and NSTA Vernier Technology Award. She has published multiple articles and 10 books about teaching of mathematics and science.

Ronald J. MacDonald teaches science methods, technology integration and research methods at the University of Prince Edward Island, Prince Edward Island, Canada. He has been a junior and senior high school science teacher in Nova Scotia and Ontario, Canada, for 15 years. He has also been an information technology integration specialist and professional development facilitator. His PhD dissertation addressed the intersections between teacher attitudes toward technology, leadership and professional development for technology integration. His current research focuses on the development of communities of practice of science teachers who want to increase student inquiry through the integration of technologies, such as data logging technologies. Other current research being investigate includes: gender differences in attitudes toward science brought about when technologies are integrated in the classroom/laboratory; how New Learners (first year university students) learn with new technologies; and how to improve teacher education through building stronger links between university coursework and schools.

Miika Marttunen (D.Ed.) is working as a professor at the Department of Educational Sciences in the University of Jyväskylä, Finland. Previously he has been working as a senior researcher of the Academy of Finland. He started his research activity in 1990, and completed his dissertation in 1997 on the use of e-mail in teaching argumentation skills in higher education. Currently his main research interests include collaborative learning, argumentation, and network interaction both in secondary and higher education studies.

Virginia McCormack is an Associate Professor of Education. She is a certified/licensed P-12 classroom teacher and administrator, has served as chair of Ohio Dominican University's Education Division and Director of the M.Ed. program and is currently teaching undergraduate and graduate students. Some of her publications and presentations include "Content Area Literacy for Diverse Learners," "Guiding Truth Seekers in Examining Technological Innovations that Promote Ethical Values and Decision Making" and "Free Web 2.0 Tools for Easily Created Course Activities." She holds a Bachelor of Science in Education from St. Bonaventure University; a Master of Science in Educational Administration from the University of Dayton; and a Doctor of Education from Nova Southeastern University. She is a member of organizations devoted to education and curriculum development such as the Association for Supervision and Curriculum Development, International Technology Education Association, Teachers of English to Speakers of Other Languages, and the National Middle School Association.

Charalambos Mouzakis is a part-time lecturer in the Department of Primary Education at National and Kapodistrian Univeristy of Athens. After the undergraduate studies, he earned his M.Ed. in the field of Informatics and Communication Technologies from the University of Athens. He received his Ph.D. in educational use of synchronous learning technologies from the University of Athens. His main interest is the study of the applications of Information and Communication Technologies in distance education and the evaluation of blended learning environments. He has been involved in a number of European and National research projects and he has carried out extensive research on a range of topics in e-learning and blended learning.

Kimberely Fletcher Nettleton has taught at both the middle and elementary school level and loved every minute in the classroom. She was a principal at a K-8 school before becoming an instructor at Morehead State University, where she teaches Classroom Management and Assessment. She is a firm believer in the healing power of chocolate. She is the Co-Director of the Professional Development School at Morehead. She received her BA from the University of Kentucky, an MA in elementary education from Georgetown College, and a second MA fin School Administration from Morehead State University. She is finishing her doctoral work in Instructional Design and Technology at the University of Kentucky.

Matthew Niemitz is the Curriculum Manager on the Worldwide Education team at Adobe Systems, Inc. in San Francisco. In this position, he creates instructional resources that help K-12 and Higher Education faculty use Adobe software in classrooms, schools, and universities. Niemitz has a dual background in earth science and educational technology, earning a Bachelor's degree in geology from the College of William and Mary and a Master's of Education from the Technology, Innovation, and Education program at the Harvard Graduate School of Education. His research interests in geology have focused on the paleoceanography of the equatorial Atlantic during the early Pliocene, utilizing ODP samples and data. Niemitz directed the School of Rock expedition website and ship to shore communications activities and his subsequent research interests in educational technology have focused on using communication technologies to establish real-time links between practicing scientists and students in the classroom.

Leslie Peart became director of the Deep Earth Academy (I-DEA), a program of the Consortium for Ocean Leadership, in 2004 after 21 years in South Texas classrooms and public aquaria including the Texas State Aquarium, Alaska SeaLife Center, and John G. Shedd Aquarium. I-DEA facilitates and develops activities and materials based on authentic data from shipboard research expeditions to strengthen students' mathematics, science, and analytical skills for a lifetime of learning. As director, Peart oversees I-DEA's immersive School of Rock professional development program, curriculum design and dissemination through a searchable database on the I-DEA website (<http://www.deepearthacademy.org>), and education planning for IODP expeditions, including the creation of a new website (<http://www.joidesresolution.org>), ship-to-shore broadcasts, educators-at-sea, and the use of social networking tools.

Kevin J. Reins is an associate professor of mathematics education in the Department of Curriculum and Instruction at The University of South Dakota, teaching courses in elementary, middle and secondary mathematics methods at the graduate and undergraduate levels. He reviews manuscripts and related works for Mathematics Teacher, Mathematics Teaching in the Middle School, and Allyn & Bacon. Currently he serves as a liaison for the partnership between the South Dakota Discovery Center and USD and is the State of South Dakota's team leader for the Association of State Supervisors of Mathematics (ASSM). His research and service foci are digital inking practices and pen-based computing, the use of Lesson Study with preservice and inservice mathematics teachers, instructional strategies and technology-mediated teaching and learning in mathematics.

Manuel Santos-Trigo is a professor of mathematics education at the Center for Research and Advanced Studies (Cinvestav-IPN) in Mexico City. He completed his doctorate in mathematics education at the University of British Columbia, Canada. He teaches graduate courses and does research in mathematical problem solving. He is interested in analyzing and documenting mathematical processes, resources, strategies, and conceptualizations that teachers and students develop as a result of using various computational tools in problem solving activities. He has coordinated several research projects that involve the use of computational tools in problem solving approaches.

Scott Slough, EdD, is an Associate Professor of Science Education in the Department of Teaching, Learning, and Culture at Texas A&M University. His research interests include technology-enhanced instructional design in science and mathematics: Project-Based Learning (PBL); program evaluation; geoscience education; integration of graphics and text; and change in schools, especially as it relates to technology. He is author/co-author of over 45 peer-reviewed articles, including articles in journals such as School Science and Mathematics, Journal of Computers in Mathematics and Science Teaching, Reading Psychology, Journal of Educational Multimedia and Hypermedia, and Physics Education. He is also co-editor of a recent book Project-Based Learning: An Integrated Science, Technology, Engineering, and Mathematics (STEM) Approach.

Kristen St. John is Associate Professor of Geology and Environmental Science at James Madison University. She co-led the scientific instruction of the JOI/IODP School of Rock expedition and is the lead on an NSF-funded project "Building Core Knowledge" which aims to develop active-learning exercises using scientific ocean drilling data for the undergraduate classroom. St. John is a marine sedimentologist, specializing in high latitude paleoclimate records, particularly reconstructing ice-rafting histories, and has published >15 peer reviewed papers in this field. She has participated in 4 ODP/IODP scientific expeditions, most recently as a sedimentologist with the Arctic Coring Expedition. St. John is the former chair of the Education Subcommittee of the U.S. Science Advisory Committee on Scientific Ocean Drilling (USAC), the executive associate editor of the Journal of Geoscience Education, and past-president of the Geoscience Education Division of GSA. Her teaching responsibilities include: Introductory Oceanography; Earth Systems and Climate Change; Earth Science for Teachers, and Physical Geology.

Hasan Tinmaz is a doctoral student in the "Computer Education and Instructional Technology" program at Middle East Technical University, Turkey. His dissertation topic is "utilization of social network web sites in education; a case of Facebook.com". His research interests include educational technologies, instructional design, instructional technology planning, social networks, adult education and e-learning environments. He received his B.S. degree (2001) in Computer Education from Middle East Technical University, Faculty of Education, and his M.Sc. degree (2004) in Curriculum and Instruction Program of Department of Educational Sciences from Middle East Technical University. His master thesis is entitled as "An Assessment of Preservice Teachers' Technology Perception in Relation to Their Subject Area."

Nelly Tournaki has a Ph.D. in educational psychology from New York University and is currently an associate professor at the Department of Education at the College of Staten Island, the City University of New York. Her two longstanding areas of inquiry include first, the examination of issues of teacher efficacy and effectiveness and second, the effectiveness of a variety of teaching strategies in the classroom (most notably in mathematics).

Kati Vapalahti (M.Ed.) is preparing her doctoral thesis on argumentation in collaborative learning. She has been working as a researcher in the Department of Educational Sciences at the University of Jyväskylä, Finland. Her doctoral thesis deals with methods for supporting argumentative problem-solving skills in social work education. In addition to her research work, she works as a teacher at Mikkeli University of Applied Sciences, Finland. Her main teaching subjects are education and social pedagogy.

Junko Yamamoto teaches Instructional Technology, World Language Teaching Methodology, and English Language Learners Teaching Methodology at Secondary Education/ Foundations of Education Department, Slippery Rock University. She also supervises student teachers. She earned her doctorate degree in Instructional Technology from Duquesne University. She is a reviewer for the American

Council on the Teaching of Foreign Languages / National Council for Accreditation of Teacher Education institutional accreditation for teacher education programs. She also reviews papers for multiple international conferences.

Ilker Yakin was graduated from Gazi University, Faculty of Education, department of Secondary Science and Mathematics Education in 2003. He is now a Ph.D. candidate in Middle East Technical University, department of Computer Education and Instructional Technology. He is a research assistant of Computer Education and Instructional Technology at Middle East Technical University. His dissertation is about design and evaluation of EPSS for forensic personnel. His research interests include human performance technology, electronic performance support systems (EPSS), technology training of preservice teacher education, technology planning and case-based learning.

Index

Copyright © 2010, IGI Global, distributing in print or electronic forms without written permission of IGI Global is prohibited.

D

G

H

I

Q

R

S

T

U

V

W

Y

Z